Diets, Foods and Food Components Effect on Dyslipidemia

Diets, Foods and Food Components Effect on Dyslipidemia

Editors

Federica Fogacci
Arrigo F.G. Cicero
Claudio Borghi

MDPI • Basel • Beijing • Wuhan • Barcelona • Belgrade • Manchester • Tokyo • Cluj • Tianjin

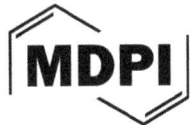

Editors

Federica Fogacci
University of Bologna
Italy

Arrigo F.G. Cicero
University of Bologna
Italy

Claudio Borghi
University of Bologna
Italy

Editorial Office
MDPI
St. Alban-Anlage 66
4052 Basel, Switzerland

This is a reprint of articles from the Special Issue published online in the open access journal *Nutrients* (ISSN 2072-6643) (available at: http://www.mdpi.com).

For citation purposes, cite each article independently as indicated on the article page online and as indicated below:

LastName, A.A.; LastName, B.B.; LastName, C.C. Article Title. *Journal Name* **Year**, *Volume Number*, Page Range.

ISBN 978-3-0365-1238-9 (Hbk)
ISBN 978-3-0365-1239-6 (PDF)

© 2021 by the authors. Articles in this book are Open Access and distributed under the Creative Commons Attribution (CC BY) license, which allows users to download, copy and build upon published articles, as long as the author and publisher are properly credited, which ensures maximum dissemination and a wider impact of our publications.

The book as a whole is distributed by MDPI under the terms and conditions of the Creative Commons license CC BY-NC-ND.

Contents

About the Editors ix

Federica Fogacci, Claudio Borghi and Arrigo F. G. Cicero
Diets, Foods and Food Components' Effect on Dyslipidemia
Reprinted from: *Nutrients* **2021**, *13*, 741, doi:10.3390/nu13030741 1

Eliana B. Souto, Raquel da Ana, Selma B. Souto, Aleksandra Zielińska, Conrado Marques, Luciana N. Andrade, Olaf K. Horbańczuk, Atanas G. Atanasov, Massimo Lucarini, Alessandra Durazzo, Amélia M. Silva, Ettore Novellino, Antonello Santini and Patricia Severino
In Vitro Characterization, Modelling, and Antioxidant Properties of Polyphenon-60 from Green Tea in Eudragit S100-2 Chitosan Microspheres
Reprinted from: *Nutrients* **2020**, *12*, 967, doi:10.3390/nu12040967 5

Suresh Khadke, Pallavi Mandave, Aniket Kuvalekar, Vijaya Pandit, Manjiri Karandikar and Nitin Mantri
Synergistic Effect of Omega-3 Fatty Acids and Oral-Hypoglycemic Drug on Lipid Normalization through Modulation of Hepatic Gene Expression in High Fat Diet with Low Streptozotocin-Induced Diabetic Rats
Reprinted from: *Nutrients* **2020**, *12*, 3652, doi:10.3390/nu12123652 21

Jong Cheol Shon, Won Cheol Kim, Ri Ryu, Zhexue Wu, Jong-Su Seo, Myung-Sook Choi and Kwang-Hyeon Liu
Plasma Lipidomics Reveals Insights into Anti-Obesity Effect of *Chrysanthemum morifolium* Ramat Leaves and Its Constituent Luteolin in High-Fat Diet-Induced Dyslipidemic Mice
Reprinted from: *Nutrients* **2020**, *12*, 2973, doi:10.3390/nu12102973 41

Marcio A. A. de Mendonça, Ana R. S. Ribeiro, Adriana K. de Lima, Gislaine B. Bezerra, Malone S. Pinheiro, Ricardo L. C. de Albuquerque-Júnior, Margarete Z. Gomes, Francine F. Padilha, Sara M. Thomazzi, Ettore Novellino, Antonello Santini, Patricia Severino, Eliana B. Souto and Juliana C. Cardoso
Red Propolis and Its Dyslipidemic Regulator Formononetin: Evaluation of Antioxidant Activity and Gastroprotective Effects in Rat Model of Gastric Ulcer
Reprinted from: *Nutrients* **2020**, *12*, 2951, doi:10.3390/nu12102951 57

Taehwan Lim, Juhee Ryu, Kiuk Lee, Sun Young Park and Keum Taek Hwang
Protective Effects of Black Raspberry (*Rubus occidentalis*) Extract against Hypercholesterolemia and Hepatic Inflammation in Rats Fed High-Fat and High-Choline Diets
Reprinted from: *Nutrients* **2020**, *12*, 2448, doi:10.3390/nu12082448 75

Naoki Nanashima, Kayo Horie, Kanako Yamanouchi, Toshiko Tomisawa, Maiko Kitajima, Indrawati Oey and Hayato Maeda
Blackcurrant (*Ribes nigrum*) Extract Prevents Dyslipidemia and Hepatic Steatosis in Ovariectomized Rats
Reprinted from: *Nutrients* **2020**, *12*, 1541, doi:10.3390/nu12051541 89

Maria Pia Adorni, Francesca Zimetti, Maria Giovanna Lupo, Massimiliano Ruscica and Nicola Ferri
Naturally Occurring PCSK9 Inhibitors
Reprinted from: *Nutrients* **2020**, *12*, 1440, doi:10.3390/nu12051440 99

Cristina Carresi, Micaela Gliozzi, Vincenzo Musolino, Miriam Scicchitano, Federica Scarano, Francesca Bosco, Saverio Nucera, Jessica Maiuolo, Roberta Macrì, Stefano Ruga, Francesca Oppedisano, Maria Caterina Zito, Lorenza Guarnieri, Rocco Mollace, Annamaria Tavernese, Ernesto Palma, Ezio Bombardelli, Massimo Fini and Vincenzo Mollace
The Effect of Natural Antioxidants in the Development of Metabolic Syndrome: Focus on Bergamot Polyphenolic Fraction
Reprinted from: *Nutrients* 2020, *12*, 1504, doi:10.3390/nu12051504 129

Elke A. Trautwein and Sue McKay
The Role of Specific Components of a Plant-Based Diet in Management of Dyslipidemia and the Impact on Cardiovascular Risk
Reprinted from: *Nutrients* 2020, *12*, 2671, doi:10.3390/nu12092671 153

Heitor O. Santos, James C. Price and Allain A. Bueno
Beyond Fish Oil Supplementation: The Effects of Alternative Plant Sources of Omega-3 Polyunsaturated Fatty Acids upon Lipid Indexes and Cardiometabolic Biomarkers—An Overview
Reprinted from: *Nutrients* 2020, *12*, 3159, doi:10.3390/nu12103159 175

Li-Juan Tan, Seong-Ah Kim and Sangah Shin
Association between Three Low-Carbohydrate Diet Scores and Lipid Metabolism among Chinese Adults
Reprinted from: *Nutrients* 2020, *12*, 1307, doi:10.3390/nu12051307 195

Sara Al-Musharaf, Ghadeer S. Aljuraiban, Syed Danish Hussain, Abdullah M. Alnaami, Ponnusamy Saravanan and Nasser Al-Daghri
Low Serum Vitamin B12 Levels Are Associated with Adverse Lipid Profiles in Apparently Healthy Young Saudi Women
Reprinted from: *Nutrients* 2020, *12*, 2395, doi:10.3390/nu12082395 213

Arrigo F.G. Cicero, Federica Fogacci, Maddalena Veronesi, Enrico Strocchi, Elisa Grandi, Elisabetta Rizzoli, Andrea Poli, Franca Marangoni and Claudio Borghi
A Randomized Placebo-Controlled Clinical Trial to Evaluate the Medium-Term Effects of Oat Fibers on Human Health: The Beta-Glucan Effects on Lipid Profile, Glycemia and inTestinal Health (BELT) Study
Reprinted from: *Nutrients* 2020, *12*, 686, doi:10.3390/nu12030686 225

Sumia Enani, Suhad Bahijri, Manal Malibary, Hanan Jambi, Basmah Eldakhakhny, Jawaher Al-Ahmadi, Rajaa Al Raddadi, Ghada Ajabnoor, Anwar Boraie and Jaakko Tuomilehto
The Association between Dyslipidemia, Dietary Habits and Other Lifestyle Indicators among Non-Diabetic Attendees of Primary Health Care Centers in Jeddah, Saudi Arabia
Reprinted from: *Nutrients* 2020, *12*, 2441, doi:10.3390/nu12082441 237

Arrigo F.G. Cicero, Sergio D'Addato and Claudio Borghi
A Randomized, Double-Blinded, Placebo-Controlled, Clinical Study of the Effects of a Nutraceutical Combination (LEVELIP DUO®) on LDL Cholesterol Levels and Lipid Pattern in Subjects with Sub-Optimal Blood Cholesterol Levels (NATCOL Study)
Reprinted from: *Nutrients* 2020, *12*, 3127, doi:10.3390/nu12103127 261

Arrigo F. G. Cicero, Cormac Kennedy, Tamara Knežević, Marilisa Bove, Coralie M. G. Georges, Agnė Šatrauskienė, Peter P. Toth and Federica Fogacci
Efficacy and Safety of Armolipid Plus®: An Updated PRISMA Compliant Systematic Review and Meta-Analysis of Randomized Controlled Clinical Trials
Reprinted from: *Nutrients* **2021**, *13*, 638, doi:10.3390/nu13020638 . . . . **271**

About the Editors

Federica Fogacci, MDc is a Clinical Meta-analyst, a Research assistant affiliated with the University of Bologna (Italy) and an author of more than 80 articles focused on dyslipidaemia and its relationship with cardiovascular disease published in peer-reviewed and indexed international journals. She is a member of the Editorial Board of several International Journals concerned with population pharmacotherapy and investigation on atherosclerosis, its risk factors and clinical manifestations.

Arrigo F.G. Cicero, MD, PhD, is a Clinical Pharmacologist, a Professor of Human Nutrition at the University of Bologna (Italy), President of the Italian Nutraceutical Society and an author of more than 400 full papers published in international peer-reviewed indexed journals, mainly focused on nutraceuticals, dyslipidaemia, and other cardiovascular disease risk factors. He is a member of the Editorial Board of several International Journals concerned with population pharmacotherapy and investigation on atherosclerosis, its risk factors and clinical manifestations.

Claudio Borghi, MD, Inernist, is a Full professor of Internal Medicine, a PhD Director, and Emergency Medicine post-graduated school Director. He is author of more than 600 full papers published in international peer-reviewed indexed journals, mainly focused on cardiovascular disease risk factor, their interactions and management, Member of the Editorial Board of several International Journals concerned with population pharmacotherapy and investigation on atherosclerosis, its risk factors and clinical manifestations.

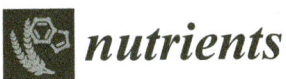

Editorial

Diets, Foods and Food Components' Effect on Dyslipidemia

Federica Fogacci [1,2,3,*], Claudio Borghi [1,2] and Arrigo F. G. Cicero [1,2,3]

1. Medical and Surgical Science Department, University of Bologna, 40138 Bologna, Italy; claudio.borghi@unibo.it (C.B.); arrigo.cicero@unibo.it (A.F.G.C.)
2. IRCCS Azienda Ospedaliero, Universitaria di Bologna, 40138 Bologna, Italy
3. Italian Nutraceutical Society (SINut), 40138 Bologna, Italy
* Correspondence: federica.fogacci@studio.unibo.it

Hypercholesterolemia is a well-known independent risk factor for cardiovascular disease and a recognized target of pharmacological therapeutic agents in both primary and secondary prevention [1]. There is increasing interest in the use of natural lipid-lowering compounds that may delay or circumvent drug therapy. These compounds could be included as part of a diet pattern, as single foods or as food components transformed into dietary supplements [2].

To date, there is a strong evidence showing that dietary factors are able to influence atherogenesis. In particular, the Mediterranean diet is particularly rich in active vegetable compounds, contributing to its positive effect on human health [3]. However, other active compounds could be isolated and concentrated from non-nutrient vegetable sources, such as medicinal plants [4]. Finally, natural dietary and non-dietary lipid-lowering compound could have pleiotropic effect on lipids and on other cardiovascular risk factors, for instance increasing the cholesterol resistance to oxidative stress, reducing microinflammation, improving the endothelial health, etc. [5].

Based on this background, the volume entitled *"Diets, Foods and Food Components' Effect on Dyslipidemia"* samples the contributions of a number of recognized experts in the field.

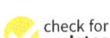

An interesting review summarizes the number of natural compounds reducing the plasma level of Proprotein convertase subtilisin/kexin type 9 (PCSK9), a key enzyme in the metabolism of LDL-cholesterol receptors on the liver cell surface [6].

Trautwein and McKay reviewed the effect of plant-based diet on dyslipidemia and cardiovascular risk [7]. Carresi et al. considered the potential effect of bergamot polyphenolic fraction on the prevention of metabolic syndrome [8] and Santos et al. critically appraised the efficacy of plant-derived omega-3 polyunsaturated fatty acids from foodstuffs and supplements upon lipid profile and several cardiometabolic markers [9].

A range of preclinical evidence highlights the antiobesity effect of *Chrysanthemum morifolium* [10], the antioxidant effect of red propolis [11], the cholesterol-lowering and hepatoprotective effects of black raspberry [12], the effect of blackcurrant in preventing dyslipidemia and hepatic steatosis [13], the antioxidant activity of polyphenon-60 from green tea in chitosan microspheres [14], and the combined effect of omega-3 fatty acids and glibenclamide on abnormal lipid profile, increased blood glucose and impaired liver and kidney functions [15].

New epidemiological evidence supports a link between different dietary patterns [16], charbohydrate intake [17], fructose intake [18], vitamin B12 serum levels [19] and lipid profile and other markers of cardiovascular disease risk. Findings from the randomized clinical trials included in the Special Issue support the use of new nutraceutical formulations with lipid-lowering effects. The BELT (Beta-glucan Effects on Lipid profile, glycemia and inTestinal health) study evaluated the medium-term effects of dietary supplementation with oat fibers in a sample of healthy subjects [20], and the NATCOL (NutrAceuTical COmbination on Low-density lipoprotein cholesterol) study tested the effect of dietary

Citation: Fogacci, F.; Borghi, C.; Cicero, A.F.G. Diets, Foods and Food Components' Effect on Dyslipidemia. *Nutrients* 2021, *13*, 741. https://doi.org/10.3390/nu13030741

Received: 22 February 2021
Accepted: 25 February 2021
Published: 26 February 2021

Publisher's Note: MDPI stays neutral with regard to jurisdictional claims in published maps and institutional affiliations.

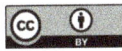

Copyright: © 2021 by the authors. Licensee MDPI, Basel, Switzerland. This article is an open access article distributed under the terms and conditions of the Creative Commons Attribution (CC BY) license (https://creativecommons.org/licenses/by/4.0/).

supplementation with Levelip Duo® on low-density lipoprotein cholesterol concentrations and lipid profile in subjects with suboptimal blood cholesterol levels [21]. Finally, a systematic review and meta-analysis of randomized controlled clinical studies included in the Special Issue supports the use of Armolipid Plus® in clinical practice [22].

In this context, the volume is a source of new knowledge on the effect of diets, foods and food components on dyslipidemia.

Funding: This research received no external funding.

Conflicts of Interest: The authors declare no conflict of interest.

References

1. Cicero, A.; Landolfo, M.; Ventura, F.; Borghi, C. Current pharmacotherapeutic options for primary dyslipidemia in adults. *Expert Opin. Pharm.* **2019**, *20*, 1277–1288. [CrossRef]
2. Cicero, A.F.G.; Fogacci, F.; Zambon, A. Red Yeast Rice for Hypercholesterolemia: JACC Focus Seminar. *J. Am. Coll. Cardiol.* **2021**, *77*, 620–628. [CrossRef]
3. Zhubi-Bakija, F.; Bajraktari, G.; Bytyçi, I.; Mikhailidis, D.P.; Henein, M.Y.; Latkovskis, G.; Rexhaj, Z.; Zhubi, E.; Banach, M.; International Lipid Expert Panel (ILEP). The impact of type of dietary protein, animal versus vegetable, in modifying cardiometabolic risk factors: A position paper from the International Lipid Expert Panel (ILEP). *Clin. Nutr.* **2021**, *40*, 255–276. [CrossRef]
4. Poli, A.; Barbagallo, C.M.; Cicero, A.; Corsini, A.; Manzato, E.; Trimarco, B.; Bernini, F.; Visioli, F.; Bianchi, A.; Canzone, G.; et al. Nutraceuticals and functional foods for the control of plasma cholesterol levels. An intersociety position paper. *Pharm. Res.* **2018**, *134*, 51–60. [CrossRef]
5. Cicero, A.; Colletti, A.; Bajraktari, G.; Descamps, O.; Djuric, D.M.; Ezhov, M.; Fras, Z.; Katsiki, N.; Langlois, M.; Latkovskis, G.; et al. Lipid-lowering nutraceuticals in clinical practice: Position paper from an International Lipid Expert Panel. *Nutr. Rev.* **2017**, *75*, 731–767. [CrossRef] [PubMed]
6. Adorni, M.P.; Zimetti, F.; Lupo, M.G.; Ruscica, M.; Ferri, N. Naturally Occurring PCSK9 Inhibitors. *Nutrients* **2020**, *12*, 1440. [CrossRef]
7. Trautwein, E.A.; McKay, S. The Role of Specific Components of a Plant-Based Diet in Management of Dyslipidemia and the Impact on Cardiovascular Risk. *Nutrients* **2020**, *12*, 2671. [CrossRef]
8. Carresi, C.; Gliozzi, M.; Musolino, V.; Scicchitano, M.; Scarano, F.; Bosco, F.; Nucera, S.; Maiuolo, J.; Macrì, R.; Ruga, S.; et al. The Effect of Natural Antioxidants in the Development of Metabolic Syndrome: Focus on Bergamot Polyphenolic Fraction. *Nutrients* **2020**, *12*, 1504. [CrossRef]
9. Santos, H.O.; Price, J.C.; Bueno, A.A. Beyond Fish Oil Supplementation: The Effects of Alternative Plant Sources of Omega-3 Polyunsaturated Fatty Acids upon Lipid Indexes and Cardiometabolic Biomarkers—An Overview. *Nutrients* **2020**, *12*, 3159. [CrossRef] [PubMed]
10. Shon, J.C.; Kim, W.C.; Ryu, R.; Wu, Z.; Seo, J.-S.; Choi, M.-S.; Liu, K.-H. Plasma Lipidomics Reveals Insights into Anti-Obesity Effect of *Chrysanthemum morifolium* Ramat Leaves and Its Constituent Luteolin in High-Fat Diet-Induced Dyslipidemic Mice. *Nutrients* **2020**, *12*, 2973. [CrossRef] [PubMed]
11. Mendonça, M.A.A.d.; Ribeiro, A.R.S.; Lima, A.K.d.; Bezerra, G.B.; Pinheiro, M.S.; Albuquerque-Júnior, R.L.C.d.; Gomes, M.Z.; Padilha, F.F.; Thomazzi, S.M.; Novellino, E.; et al. Red Propolis and Its Dyslipidemic Regulator Formononetin: Evaluation of Antioxidant Activity and Gastroprotective Effects in Rat Model of Gastric Ulcer. *Nutrients* **2020**, *12*, 2951. [CrossRef]
12. Lim, T.; Ryu, J.; Lee, K.; Park, S.Y.; Hwang, K.T. Protective Effects of Black Raspberry (*Rubus occidentalis*) Extract against Hypercholesterolemia and Hepatic Inflammation in Rats Fed High-Fat and High-Choline Diets. *Nutrients* **2020**, *12*, 2448. [CrossRef] [PubMed]
13. Nanashima, N.; Horie, K.; Yamanouchi, K.; Tomisawa, T.; Kitajima, M.; Oey, I.; Maeda, H. Blackcurrant (*Ribes nigrum*) Extract Prevents Dyslipidemia and Hepatic Steatosis in Ovariectomized Rats. *Nutrients* **2020**, *12*, 1541. [CrossRef] [PubMed]
14. Souto, E.B.; da Ana, R.; Souto, S.B.; Zielińska, A.; Marques, C.; Andrade, L.N.; Horbańczuk, O.K.; Atanasov, A.G.; Lucarini, M.; Durazzo, A.; et al. In Vitro Characterization, Modelling, and Antioxidant Properties of Polyphenon-60 from Green Tea in Eudragit S100-2 Chitosan Microspheres. *Nutrients* **2020**, *12*, 967. [CrossRef] [PubMed]
15. Khadke, S.; Mandave, P.; Kuvalekar, A.; Pandit, V.; Karandikar, M.; Mantri, N. Synergistic Effect of Omega-3 Fatty Acids and Oral-Hypoglycemic Drug on Lipid Normalization through Modulation of Hepatic Gene Expression in High Fat Diet with Low Streptozotocin-Induced Diabetic Rats. *Nutrients* **2020**, *12*, 3652. [CrossRef]
16. Enani, S.; Bahijri, S.; Malibary, M.; Jambi, H.; Eldakhakhny, B.; Al-Ahmadi, J.; Al Raddadi, R.; Ajabnoor, G.; Boraie, A.; Tuomilehto, J. The Association between Dyslipidemia, Dietary Habits and Other Lifestyle Indicators among Non-Diabetic Attendees of Primary Health Care Centers in Jeddah, Saudi Arabia. *Nutrients* **2020**, *12*, 2441. [CrossRef]
17. Tan, L.-J.; Kim, S.-A.; Shin, S. Association between Three Low-Carbohydrate Diet Scores and Lipid Metabolism among Chinese Adults. *Nutrients* **2020**, *12*, 1307. [CrossRef]
18. Cicero, A.; Fogacci, F.; Desideri, G.; Grandi, E.; Rizzoli, E.; D'Addato, S.; Borghi, C. Arterial Stiffness, Sugar-Sweetened Beverages and Fruits Intake in a Rural Population Sample: Data from the Brisighella Heart Study. *Nutrients* **2019**, *11*, 2674. [CrossRef]

19. Al-Musharaf, S.; Aljuraiban, G.S.; Danish Hussain, S.; Alnaami, A.M.; Saravanan, P.; Al-Daghri, N. Low Serum Vitamin B12 Levels Are Associated with Adverse Lipid Profiles in Apparently Healthy Young Saudi Women. *Nutrients* **2020**, *12*, 2395. [CrossRef]
20. Cicero, A.F.G.; Fogacci, F.; Veronesi, M.; Strocchi, E.; Grandi, E.; Rizzoli, E.; Poli, A.; Marangoni, F.; Borghi, C. A Randomized Placebo-Controlled Clinical Trial to Evaluate the Medium-Term Effects of Oat Fibers on Human Health: The Beta-Glucan Effects on Lipid Profile, Glycemia and inTestinal Health (BELT) Study. *Nutrients* **2020**, *12*, 686. [CrossRef]
21. Cicero, A.F.G.; D'Addato, S.; Borghi, C. A Randomized, Double-Blinded, Placebo-Controlled, Clinical Study of the Effects of a Nutraceutical Combination (LEVELIP DUO®) on LDL Cholesterol Levels and Lipid Pattern in Subjects with Sub-Optimal Blood Cholesterol Levels (NATCOL Study). *Nutrients* **2020**, *12*, 3127. [CrossRef] [PubMed]
22. Cicero, A.F.G.; Kennedy, C.; Knežević, T.; Bove, M.; Georges, C.M.G.; Šatrauskienė, A.; Toth, P.P.; Fogacci, F. Efficacy and Safety of Armolipid Plus®: An Updated PRISMA Compliant Systematic Review and Meta-Analysis of Randomized Controlled Clinical Trials. *Nutrients* **2021**, *13*, 638. [CrossRef]

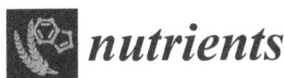

Article

In Vitro Characterization, Modelling, and Antioxidant Properties of Polyphenon-60 from Green Tea in Eudragit S100-2 Chitosan Microspheres

Eliana B. Souto [1,2,*], Raquel da Ana [1], Selma B. Souto [3], Aleksandra Zielińska [1], Conrado Marques [4,5,6], Luciana N. Andrade [7], Olaf K. Horbańczuk [8], Atanas G. Atanasov [9,10,11,12], Massimo Lucarini [13], Alessandra Durazzo [13], Amélia M. Silva [14,15], Ettore Novellino [16,*], Antonello Santini [16,*] and Patricia Severino [4,5,6]

1. Department of Pharmaceutical Technology, Faculty of Pharmacy, University of Coimbra, Pólo das Ciências da Saúde, Azinhaga de Santa Comba, 3000-548 Coimbra, Portugal; quele.ana@gmail.com (R.d.A.); zielinska-aleksandra@wp.pl (A.Z.)
2. CEB—Centre of Biological Engineering, University of Minho, Campus de Gualtar, 4710-057 Braga, Portugal
3. Department of Endocrinology, Hospital de São João, Alameda Prof. Hernâni Monteiro, 4200-319 Porto, Portugal; sbsouto.md@gmail.com
4. Laboratory of Nanotechnology and Nanomedicine (LNMED), Institute of Technology and Research (ITP), Av. Murilo Dantas, 300, Aracaju 49010-390, Brazil; conrado.marques@souunit.com.br (C.M.); pattypharma@gmail.com (P.S.)
5. Industrial Biotechnology Program, University of Tiradentes (UNIT), Av. Murilo Dantas 300, Aracaju 49032-490, Brazil
6. Tiradentes Institute, 150 Mt Vernon St, Dorchester, MA 02125, USA
7. Department of Physiology, Federal University of Sergipe, CEP São Cristóvão 49100-000, Sergipe, Brazil; luciana.nalone@hotmail.com
8. Department of Technique and Food Product Development, Warsaw University of Life Sciences (WULS-SGGW) 159c Nowoursynowska, 02-776 Warsaw, Poland; olaf_horbanczuk@sggw.pl
9. The Institute of Genetics and Animal Breeding, Polish Academy of Sciences, Jastrzębiec, 05-552 Magdalenka, Poland; atanas.atanasov@univie.ac.at
10. Institute of Neurobiology, Bulgarian Academy of Sciences, 23 Acad. G. Bonchev str., 1113 Sofia, Bulgaria
11. Department of Pharmacognosy, University of Vienna, 1090 Vienna, Austria
12. Ludwig Boltzmann Institute for Digital Health and Patient Safety, Medical University of Vienna, Spitalgasse 23, 1090 Vienna, Austria
13. CREA-Research Centre for Food and Nutrition, Via Ardeatina 546, 00178 Rome, Italy; massimo.lucarini@crea.gov.it (M.L.); alessandra.durazzo@crea.gov.it (A.D.)
14. Department of Biology and Environment, University of Trás-os-Montes e Alto Douro (UTAD), Quinta de Prados, 5001-801 Vila Real, Portugal; amsilva@utad.pt
15. Centre for Research and Technology of Agro-Environmental and Biological Sciences (CITAB), University of Trás-os-Montes e Alto Douro (UTAD), 5001-801 Vila Real, Portugal
16. Department of Pharmacy, University of Napoli Federico II, 80131 Napoli, Italy
* Correspondence: ebsouto@ff.uc.pt (E.B.S.); ettore.novellino@unina.it (E.N.); asantini@unina.it (A.S.); Tel.: +351-239-488-400 (E.B.S.); Tel.: +39-81- 678-643 (E.N.); Tel.: +39-81-253-9317 (A.S.)

Received: 27 February 2020; Accepted: 30 March 2020; Published: 31 March 2020

Abstract: Eudragit S100-coated chitosan microspheres (S100Ch) are proposed as a new oral delivery system for green tea polyphenon-60 (PP60). PP60 is a mixture of polyphenolic compounds, known for its active role in decreasing oxidative stress and metabolic risk factors involved in diabetes and in other chronic diseases. Chitosan-PP60 microspheres prepared by an emulsion cross-linking method were coated with Eudragit S100 to ensure the release of PP60 in the terminal ileum. Different core–coat ratios of Eudragit and chitosan were tested. Optimized chitosan microspheres were obtained with a chitosan:PP60 ratio of 8:1 (Ch-PP60$_{8:1}$), rotation speed of 1500 rpm, and surfactant concentration of 1.0% (m/v) achieving a mean size of 7.16 μm. Their coating with the enteric polymer (S100Ch-PP60) increased the mean size significantly (51.4 μm). The in vitro modified-release of PP60 from S100Ch-PP60 was confirmed in simulated gastrointestinal conditions. Mathematical fitting models were used to characterize the release mechanism showing that both Ch-PP60$_{8:1}$ and S100Ch-PP60 fitted the Korsmeyers–Peppas model. The antioxidant activity of PP60 was kept in glutaraldehyde-crosslinked chitosan microspheres before and after their coating, showing an IC$_{50}$ of 212.3 µg/mL and 154.4 µg/mL, respectively. The potential of chitosan microspheres for the delivery of catechins was illustrated, with limited risk of cytotoxicity as shown in Caco-2 cell lines using the 3-(4,5-dimethylthiazole-2-yl)-2,5-diphenyltetrazolium bromide (MTT) assay. The beneficial effects of green tea and its derivatives in the management of metabolic disorders can be exploited using mucoadhesive chitosan microspheres coated with enteric polymers for colonic delivery.

Keywords: green tea; epigallocatechin gallate; chitosan; microspheres; Eudragit; metabolic diseases

1. Introduction

Green tea is obtained from the fresh leaves of *Camellia sinensis*, a plant from the *Theaceae* family which has been used for centuries as a natural antioxidating beverage. Its polyphenolic constituents provide it with additional therapeutic benefits in the modulation of oxidative stress-induced cardiovascular diseases associated with diabetes, already confirmed in clinical trials [1–6]. Green tea extracts, rich in antioxidant polyphenols (e.g., epigallocatechin-3-gallate), have been reported for reducing lipid peroxidation, oxidized low-density lipoproteins (LDL), cholesterol levels, and anti-hypertensive effects, factors that are relevant to reduce cardio-metabolic disease risk [7]. A catechin extract from green tea, containing a mixture of the main active green tea polyphenols components, named polyphenon-60 [8], has recently drawn attention. Indeed, the role of green tea polyphenon-60 (PP60) in decreasing metabolic risk factors, oxidative stress, inflammation, and in the amelioration of cardiac apoptosis in experimentally induced diabetes has been described [9]. Among the naturally derived catechins (flavonoids composing the majority of soluble solids of green tea extracts), epigallocatechin gallate (EGCG) has already been proposed as active ingredient in polymeric nanoparticles for oral administration [10], and as lipid nanoparticles for ocular administration [11,12].

From a quick search using as keywords "epigallocatechin and nanoparticles" 376 publications appeared indexed in the Web of Science dated between 2000 and 2020, while "green tea and nanoparticles" resulted in the list of 780 publications. When associating epigallocatechin and dyslipidemia/dyslipidemia [13], only 33 works were listed as published over the last 20 years.

While the molecular mechanisms involved in the effect of catechins on the metabolism of lipids and sugars remains to be fully described, catechins are known to induce antioxidant enzymes, inhibit pro-oxidant enzymes and scavenge reactive oxygen species (ROS), and to chelate metals [14–16]. EGCG has been reported to improve insulin-resistance and metabolic profiles, as well as to reduce adipocyte area as a consequence of lipolytic action [17]. Anti-obesity effects, such as inhibition of fatty acid absorption and reduction in leptin levels were reported in a high-fat diet rat model combined with green tea extract administration [18]. Green tea and its polyphenols have been widely reported to exhibit positive effects against inflammation, cancer, aging, and others [11,19].

Casanova et al. [20] reviewed the effect of epigallocatechin gallate (EGCG) on oxidative stress and inflammation linked to the metabolic dysfunction of skeletal muscle in obesity and their underlying mechanisms and highlighted that in order to overcome the problem of EGCG instability and low bioavailability, future direction is the use of nanocarriers [20]. Chitosan is a biodegradable linear biopolyaminosaccharide obtained by alkaline deacetylation of chitin, with several advantages for oral drug delivery. It is a non-toxic, mucoadhesive natural polymer, with a high charge density, showing not only the capacity to improve dissolution of drugs, but also to improve the fat metabolism in the body [21,22]. Chitosan is being extensively used in the production of drug delivery systems (e.g., silica nanoparticles, microspheres) for oral administration [22–26]. The production of microspheres can be achieved by the electrostatic interaction between the biopolyaminosaccharide and the low molecular counterions such as polyphosphates, sulphates, and cross-linking with glutaraldehyde producing a gel [27–29].

To be effective in the management of metabolic diseases, the oral administration route is of preference due to higher convenience and higher patient compliance. Polyphenon-60 contains pure catechins, mainly EGCG, and has been selected for the present work as the active ingredient to be loaded into chitosan microspheres coated with Eudragit S-100 for delayed release in the gut. The choice of the oral route is primarily due to it being non-invasive and appropriate for self-administration, which increases the success of the therapeutic outcome. However, the hydrophilic environment of the gastrointestinal tract (GIT) compromises the absorption of many sensitive drugs [22].

The aim of this work was the development of a delayed release oral formulation for PP60. Chitosan microspheres produced by the ionic cross-linking method was been loaded with PP60 and further coated with methacrylic anionic copolymers (Eudragit S-100) to obtain an enteric dosage form, capable of releasing the active in the ileum with improved bioavailability aiming the prevention of metabolic diseases.

2. Materials and Methods

2.1. Materials

Polyphenon-60 (PP60, yellow powder with a total cathecin content >60%), chitosan from shrimp shells (molecular weight 150 kDa, 95% deacetylated, low viscosity <200 mPa·s), glutaraldehyde, ascorbic acid, and Span 80 (sorbitan monooleate) were purchased from Sigma-Aldrich (Saint Louis, Missouri, USA). Eudragit S-100 (poly(methacylic acid-co-methyl methacrylate) 1:2) was received as a kind gift from Evonik (São Paulo, Brazil). Liquid paraffin was obtained from VWR Chemicals (Lisbon, Portugal). All other reagents (glacial acetic acid, monobasic potassium phosphate, sodium dihydrogen phosphate, sodium hydroxide, toluene, petroleum ether, acetone, ethanol, and methanol) were obtained from Reagente-5 (Porto, Portugal). For cell culture, Dulbecco's modified Eagle's medium (DMEM), fetal bovine serum (FBS), Minimum Essential Medium Eagle's (MEME), Trypsin-0.3% EDTA, phosphate buffered saline (PBS), L-glutamine, non-essential amino acids (NEAA), sodium dodecyl sulfate (SDS), dimethylformamide (DMF), 3-(4,5-dimethylthiazol-2-yl)-2,5-diphenyltetrazolium bromide (MTT), Triton® X, and gentamicin were purchased from Sigma-Aldrich (Saint Louis, MO, USA). Caco-2 cell line was purchased from American Type Culture Collection (ATCC, Pensabio Biotecnologia, São Paulo, Brazil). The water used in all experiments was ultrapure, obtained from a MilliQ® Plus, Millipore® (Germany).

2.2. Production of Chitosan Microspheres

Chitosan microspheres were produced by emulsion cross-linking, at room temperature and following the method described by Jose et al. [26]. Briefly, PP60 was added to a solution of 2% (m/v) chitosan prepared in 1% (w/v) of glacial acetic acid aqueous solution. From the obtained solution, a volume of 3 mL was sampled and injected into 20 mL of oil phase of paraffin containing Span 80 with a syringe (No. 23) under mechanical stirring (Ultra-Turrax, T18, IKA, Staufen, Germany) for 30 min to form a w/o emulsion. A volume of 1.5 mL of toluene-saturated glutaraldehyde (8:1) was then added to the obtained emulsion, which was left to stabilize and to cross-link over a period of 5.5 hours. The obtained microspheres were centrifuged at 4000 rpm, the precipitate washed with petroleum ether and acetone and dried in a laboratory hot air oven (Binder Inc, Germany) at 50 °C. A total of 10 batches were produced by varying the processing parameters as shown in Table 1. For the first set of batches (Ch-PP60$_{2:1}$, Ch-PP60$_{4:1}$, Ch-PP60$_{8:1}$, and Ch-PP60$_{10:1}$), the rotational speed was kept constant at 1500 rpm and the concentration of Span 80 in liquid paraffin was kept at 1% (m/v), and varying the chitosan:PP60 ratios. For the second set of batches (Speed$_{10}$, Speed$_{15}$, and Speed$_{20}$), the chitosan:PP60 ratio was maintained at 4:1, the concentration of Span 80 in liquid paraffin was kept at 1% (m/v), and the rotational speed varied from 1000–2000 rpm. For the third set of batches (S80$_{0.5}$,

S80$_{1.0}$, and S80$_{1.5}$), the chitosan:PP60 ratio was maintained at 4:1, the rotational speed at 1500 rpm, while the concentration of surfactant (Span 80) in liquid paraffin ranged from 0.5%–1.5% (m/v).

Table 1. Variable parameters of chitosan microspheres produced by emulsion cross-linking method (PP60, polyphenon 60; rpm, rotations per minute; % (w/v), percentage weight per volume).

Constant Parameters	Processing Variables	Formulation Code
Rotational speed: 1500 rpm Concentration of Span 80: 1%	Chitosan:PP60 ratio 2:1 4:1 8:1 10:1	Ch-PP60$_{2:1}$ Ch-PP60$_{4:1}$ Ch-PP60$_{8:1}$ Ch-PP60$_{10:1}$
Chitosan:PP60 ratio: 4:1 Concentration of Span 80: 1%	Rotational speed 1000 rpm 1500 rpm 2000 rpm	Speed$_{10}$ Speed$_{15}$ Speed$_{20}$
Chitosan:PP60 ratio: 4:1 Rotational speed: 1500 rpm	Span 80 0.5% 1.0% 1.5%	S80$_{0.5}$ S80$_{1.0}$ S80$_{1.5}$

2.3. Eudragit S-100 Coating of PP60-Loaded Chitosan Microspheres

The coating of Ch-PP60 microspheres with Eudragit S-100 to obtain S100Ch-PP60 was done by emulsion-solvent evaporation technique, as described by Jose et al. [26]. Ch-PP60 microspheres were suspended in a 10% (w/v) of Eudragit S-100 in ethanol (2.5 mL) and then emulsified in light liquid paraffin (40 mL) containing 1.0% (w/v) Span 80. To form a stable emulsion, 2 mL of ethanol was added drop wise. The emulsion was kept for 3 h under mechanical stirrer (Ultra-Turrax, T18, IKA, Staufen, Germany) at 1000 rpm. The S100Ch-PP60 was collected, rinsed with petroleum ether, and dried in a laboratory hot air oven (Binder Inc., Germany) at 50 °C.

2.4. Particle Size Analysis

The particle size of Ch-PP60 (uncoated) and S100Ch-PP60 (coated) microspheres was measured in an optical Zeiss microscope (Oberkochen, Germany) fitted with a calibrated eyepiece micrometer under a magnification of 40×. The diameter of about 100 microspheres was measured randomly and the average size (D_{mean}) determined using the Edmondson's equation [26]:

$$D_{mean} = \frac{\sum nd}{n} \quad (1)$$

where n is the number of counted microspheres and d is the mean size range.

2.5. Yield of Production, Loading Capacity, and Encapsulation Efficiency

The yield of production (YP%) was calculated based on the dry weight of microspheres, applying the following equation:

$$YP\% = \frac{W_m}{W_{PP60} + W_c} \times 100 \quad (2)$$

where W_m is the mass of produced microspheres, and W_{PP60} and W_c are the mass of PP60 and chitosan, respectively, initially taken for the production of the microspheres. For the determination of the loading capacity (LC%) and encapsulation efficiency (EE%), 10 mg of microspheres were weighted and triturated in a mortar and pestle with 20 mL methanol. The mixture was kept overnight for the extraction of the active from chitosan. After filtration and proper dilution with methanol, the absorbance was read in a UV spectrophotometer Shimadzu UV-1601 (Shimadzu Italy, Cornaredo, Italy) at 280 nm against a calibration curve for the quantification of EGCG ($W_{EGCG\ read\ \lambda 280nm}$) [30]. The LC% and EE% were calculated using the following equations:

$$LC\% = \frac{W_{EGCG\ read\ \lambda 280nm}}{W_m} \times 100 \qquad (3)$$

$$EE\% = \frac{W_{EGCG\ read\ \lambda 280nm}}{Wm} \times 100 \qquad (4)$$

2.6. In Vitro Release Assay

The in vitro release of PP60 from Ch-PP60 (uncoated) and S100Ch-PP60 (coated) microspheres was evaluated in simulated gastrointestinal (GI) conditions using the United States Pharmacopoeia (USP) rotating paddle dissolution apparatus at 100 rpm and at 37 ± 0.5 °C, as described by Jose et al. [26]. Accurately weighed mass of microspheres, equivalent to 30 mg of PP60, was added to 450 mL of dissolution medium and GI conditions simulated over time by modifying the pH at pre-determined time intervals. From 0–2 h, the pH was kept at 1.2 by adding HCl (0.1 N). From 2–4 hours, 1.7 g of KH_2PO_4 and 2.225 g of $Na_2HPO_4 \cdot 2H_2O$ were added to the medium and the pH adjusted to 4.5 with NaOH (1.0 M). From 4–12 h, NaOH (1.0 M) was added to adjust the pH to 7.4. Over the course of the assay, and at pre-determined time intervals up to 12 hours, a volume of 2 mL was withdrawn from the medium and replaced with fresh dissolution medium to ensure sink conditions over the entire experiment. Samples were analyzed by reading the absorbance in a spectrophotometer Shimadzu UV-1601 (Shimadzu Italy, Cornaredo, Italy) at 280 nm against a calibration curve for the quantification of EGCG [30]. The effect of the chitosan:PP60 ratio on the in vitro drug release was analyzed and the best ratio compared to the coated formulation. All measurements were done in triplicate. The in vitro drug release data of the coated S100Ch-PP60 formulation was fitted to four kinetic models i.e., zero order, first order, Higuchi, and Korsemeyer–Peppas models [25], selecting the most appropriate model based on the obtained R^2 values.

2.7. Antioxidant Activity

2.7.1. DPPH Assay

The antioxidant activity of PP60 was measured when loaded into chitosan microspheres, and the effect of the enteric Eudragit S-100 coating (Ch-PP60 versus S100Ch-PP60) was compared. The assay evaluated the ability of the loaded PP60 to scavenge the stable DPPH• radical [31]. Briefly, microspheres (Ch-PP60; S100Ch-PP60) were dissolved in 0.1 mM DPPH methanolic solution. Then, a volume of 20 µL of sample was placed in the microplate wells to which 200 µL DPPH methanolic solution (0.1 mM) was added. Methanol was used as negative control and butylated hydroxytoluene (BHT, 0–6 µg/mL) was used as the positive control. The microplates were incubated at 25 °C for 30 min, and then read at 517 nm in a multiplate reader (DTX 880 Multimode Detector, Beckman Coulter Inc.). The percentage of the antioxidant activity (AA (%)) was calculated from the recorded optical densities (OD), using the following equation:

$$AA(\%) = \frac{OD\ of\ negative\ control\ -\ OD\ of\ sample}{OD\ of\ negative\ control} \times 100 \qquad (5)$$

The linear regression equation was obtained by plotting the concentration in the X-axis (µg/mL) against AA(%) in the Y-axis (% inhibition), from which the IC_{50} value could be calculated.

2.7.2. In Vitro Caco-2 Cells Proliferation Assay

The MTT assay was used for the evaluation of the proliferative capacity of Caco-2 cells when treated with Ch-PP60 (uncoated) and S100Ch-PP60 (coated) microspheres [32]. Caco-2 cell lines were firstly seeded in 96-well microtiter plates (0.1×10^6 cells/mL; 100 µL/well). After 24 h of incubation, serum DMEM was replaced with serum free DMEM. The next day, cells were treated with the microspheres. Solutions of Ch-PP60 and S100Ch-PP60 in dimethyl sulfoxide (DMSO 0.7%) at gradient concentrations (0.5, 2.5, 5, 10, and 15 µg/mL of microspheres) were prepared in serum free DMEM, added to each well and incubated for more 24 and 48 h at 37 °C in a 5% CO_2 atmosphere. A solution of DMSO 1% was set as the negative control, whereas a doxorubicin solution (100 µg/mL) was set as the positive control. At the end of the incubation period, test solutions were removed. MTT solution (150 µL) at 0.5 mg/mL was added to each well and incubated in the dark for 4 h at 37 °C in a 5% CO_2 atmosphere. The experiments were repeated three times, and quadruplicates were done for each condition in each assay. Cell viability was determined as the ability of viable cells to reduce the yellow dye MTT to the purple formazan. The obtained precipitate was dissolved in 150 µL DMSO and the absorbance was read at 595 nm using a multiplate reader (DTX 880 Multimode Detector, Beckman Coulter Inc.). The results were expressed as percentage of cell viability in relation to the negative control as follows:

$$Cell\ viability[\%] = \left[\frac{Abs_{Test}}{Abs_{Negative\ Control}} \times 100\right] \quad (6)$$

2.8. Statistical Analysis

All measurements were performed in triplicate, and results expressed as the mean ± S.D. Statistical significance was established at $p < 0.05$ and was calculated using a one-way analysis of variance ANOVA followed by the Tukeys Test. Values of $p < 0.05$ were considered significant. All statistical analyses were carried out using the GraphPad program 5.0® (Intuitive Software for Science, San Diego, CA, USA).

3. Results

The microspheres produced by emulsion cross-linking between chitosan and glutaraldehyde to load PP60 were yellowish because of the natural color of the active ingredient. To select the best combination of chitosan and PP60, and the production parameters, the particle size (D_{mean}), yield of production (YP%), loading capacity (LC%), and encapsulation efficiency (EE%) were determined for the different batches (as shown in Table 1), and the results of the physicochemical characterization are given in Table 2.

Table 2. Particle size, percentage yield, percent drug content, and entrapment efficiency of uncoated and Eudragit coated chitosan microspheres. The results were subjected to one-way ANOVA (Tukeys Test. Data are presented as mean ± SD (standard deviation); n = 3.

Formulation code	D_{mean} (µm)	YP% (%)	LC (%)	EE (%)
Ch-PP60$_{2:1}$	5.57	69.73 ± 0.27	18.36 ± 0.71	75.26 ± 0.27
Ch-PP60$_{4:1}$	6.23	78.64 ± 0.76	13.91 ± 0.22	76.81 ± 0.55
Ch-PP60$_{8:1}$	7.16	86.15 ± 0.88	7.72 ± 0.11	87.21 ± 0.33
Ch-PP60$_{10:1}$	7.83	89.99 ± 0.70	6.99 ± 0.53	85.61 ± 0.14
Speed$_{10}$	9.22	89.27 ± 0.45	12.91 ± 0.27	77.82 ± 0.91
Speed$_{15}$	7.68	91.25 ± 0.34	13.84 ± 0.61	79.33 ± 0.17
Speed$_{20}$	6.97	90.11 ± 0.56	13.25 ± 0.12	76.16 ± 0.73
S80$_{0.5}$	11.82	88.37 ± 0.66	9.36 ± 0.11	81.11 ± 0.49
S80$_{1.0}$	6.45	92.27 ± 0.55	11.32 ± 0.41	83.55 ± 0.81
S80$_{1.5}$	6.11	90.28 ± 0.47	10.51 ± 0.27	82.24 ± 0.77

Both Ch-PP60$_{8:1}$ and S100Ch-PP60 were tested for their release profile in simulated gastrointestinal fluids using USP dissolution test apparatus at 37 ± 0.5 °C (Figure 1). The release profile of epigallocatechin gallate (EGCG) from non-coated microspheres (Ch-PP60$_{8:1}$) and Eudragit S-100 coated microspheres (S100Ch-PP60) formulations were compared over the pH range from 1.2 (simulated gastric fluid) in acid buffer solution for 2 h, to pH 4.5 (simulated duodenum) for another 2 h, to pH 7.4 (simulated distal ileum and colon) for the remaining 20 h.

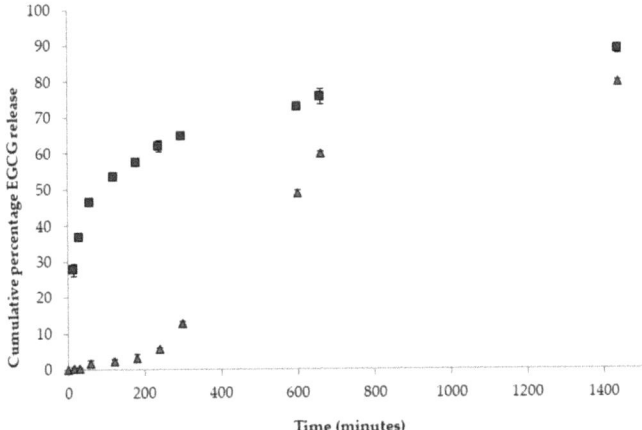

Figure 1. Cumulative percentage of epigallocatechin gallate (EGCG) release from non-coated microspheres (Ch-PP60$_{8:1}$, ■) and Eudragit S-100 coated microspheres (S100Ch-PP60, ▲) in simulated gastrointestinal conditions. Error bars ± standard deviation (SD); $n = 3$.

Mathematical fitting models (Higuchi model, Korsmeyer–Peppas model, zero order, and first order) have been used to describe the recorded profiles from both tested batches and results are shown in Figures 2 and 3, respectively.

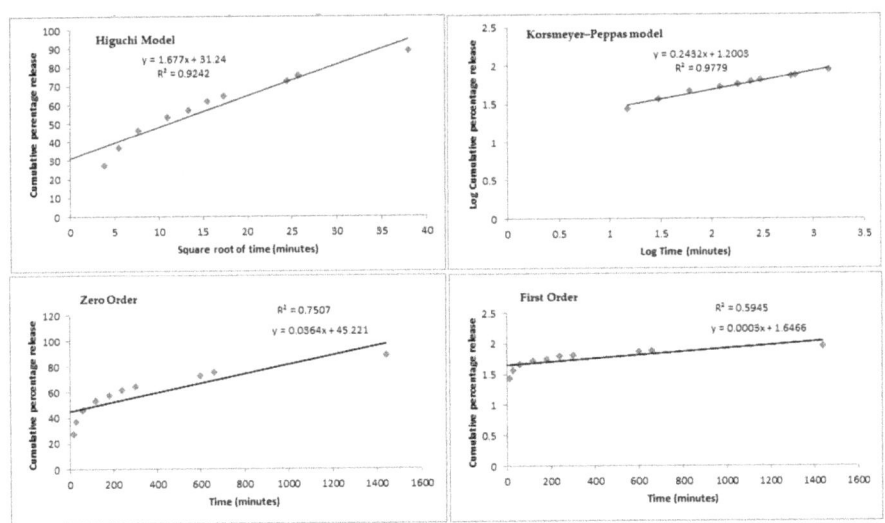

Figure 2. Mathematical fitting models (Higuchi model, Korsmeyer–Peppas model, zero order, and first order) of the cumulative percentage of EGCG release from non-coated microspheres (Ch-PP60$_{8:1}$) in simulated gastrointestinal conditions.

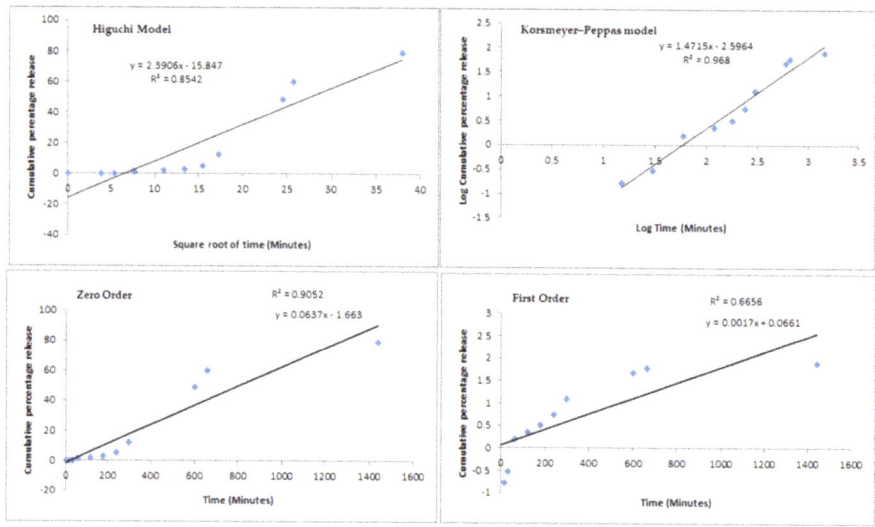

Figure 3. Mathematical fitting models (Higuchi model, Korsmeyer–Peppas model, zero order, and first order) of the cumulative percentage of EGCG release from Eudragit S-100 coated microspheres (S100Ch-PP60) in simulated gastrointestinal conditions.

The capacity of S100Ch-PP60 to neutralize reactive oxygen species (ROS) was evaluated using the DPPH scavenging assay, which was shown to be concentration dependent. The absorbance decay of the control test was compared with the recorded absorbance decay of Ch-PP60$_{8:1}$ versus S100Ch-PP60, resulting in the percentage scavenging of free radicals translated as the antioxidant activity (Table 3) [33]. Differences were shown to be statistically significant. For the positive control (BHT) 78.11% scavenging of DPPH radical was recorded at the highest tested concentration (6.0 µg/mL) [33,34]. For the Ch-PP60$_{8:1}$, the linear regression of $R^2 = 0.9941$ (y = 4.2743x − 1.45) was obtained and the IC$_{50}$ calculated as 212.3 µg/mL, which confirms the cross-linking of chitosan with glutaraldehyde did not compromise the antioxidant activity of catechin. The coating with Eudragit (S100Ch-PP60) resulted in the linear regression of $R^2 = 0.9895$ (y = 3.1023x − 0.728) with the IC$_{50}$ of 154.4 µg/mL.

Table 3. Percentage of scavenging of free radical DPPH (antioxidant activity; AA (%)) by Ch-PP60$_{8:1}$ and S100Ch-PP60. Values are mean ± SD ($n = 3$).

µg/mL	AA(%)	
	Ch-PP60$_{8:1}$	S100Ch-PP60
1	2.23 ± 0.98	1.83 ± 1.10
2	7.15 ± 0.03	5.24 ± 1.04
3	12.38 ± 1.04	9.44 ± 0.23
4	15.87 ± 1.02	12.29 ± 1.67
5	19.22 ± 0.33	14.65 ± 0.91
10	24.21 ± 0.75	17.33 ± 0.82

From the MTT assay (Figure 4), we can see that there was no significant difference in cell viability, over the concentration range tested, i.e., between 0.5 and 15 µg/mL. Despite the statistical ($p < 0.05$) significant reduction in cell viability observed in all tested concentrations and at both time-points (compared to the control), the cell viability remained above 70% at all tested concentrations for the non-coated microspheres, indicating limited risk of cytotoxic events. The Eudragit coating slightly reduced the cell viability. At the end of the 48 h, the reduction in cell viability was 35.41% and 40.63% for Ch-PP60$_{8:1}$ and S100Ch-PP60, respectively, at the highest tested concentration.

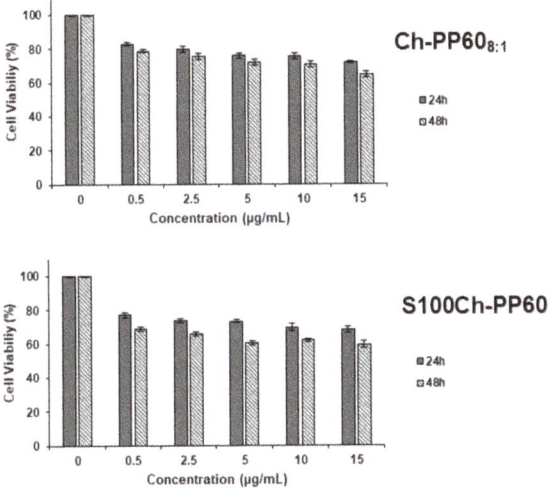

Figure 4. Evaluation of the cytotoxic activity of Ch-PP60$_{8:1}$ and S100Ch-PP60 in Caco-2 cell line using the MTT assay at 24 and 48 h. The data represent the mean values ± SD (n = 3).

4. Discussion

When varying the chitosan:PP60 ratio from 2:1 to 10:1, the mean diameter of microspheres increased from 5.57 µm to 7.83 µm (Table 2), which was an expected result as the increase of polymer concentration contributes to an increase the mean particle size. The higher encapsulation efficiency was obtained for the ratio 8:1 (Ch-PP60$_{8:1}$, 87.21 ± 0.33%) with a loading capacity of 7.72 ± 0.11%. Increasing the amount of chitosan also resulted in the increase of the yield of production up to 89.99 ± 0.70%. When increasing the speed rotation from 1000 rpm to 2000 rpm, the size decreased from 9.22 µm down to 6.97 µm. This is attributed to the improved distribution of small emulsion droplets within the aqueous phase, which are then stabilized with the surfactant molecules. The highest yield of production (92.27 ± 0.55%), loading capacity (11.32 ± 0.41%), and encapsulation efficiency (83.55 ± 0.81%) were achieved with 1% (m/v) of surfactant concentration, with this amount suitable to cover all new particle surfaces being formed upon emulsion cross-linking. When varying the speed, no significant changes were seen for the loading capacity as the chitosan:PP60 ratio remained 4:1 (Table 1). The best results (highest YP%, LC%, and EE%) were obtained with the 1.0% (w/v) of Span 80, resulting in microspheres with a mean diameter of 6.45 µm. The formulations produced with a chitosan:PP60 ratio of 8:1 (Ch-PP60$_{8:1}$) dispersed in 1% (m/v) Span 80 at 1500 rpm have been selected for further studies. The obtained microspheres (Ch-PP60$_{8:1}$) were coated with Eudragit S-100 (S100Ch-PP60) and showed a significant increase of the D_{mean} (51.4 µm). Eudragit S-100 is an anionic copolymer based on methacrylic acid and methyl methacrylate, both polymers contributing for the increase of the particles diameter which demonstrate that particles are coated with the enteric copolymer.

When comparing the release profile between Ch-PP60$_{8:1}$ and S100Ch-PP60 in simulated gastrointestinal conditions, the results depicted a delayed release of the active ingredient when coating the chitosan microspheres with the enteric polymer. Within the first 2 h, about 53.45 ± 0.28% of EGCG released from non-coated microspheres was quantified in the dissolution medium, whereas only ca. 2.24 ± 0.52% was released from the coated microspheres. The increase of the pH to 4.5 induced the further release up to 61.90 ± 1.59% and 5.51 ± 0.22% by the end of the 4th hour from non-coated and Eudragit S-100 coated microspheres, respectively. After 24 h of assay, the cumulative amount reached 88.56 ± 1.24% and 79.54 ± 0.52% when released from non-coated and Eudragit S-100 coated microspheres, respectively. These results also demonstrate that S100Ch-PP60 was effectively coated with polyacrylic polymer and this is able to ensure an enteric resistance of the microspheres until they reach the colon.

Comparing the R^2 values recorded for the different fitting models, the release plots of both profiles followed the Korsmeyer–Peppas model with the highest correlation coefficient values of 0.9779 (Ch-PP60$_{8:1}$) and 0.9680 (S100Ch-PP60). When coating the microspheres with Eudragit S-100, the release mechanism fitted to the Power Law profile which follows the equation $M_t/M_\infty = k't^n$, where M_t is the cumulative amount of active released at time t, M_∞ is the cumulative amount of active released at infinite time, k' is the Korsmeyers–Peppas constant that is governed by the physicochemical properties of the microspheres. The diffusional exponent n translates the release mechanism, i.e., if n = 0.5 the release follows the Fickian diffusion, and if $0.5 < n < 1.0$ it follows a non-Fickian diffusion. A Case II transport is seen as n approaches 1.0 when the release independent of time and reaches zero-order release; a super Case II transport is followed when $n > 1.0$ [35]. Interestingly the Eudragit coating significantly changed the transport mechanism; for the non-coated microspheres the release followed the Fickian diffusion, which means that the active was released from the glutaraldehyde cross-linked chitosan microspheres by the usual molecular diffusion attributed to a chemical potential gradient. With the enteric coating, a super Case II was approached, in which the transport mechanism of the active from the microspheres is associated with the erosion of polymeric coating, as seen with the increase of the pH up to 7.4 (Figure 1). The second-best fitting model for the coated microspheres was the zero-order release. The obtained profiles seem to be appropriate to the proposed colonic delivery of PP60. Indeed, it is expected that the release of the active is kept at minimum through the transport of the microspheres through the stomach and small intestine before they reach colon. Eudragit S-100 is soluble at pH above 7; when reaching pH 7.4 the amount of active being released increased almost 40%. The presence of a modified release profile in both formulations could be confirmed, with a drug protective effect promoted by the enteric coating.

The antioxidant activity represents the first step for the evaluation of health benefits [36–38]. For an effective activity against metabolic diseases, the well-known antioxidant activity of green tea should be kept until it is released from the microspheres. The DPPH test demonstrated that the scavenging capacity of S100Ch-PP60 was dependent on the concentration, i.e., the higher the concentration the higher the scavenging activity. The coating of the microspheres with the polyacrylic polymer did not compromise the antioxidant activity of the loaded PP60, a property that can be further exploited for the treatment/prophylaxis of metabolic diseases.

Prior to any in vivo experiment, toxicological studies should be first performed in vitro, using cell models that mimic the body conditions, in order to minimize the number of animal studies and to have an idea of the cytotoxicity of the drug delivery system at an early stage. Although known to be biocompatible and biodegradable, glutaraldehyde-cross-linked chitosan microspheres should be characterized for their capacity to maintain the viability of cells in vitro. For oral delivery, the main barrier of drug absorption is the intestinal epithelium. The Caco-2 cell line is a human colon epithelial cancer cell line often used as a model to mimic the gastrointestinal conditions. While other cell lines are available for cyto/geno-toxicity assessment [39,40], this model seems to be the most realistic cell culture to test oral drug delivery systems. Cytotoxicity of drug delivery systems in the gut is frequently estimated by colorimetric methods in Caco-2 cells [27,41,42]. Among these methods, the most frequently used is the MTT assay. In the MTT assay, the mitochondrial function of the cells is tested. Only live cells will produce the enzymes capable to reduce the MTT reagent. The cytotoxicity of Ch-PP60$_{8:1}$ was checked in the Caco-2 cell line, in comparison to the Eudragit-coated microspheres (S100Ch-PP60). From the obtained results, cells remained viable when treated with both Ch-PP60$_{8:1}$ and S100Ch-PP60 over the tested concentration range over a period of 24 h or 48 h. The coating of the chitosan microspheres with the acrylic polymer reduced the cell viability down to approximately 60% at the highest tested concentration (15 µg/mL) after 48 h. The effect of size and concentration of particles on cell viability is well-described in scientific literature, being also very much dependent on the type of cell lines [43]. Monolayer type adherent cells, i.e., cells that adhere onto the surface of the culture dish as happens with Caco-2, are more sensitive to the effect of size and concentration as more surface area is exposed. The smaller the size and the lower the concentration, the higher the cell uptake which in principle would induce higher cytotoxicity [44]. Our results show that cell viability was slightly compromised by the coating with the polyacrylic polymer attributed to the density of particles onto the surface of the cell's monolayer.

It is expected that S100Ch-PP60 microspheres can be further processed in foodstuff and in beverages to provide an alternative approach for the administration and delivery of phytochemicals with nutraceutical value. Indeed, micro/nano-nutraceuticals represent a useful tool in managing health conditions, particularly in patients not eligible for conventional therapy [45,46]. Follow up studies, use, and compliance [47–50], as well as communication strategies and assessment [51], should be applied also to nutraceuticals. This approach will allow the management of different health conditions, as happens with the metabolic syndrome [52,53], obesity, and dysmetabolism [54–58], which are often related to the food intake/dietary habits. Given its high levels of antioxidants and polyphenols, green tea is sometimes seen as the healthiest beverage on earth. It has recognized health benefits in metabolic syndrome, e.g., against fat gain, in preventing and managing type 2 diabetes, besides lowering the risk of cancer among others biological effects. Metabolic syndrome is a combination of risk factors ending up in chronic diseases, such as obesity, and is intimately related to oxidative stress and inflammation. As a prophylactic measure, antioxidants, such as those of green tea, can further be exploited in foodstuff as nutraceutical. The smart delivery of nutraceuticals [3,5,6,59–65], through their encapsulation in micro/nanoparticles, can offer an approach to increase their bioavailability. Besides, chitosan microspheres coated with an enteric polymer can be formulated in different food matrices for a modified release in the gut, offering the opportunity to enrich the nutraceutical value of food, supplements, and beverages recommended for the prevention and/or treatment of health conditions linked to dysmetabolism. Such micro/nano-based products should become part of an improved lifestyle as a prophylactic approach against metabolic disorders.

5. Conclusions

Polyphenon-60-loaded chitosan microspheres cross-linked with glutaraldehyde were successfully prepared. The microspheres were then coated with Eudragit and tested for their modified release in simulated gastrointestinal conditions. The delayed release of green tea was confirmed; both non-coated and Eudragit coated microspheres followed the Korsmeyers–Peppas release model, demonstrating capacity to retain the antioxidant activity of the active ingredient. The coated microspheres increased their size significantly, however without significantly compromising their biocompatibility with the intestinal epithelial Caco-2 cells. The potential for this formulation to deliver poorly water-soluble drugs, such as catechins, was illustrated and can be exploited for the management of metabolic diseases, exploiting the biological effects of green tea, as well as being applied to other matrices of vegetal origin and mucoadhesive chitosan microspheres.

Author Contributions: R.d.A., S.B.S., A.Z., C.M., L.N.A., O.K.H., A.G.A., M.L., and E.N. contributed to the methodology, formal analysis, investigation, resources, and data curation; production of non-coated and coated microspheres and the study of optimized parameters have been carried out by R.d.A., A.Z., C.M., and M.L.; physicochemical characterization of the microspheres and quantification of the catechin have been performed by A.D., E.N., and A.S.; the in vitro release assay and mathematical modelling have been done by E.B.S., S.B.S., L.K.H., and A.G.A.; the antioxidant activity and cell line studies have been carried out by L.N.A., P.S., and A.M.S.; writing of the original manuscript was contributed to by E.B.S., S.B.S., R.d.A., A.D., A.S., and P.S.; conceptualization, review, and editing of the manuscript, as well as project administration, supervision, and funding acquisition was contributed to by E.B.S., A.M.S., A.S., and P.S. All authors have read and agreed to the published version of the manuscript.

Funding: This research was supported by the Coordenação Aperfeiçoamento de Pessoal de Nivel Superior (CAPES), Fundação de Amparo à Pesquisa do Estado de Sergipe (FAPITEC) CHAMADA MS/CNPq/FAPITEC/SE/SES N° 06/2018 – PROGRAMA DE PESQUISA PARA O SUS: GESTÃO COMPARTILHADA EM SAÚDE – PPSUS

SERGIPE 2017/2018, and Conselho Nacional de Desenvolvimento Científico e Tecnológico (CNPq). This work was also financed through the projects M-ERA-NET/0004/2015-PAIRED, UIDB/04469/2020 (strategic fund) and PEst-OE/UID/AGR/04033/2019 (CITAB strategic fund), receiving support from the Portuguese Science and Technology Foundation, Ministry of Science and Education (FCT/MEC) through national funds, and co-financed by FEDER, under the Partnership Agreement PT2020. The authors acknowledge the support of the research project: Nutraceutica come supporto nutrizionale nel paziente oncologico, CUP: B83D18000140007.

Conflicts of Interest: The authors declare no conflict of interest.

References

1. El-Mowafy, A.M.; Al-Gayyar, M.M.; Salem, H.A.; El-Mesery, M.E.; Darweish, M.M. Novel chemotherapeutic and renal protective effects for the green tea (EGCG): Role of oxidative stress and inflammatory-cytokine signaling. *Phytomedicine* **2010**, *17*, 1067–1075. [CrossRef] [PubMed]
2. Khan, N.; Mukhtar, H. Tea Polyphenols in Promotion of Human Health. *Nutrients* **2018**, *11*, 39. [CrossRef] [PubMed]
3. Durazzo, A.; Lucarini, M.; Souto, E.B.; Cicala, C.; Caiazzo, E.; Izzo, A.A.; Novellino, E.; Santini, A. Polyphenols: A concise overview on the chemistry, occurrence, and human health. *Phytother. Res.* **2019**, *33*, 2221–2243. [CrossRef]
4. Rothenberg, D.O.N.; Zhou, C.; Zhang, L. A Review on the Weight-Loss Effects of Oxidized Tea Polyphenols. *Molecules* **2018**, *23*, 1176. [CrossRef] [PubMed]
5. Santini, A.; Novellino, E. Nutraceuticals: Beyond the diet before the drugs. *Curr. Bioact. Compd.* **2014**, *10*, 1–12. [CrossRef]
6. Santini, A.; Novellino, E. To Nutraceuticals and Back: Rethinking a Concept. *Foods* **2017**, *6*, 74. [CrossRef]
7. Cicero, A.F.G.; Fogacci, F.; Colletti, A. Food and plant bioactives for reducing cardiometabolic disease risk: An evidence based approach. *Food Funct.* **2017**, *8*, 2076–2088. [CrossRef]
8. Ramis, M.R.; Sarubbo, F.; Tejada, S.; Jiménez, M.; Esteban, S.; Miralles, A.; Moranta, D. Chronic Polyphenon-60 or Catechin Treatments Increase Brain Monoamines Syntheses and Hippocampal SIRT1 LEVELS Improving Cognition in Aged Rats. *Nutrient* **2020**, *12*, 326. [CrossRef]
9. El-Missiry, M.A.; Amer, M.A.; Othman, A.I.; Yaseen, k. Polyphenon-60 ameliorates metabolic risk factors, oxidative stress, and proinflammatory cytokines and modulates apoptotic proteins to protect the heart against streptozotocin-induced apoptosis. *Egypt. J. Basic Appl. Sci.* **2015**, *2*, 120–131. [CrossRef]
10. Cano, A.; Ettcheto, M.; Chang, J.H.; Barroso, E.; Espina, M.; Kuhne, B.A.; Barenys, M.; Auladell, C.; Folch, J.; Souto, E.B.; et al. Dual-drug loaded nanoparticles of Epigallocatechin-3-gallate (EGCG)/Ascorbic acid enhance therapeutic efficacy of EGCG in a APPswe/PS1dE9 Alzheimer's disease mice model. *J. Control. Release* **2019**, *301*, 62–75. [CrossRef]
11. Fangueiro, J.F.; Andreani, T.; Fernandes, L.; Garcia, M.L.; Egea, M.A.; Silva, A.M.; Souto, E.B. Physicochemical characterization of epigallocatechin gallate lipid nanoparticles (EGCG-LNs) for ocular instillation. *Colloids Surf. B Biointerfaces* **2014**, *123*, 452–460. [CrossRef] [PubMed]
12. Fangueiro, J.F.; Calpena, A.C.; Clares, B.; Andreani, T.; Egea, M.A.; Veiga, F.J.; Garcia, M.L.; Silva, A.M.; Souto, E.B. Biopharmaceutical evaluation of epigallocatechin gallate-loaded cationic lipid nanoparticles (EGCG-LNs): In vivo, in vitro and ex vivo studies. *Int. J. Pharm.* **2016**, *502*, 161–169. [CrossRef] [PubMed]
13. Kopin, L.; Lowenstein, C.J. Dyslipidemia. *Ann. Intern. Med.* **2017**, *167*, ITC81–ITC96. [CrossRef] [PubMed]
14. Bernatoniene, J.; Kopustinskiene, D.M. The Role of Catechins in Cellular Responses to Oxidative Stress. *Molecules* **2018**, *23*, 965. [CrossRef]
15. Caro, A.A.; Davis, A.; Fobare, S.; Horan, N.; Ryan, C.; Schwab, C. Antioxidant and pro-oxidant mechanisms of (+) catechin in microsomal CYP2E1-dependent oxidative stress. *Toxicol. In Vitro* **2019**, *54*, 1–9. [CrossRef]
16. Lucarini, M.; Sciubba, F.; Capitani, D.; Di Cocco, M.E.; D'Evoli, L.; Durazzo, A.; Delfini, M.; Lombardi Boccia, G. Role of catechin on collagen type I stability upon oxidation: A NMR approach. *Nat. Prod. Res.* **2020**, *34*, 53–62. [CrossRef]
17. Santana, A.; Santamarina, A.; Souza, G.; Mennitti, L.; Okuda, M.; Venancio, D.; Seelaender, M.; do Nascimento, C.O.; Ribeiro, E.; Lira, F.; et al. Decaffeinated green tea extract rich in epigallocatechin-3-gallate improves insulin resistance and metabolic profiles in normolipidic diet—But not high-fat diet-fed mice. *J. Nutr. Biochem.* **2015**, *26*, 893–902. [CrossRef]

18. Xu, Y.; Zhang, M.; Wu, T.; Dai, S.; Xu, J.; Zhou, Z. The anti-obesity effect of green tea polysaccharides, polyphenols and caffeine in rats fed with a high-fat diet. *Food Funct.* **2015**, *6*, 297–304. [CrossRef]
19. Santos, I.S.; Ponte, B.M.; Boonme, P.; Silva, A.M.; Souto, E.B. Nanoencapsulation of polyphenols for protective effect against colon-rectal cancer. *Biotechnol. Adv.* **2013**, *31*, 514–523. [CrossRef]
20. Casanova, E.; Salvadó, J.; Crescenti, A.; Gibert-Ramos, A. Epigallocatechin Gallate Modulates Muscle Homeostasis in Type 2 Diabetes and Obesity by Targeting Energetic and Redox Pathways: A Narrative Review. *Int. J. Mol. Sci.* **2019**, *20*, 532. [CrossRef]
21. Sinha, V.R.; Singla, A.K.; Wadhawan, S.; Kaushik, R.; Kumria, R.; Bansal, K.; Dhawan, S. Chitosan microspheres as a potential carrier for drugs. *Int. J. Pharm.* **2004**, *274*, 1–33. [CrossRef] [PubMed]
22. Teixeira, M.D.C.; Santini, A.; Souto, E.B. Delivery of Antimicrobials by Chitosan-Composed Therapeutic Nanostructures. In *Nanostructures for Antimicrobial Therapy*; Anton, F., Alexandru, G., Eds.; Chapter 8; Elsevier: Amsterdam, The Netherlands, 2017; pp. 203–222. [CrossRef]
23. Ataide, J.A.; Gerios, E.F.; Cefali, L.C.; Fernandes, A.R.; Teixeira, M.D.C.; Ferreira, N.R.; Tambourgi, E.B.; Jozala, A.F.; Chaud, M.V.; Oliveira-Nascimento, L.; et al. Effect of Polysaccharide Sources on the Physicochemical Properties of Bromelain-Chitosan Nanoparticles. *Polymers* **2019**, *11*, 1618. [CrossRef] [PubMed]
24. Jose, S.; Fangueiro, J.F.; Smitha, J.; Cinu, T.A.; Chacko, A.J.; Premaletha, K.; Souto, E.B. Cross-linked chitosan microspheres for oral delivery of insulin: Taguchi design and in vivo testing. *Colloids Surf. B Biointerfaces* **2012**, *92*, 175–179. [CrossRef] [PubMed]
25. Jose, S.; Fangueiro, J.F.; Smitha, J.; Cinu, T.A.; Chacko, A.J.; Premaletha, K.; Souto, E.B. Predictive modeling of insulin release profile from cross-linked chitosan microspheres. *Eur. J. Med. Chem.* **2013**, *60*, 249–253. [CrossRef]
26. Jose, S.; Prema, M.T.; Chacko, A.J.; Thomas, A.C.; Souto, E.B. Colon specific chitosan microspheres for chronotherapy of chronic stable angina. *Colloids Surf. B Biointerfaces* **2011**, *83*, 277–283. [CrossRef]
27. Andreani, T.; Fangueiro, J.F.; Severino, P.; Souza, A.L.R.; Martins-Gomes, C.; Fernandes, P.M.V.; Calpena, A.C.; Gremiao, M.P.; Souto, E.B.; Silva, A.M. The Influence of Polysaccharide Coating on the Physicochemical Parameters and Cytotoxicity of Silica Nanoparticles for Hydrophilic Biomolecules Delivery. *Nanomaterials* **2019**, *9*, 81. [CrossRef]
28. Andreani, T.; Kiill, C.P.; de Souza, A.L.; Fangueiro, J.F.; Fernandes, L.; Doktorovova, S.; Santos, D.L.; Garcia, M.L.; Gremiao, M.P.; Souto, E.B.; et al. Surface engineering of silica nanoparticles for oral insulin delivery: Characterization and cell toxicity studies. *Colloids Surf. B Biointerfaces* **2014**, *123*, 916–923. [CrossRef]
29. Andreani, T.; Miziara, L.; Lorenzon, E.N.; de Souza, A.L.; Kiill, C.P.; Fangueiro, J.F.; Garcia, M.L.; Gremiao, P.D.; Silva, A.M.; Souto, E.B. Effect of mucoadhesive polymers on the in vitro performance of insulin-loaded silica nanoparticles: Interactions with mucin and biomembrane models. *Eur. J. Pharm. Biopharm.* **2015**, *93*, 118–126. [CrossRef]
30. Fangueiro, J.F.; Parra, A.; Silva, A.M.; Egea, M.A.; Souto, E.B.; Garcia, M.L.; Calpena, A.C. Validation of a high performance liquid chromatography method for the stabilization of epigallocatechin gallate. *Int. J. Pharm.* **2014**, *475*, 181–190. [CrossRef]
31. Aksoy, L.; Kolay, E.; Ağılönü, Y.; Aslan, Z.; Kargıoğlu, M. Free radical scavenging activity, total phenolic content, total antioxidant status, and total oxidant status of endemic Thermopsis turcica. *Saudi J. Biol. Sci.* **2013**, *20*, 235–239. [CrossRef]
32. Rigon, R.B.; Goncalez, M.L.; Severino, P.; Alves, D.A.; Santana, M.H.A.; Souto, E.B.; Chorilli, M. Solid lipid nanoparticles optimized by 2(2) factorial design for skin administration: Cytotoxicity in NIH3T3 fibroblasts. *Colloids Surf. B Biointerfaces* **2018**, *171*, 501–505. [CrossRef]
33. Souto, E.B.; Zielinska, A.; Souto, S.B.; Durazzo, A.; Lucarini, M.; Santini, A.; Silva, A.M.; Atanasov, A.G.; Marques, C.; Andrade, L.N.; et al. (+)-Limonene 1,2-epoxide-loaded SLN: Evaluation of drug release, antioxidant activity and cytotoxicity in HaCaT cell line. *Int. J. Mol. Sci.* **2020**, *21*, E1449. [CrossRef] [PubMed]
34. Souto, E.B.; Souto, S.B.; Zielinska, A.; Durazzo, A.; Lucarini, M.; Santini, A.; Horbańczuk, O.K.; Atanasov, A.G.; Marques, C.; Andrade, L.N.; et al. Perillaldehyde 1,2-epoxide loaded SLN-tailored mAb: Production, physicochemical characterization and in vitro cytotoxicity profile in MCF-7 cell lines. *Pharmaceutics* **2020**, *12*, 161. [CrossRef] [PubMed]

35. Nita, L.E.; Chiriac, A.P.; Nistor, M. An in vitro release study of indomethacin from nanoparticles based on methyl methacrylate/glycidyl methacrylate copolymers. *J. Mater. Sci. Mater. Med.* **2010**, *21*, 3129–3140. [CrossRef] [PubMed]
36. Durazzo, A.; Lucarini, M. Extractable and Non-Extractable Antioxidants. *Molecules* **2019**, *24*, 1933. [CrossRef] [PubMed]
37. Durazzo, A. Extractable and Non-extractable polyphenols: An overview. In *Non-Extractable Polyphenols and Carotenoids: Importance in Human Nutrition and Health*; Saura-Calixto, F., Pérez-Jiménez, J., Eds.; Royal Society of Chemistry: London, UK, 2018; pp. 1–37.
38. Durazzo, A.; Lucarini, M. A Current shot and re-thinking of antioxidant research strategy. *Braz. J. Anal. Chem.* **2018**, *5*, 9–11. [CrossRef]
39. Silva, A.M.; Alvarado, H.L.; Abrego, G.; Martins-Gomes, C.; Garduno-Ramirez, M.L.; Garcia, M.L.; Calpena, A.C.; Souto, E.B. In Vitro Cytotoxicity of Oleanolic/Ursolic Acids-Loaded in PLGA Nanoparticles in Different Cell Lines. *Pharmaceutics* **2019**, *11*, 362. [CrossRef]
40. Souto, E.B.; Campos, J.R.; Da Ana, R.; Martins-Gomes, C.; Silva, A.M.; Souto, S.B.; Lucarini, M.; Durazzo, A.; Santini, A. Ocular Cell Lines and Genotoxicity Assessment. *Int. J. Environ. Res. Public Health* **2020**, *17*, 46. [CrossRef]
41. Silva, A.M.; Martins-Gomes, C.; Fangueiro, J.F.; Andreani, T.; Souto, E.B. Comparison of antiproliferative effect of epigallocatechin gallate when loaded into cationic solid lipid nanoparticles against different cell lines. *Pharm. Dev. Technol.* **2019**, *24*, 1243–1249. [CrossRef]
42. Campos, J.R.; Fernandes, A.R.; Sousa, R.; Fangueiro, J.F.; Boonme, P.; Garcia, M.L.; Silva, A.M.; Naveros, B.C.; Souto, E.B. Optimization of nimesulide-loaded solid lipid nanoparticles (SLN) by factorial design, release profile and cytotoxicity in human Colon adenocarcinoma cell line. *Pharm. Dev. Technol.* **2019**, *24*, 616–622. [CrossRef]
43. Zauner, W.; Farrow, N.A.; Haines, A.M.R. In vitro uptake of polystyrene microspheres: Effect of particle size, cell line and cell density. *J. Control. Release* **2001**, *71*, 39–51. [CrossRef]
44. Sahu, D.; Kannan, M.; Tailang, M.; Vijayaraghavan, R. In Vitro Cytotoxicity of Nanoparticles: A Comparison between Particle Size and Cell Type. *J. Nanosci.* **2016**, *2016*. [CrossRef]
45. Souto, E.B.; Silva, G.F.; Dias-Ferreira, J.; Zielinska, A.; Ventura, F.; Durazzo, A.; Lucarini, M.; Novellino, E.; Santini, A. Nanopharmaceutics: Part I—Clinical Trials Legislation and Good Manufacturing Practices (GMP) of Nanotherapeutics in the EU. *Pharmaceutics* **2020**, *12*, 146. [CrossRef] [PubMed]
46. Souto, E.B.; Silva, G.F.; Dias-Ferreira, J.; Zielinska, A.; Ventura, F.; Durazzo, A.; Lucarini, M.; Novellino, E.; Santini, A. Nanopharmaceutics: Part II—Production scales and clinically compliant production methods. *Nanomaterials* **2020**, *10*, 455. [CrossRef]
47. Menditto, E.; Cahir, C.; Aza-Pascual-Salcedo, M.; Bruzzese, D.; Poblador-Plou, B.; Malo, S.; Costa, E.; González-Rubio, F.; Gimeno-Miguel, A.; Orlando, V.; et al. Adherence to chronic medication in older populations: Application of a common protocol among three European cohorts. *Patient Prefer. Adherence* **2018**, *12*, 1975–1987. [CrossRef]
48. Menditto, E.; Guerriero, F.; Orlando, V.; Crola, C.; Di Somma, C.; Illario, M.; Morisky, D.E.; Colao, A. Self-Assessment of Adherence to Medication: A Case Study in Campania Region Community-Dwelling Population. *J. Aging Res.* **2015**, *2015*, 682503. [CrossRef]
49. Putignano, D.; Bruzzese, D.; Orlando, V.; Fiorentino, D.; Tettamanti, A.; Menditto, E. Differences in drug use between men and women: An Italian cross sectional study. *BMC Womens Health* **2017**, *17*, 73. [CrossRef]
50. Iolascon, G.; Gimigliano, F.; Moretti, A.; Riccio, I.; Di Gennaro, M.; Illario, M.; Monetti, V.M.; Orlando, V.; Menditto, E. Rates and reasons for lack of persistence with anti-osteoporotic drugs: Analysis of the Campania region database. *Clin. Cases Miner. Bone Metab.* **2016**, *13*, 127–130. [CrossRef]
51. Scala, D.; Menditto, E.; Armellino, M.F.; Manguso, F.; Monetti, V.M.; Orlando, V.; Antonino, A.; Makoul, G.; De Palma, M. Italian translation and cultural adaptation of the communication assessment tool in an outpatient surgical clinic. *BMC Health Serv. Res.* **2016**, *16*, 163. [CrossRef]
52. Sherling, D.H.; Perumareddi, P.; Hennekens, C.H. Metabolic Syndrome:Clinical and Policy Implications of the New Silent Killer. *J. Cardiovasc. Pharmacol. Ther.* **2017**, *22*, 365–367. [CrossRef]
53. Schnack, L.L.; Romani, A.M.P. The Metabolic Syndrome and the Relevance of Nutrients for its Onset. *Recent Pat. Biotechnol.* **2017**, *11*, 101–119. [CrossRef] [PubMed]

54. Souto, E.B.; Souto, S.B.; Campos, J.R.; Severino, P.; Pashirova, T.N.; Zakharova, L.Y.; Silva, A.M.; Durazzo, A.; Lucarini, M.; Izzo, A.A.; et al. Nanoparticle Delivery Systems in the Treatment of Diabetes Complications. *Molecules* **2019**, *24*, 4209. [CrossRef] [PubMed]
55. Vieira, R.; Souto, S.B.; Sanchez-Lopez, E.; Machado, A.L.; Severino, P.; Jose, S.; Santini, A.; Fortuna, A.; Garcia, M.L.; Silva, A.M.; et al. Sugar-Lowering Drugs for Type 2 Diabetes Mellitus and Metabolic Syndrome-Review of Classical and New Compounds: Part-I. *Pharmaceuticals* **2019**, *12*, 152. [CrossRef] [PubMed]
56. Vieira, R.; Souto, S.B.; Sánchez-López, E.; Machado, A.L.; Severino, P.; Jose, S.; Santini, A.; Silva, A.M.; Fortuna, A.; García, M.L.; et al. Sugar-Lowering Drugs for Type 2 Diabetes Mellitus and Metabolic Syndrome-Strategies for In Vivo Administration: Part-II. *J. Clin. Med.* **2019**, *8*, 1332. [CrossRef]
57. Hossen, M.N.; Kajimoto, K.; Akita, H.; Hyodo, M.; Harashima, H. A comparative study between nanoparticle-targeted therapeutics and bioconjugates as obesity medication. *J. Control. Release* **2013**, *171*, 104–112. [CrossRef]
58. Vieira, R.; Severino, P.; Nalone, L.A.; Souto, S.B.; Silva, A.M.; Lucarini, M.; Durazzo, A.; Santini, A.; Souto, E.B. Sucupira Oil-Loaded Nanostructured Lipid Carriers (NLC): Lipid Screening, Factorial Design, Release Profile, and Cytotoxicity. *Molecules* **2020**, *25*, 685. [CrossRef]
59. Abenavoli, L.; Izzo, A.A.; Milic, N.; Cicala, C.; Santini, A.; Capasso, R. Milk thistle (*Silybum marianum*): A concise overview on its chemistry, pharmacological, and nutraceutical uses in liver diseases. *Phytother. Res.* **2018**, *32*, 2202–2213. [CrossRef]
60. Santini, A.; Tenore, G.C.; Novellino, E. Nutraceuticals: A paradigm of proactive medicine. *Eur. J. Pharm. Sci.* **2017**, *96*, 53–61. [CrossRef]
61. Daliu, P.; Santini, A.; Novellino, E. From pharmaceuticals to nutraceuticals: Bridging disease prevention and management. *Expert Rev. Clin. Pharmacol.* **2019**, *12*, 1–7. [CrossRef]
62. Daliu, P.; Santini, A.; Novellino, E. A decade of nutraceutical patents: Where are we now in 2018? *Expert Opin. Ther. Pat.* **2018**, *28*, 875–882. [CrossRef]
63. Durazzo, A.; D'Addezio, L.; Camilli, E.; Piccinelli, R.; Turrini, A.; Marletta, L.; Marconi, S.; Lucarini, M.; Lisciani, S.; Gabrielli, P.; et al. From Plant Compounds to Botanicals and Back: A Current Snapshot. *Molecules* **2018**, *23*, 1844. [CrossRef] [PubMed]
64. Santini, A.; Novellino, E. Nutraceuticals—Shedding light on the grey area between pharmaceuticals and food. *Expert Rev. Clin. Pharmacol.* **2018**, *11*, 545–547. [CrossRef] [PubMed]
65. Santini, A.; Cammarata, S.M.; Capone, G.; Ianaro, A.; Tenore, G.C.; Pani, L.; Novellino, E. Nutraceuticals: Opening the debate for a regulatory framework. *Br. J. Clin. Pharmacol.* **2018**, *84*, 659–672. [CrossRef] [PubMed]

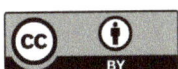

© 2020 by the authors. Licensee MDPI, Basel, Switzerland. This article is an open access article distributed under the terms and conditions of the Creative Commons Attribution (CC BY) license (http://creativecommons.org/licenses/by/4.0/).

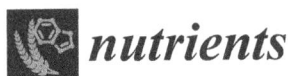

Article

Synergistic Effect of Omega-3 Fatty Acids and Oral-Hypoglycemic Drug on Lipid Normalization through Modulation of Hepatic Gene Expression in High Fat Diet with Low Streptozotocin-Induced Diabetic Rats

Suresh Khadke [1], Pallavi Mandave [1], Aniket Kuvalekar [1], Vijaya Pandit [2], Manjiri Karandikar [3] and Nitin Mantri [4,*]

[1] Interactive Research School for Health Affairs, Bharati Vidyapeeth, Deemed to be University, Pune-Satara Road, Pune 411043, Maharashtra, India; spkhadke@gmail.com (S.K.); mandavepallavi@gmail.com (P.M.); kuaniket@gmail.com (A.K.)
[2] Department of Pharmacology, Bharati Vidyapeeth Medical College, Bharati Vidyapeeth, Deemed to be University, Pune-Satara Road, Pune 411043, Maharashtra, India; vijaya.pandit@bharatividyapeeth.edu
[3] Department of Pathology, Bharati Vidyapeeth Medical College, Bharati Vidyapeeth, Deemed to Be University, Pune-Satara Road, Pune 411043, Maharashtra, India; manjiri.karandikar@bharatividyapeeth.edu
[4] The Pangenomics Lab, School of Science, RMIT University, Melbourne, VIC 3000, Australia
* Correspondence: nitin.mantri@rmit.edu.au; Tel.: +61-399-257-152

Received: 26 October 2020; Accepted: 23 November 2020; Published: 27 November 2020

Abstract: Type 2 diabetes mellitus, which an outcome of impaired insulin action and its secretion, is concomitantly associated with lipid abnormalities. The study was designed to evaluate the combinational effect of omega-3 fatty acids (flax and fish oil) and glibenclamide on abnormal lipid profiles, increased blood glucose, and impaired liver and kidney functions in a high fat diet with low streptozotocin (STZ)-induced diabetic rats, including its probable mechanism of action. The male Wistar rats (n = 48) were distributed into eight groups. All animal groups except the healthy received a high fat diet (HFD) for 90 days. Further, diabetes was developed by low dose STZ (35 mg/kg). Diabetic animals received, omega-3 fatty acids (500 mg/kg), along with glibenclamide (0.25 mg/kg). Both flax and fish oil intervention decreased ($p \leq 0.001$) serum triglycerides and very low density lipoprotein and elevated ($p \leq 0.001$) high density lipoprotein levels in diabetic rats. Total cholesterol and low-density lipoprotein level was decreased ($p \leq 0.001$) in fish oil-treated rats. However, it remained unaffected in the flax oil treatment group. Both flax and fish oil intervention downregulate the expression of fatty acid metabolism genes, transcription factors (sterol regulatory element-binding proteins-1c and nuclear factor-$\kappa\beta$), and their regulatory genes i.e., acetyl-coA carboxylase alpha, fatty acid synthase, and tumor necrosis factors-α. The peroxisome proliferator-activated receptor gamma gene expression was upregulated ($p \leq 0.001$) in the fish oil treatment group. Whereas, carnitine palmitoyltransferase 1 and fatty acid binding protein gene expression were upregulated ($p \leq 0.001$) in both flax and fish oil intervention group.

Keywords: type 2 diabetes mellitus; glibenclamide; omega-3 fatty acids; high fat diet; transcription factors; streptozotocin

1. Introduction

Type 2 diabetes mellitus (T2DM) is a metabolic disorder characterized by an increase in blood glucose due to impaired insulin secretion and its action [1]. The consistent hyperglycemia, insulin resistance, and insulin deficiency contribute to lipid abnormalities in T2DM [2]. The lipid abnormality is an independent risk factor for cardiovascular disease (CVD) development and commonly found in T2DM individuals [3]. Diabetic dyslipidemia is significantly associated with mortality and morbidity due to cardiovascular complications [4]. It accounts for 80% of deaths in diabetic individuals due to CVD [5]. The hyperglycemia, along with lipid abnormalities, is a modifiable risk factor for CVD, and remains uncontrolled in T2DM individuals [4,6]. In spite of advancements in therapeutic strategies, there has been no significant decrease in the mortality related to CVD [7]. The majority of T2DM individuals failed to achieve all standard goals for lipid management, and, therefore, aggressive management strategies are required to lower lipid abnormalities in T2DM individuals [7,8].

Omega-3 fatty acids are a principle component of cell membranes, which serve several important physiological functions, including as signaling molecules, transporters, and modulators of gene expression [9,10]. Previous studies reported several pharmacological activities of omega-3 fatty acids such as anti-hyperlipidemic, anti-inflammatory, and vasodilatory effects [9,11,12]. They have benefited the management of numerous chronic diseases like diabetes, CVD, and autoimmune disorders [9,13,14]. Over a period of three decades, epidemiological studies also reported that omega-3 fatty acids dietary intake provides beneficial effects in cardiovascular diseases [15,16]. Although statin drug treatment lowered the CVD incidence and its associated mortality, increased triglyceride (TG) levels and residual CVD risk remains in diabetic dyslipidemic individuals despite a decrease in LDL levels [16,17]. Therefore, adjunctive therapy is needed to lower the CVD risk. This study was designed to examine the synergistic effect of omega-3 fatty acids and oral hypoglycemic drugs i.e., glibenclamide compared with glibenclamide alone and in combination with statin drug treatment.

Various animal models have been used to assess the pathogenesis of diabetes and its associated complications [18–20]. High fat diet with low dose streptozotocin induces insulin resistance, hyperglycemia, hyperinsulinemia, and hyperlipidemia, which are characteristics of T2DM [21,22]. With this background, we investigated the effect of omega-3 fatty acids i.e., flax and fish oil, along with glibenclamide, against diabetic dyslipidemia by using a high fat diet with low dose streptozotocin-induced diabetic rat model.

2. Materials and Methods

2.1. Chemicals and Reagents

Flax oil capsules were procured from the Real World Nutritional Laboratory, Pune, India (Alvel-500). Fish oil capsules purchased from a local pharmacy (Merck Ltd., Pune, India) (Maxepa-500). Streptozotocin (STZ) (Sigma-Aldrich St. Louis, Missouri, USA), and glibenclamide tablets (Daonil-5 mg; Aventis Pharma, Pune, MH, India) were procured from a local pharmacy. The lard oil was purchased from the local market. The standard chow diet was procured from Nutrivet life sciences (Pune, MH, India).

2.2. Animals

Design of experiment, along with their procedures and techniques, was sanctioned by the Institutional Animal Ethics Committee (IAEC) of Bharati Vidyapeeth University, Pune, India. The study was approved through sanction number: (BVDUMC/2881/2016/001/001). Forty-eight male Wistar rats weighing (120–150 gm, 10 weeks old) which were received from Medical College of Bharati Vidyapeeth, Pune, India. The animals were kept in standard animal house conditions (temperature 22 ± 2 °C and 12:12 hr light and dark cycle condition with 55 ± 5% humidity, about 3 animals per cage). The high fat diet (HFD) composition is represented in Table 1.

Table 1. High fat diet (HFD) composition.

Sr. No.	Ingredients	Weight (gm/Kg)
1	Powdered normal pellet diet	700
2	Lard oil	300

After acclimatization, rats were randomly distributed into eight groups ($n = 6$) and treatment protocol as follows:

All groups of animals except healthy control received high fat diet (HFD) and water *ad libitum* during the experimental period. Group I (HC): healthy control; received standard chow diet for 90 days; group II (HFDC): high fat diet control; group III (DC): diabetic control received low dose streptozotocin (35 mg/kg); group IV (GC): glibenclamide control treated with STZ and glibenclamide; group V (SC): statin control treated with STZ and statin; group VI (GSC): glibenclamide—statin control given glibenclamide and statin; group VII (flax oil): received flax oil and glibenclamide; group VIII (fish oil): received fish oil and glibenclamide.

The glibenclamide and statin was given at 0.25 mg/kg and 10 mg/kg body weight (b.w.)/day, p.o. respectively. All standard drug interventions were given after the development of stable hyperglycemia. The flax and fish oil were given daily at a dose 500 mg/kg body weight (b.w.), p.o. The flax and fish oil intervention was given throughout the experiment i.e., from 1st day to 90th day. However, after the confirmation of stable hyperglycemia, flax and fish oil interventions were continued with glibenclamide (0.25 mg/kg b.w./day, p.o.) till completion of the experiment.

2.3. Experimental Design

All animals were kept on a respective diet for 90 days. Intraperitoneal glucose tolerance test (IPGTT) was done on 51st day for the detection of glucose intolerance in animals. After confirmation of glucose intolerance, rats from different groups (III-VIII) were injected with a single dose of STZ (35 mg/kg body weight (b.w., i.p.) and wait for the development of stable hyperglycemia. The design of the experiment is demonstrated in Figure 1. The intake of food and water intake was recorded daily. At the end of the experiment, all animals were sacrificed. For various biochemical estimations, the blood was collected at 0 (before providing HFD), 52nd (before STZ induction) and 90th day (at end of the experiment). The different tissues like liver, kidney, pancreas, visceral adipose tissue near kidney, gastrocnemius muscle (hindlimb muscle), and heart were excised, snap-frozen immediately in liquid nitrogen and kept at −80 °C. The liver was used for gene expression studies. A small parts of the tissues (liver, pancreas, and kidney) were kept in neutral buffered formalin (10%) for the histopathological examination.

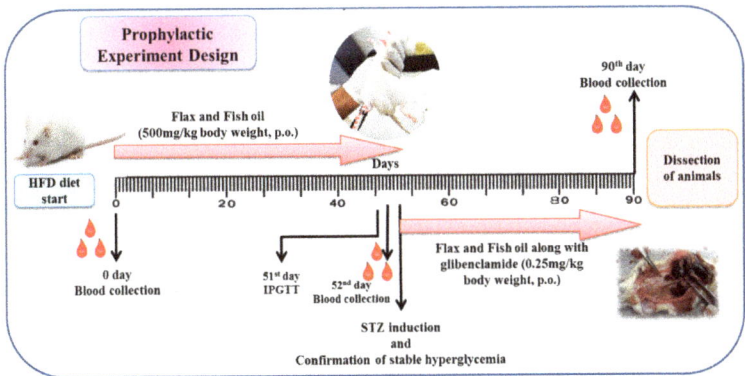

Figure 1. Design of the experiment. HFD: High fat diet, IPGTT: Intraperitoneal glucose tolerance test, STZ: streptozotocin; p.o. per os.

2.4. Intraperitoneal Glucose Tolerance Test (IPGTT)

After seven weeks of HFD, supplementation, all animal groups were fasted for 6 hrs. Initial blood glucose levels (0 min) were assessed. The glucose (2 gm/kg b.w.) solution was injected (i.p.) to all animals. Blood glucose levels were assessed using Accu-Chek monitor (Roche Diagnostics Pty. Ltd., Basel, Switzerland) at different time points (i.e., 0, 15, 30, 60, 90, and 120 min) from tail vein.

2.5. Assessment of Insulin Resistance

Insulin was estimated through rat-specific ELISA assay kits (Ray Biotech, GA, USA) after confirmation of glucose tolerance by IPGTT. The HOMA-IR (homeostasis model assessment of insulin resistance) was calculated as per the formula from Uma [23]:

$$\text{HOMA-IR} = \text{Insulin} (\mu U/mL) \times \text{glucose} (mM)/22.5$$

2.6. Biochemical Parameters

The biochemical assessments were done by commercially available kits (Coral Clinical Systems, Goa, India). The glucose, lipid profile, liver, and kidney function markers were estimated from serum at 0 day (before providing HFD), 52nd (before STZ induction) and 90th day. Triglycerides (TGs), total cholesterol (TC), very low density lipoprotein (VLDL), low-density lipoprotein (LDL), and high density lipoprotein (HDL) were measured. In the liver function tests, serum glutamic oxaloacetic transaminase (SGOT) and serum glutamic pyruvic transaminase (SGPT) were also assessed. Urea and creatinine markers were estimated to assess the kidney function.

2.7. Selection of Gene for Quantitative Real-Time Polymerase Chain Reaction (qRT-PCR) Analysis

In this study, 3 transcription factors [Sterol Regulatory Element-Binding Protein-1c (SREBP-1c), Nuclear Factor-κβ (NFκβ) and Peroxisome Proliferator-Activated Receptor Gamma (PPAR-γ)] were selected, which regulates the expression of target genes, such as Fatty Acid Synthase (FASN), Acetyl-CoA Carboxylase Alpha (ACACA), Carnitine Palmitoyltransferase 1 (CPT1) and inflammatory marker [Tumor Necrosis Factor—Alpha (TNF-α)]. The Fatty Acid Binding Proteins (FABP) gene was also studied. KicqStart® Primers were procured from Sigma Aldrich (New York, USA). The selected genes and their primer sequences are depicted in Table 2.

2.8. Assessment of Hepatic Gene Expression by qRT-PCR

Total RNA was extracted from liver by TRIZOL method (Invitrogen, Carlsbad, CA, USA). The quality of RNA was assessed by agarose gel electrophoresis (BioRad, Hercules, CA, USA). The RNA quantification was achieved by ND-1000 UV spectrophotometer (Nanodrop Technologies, Wilmington, DE, USA). For qRT-PCR assessment, the isolated RNA (2 µg) was used to synthesize cDNA by using SuperScriptTM first strand synthesis kit (Invitrogen).

The Real-time PCR analysis was done by SYBr green assays (Applied Biosystems, Waltham, Massachusetts, CA, USA) on StepOne real-time PCR system (Applied Biosystems, Waltham, Massachusetts, CA, USA). The following qRT-PCR protocol was used: initial denaturation step was done at 95 °C for 10 min. This step was followed by the 40 cycles of denaturation (95 °C for 3 s); annealing (60 °C for 30 s) and extension (95 °C for 15 s). The final extension step was achieved at 60 °C for 15 s. Three biological replicates were analyzed from each group. The reaction was carried out in duplicate and the Ct (cycle threshold) values of all samples were normalized by using Glyceraldehyde-3-Phosphate Dehydrogenase (GAPDH) (endogenous housekeeping control).

Table 2. The selected genes and their primer sequences.

Sr No	Target Genes	Primers	Sequences
	Housekeeping Gene		
1	Glyceraldehyde-3-phosphate dehydrogenase	Forward Reverse	AGTTCAACGGCACAGTCAAG TACTCAGCACCAGCATCACC
	Transcription Factors		
1	Sterol Regulatory Element-Binding Proteins-1c	Forward Reverse	AAACCTGAAGTGGTAGAAAC TTATCCTCAAAGGCTGGG
2	Peroxisome Proliferator-Activated Receptor Gamma	Forward Reverse	AAGACAACAGACAAATCACC CAGGGATATTTTTGGCATACTC
3	Nuclear Factor-$\kappa\beta$	Forward Reverse	AAAAACGAGCCTAGAGATTG ACATCCTCTTCCTTGTCTTC
	Fatty Acid Metabolism Genes		
1	Fatty Acid Synthase	Forward Reverse	AAAAGGAAAGTAGAGTGTGC GACACATTCTGTTCACTACAG
2	Acetyl-CoA Carboxylase Alpha	Forward Reverse	AGCAGTATTTGAACACATGG CAGTTCCAAGAAGTAGAAGC
3	Carnitine Palmitoyltransferase 1	Forward Reverse	CACTGATGAAGGAAGAAGAC CCAGTCACTCACGTAATTTG
4	Fatty Acid Binding Protein	Forward Reverse	TGGAGGGTGACAATAAAATG TCATGGTATTGGTGATTGTG
	Inflammatory Marker		
1	Tumor Necrosis Factors-α	Forward Reverse	CTCACACTCAGATCATCTTC GAGAACCTGGGAGTAGATAAG

2.9. Histological Examination

All animals were sacrificed and different tissues (liver, pancreas, kidney, adipose tissue, muscle and heart) were collected for further analysis. The part of liver, pancreas, and kidney were fixed in buffered formalin solution (10%, pH 7). Then all tissues were embedded in paraffin for block preparation. The tissue sections were cut to 4 µm thickness and stained by Hematoxylin and Eosin. The slides were observed under the light microscope (EVOS™ FL Auto 2 Imaging System, Invitrogen, Carlsbad, CA, USA).

2.10. Statistical Analysis

The data are represented as Mean ± standard error (SE). Statistical analysis was carried out by using one-way analysis of variance (ANOVA) followed by Dunnett's Multiple Comparison Test using GraphPad Instat (Version 5, GraphPad Software Inc., San Diego, CA, USA).

3. Results

3.1. Assessment of Average Body Weight, Feed and Water Consumption

The feed and water intake and body weight of experimental groups is represented in Table 3. The water and feed intake increased ($p \leq 0.001$) in the diabetic rats (DC) as compared to the healthy control rats (HC). Initially, the average body weight of all animals was between 120–150 gm. The body weight was not statistically significant between diabetic and healthy rats. The flax oil-treated rats showed an increase ($p \leq 0.001$) in feed consumption as compared to the diabetic rats. The omega-3 fatty acid intervention groups showed decreased ($p \leq 0.001$) water intake as compared to the diabetic group. Whereas, body weight was significantly ($p \leq 0.001$) elevated in flax and fish oil treatment groups as compared to the diabetic group.

Table 3. Average body weight, feed, and water intake of the experimental groups.

Groups	Weight (gm)	Feed Intake (gm)	Water Intake (mL)
HC	199 ± 2.73	102 ± 0.09 ***	209.1 ± 1.1 ***
HFDC	279 ± 4.66 ***	181.8 ± 0.79 ***	136.4 ± 0.9 ***
DC	199 ± 2.73	110.2 ± 0.36	347.4 ± 0.3
GC	286 ± 9.11 ***	162.1 ± 1.53 ***	141.6 ± 0.5 ***
SC	275 ± 3.62 ***	143.9 ± 0.59 ***	139.8 ± 1.1 ***
GSC	267 ± 3.35 ***	169.9 ± 1.22 ***	133 ± 0.4 ***
Flax	253 ± 4.96 ***	114.9 ± 0.28 ***	144.5 ± 0.6 ***
Fish	315 ± 12.15 ***	110.6 ± 0.94	142.6 ± 0.3 ***

Results are denoted as Mean ± SE (standard error) ($n = 6$ for each group). *** $p \leq 0.001$, when compared with the diabetic control group (Dunnett's Multiple Comparisons Test). HC: Healthy control, HFDC: High fat diet control, DC: Diabetes control, GC: Glibenclamide control, SC: Statin control, GSC: Glibenclamide statin control.

3.2. Estimation of Organ Weight

Organ weight of all experimental animals are shown in Table 4. Diabetic rats showed increased liver, adipose tissue and muscle tissue weight ($p < 0.001$) increased as compared to the HC rats. Whereas, kidney ($p < 0.001$) and heart weight was decreased in the DC group as compared to the healthy group.

Table 4. Measurement organ weight (gm).

Groups	Liver	Kidney	Adipose Tissue	Muscle	Heart
HC	8.16 ± 0.17 ***	2.14 ± 0.05 ***	3.99 ± 0.09 ***	2.51 ± 0.07 ***	1.65 ± 0.05
HFDC	12.43 ± 0.19	1.64 ± 0.08	15.17 ± 0.71	4.84 ± 0.33	1.90 ± 0.03 ***
DC	11.31 ± 1.12	1.81 ± 0.04	14.43 ± 0.74	4.94 ± 0.72	1.52 ± 0.09
GC	10.85 ± 0.34	2.67 ± 0.05 ***	4.39 ± 0.39 ***	4.12 ± 0.15	1.75 ± 0.09
SC	9.75 ± 0.36	2.27 ± 0.07 **	3.47 ± 0.15 ***	5.58 ± 0.25	1.50 ± 0.08
GSC	10.37 ± 0.28	2.28 ± 0.14 **	3.90 ± 0.46 ***	5.34 ± 0.35	1.43 ± 0.03
Flax	8.55 ± 0.19 ***	2.43 ± 0.03 ***	1.75 ± 0.04 ***	4.29 ± 0.08	1.39 ± 0.01
Fish	8.59 ± 0.05 **	2.44 ± 0.13 ***	2.88 ± 0.18 ***	2.85 ± 0.08 ***	1.90 ± 0.01 ***

Results are recorded as Mean ± SE ($n = 6$ for each group). ** $p \leq 0.01$ and *** $p \leq 0.001$, when compared with the diabetic control group (Dunnett's Multiple Comparisons Test). HC: Healthy control, HFDC: High fat diet control, DC: Diabetes control, GC: Glibenclamide control, SC: Statin control, GSC: Glibenclamide statin control.

The flax ($p < 0.001$) and fish ($p < 0.01$) oil intervention group showed decreased liver weight as compared to the diabetic group. Similarly, adipose tissue weight also decreased ($p < 0.001$) in flax and fish oil intervention groups as compared to DC group. Whereas, muscle weight was decreased in both flax and fish ($p < 0.001$) oil treatment groups as compared to DC group. The flax and fish oil intervention groups showed increase in kidney weight ($p < 0.001$) as compared to DC group. The heart weight was decreased in flax oil treatment group and elevated ($p < 0.001$) in fish oil treatment group as compared to the DC.

3.3. Assessment of Biochemical Parameters at Zero Day

Biochemical estimations of all experimental animals before providing HFD are shown in Table 5. Serum glucose, lipid profile (total cholesterol, triglycerides, VLDL, LDL and HDL) liver (SGOT and SGPT) and kidney function tests (creatinine and urea) were found not significantly different among all experimental groups before providing of respective diet.

3.4. IPGTT and Area under the Curve (AUC) for the Experimental Groups

Figure 2A,B depicts the glucose clearance and area under the curve (AUC) of IPGTT. The blood glucose levels at 0 and 120 min was elevated in all the experimental group as compared to the healthy group (Figure 2A). All experimental groups showed increase ($p \leq 0.001$) in AUC as compared to the healthy control group. The glucose clearance was not statistically significant between HFDC, flax, and fish oil intervention groups.

Table 5. Biochemical assessment before initiation of HFD.

Parameters	HC	HFDC	DC	GC	SC	GSC	Flax	Fish
Glu (mg/dl)	67.95 ± 6.05	68.33 ± 4.38	66.20 ± 9.09	61.18 ± 8.61	73.10 ± 4.34	53.97 ± 3.18	60.85 ± 2.03	56.08 ± 4.17
Lipid profile (mg/dl)								
TC	43.58 ± 4.37	57.63 ± 5.97	51.07 ± 3.15	49.70 ± 6.35	42.30 ± 2.63	44.48 ± 4.52	41.13 ± 4.76	47.97 ± 3.35
TGs	30.58 ± 5.71	47.40 ± 2.20	46.72 ± 2.63	36.62 ± 6.48	35.8 ± 6.63	26.47 ± 3.67	22.49 ± 0.76	33.90 ± 4.66
HDL	17.95 ± 0.20	22.19 ± 2.35	23.70 ± 1.82	23.95 ± 0.95	23.20 ± 2.50	26.83 ± 0.00	22.49 ± 0.76	21.78 ± 3.30
LDL	17.56 ± 0.10	13.37 ± 1.47	12.27 ± 2.17	16.50 ± 0.25	14.50 ± 0.66	13.80 ± 2.21	12.43 ± 0.89	12.43 ± 0.53
VLDL	6.12 ± 1.13	9.50 ± 0.44	9.31 ± 0.52	7.33 ± 1.28	7.17 ± 1.32	5.30 ± 0.74	8.36 ± 1.26	6.78 ± 0.92
Liver Function Test (Unit/mL)								
SGOT	41.60 ± 2.57	39.30 ± 5.09	55.87 ± 1.50	57.63 ± 4.87	45.52 ± 6.17	44.03 ± 2.05	44.68 ± 2.63	46.40 ± 5.20
SGPT	31.35 ± 3.90	34.45 ± 2.12	25.51 ± 2.53	26.60 ± 3.10	38.82 ± 2.52	34.03 ± 4.02	34.66 ± 2.89	33.75 ± 1.13
Kidney Function Test (mg/dl)								
Creatinine	0.60 ± 0.08	0.70 ± 0.07	0.57 ± 0.07	0.54 ± 0.07	0.55 ± 0.09	0.46 ± 0.12	0.55 ± 0.08	0.57 ± 0.06
Urea	26.49 ± 3.05	26.24 ± 0.59	25.05 ± 3.82	29.22 ± 1.04	27.55 ± 3.25	30.48 ± 0.45	28.19 ± 1.07	22.53 ± 1.53

Results are represented as Mean ± SE ($n = 6$ for each group and reactions were carried out in triplicates). All values for experimental groups were non-significantly different as compared with the healthy control group (Dunnett's Multiple Comparisons Test). Glu: Glucose, TC: Total cholesterol, TGs: Triglycerides, LDL: Low-density lipoprotein, VLDL: Very low-density lipoprotein, HDL: High-density lipoprotein, SGOT: Serum glutamic oxaloacetic transaminase, SGPT: Serum glutamic pyruvic transaminase.

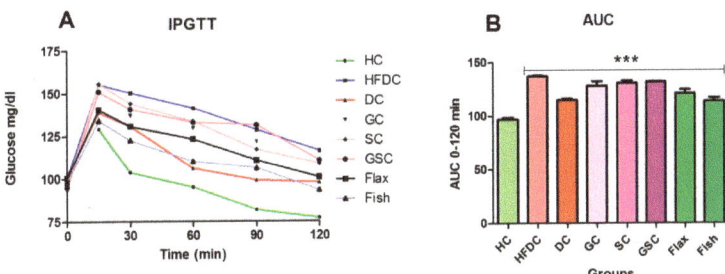

Figure 2. IPGTT and area under the curve (AUC) for the experimental groups. (**A**) Variations in blood glucose levels during IPGTT; (**B**) Area under the curve (AUC) for IPGTT. Results are represented as Mean ± SE ($n = 6$ for each group). *** $p \leq 0.001$, when compared with the HC animals (Dunnett's Multiple Comparisons Test). HC: Healthy control, HFDC: High fat diet control, DC: Diabetes control, GC: Glibenclamide control, SC: Statin control, GSC: Glibenclamide statin control.

3.5. Insulin Resistance

Serum glucose and insulin levels are shown in Table 6. Serum glucose level was significantly elevated ($p \leq 0.001$) in HFD fed rats (all groups except HC) as compared to healthy control rats. Flax and fish oil-treated rats showed non-significant difference in serum insulin level as compared to the healthy rats. HOMA-IR of all the experimental groups is represented in Figure 3. All animals from HFDC, DC and treatment groups of (GC, SC, GSC, flax and fish oil groups) rats showed a significantly increased ($p \leq 0.001$) HOMA-IR as compared to the healthy control group. Prophylactically, omega-3 fatty acids significantly lowered lipid profile, liver function markers (SGOT and SGPT), and kidney function markers (creatinine and urea) (supplementary Figures S1 and S2).

Table 6. Serum glucose and insulin for HOMA-IR assessment.

Experimental Groups	Glucose (mM)	Insulin (µU/mL)
HC	3.682 ± 0.10	6.293 ± 0.04
HFDC	5.208 ± 0.14 ***	7.248 ± 0.11 ***
DC	4.81 ± 0.15 ***	7.21 ± 0.10 ***
GC	4.995 ± 0.08 ***	6.822 ± 0.17 *
SC	5.134 ± 0.15 ***	6.852 ± 0.17 *
GSC	4.875 ± 0.02 ***	6.788 ± 0.14 *
Flax	6.105 ± 0.30 ***	6.418 ± 0.12
Fish	5.458 ± 0.12 ***	6.315 ± 0.03

Results are represented as Mean ± SE ($n = 6$ for each group). * $p \leq 0.05$ and *** $p \leq 0.001$, when compared with the HC (Dunnett's Multiple Comparisons Test). HC: Healthy control, HFDC: High fat diet control, DC: Diabetes control, GC: Glibenclamide control, SC: Statin control, GSC: Glibenclamide statin control, HOMA-IR: Homeostasis model assessment of insulin resistance.

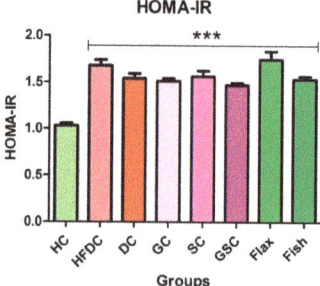

Figure 3. HOMA-IR of different experimental groups Results are represented as Mean ± SE ($n = 6$ for each group). *** $p \leq 0.001$, when compared with the HC (Dunnett's Multiple Comparisons Test). HC: Healthy control, HFDC: High fat diet control, DC: Diabetes control, GC: Glibenclamide control, SC: Statin control, GSC: Glibenclamide statin control, HOMA-IR: Homeostasis model assessment of insulin resistance.

3.6. Estimation of Biochemical Parameters

3.6.1. Fish Oil Treatment Significantly Lowered Serum Glucose

Figure 4 represents the serum glucose levels of all the experimental groups. Serum glucose level was significantly elevated ($p \leq 0.001$) in diabetic rats as compared to healthy control rats. Fish oil-treated rats had significantly lower ($p \leq 0.001$) serum glucose levels as compared to the diabetic rats.

3.6.2. Fish Oil Treatment Lowered Abnormal Lipid Profile

Figure 5A–E depicts the serum lipid profile of all experimental groups. Diabetic animals showed significantly ($p \leq 0.001$) increased serum TC, TGs, LDL, and VLDL levels as compared to the healthy control animals. The HDL level was significantly ($p \leq 0.001$) decreased in diabetic animals as compared to healthy control animals. Flax and fish ($p \leq 0.001$) oil treatment group showed decreased serum TC level as compared with diabetic group. Serum TG and VLDL levels were significantly ($p \leq 0.001$) decreased in flax and fish oil-treated animals as compared to the diabetic animals. Serum LDL level was decreased ($p \leq 0.001$) in fish oil-treated animals as compared to the diabetic animals. Flax and fish oil intervention elevated ($p \leq 0.001$) serum HDL levels as compared to the DC group. Flax oil-treated animals showed significant ($p \leq 0.001$) increase in TC, TGs, LDL, VLDL and HDL as compared to SC and GSC-treated animals. The serum TC level found to be comparable among SC, GSC and fish oil-treated groups. Serum LDL level increased in fish oil group as compared to SC and GSC group. Serum TGs, VLDL and HDL levels were significantly increased ($p \leq 0.001$) in fish oil intervention group as compared to SC and GSC group. The fish oil treatment showed a significant decrease in abnormal lipid profile and increase serum HDL.

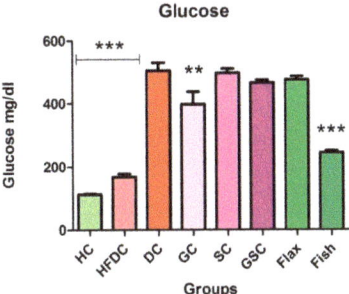

Figure 4. Fish oil intervention lowered serum glucose Results are represented as Mean ± SE ($n = 6$ for each group). ** $p \leq 0.01$ and *** $p \leq 0.001$, when compared with the DC group (Dunnett's Multiple Comparisons Test). HC: Healthy control, HFDC: High fat diet control, DC: Diabetes control, GC: Glibenclamide control, SC: Statin control, GSC: Glibenclamide statin control.

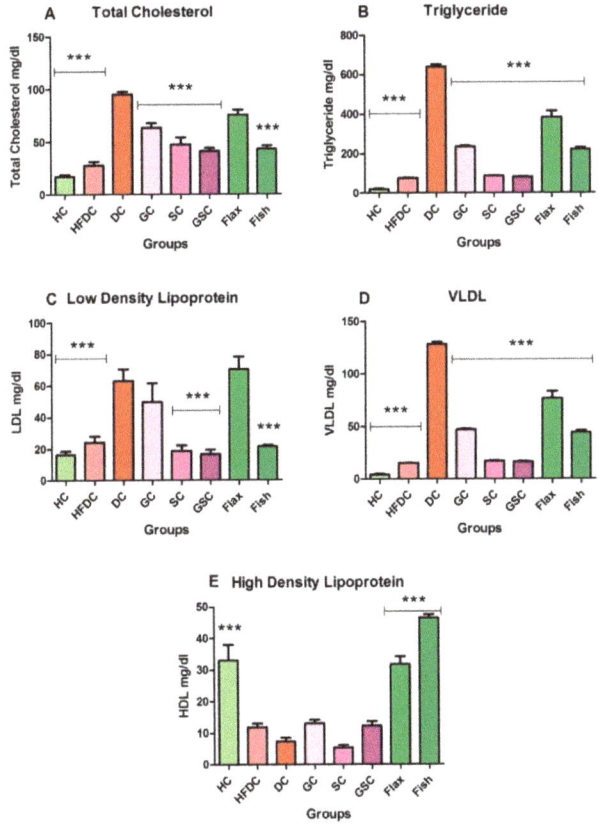

Figure 5. Assessment of lipid profile from experimental groups. Results are represented as Mean ± SE ($n = 6$ for each group). *** $p \leq 0.001$, when compared with the DC group (Dunnett's Multiple Comparisons Test). (**A**) Serum total cholesterol level, (**B**) Serum triglycerides level, (**C**) Serum low-density lipoprotein level, (**D**) Serum very low-density lipoprotein level, (**E**) Serum high-density lipoprotein level. HC: Healthy control, HFDC: High fat diet control, DC: Diabetes control, GC: Glibenclamide control, SC: Statin control, GSC: Glibenclamide statin control, LDL: Low-density lipoprotein, VLDL: Very low-density lipoprotein, HDL: High-density lipoprotein,.

3.6.3. Flax and Fish Oil Interventions Decreases Level of Hepatic Enzymes

In diabetic rats, serum SGOT and SGPT levels were elevated ($p \leq 0.001$) as compared to the healthy rats. Flax and fish oil-treated group showed significant decrease ($p \leq 0.001$) in serum SGOT and SGPT level as compared to the diabetic group. The SGOT level was increased in flax ($p \leq 0.001$) and fish oil intervention groups as compared to SC and GSC. Serum SGPT level decreased in both flax and fish oil groups as compared to SC and GSC. Serum SGOT and SGPT levels of all the experimental groups are represented in Figure 6A,B.

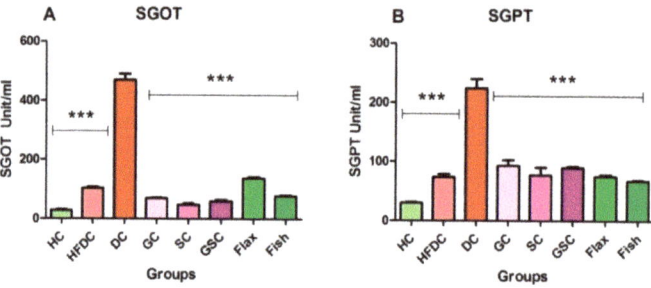

Figure 6. Flax and fish oil interventions lowered level of hepatic enzymes. Results are represented as Mean ± SE (n = 6 for each group). *** $p \leq 0.001$, when compared with the DC group (Dunnett's Multiple Comparisons Test). (**A**) Serum glutamic oxaloacetic transaminase level (**B**) Serum glutamic pyruvic transaminase level. HC: Healthy control, HFDC: High fat diet control, DC: Diabetes control, GC: Glibenclamide control, SC: Statin control, GSC: Glibenclamide statin control, SGOT: Serum glutamic oxaloacetic transaminase, SGPT: Serum glutamic pyruvic transaminase.

3.6.4. Flax and Fish Oil Intervention Improved Kidney Function

Serum creatinine and urea levels of all experimental groups were depicted in Figure 7A,B. Diabetic animals showed significantly ($p \leq 0.001$) increased serum creatinine and urea levels as compared to the healthy control animals. Flax oil intervention groups showed decreased serum creatinine and urea ($p \leq 0.001$) levels as compared to the diabetic group. While fish oil intervention significantly ($p \leq 0.001$) lowered both serum creatinine and urea levels as compared to the diabetic group. Serum creatinine and urea levels were non-significantly decreased in flax oil intervention groups as compared to SC and GSC. The serum creatinine level was decreased in fish oil intervention groups as compared to SC ($p \leq 0.001$) and GSC. Serum urea was not significantly different among SC, GSC, and fish oil groups. Fish oil intervention effectively improved kidney function.

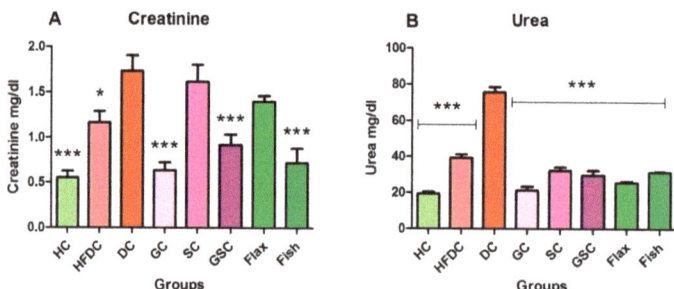

Figure 7. Flax and fish oil interventions improved kidney function. Results are represented as Mean ± SE (n = 6 for each group). * $p \leq 0.05$ and *** $p \leq 0.001$, when compared with the DC group (Dunnett's Multiple Comparisons Test). (**A**) Serum creatinine level, (**B**) Serum urea level. HC: Healthy control, HFDC: High fat diet control, DC: Diabetes control, GC: Glibenclamide control, SC: Statin control, GSC: Glibenclamide statin control.

3.7. Expression of Transcription Factors and Their Regulatory Genes

In the present study, we have examined the effect of flax and fish oil along with glibenclamide against diabetic dyslipidemia. For gene expression studies, three transcription factors and five regulatory genes were examined. The expression profiles are shown in (Figures 8–10). qRT-PCR amplification efficiencies are depicted in Table 7.

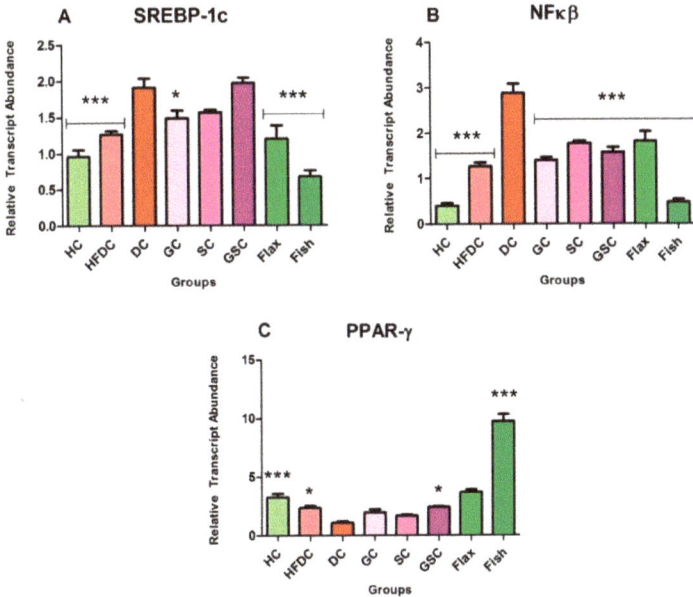

Figure 8. Expression of transcription factors are modulated after intervention of flax and fish oil. Results are represented as Mean ± SE (n = 3 for each group). * $p \leq 0.05$ and *** $p \leq 0.001$, when compared with the DC group (Dunnett's Multiple Comparisons Test). (**A**) Expression of sterol regulatory element-binding proteins-1c gene, (**B**) Expression of nuclear factor-κβ gene, (**C**) Expression of peroxisome proliferator-activated receptor gamma gene. HC: Healthy control, HFDC: High fat diet control, DC: Diabetic control, PPAR-γ: Peroxisome proliferator-activated receptor gamma, SREBP-1c: Sterol regulatory element-binding proteins-1c, NFκβ: Nuclear factor-κβ.

3.7.1. Flax and Fish Oil Interventions Modulates the Expression of Transcription Factors Resulting in Lipid Normalization

The expression of transcription factors is depicted in Figure 8A–C. In diabetic animals (DC), SREBP-1c expression was significantly ($p \leq 0.001$) upregulated by ~1.98 and ~1.51-fold as compared to the HC and HFDC animals, respectively. Comparatively, flax and fish oil intervention groups showed significant downregulation by ~1.59 and ~2.84-fold as compared to the diabetic group.

NFκβ gene expression was significantly ($p \leq 0.001$) upregulated in the diabetic animals by ~7.27 and ~2.27-fold as compared to the HC and HFDC animals, respectively. On the other hand, its expression was significantly ($p \leq 0.001$) downregulated by ~1.59 and ~6.16-fold in flax and fish oil treatment groups as compared with the diabetic group.

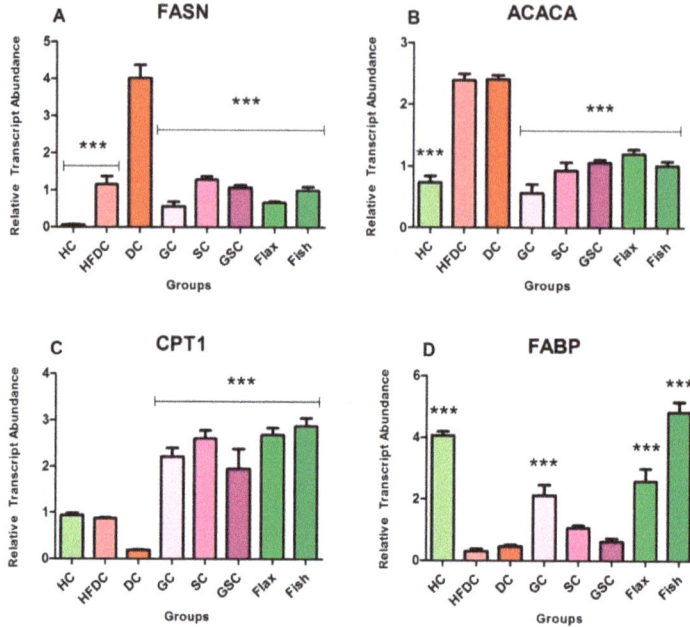

Figure 9. Expression profiles of fatty acid metabolism genes. Results are denoted as Mean ± SE (n = 3 for each group). *** $p \leq 0.001$, when compared with the DC group (Dunnett's Multiple Comparisons Test). (**A**) Expression of fatty acid synthase gene, (**B**) Expression of acetyl-CoA carboxylase alpha gene, (**C**) Expression of carnitine palmitoyl transferase 1 gene, (**D**) Expression of fatty-acid-binding proteins gene. HC: Healthy control, HFDC: High fat diet control, DC: Diabetic control, ACACA: Acetyl-CoA carboxylase alpha, FASN: Fatty acid synthase, CPT1: Carnitine palmitoyl transferase 1, FABP: Fatty-acid-binding proteins.

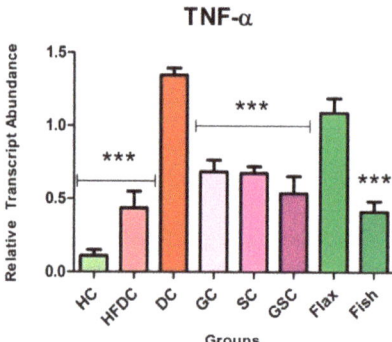

Figure 10. Expression of TNF-α in experimental groups. Results are represented as Mean ± SE (n = 3 for each group). *** $p \leq 0.001$, when compared with the DC group (Dunnett's Multiple Comparisons Test). HC: Healthy control, HFDC: High fat diet control, DC: Diabetic control group-treated STZ and TNF-α: Tumor necrosis factor-alpha.

Table 7. The qRT-PCR efficiency for absolute mRNA quantification.

No.	Target Genes	Symbol	Efficiency
	Housekeeping Gene		
1	Glyceraldehyde-3-phosphate dehydrogenase	GAPDH	97.27
	Transcription Factors		
1	Sterol Regulatory Element-Binding Proteins-1c	SREBP-1c	91.14
2	Peroxisome Proliferator-Activated Receptor Gamma	PPAR-γ	91.81
3	Nuclear Factor-κβ	NF-κβ	101.90
	Fatty Acid Metabolism Genes		
1	Fatty Acid Synthase	FASN	91.67
2	Acetyl-CoA Carboxylase Alpha	ACACA	84.87
3	Carnitine Palmitoyltransferase 1	CPT 1	101.65
4	Fatty Acid Binding Protein	FABP	92.96
	Inflammatory Marker		
1	Tumor Necrosis Factors-α	TNF-α	107.09

Efficiency is calculated from the slope of the curve as $E = 10(-1/\text{slope})^{-1}$.

Expression of PPAR-γ was significantly downregulated in diabetic animals by ~3.00 and ~2.15-fold, as compared to the HC ($p \leq 0.001$) and HFDC ($p \leq 0.05$) control animals. Flax oil-treated animals showed non-significant increased expression as compared to the diabetic group. While, fish oil-treated animals showed significant ($p \leq 0.001$) upregulation expression by ~8.95, ~4.94, ~5.84, and ~4.04-fold as compared to the diabetic animals.

3.7.2. Flax and Fish oil Intervention Modulates the Expression Fatty Acid Metabolism Genes Which Results in Decreased Lipid Abnormality

Figure 9A–D represents the expression of lipid metabolism genes. Expression of FASN genes was significantly upregulated ($p \leq 0.001$) in the diabetic animals by ~70.48 and ~3.47-fold as compared to HC and HFDC animals. Flax and fish oil-treated animals showed downregulation ($p \leq 0.001$) by ~6.01 and ~4.04-fold as compared to the diabetic animals.

ACACA gene expression was significantly ($p \leq 0.001$) upregulated in the diabetic rats by ~3.26-fold as compared to the healthy rats. Flax ($p \leq 0.001$) and fish ($p \leq 0.05$) oil-treated groups showed upregulation by ~2.12 and ~1.78-fold as compared to the diabetic group, respectively.

Expression of CPT1 genes was non-significantly downregulated in the diabetic rats by ~4.95 and ~4.63-fold as compared to the HC and HFDC rats. Flax and fish oil intervention groups showed significant upregulation ($p \leq 0.001$) by ~14.17 and ~15.20-fold as compared to the diabetic group.

FABP gene expression was significantly downregulated ($p \leq 0.001$) by ~8.87-fold in diabetic rats as compared to the healthy rat group. Both flax and fish oil intervention groups showed significant upregulation ($p \leq 0.001$) by ~5.64 and ~10.51-fold as compared to the diabetic groups, respectively.

3.7.3. Fish Oil Intervention Downregulates the Expression of TNF-α

In DC rats, TNF-α gene expression was upregulated ($p \leq 0.001$) by ~12.31 and ~3.09-fold as compared to the healthy and high fat diet control rats, respectively. Comparatively, flax and fish ($p \leq 0.001$) oil-treated groups showed downregulation by ~1.24 and ~3.28-fold as compared to the diabetic group, respectively. Figure 10 represents the inflammatory gene expression, TNF-α.

3.8. Histological Examination of Liver, Pancreas, and Kidney from Experimental Animals

Animals from experimental groups developed typical changes in liver, pancreas and kidney. Their histopathological examination is shown in Figures 11–13.

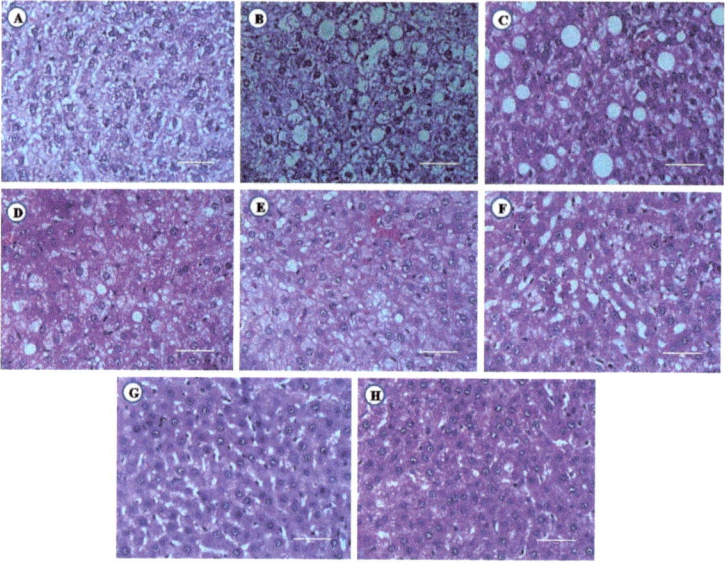

Figure 11. Histological examination of liver tissue (Scale bar 50 μm). Healthy. (**A**) Healthy control, (**B**) High fat diet control, (**C**) Diabetic control, (**D**) Glibenclamide control, (**E**) Statin control, (**F**) Glibenclamide statin control, (**G**) Flax oil (500 mg/kg), (**H**) Flax oil (500 mg/kg).

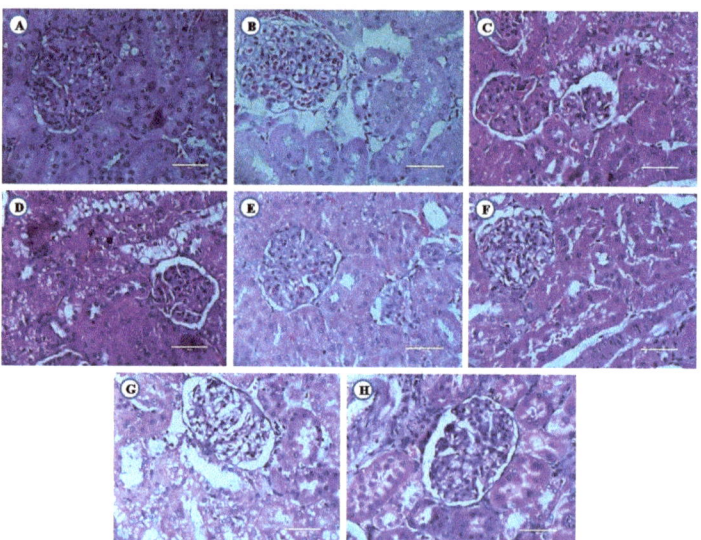

Figure 12. Histological examination of kidney (Scale bar 50 μm). (**A**) Healthy control, (**B**) High fat diet control, (**C**) Diabetic control, (**D**) Glibenclamide control, (**E**) Statin control, (**F**) Glibenclamide statin control, (**G**) Flax oil (500 mg/kg), (**H**) Flax oil (500 mg/kg).

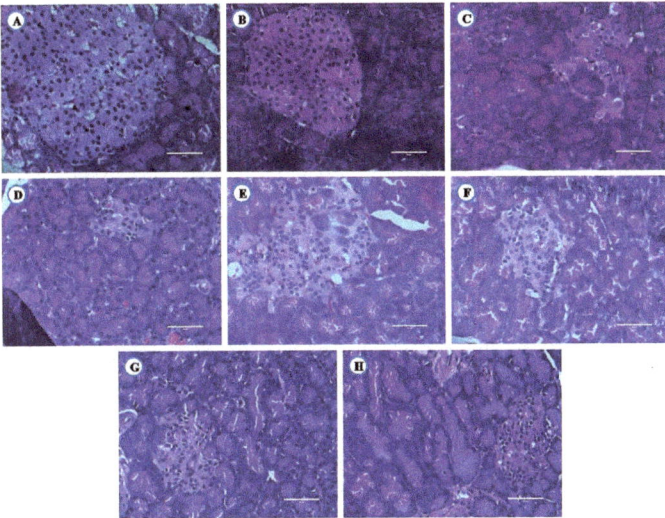

Figure 13. Histological examination of pancreas (Scale bar 50 µm). (**A**) Healthy control, (**B**) High fat diet control, (**C**) Diabetic control, (**D**) Glibenclamide control, (**E**) Statin control, (**F**) Glibenclamide statin control, (**G**) Flax oil (500 mg/kg), (**H**) Flax oil (500 mg/kg).

3.8.1. Histological Examination of Liver

Healthy animals showed normal architecture of hepatocytes (Figure 11A). High fat diet control group rats showed focal fatty changes in the liver (Figure 11B). Diabetic animals develop microvesicular fatty changes in the liver (Figure 11C). The flax oil intervention, along with glibenclamide showed focal fatty changes in the liver (Figure 11G). However, fish oil intervention, along with glibenclamide showed near-normal architecture of hepatocytes (Figure 11H).

3.8.2. Histological Examination of Kidney

Healthy and high fat diet control group animals showed normal architecture of the kidney (Figure 12A,B). Diabetic rats showed tubules with vacuolated cells (Figure 12C). The animals receiving standard drugs (GC, SC and GSC) also showed tubules with vacuolated cells (Figure 12D,F). Flax and fish oil interventions along with the combination of glibenclamide showed tubules with vacuolated cells (Figure 12G,H).

3.8.3. Histological Examination of Pancreas

Healthy and high fat diet control animals showed normal architecture of the pancreatic tissue (Figure 13A,B). Diabetic rats showed reduced number and size of islets of Langerhans and β cells (Figure 13C). Flax and fish oil intervention group showed reduced number and size of Langerhans and β cells (Figure 13G,H).

4. Discussion

The provision of HFD, along with a low dose of streptozotocin in rats, results in a condition that mimics the pathophysiology of type 2 diabetes (T2DM) in humans and is thus a suitable model for the practical investigations and testing of different natural compounds for the effective management of type 2 diabetes and its complications [20–22]. Despite advancement in the prevention and management strategies of diabetes and its associated complications in recent years, still, it has been growing alarmingly with the high rate of morbidity and mortality [24]. Therefore, aggressive management strategies for T2DM and its associated lipid abnormalities are highly recommended [4,22].

STZ-treated diabetic rats showed decreased body weights and elevated blood glucose, which are characteristic features of diabetes [18]. In the present study, a significant decrease in body weight and sustained hyperglycemia was observed in diabetic rats. The lipid abnormality is a very frequent impairment in type 2 diabetes patients [24]. For its management, they are commonly prescribed lipid-lowering drugs like statins. Therefore, one of the groups was given treatment with a normolipidemic drug just to evaluate the effect of the same drug on lipid abnormalities.

Several studies have reported the triglyceride-lowering effect of omega-3 fatty acids [9,25–27]. Some also studied cardioprotective effects of omega-3 fatty acids in animal models as well as in humans [28]. Flax oil, is a major source of alpha linolenic acid (ALA), and fish oil, predominantly contain eicosapentaenoic acid (EPA) and docosahexaenoic acid (DHA) are the principle sources of omega-3 fatty acids [9]. Previous studies showed that, flax and fish oil treatment lowered abnormal lipid profile in diabetic rats [9]. Our results are in accordance with previous findings. Both flax and fish oil exhibit beneficial effects on hepatic cholesterol metabolism in HFD-fed animals [29].

Hendrich [30] reviewed the effect of omega-3 fatty acid in human clinical trials and concluded that its effects in T2DM were not well studied [9,30]. The management of metabolic disorders (T2DM and its associated complications) recommended combining lifestyle changes with pharmacological therapy [31]. In this regard, several studies reported, the beneficial effect of omega-3 fatty acids with different allopathic drugs (thiazolidinediones, pioglitazone, rosiglitazone, etc.) in HFD-fed mice results in the increased adiponectin secretion [31,32]. With this background, we have studied the effect of flax and fish oil intervention in combination with glibenclamide in HFD with low STZ-induced diabetic dyslipidemia. The present study helps to fill the gap and investigates the combinational effect of omega-3 fatty acids and oral hypoglycemic drug on lipid abnormalities through modulation of transcription factors and their regulatory genes.

Several studies reported that flax and fish oil intervention exhibited triglyceride-lowering effect in streptozotocin-induced diabetic rats [9,27,33,34]. However, the treatment did not show any effect on serum TC and LDL levels. In the present study, flax and fish oil along with glibenclamide treatment effectively lowered serum TC, triglycerides, VLDL, and LDL levels in diabetic rats. It has been previously reported that flax and fish oil intervention significantly increase HDL levels in STZ-induced diabetic rats [9,27,33]. In our study, a similar trend was observed. Thus, effective lowering of the abnormal lipid profile was observed in fish oil and glibenclamide combinational treatment. The overall mechanism of the action of flax and fish oil on hepatic gene expression is depicted in Figure 14.

SREBP is an important transcription factor that plays a crucial role in the regulation of fatty acid and cholesterol metabolism in the liver [35]. It consists of two isoforms i.e., SREBP-1a and SREBP-1c, which are expressed highly in the liver. Its overexpression was associated with elevated levels of cholesterol and triglycerides [36,37]. Earlier studies document that upregulated lipogenic gene expression, such as for fatty acid synthase (FASN) and acetyl-CoA carboxylase (ACACA), was resulting in increased SREBP-1c expression, which leads to hepatic steatosis [38,39]. Hence, downregulation of SREBP-1c has a therapeutic value in the treatment of diabetic dyslipidemia [22,40,41]. The omega-3 fatty acid supplementation effectively lowered triglycerides level through downregulation of SREBP-1c gene expression [9,27,42]. Similarly, in our study, both flax and fish oil-treated animals showed downregulated SREBP-1c expression followed by a decrease in the expression of FASN and ACACA genes. These gene modulations may be one of the reasons for lowering the lipid abnormalities in flax and fish oil-treated rats.

CPT1 gene plays a major role in the uptake of fatty acids by the mitochondria for fatty acids β-oxidation [43]. In our study, the CPT1 expression was found to be increased in flax and fish oil-treated animals. This might be the probable reason for lowering serum triglyceride levels in diabetic rats.

Several studies reported that NF-κβ, a transcription factor (TF), plays a crucial role in insulin resistance and T2DM pathogenesis [22,41,44,45]. In diabetic conditions, upregulated NF-κβ expression leads to an increase inflammatory cytokine expression, e.g. tumor necrosis factor-α (TNF-α) [22,46,47]. In turn, it is associated with atherosclerotic lesions, lipolysis, and lipogenesis. Overall, this may result in an increased risk of cardiovascular complications in T2DM individuals [46,47]. In the present study, both TNF-α expression and its transcription factor NF-κβ were found to be downregulated in flax and fish oil-treated groups.

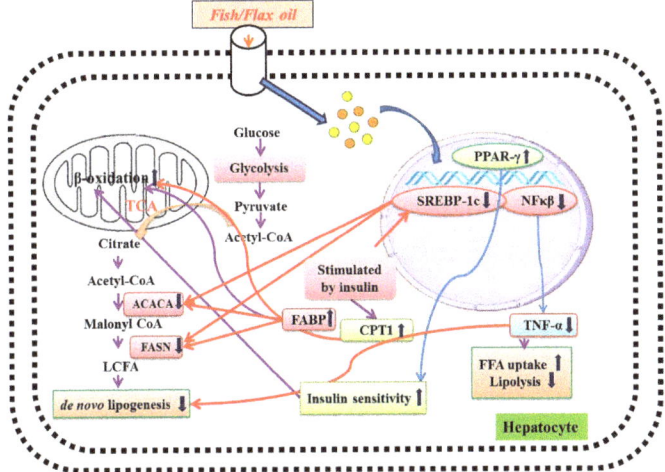

Figure 14. Mechanism of action of flax and fish oil intervention. PPAR-γ: Peroxisome proliferator-activated receptor gamma, SREBP-1c: Sterol regulatory element-binding proteins-1c, NFκβ: Nuclear factor-κβ, ACACA: Acetyl-CoA carboxylase alpha, FASN: Fatty acid synthase, CPT1: Carnitine palmitoyl transferase 1, FABP: Fatty-acid-binding proteins, TNF-α: Tumor necrosis factor-alpha, TCA: Tricarboxylic acid cycle, FFA: Free fatty acids, LCFA: Long chain fatty acids.

PPAR-γ, a transcription factor, is a member of the nuclear receptor family PPARs [48]. It plays an important role in carbohydrate and lipid homeostasis [48]. The activation of PPAR-γ stimulates β-oxidation of fatty acids and it results in lower serum triglyceride levels [49]. In the present study, flax and fish oil treatment upregulated the expression of PPAR-γ, and this may result in decreased serum triglyceride levels.

The FABP are members of a multigene family of cytoplasmic lipid transport proteins [50]. It is a potential target in the treatment of insulin resistance, lipid abnormalities, and atherosclerosis [50]. It facilitates fatty acid oxidation in the liver and may be beneficial for normalizing the hyperlipidemic condition [51]. Newberry et al. [52] reported that the L-FABP-null mice exhibit poor triglyceride accumulation in the liver, which leads to an increased serum triglyceride level [52]. A Wolfrum et al. [53] study shows that L-FABP acts as a gateway for the hypolipidemic drug and polyunsaturated fatty acids, which acts as a PPAR agonists [53]. Thus, upregulation of L-FABP expression would enhance the activation of PPAR through these agonists. In the present study, both flax and fish oil supplementation upregulated the expression of L-FABP in diabetic rats and this might be one of the reasons behind lowering serum triglyceride levels. FABPs are also associated with the docosahexaenoic acid (DHA) uptake and this might be the reason behind accelerating β-oxidation of fatty acids through higher activation of PPAR. This ultimately results in lowering serum triglyceride levels [54]. Our results are in accordance with the above findings [53,54].

5. Conclusions

The combinational treatment of glibenclamide and flax/fish oil intervention prophylactically against diabetic dyslipidemic rats exhibited potential effects on improving lipid abnormalities through modulating the expression of transcription factors (SREBP1-c, NF-kβ and PPAR-γ) and their regulatory genes i.e., ACACA, FASN, CPT1, FABP, and TNF-α. In the future, combination therapy of glibenclamide and omega-3 fatty acid intervention at a therapeutic level is worth investigation in the diabetic dyslipidemic condition.

Supplementary Materials: The following are available online at http://www.mdpi.com/2072-6643/12/12/3652/s1, Figure S1: Assessment of glucose and lipid profile before diabetes development, Figure S2: LFT and KFT before diabetes development.

Author Contributions: Conceptualization, A.K. and N.M.; Data curation and analysis, S.K.; Investigation, S.K.; Methodology, A.K., V.P., and N.M.; Performed the assays and acquisition of data, S.K. and P.M.; Project administration, A.K.; Supervision, A.K. and N.M.; Histological examination, M.K.; Experimental design, V.P.; Writing—original draft, S.K.; Writing—review & editing, A.K. and N.M. All authors have read and agreed to the published version of the manuscript.

Funding: This research received no external funding.

Acknowledgments: The authors are grateful to Bharati Vidyapeeth Deemed University for the financial support of this research.

Conflicts of Interest: The authors declare no conflict of interest.

References

1. Brown, T.J.; Brainard, J.; Song, F.; Wang, X.; Abdelhamid, A.; Hooper, L. Omega-3, omega-6, and total dietary polyunsaturated fat for prevention and treatment of type 2 diabetes mellitus: Systematic review and meta-analysis of randomised controlled trials. *BMJ* **2019**, *366*, l4697. [CrossRef]
2. Adiels, M.; Olofsson, S.O.; Taskinen, M.R.; Boren, J. Diabetic dyslipidaemia. *Curr. Opin. Lipidol.* **2006**, *17*, 238–246. [CrossRef]
3. Narindrarangkura, P.; Bosl, W.; Rangsin, R.; Hatthachote, P. Prevalence of dyslipidemia associated with complications in diabetic patients: A nationwide study in thailand. *Lipids Health Dis.* **2019**, *18*, 90. [CrossRef] [PubMed]
4. Krishnaswami, V. Treatment of dyslipidemia in patients with type 2 diabetes. *Lipids Health Dis.* **2010**, *9*, 144.
5. Mithal, A.; Majhi, D.; Shunmugavelu, M.; Talwarkar, P.G.; Vasnawala, H.; Raza, A.S. Prevalence of dyslipidemia in adult Indian diabetic patients: A cross sectional study (SOLID). *Indian J. Endocrinol. Metab.* **2014**, *18*, 642–647.
6. Saydah, S.H.; Fradkin, J.; Cowie, C.C. Poor control of risk factors for vascular disease among adults with previously diagnosed diabetes. *JAMA* **2004**, *291*, 335–342. [CrossRef]
7. Parikh, R.M.; Joshi, S.R.; Menon, P.S.; Shah, N.S. Prevalence and pattern of diabetic dyslipidemia in Indian type 2 diabetic patients. *Diabetes Metab. Syndr. Clin. Res. Rev.* **2010**, *4*, 10–12. [CrossRef]
8. Goff, D.C.; Gerstein, H.C.; Ginsberg, H.N.; Cushman, W.C.; Margolis, K.L.; Byington, R.P.; Buse, J.B.; Genuth, S.; Probstfield, J.L.; Simons-Morton, D.G. Prevention of cardiovascular disease in persons with type 2 diabetes mellitus: Current knowledge and rationale for the Action to Control Cardiovascular Risk in Diabetes (ACCORD) trial. *Am. J. Cardiol.* **2007**, *99*, 4i–20i. [CrossRef]
9. Devarshi, P.P.; Jangale, N.M.; Ghule, A.E.; Bodhankar, S.L.; Harsulkar, A.M. Beneficial effects of flaxseed oil and fish oil diet are through modulation of different hepatic genes involved in lipid metabolism in streptozotocin-nicotinamide induced diabetic rats. *Genes Nutr.* **2013**, *8*, 329–342. [CrossRef]
10. Liu, J.; Ma, D.W. The role of n-3 polyunsaturated fatty acids in the prevention and treatment of breast cancer. *Nutrients* **2014**, *18*, 5184–5223. [CrossRef]
11. Jangale, N.M.; Devarshi, P.P.; Dubal, A.A.; Ghule, A.E.; Koppikar, S.J.; Bodhankar, S.L.; Chougale, A.D.; Kulkarni, M.J.; Harsulkar, A.M. Dietary flaxseed oil and fish oil modulates expression of antioxidant and inflammatory genes with alleviation of protein glycation status and inflammation in liver of streptozotocin-nicotinamide induced diabetic rats. *Food Chem.* **2013**, *141*, 187–195. [CrossRef] [PubMed]
12. Connor, W.E. Importance of n-3 fatty acids in health and disease. *Am. J. Clin. Nutr.* **2000**, *71* (Suppl. 1), 171S–175S. [CrossRef] [PubMed]
13. Simopoulos, A.P. Omega-3 fatty acids in inflammation and autoimmune diseases. *J. Am. Coll. Nutr.* **2002**, *21*, 495–505. [CrossRef] [PubMed]
14. Wu, J.H.; Micha, R.; Imamura, F.; Pan, A.; Biggs, M.L.; Ajaz, O.; Djousse, L.; Hu, F.B.; Mozaffarian, D. Omega-3 fatty acids and incident type 2 diabetes: A systematic review and meta-analysis. *Br. J. Nutr.* **2012**, *107*, 214–227. [CrossRef]

15. Bang, H.O.; Dyerberg, J.; Nielsen, A.B. Plasma lipid and lipoprotein pattern in Greenlandic West-coast Eskimos. *Lancet* **1971**, *1*, 1143–1145. [CrossRef]
16. Fialkow, J. Omega-3 fatty acid formulations in cardiovascular disease: Dietary supplements are not substitutes for prescription products. *Am. J. Cardiovasc. Drugs* **2016**, *16*, 229–239. [CrossRef]
17. Kim, C.H.; Han, K.A.; Yu, J.; Lee, S.H.; Jeon, H.K.; Kim, S.H.; Kim, S.Y.; Han, K.H.; Won, K.; Kim, D.B.; et al. Efficacy and safety of adding omega-3 fatty acids in statin-treated patients with residual hypertriglyceridemia: ROMANTIC (Rosuvastatin-Omacor in residual hypertriglyceridemia), a randomized, double-blind, and placebo-controlled trial. *Clin. Ther.* **2018**, *40*, 83–94. [CrossRef]
18. Srinivasan, K.; Ramarao, P. Animal models in type 2 diabetes research: An overview. *Indian J. Med. Res.* **2007**, *125*, 451–472.
19. Zhang, M.; Lv, X.Y.; Li, J.; Xu, Z.G.; Chen, L. The characterization of high-fat diet and multiple low-dose streptozotocin induced type 2 diabetes rat model. *Exp. Diabetes Res.* **2008**, *2008*, 1–9. [CrossRef]
20. Binh, D.V.; Dung, N.T.K.; Thao, L.T.B.; Nhi, N.B.; Chi, P.V. Macro- and microvascular complications of diabetes induced by high-fat diet and low-dose streptozotocin injection in rats model. *Int. J. Diabetes Res.* **2013**, *2*, 50–55.
21. Srinivasan, K.; Viswanad, B.; Asrat, L.; Kaul, C.L.; Ramarao, P. Combination of high-fat diet-fed and low-dose streptozotocin-treated rat: A model for type 2 diabetes and pharmacological screening. *Pharmacol. Res.* **2005**, *52*, 313–320. [CrossRef]
22. Khadke, S.P.; Kuvalekar, A.A.; Harsulkar, A.M.; Mantri, N. High energy intake induced overexpression of transcription factors and its regulatory genes involved in acceleration of hepatic lipogenesis: A rat model for type 2 diabetes. *Biomedicines* **2019**, *7*, 76. [CrossRef]
23. Uma, B.; Hemantkumar, S.C.; Geetika, K.; Abul, K.N. Antidiabetic effects of *Embelia ribes* extract in high fat diet and low dose streptozotocin-induced type 2 diabetic rats. *Front. Life Sci.* **2013**, *7*, 186–196.
24. Arshag, D.M. Dyslipidemia in type 2 diabetes mellitus. *Nat. Clin. Pract. Endocrinol. Metab.* **2009**, *5*, 3150–3159.
25. Rivellese, A.A.; Maffettone, A.; Iovine, C.; Di Marino, L.; Annuzzi, G.; Mancini, M.; Riccardi, G. Long-term effects of fish oil on insulin resistance and plasma lipoproteins in NIDDM patients with hypertriglyceridemia. *Diabetes Care* **1996**, *19*, 1207–1213. [CrossRef]
26. Montori, V.M.; Farmer, A.; Wollan, P.C.; Dinneen, S.F. Fish oil supplementation in type 2 diabetes: A quantitative systematic review. *Diabetes Care* **2000**, *23*, 1407–1415. [CrossRef]
27. Ghadge, A.; Harsulkar, A.; Karandikar, M.; Pandit, V.; Kuvalekar, A. Comparative anti-inflammatory and lipid-normalizing effects of metformin and omega-3 fatty acids through modulation of transcription factors in diabetic rats. *Genes Nutr.* **2016**, *11*, 10. [CrossRef]
28. Bassett, C.M.; Rodriguez-Leyva, D.; Pierce, G.N. Experimental and clinical research findings on the cardiovascular benefits of consuming flaxseed. *Appl. Physiol. Nutr. Metab.* **2009**, *34*, 965–974. [CrossRef]
29. Vijaimohan, K.; Jainu, M.; Sabitha, K.E.; Subramaniyam, S.; Anandhan, C.; Shyamala, D.C.S. Beneficial effects of alpha linolenic acid rich flaxseed oil on growth performance and hepatic cholesterol metabolism in high fat diet fed rats. *Life Sci.* **2006**, *79*, 448–454. [CrossRef]
30. Hendrich, S. (n-3) Fatty acids: Clinical trials in people with type 2 diabetes. *Adv. Nutr.* **2010**, *1*, 3–7. [CrossRef]
31. Kus, V.; Flachs, P.; Kuda, O.; Bardova, K.; Janovska, P.; Svobodova, M.; Jilkova, Z.M.; Rossmeisl, M.; Wang-Sattler, R.; Yu, Z.; et al. Unmasking differential effects of rosiglitazone and pioglitazone in the combination treatment with n-3 fatty acids in mice fed a high-fat diet. *PLoS ONE* **2011**, *6*, e27126. [CrossRef]
32. Laila, A.E.; Noha, A.R.; Salma, M. Effects of omega-3 fatty acids and pioglitazone combination on insulin resistance through fibroblast growth factor 21 in type 2 diabetes mellitus. *EJBAS* **2015**, *2*, 75–86.
33. Kaithwas, G.; Majumdar, D. In-vitro antioxidant and in vivo antidiabetic, antihyperlipidemic activity of linseed oil against streptozotocin-induced toxicity in albino rats. *Eur. J. Lipid. Sci. Technol.* **2012**, *114*, 1237–1245. [CrossRef]
34. Mahmud, I.; Hossain, A.; Hossain, S.; Hannan, A.; Ali, L.; Hashimoto, M. Effects of Hilsa ilisa fish oil on the atherogenic lipid profile and glycaemic status of streptozotocin-treated type 1 diabetic rats. *Clin. Exp. Pharmacol. Physiol.* **2004**, *31*, 76–81. [CrossRef]
35. Horton, J.D.; Goldstein, J.L.; Brown, M.S. SREBPs: Activators of the complete program of cholesterol and fatty acid synthesis in the liver. *J. Clin. Investig.* **2002**, *109*, 1125–1131. [CrossRef]
36. Shimano, H.; Horton, J.D.; Hammer, R.E.; Shimomura, I.; Brown, M.S.; Goldstein, J.L. Overproduction of cholesterol and fatty acids causes massive liver enlargement in transgenic mice expressing truncated SREBP-1a. *J. Clin. Investig.* **1996**, *98*, 1575–1584. [CrossRef]

37. Shimano, H.; Horton, J.D.; Shimomura, I.; Hammer, R.E.; Brown, M.S.; Goldstein, J.L. Isoform 1c of sterol regulatory element binding protein is less active than isoform 1a in livers of transgenic mice and in cultured cells. *J. Clin. Investig.* **1997**, *99*, 846–854. [CrossRef]
38. Shimomura, I.; Bashmakov, Y.; Horton, J.D. Increased levels of nuclear SREBP-1c associated with fatty livers in two mouse models of diabetes mellitus. *J. Biol. Chem.* **1999**, *274*, 30028–30032. [CrossRef]
39. Higuchi, N.; Kato, M.; Shundo, Y.; Tajiri, H.; Tanaka, M.; Yamashita, N.; Kohjima, M.; Kotoh, K.; Nakamuta, M.; Takayanagi, R.; et al. Liver X receptor in cooperation with SREBP-1c is a major lipid synthesis regulator in nonalcoholic fatty liver disease. *Hepatol. Res.* **2008**, *38*, 1122–1129. [CrossRef]
40. Moon, Y.A.; Liang, G.; Xie, X.; Frank-Kamenetsky, M.; Fitzgerald, K.; Koteliansky, V.; Brown, M.S.; Goldstein, J.L.; Horton, J.D. The Scap/SREBP pathway is essential for developing diabetic fatty liver and carbohydrate-induced hypertriglyceridemia in animals. *Cell Metab.* **2012**, *15*, 240–246. [CrossRef]
41. Mandave, P.; Khadke, S.; Karandikar, M.; Pandit, V.; Ranjekar, P.; Kuvalekar, A.; Mantri, N. Antidiabetic, lipid normalizing, and nephroprotective actions of the strawberry: A potent supplementary fruit. *Int. J. Mol. Sci.* **2017**, *18*, 124. [CrossRef]
42. Davidson, M.H. Mechanisms for the hypotriglyceridemic effect of marine omega-3 fatty acids. *Am. J. Cardiol.* **2006**, *98*, 27–33. [CrossRef]
43. Sharma, S.; Black, S.M. Carnitine homeostasis, mitochondrial function, and cardiovascular disease. *Drug Discov. Today Dis. Mech.* **2009**, *6*, 31–39. [CrossRef]
44. Cai, D.; Yuan, M.; Frantz, D.F.; Melendez, P.A.; Hansen, L.; Lee, J.; Shoelson, S.E. Local and systemic insulin resistance resulting from hepatic activation of IKK-β and NF-κβ. *Nat. Med.* **2005**, *11*, 183–190. [CrossRef]
45. Arkan, M.C.; Hevener, A.L.; Greten, F.R.; Maeda, S.; Li, Z.W.; Long, J.M.; Wynshaw-Boris, A.; Poli, G.; Olefsky, J.; Karin, M. IKK-β links inflammation to obesity-induced insulin resistance. *Nat. Med.* **2005**, *11*, 191–198. [CrossRef]
46. Popa, C.; Netea, M.G.; van Riel, P.L.; van der Meer, J.W.; Stalenhoef, A.F. The role of TNF-α in A in chronic inflammatory conditions, intermediary metabolism, and cardiovascular risk. *J. Lipid Res.* **2007**, *48*, 751–762. [CrossRef]
47. Jagannathan-Bogdan, M.; McDonnell, M.E.; Shin, H.; Rehman, Q.; Hasturk, H.; Apovian, C.M.; Nikolajczyk, B.S. Elevated proinflammatory cytokine production by a skewed T cell compartment requires monocytes and promotes inflammation in type 2 diabetes. *J. Immunol.* **2011**, *186*, 1162–1172. [CrossRef]
48. Keller, H.; Wahli, W. Peroxisome proliferator-activated receptors—A link between endocrinology and nutrition? *Trends Endocrinol. Metab.* **1993**, *4*, 291–296. [CrossRef]
49. Schoonjans, K.; Staels, B.; Auwerx, J. The peroxisome proliferator activated receptors (PPARS) and their effects on lipid metabolism and adipocyte differentiation. *Biochim. Biophys. Acta* **1996**, *1302*, 93–109. [CrossRef]
50. Boord, J.B.; Fazio, S.; Linton, M.F. Cytoplasmic fatty acid-binding proteins: Emerging roles in metabolism and atherosclerosis. *Curr. Opin. Lipidol.* **2002**, *13*, 141–147. [CrossRef]
51. Veerkamp, J.H.; van Moerkerk, H.T. Fatty acid-binding protein and its relation to fatty acid oxidation. *Mol. Cell. Biochem.* **1993**, *123*, 101–106. [CrossRef]
52. Newberry, E.P.; Xie, Y.; Kennedy, S.; Han, X.; Buhman, K.K.; Luo, J.; Gross, R.W.; Davidson, N.O. Decreased hepatic triglyceride accumulation and altered fatty acid uptake in mice with deletion of the liver fatty acid-binding protein gene. *J. Biol. Chem.* **2003**, *278*, 51664–51672. [CrossRef]
53. Wolfrum, C.; Borrmann, C.M.; Borchers, T.; Spener, F. Fatty acids and hypolipidemic drugs regulate peroxisome proliferator-activated receptors alpha—and gamma-mediated gene expression via liver fatty acid binding protein: A signaling path to the nucleus. *Proc. Natl. Acad. Sci. USA* **2001**, *98*, 2323–2328. [CrossRef]
54. Dutta-Roy, A.K. Transport mechanisms for long-chain polyunsaturated fatty acids in the human placenta. *Am. J. Clin. Nutr.* **2000**, *71* (Suppl. 1), 315S–322S. [CrossRef]

Publisher's Note: MDPI stays neutral with regard to jurisdictional claims in published maps and institutional affiliations.

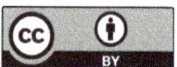

© 2020 by the authors. Licensee MDPI, Basel, Switzerland. This article is an open access article distributed under the terms and conditions of the Creative Commons Attribution (CC BY) license (http://creativecommons.org/licenses/by/4.0/).

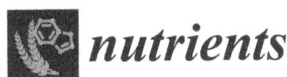

Article

Plasma Lipidomics Reveals Insights into Anti-Obesity Effect of *Chrysanthemum morifolium* Ramat Leaves and Its Constituent Luteolin in High-Fat Diet-Induced Dyslipidemic Mice

Jong Cheol Shon [1,2], Won Cheol Kim [2], Ri Ryu [3], Zhexue Wu [2], Jong-Su Seo [1], Myung-Sook Choi [4,*] and Kwang-Hyeon Liu [2,*]

1. Environmental Chemistry Research Group, Korea Institute of Toxicology, Jinju 52834, Korea; sleier7640@naver.com (J.C.S.); jsseo@kitox.re.kr (J.-S.S.)
2. College of Pharmacy and Research Institute of Pharmaceutical Sciences, Kyungpook National University, Daegu 41566, Korea; wk3012@naver.com (W.C.K.); wuzhexue527@gmail.com (Z.W.)
3. Research Institute of Eco-Friendly Livestock Science, Institute of Green-Bio Science and Technology, Seoul National University, Pyeongchang 25354, Korea; sangsang0119@gmail.com
4. Center for Food and Nutritional Genomics Research, Kyungpook National University, Daegu 41566, Korea
* Correspondence: mschoi@knu.ac.kr (M.-S.C.); dstlkh@knu.ac.kr (K.-H.L.); Tel.: +82-53-950-6232 (M.-S.C.); +82-53-950-8567 (K.-H.L.); Fax: +82-53-950-8557 (M.-S.C. & K.-H.L.)

Received: 2 September 2020; Accepted: 26 September 2020; Published: 29 September 2020

Abstract: The *Chrysanthemum morifolium* Ramat (CM) is widely used as a traditional medicine and herbal tea by the Asian population for its health benefits related to obesity. However, compared to the flowers of CM, detailed mechanisms underlying the beneficial effects of its leaves on obesity and dyslipidemia have not yet been elucidated. Therefore, to investigate the lipidomic biomarkers responsible for the pharmacological effects of CM leaf extract (CLE) in plasma of mice fed a high-fat diet (HFD), the plasma of mice fed a normal diet (ND), HFD, HFD plus CLE 1.5% diet, and HFD plus luteolin 0.003% diet (LU) for 16 weeks were analyzed using liquid chromatography-tandem mass spectrometry (LC-MS/MS) combined with multivariate analysis. In our analysis, the ND, HFD, CLE, and LU groups were clearly differentiated by partial least-squares discriminant analysis (PLS-DA) score plots. The major metabolites contributing to this differentiation were cholesteryl esters (CEs), lysophosphatidylcholines (LPCs), phosphatidylcholines (PCs), ceramides (CERs), and sphingomyelins (SMs). The levels of plasma CEs, LPCs, PCs, SMs, and CERs were significantly increased in the HFD group compared to those in the ND group, and levels of these lipids recovered to normal after administration of CLE or LU. Furthermore, changes in hepatic mRNA expression levels involved in the Kennedy pathway and sphingolipid biosynthesis were also suppressed by treatment with CLE or LU. In conclusion, this study examined the beneficial effects of CLE and LU on obesity and dyslipidemia, which were demonstrated as reduced synthesis of lipotoxic intermediates. These results may provide valuable insights towards evaluating the therapeutic effects of CLE and LU and understanding obesity-related diseases.

Keywords: *Chrysanthemum morifolium* Ramat leaves; obesity; lipidomics; liquid chromatography tandem mass spectrometry; phospholipid; sphingolipid

1. Introduction

Obesity, one of the major worldwide health problems in recent years, is usually caused by an imbalance in food intake and energy expenditure, with overconsumption of energy intake or decrease in physical activity. Among the various models of inducing obesity in animals, the high-fat diet

(HFD)-induced obesity model alters diverse biochemical factors, such as insulin, eventually leading to abnormal lipid metabolism. HFD-induced obesity is characterized by abnormally high levels of blood lipids, such as cholesterol, low-density lipoprotein (LDL), and triacylglycerol (TAG), leading to progressive weight gain in various tissues of the body (e.g., liver and fat tissues) due to excess fat accumulation [1,2]. It is also associated with an increase in the prevalence and risk of metabolic syndrome-related diseases, including type 2 diabetes (T2D), dyslipidemia, cardiovascular diseases (CVD), hypertension, and fatty liver [3,4]. Especially, the development of obesity by HFD indicates that it is pathophysiologically very similar to obesity in humans [5,6].

Chrysanthemum morifolium Ramat (CM) has been used for almost a hundred years in the form of a traditional medicine, beverage, and herbal tea in many Asian countries, including Japan, China, Thailand, and Korea, due to its health benefits related to inflammation, hypertension, and arteriosclerosis. The main bioactive components in the flowers of CM are flavonoids and phenolic acids, which are composed of chlorogenic acid, acacetin, apigenin, and luteolin, along with its glucoside form [7]. Previous studies have shown that CM and its components possess various biological functions, including antioxidant [8], anti-inflammatory [9], anti-tumorigenic [10], and cardiovascular-protective functions [11]. Moreover, the CM flower extract has been shown to prevent hyperlipidemic fatty liver disease by increasing hepatic peroxisome proliferator-activated receptor (PPAR)-α expression in hyperlipidemic fatty liver disease caused by high-fat milk [12]. Such beneficial effects have also been reported in HFD-induced obese mice [13] and an alloxan-induced diabetes mellitus model [14]. Almost all the studies conducted on the efficacy of CM related to health-promoting effects have been focused on its flowers. However, although not used as a traditional medicine, unlike flowers, the leaves of CM have a large amount of potential bioactive components, such as flavonoids, galuteolin, quercetin, and chlorogenic acid [15,16]. Consequently, the leaves can be used for medicinal purposes because of their high content of bioactive components. Furthermore, a recent study revealed that weight gain, fat deposition, and plasma lipid levels were significantly reduced by the administration of CM leaf extract (CLE) in HFD-fed mice [17]. However, apart from the previous approach based on the major lipids, such as cholesterol, lipoprotein, and TAG, detailed studies on lipid profiles, including changes in individual lipid species, towards the pharmacological effects of CLE in obese mice have rarely been described.

Modern lipidomics technology based on mass spectrometry provides significant insights into the metabolism and alterations in lipids through the identification and quantification of individual lipid species in a broad range of lipids [18]. This technology has been used extensively in biomedical research to evaluate toxicity and pharmacological properties of drugs [19], to discover potential biomarkers for disease states [20], and to understand the pathological mechanism of the metabolic syndrome [21]. Previous studies have shown that changes in specific lipid profiles and composition, such as ceramides and sphingomyelin species, are closely related to obesity-related diseases and metabolic disorders [22,23]. In addition, these techniques have also been used to explore the pharmacological effects of herbal medicines, such as *Cyclocarya paliurus* [24] and *Camellia sinensis* leaves [25], and *Panax ginseng* radix [26].

Thus, in this study, we conducted lipidomics analysis in HFD-induced metabolic disorders representing obesity and dyslipidemia as a pathology model. In addition, we also investigated the pharmacological effects of CLE and luteolin, which are closely related to the physiological functions and quality of CM [27], and its mechanisms against HFD-induced dyslipidemia through alterations of plasma lipid metabolites using the technique of liquid chromatography coupled with tandem mass spectrometry (LC-MS/MS).

2. Materials and Methods

2.1. Chemicals and Reagents

Methanol, isopropanol, and water were purchased from Merck (LC-MS grade, Darmstadt, Germany). Ammonium acetate, chloroform, methyl-*tert*-butyl ether (MTBE), butylhydroxytoluene

(BHT), and TAG (15:0/15:0/15:0) were purchased from Sigma-Aldrich (St. Louis, MO, USA). Lysophosphatidylcholine (LPC 17:1), lysophosphatidylethanolamine (LPE 17:1), phosphatidylcholine (PC 17:0/14:1), phosphatidylethanolamine (PE 17:0/14:1), diacylglycerol (DAG 8:0/8:0), sphingomyelin (SM d18:1/12:0), ceramide (CER d18:1/12:0), and cholesteryl ester (CE 15:0) were obtained from Avanti Polar Lipids (Alabaster, AL, USA). The lipid standards mentioned above were used as internal standards for semi-quantification of each lipid.

2.2. Preparation of Chrysanthemum morifolium Ramat Leaf Extract

CM leaves (Haihang Industry, Jinan, China) were washed, crushed to 20 mesh, and extracted by adding 10 volumes of 70% ethanol to 10 kg CLE in an extraction vessel. The extraction was performed at 65–70 °C in the roof of the pot, which had a condenser. Vapor was condensed and returned back to the pot, which was recirculated three times, and each time-period lasted for 2 h. The extracted CLE liquid was subsequently concentrated and spray-dried at 120 °C to 80 mesh. The yield obtained was 10%. The contents of flavonoids in the CLE were analyzed using liquid chromatography-tandem mass spectrometry (LC-MS/MS) as described in previous papers [28–30]. The contents (mg/g dry weight) of ten flavonoids in CLE were as follows: luteolin, 0.057; galuteolin, 0.47; luteolin-7-O-glucuronide, 0.28; luteolin-7-O-6-acetyl glucoside, 0.0047; diosmetin-7-O-rutinoside, 0.056; diosmetin-7-O-glucoside, 0.055; acacetin-7-O-rutinoside, 1.7; apigenin, 0.0062; quercetin, 0.0032; chlorogenic acid, 0.19 (Figure 1).

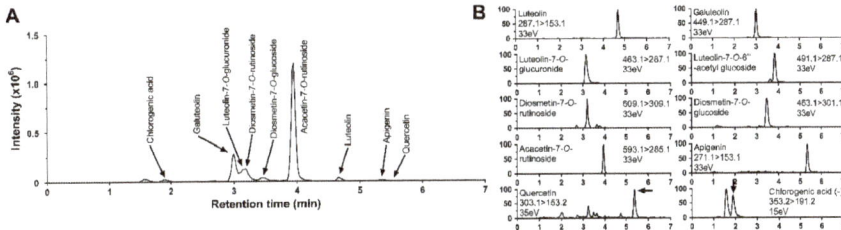

Figure 1. The total ion chromatogram (**A**) and selected reaction monitoring chromatogram (**B**) of individual flavonoids from *Chrysanthemum morifolium* Ramat leaf extracts (CLE).

2.3. Animal Experiments

Male C57BL/6J mice (4-week-old) were obtained from the Jackson Laboratory (Bar Harbor, ME, USA). All the mice were individually housed under constant temperature (24 °C) and a 12 h light/dark cycle, fed a normal chow diet for a one-week acclimation period, and subsequently, randomly divided into four groups. The mice in the different groups were fed a normal diet (ND, 12% kcal from fat, $n = 6$), high-fat diet (HFD, 45% kcal from fat, $n = 6$), HFD with 1.5% CLE (w/w) ($n = 6$), and HFD with 0.003% luteolin (w/w) (LU, $n = 6$) for 16 weeks. The mice were given free access to food and distilled water, and food intake and body weight were measured weekly. At the end of the mice experimental period, all the mice were anesthetized with isoflurane after 12 h of fasting. Blood samples were collected from the inferior vena cava in heparin-coated tubes, and plasma samples were obtained by centrifuging blood at 4000× g for 15 min at 4 °C. The liver, epididymal white adipose tissue (WAT), perirenal WAT, retroperitoneal WAT, mesentery WAT, subcutaneous WAT, interscapular WAT, interscapular brown adipose tissue, and skeletal muscle were removed, weighed, and immediately frozen in liquid nitrogen and stored at 80 °C. Animal studies were performed using protocols approved by the Kyungpook National University Industry Foundation (Approval No. KNU-2016-49).

2.4. Lipid Extraction

Lipids were extracted from mouse plasma according to the Matyash method with slight modifications [31]. In brief, a 50 µL internal standard (IS) mixture (LPC 17:1 400 ng/mL; LPE

17:1 400 ng/mL; PC 17:0/14:1 400 ng/mL; PE 17:0/14:1 400 ng/mL; DAG 8:0/8:0 40 ng/mL; SM d18:1/12:0 400 ng/mL; CER d18:1/12:0 40 ng/mL; CE 15:0 4 µg/mL; TAG 15:0/15:0/15:0 40 ng/mL) was transferred to a 2 mL Eppendorf tube and dried. Later, 5 µL plasma, 300 µL cold methanol, 100 µL water, and 1 mL MTBE along with 0.1% BHT were added to the tube. The mixture was shaken for 1 h at room temperature. Next, phase separation was induced by adding 250 µL water and incubating for 10 min at room temperature. After centrifugation (14,000× g for 15 min at 4 °C), the two phases were separately collected in 1.5 mL tubes. The upper (220 µL) and lower (110 µL) fractions were pooled and dried in a vacuum centrifuge (LABCONCO, Kansas City, MO, USA) for lipid profiling. The dried lipid extracts were reconstituted in 100 µL chloroform/methanol (1:9, v/v) prior to lipidomics analysis. Using the above method, hepatic lipids were extracted from the lyophilized samples (10 mg).

2.5. Lipidomics Study

Analysis of lipid extracts was performed using a high-performance liquid chromatography (HPLC) apparatus coupled to a Shimadzu 8040 tandem mass spectrometer (Shimadzu Corporation, Kyoto, Japan), based on a previously reported method with some modifications [32,33]. Semi-quantitative analysis of the extracted lipids from the plasma of mice was carried out using a Kinetex C18 column (100 × 2.1 mm, 2.6 µm, Phenomenex, Torrance, CA, USA) with a flow rate of 200 µL/min in positive mode. Mobile phase A was 10 mM ammonium acetate in water:methanol (1:9, v/v) and mobile phase B was 10 mM ammonium acetate in methanol:isopropanol (1:1, v/v). To achieve the best separation of the lipids, gradient elution was conducted as follows: 30% B (0 min), 95% B (15 min), 95% B (20 min), and 30% B (20–25 min). Each lipid quantitation was performed by selected reaction monitoring (SRM) of the precursor ions, ($[M + H]^+$ or $[M + NH_4]^+$), and the related product ion for each lipid. To calculate the concentration of each target lipid species, the ratio of target analyte and internal standard (IS) was multiplied by the concentration of one specific IS representing each lipid species based on single-point calibrations [34–36]. IS and SRM transition ions for each lipid class are described in a previously published paper [33].

2.6. Hepatic Gene Expression Analyses

Total RNA from the liver was extracted from three representative samples in each group according to the manufacturer's instructions (Invitrogen Life Technologies, Grand Island, NY, USA). The libraries of mRNA sequences were prepared as paired-end reads with a length of 100 bases using the TruSeq RNA Sample Preparation Kit (Illumina, CA, USA). After cDNA synthesis, the quality of these cDNA libraries was evaluated employing the Agilent 2100 Bioanalyzer (Agilent, CA, USA), and then sequenced as paired-ends using Illumina HiSeq2500 (Illumina, CA, USA). Quality control was performed using FastQC v. 0.11.2. Transcripts were assembled in Cufflinks v2.2.1 with TopHat Aligner [17,37]. Gene expression levels were estimated as fragments per kilobase of transcript per million mapped reads. Normalization factors were calculated using the differentially expressed genes (DEGES)/Empirical analysis of digital gene expression data in R (edgeR) method. Differentially expressed genes were identified based on a q-value threshold of less than 0.05. The RNA-sequence data is available at the National Center for Biotechnology Information (NCBI)'s Gene Expression Omnibus Database (http://www.ncbi.nlm.nih.gov/geo/): accession number GSE124777.

2.7. Data Processing and Statistical Analyses

To confirm stability and reproducibility of the mass spectrometric analysis, a quality control (QC) sample [National Institute of Standards and Technology (NIST) Standard Reference Material (SRM 1950 plasma)] was loaded at regular intervals (ten samples) [38,39]. Unsupervised principal component analysis (PCA) and supervised partial least squares-discriminant analysis (PLS-DA) multivariate analyses were used to construct pattern recognition models based on plasma lipidomics data with Pareto scaling, to explore the extent of differences among the four groups using the software SIMCA-P+ (version 13.0, Umetrics, Umea, Sweden). All data were reported as mean ± standard deviation

3. Results and Discussion

3.1. Animal Characteristics

Male C57BL/6J mice were fed an ND, HFD, HFD + CLE, and HFD + LU for 16 weeks. Changes in biological characteristics of these mice are shown in Figure 2. The values of body weight, liver weight, total adipose tissue weight, and total cholesterol were 28.1 ± 1.4 g, 1.0 ± 0.1 g, 1.8 ± 0.2 g, and 4.1 ± 0.6 mmol/L in the ND group, respectively; however, due to administration of HFD, these levels were significantly elevated to 46.6 ± 1.5 g, 2.8 ± 0.3 g, 7.7 ± 0.6 g, and 7.8 ± 1.7 mmol/L respectively, indicating that the obese mouse model was well-established. In contrast, supplementation with CLE or LU significantly lowered body weight ($p < 0.001$), liver weight ($p < 0.01$), and total adipose tissue weight ($p < 0.01$) compared to that in the HFD group. Recently, CLE was shown to ameliorate insulin resistance, thermogenesis, and energy expenditure along with a decrease in weight gain in white adipose tissue [17]. Liver histological analysis using Hemotoxylin and Eosin (H&E) staining was employed to evaluate the preventive effects of CLE on HFD-induced obese mice (Figure 2f). The livers of mice in the ND group did not exhibit lipid deposition and signs of steatosis, whereas those in the HFD group displayed accumulation of lipid droplets and developed hepatic steatosis. However, the CLE- or LU-treated groups exhibited a significant reduction of hepatic lipid droplets. While LU also decreased the number of lipid droplets in the liver as CLE, this effect tended to be less (Figure 2f). The hepatic TAG contents in each group were calculated by summing the contents of all quantified TAGs. The hepatic TAG contents in the ND, HFD, CLE, and LU groups were 222.3 ± 21.2, 707.0 ± 76.5, 531.6 ± 57.2, and 587.2 ± 31.0 µg/mg, respectively (Figure 2e). As expected, the hepatic TAG contents in the CLE and LU groups were lower than those in the HFD group ($p < 0.01$), and most individual TAG species in CLE tended to decrease slightly more than those in the LU group ($p > 0.05$) (Supplementary Figure S1). The more effective decrease of lipid droplet number and total hepatic triacylglycerols in the CLE treatment group compared to the LU treatment may be due to bioactive compounds such as quercetin and chlorogenic acid present with luteolin in CM leaves. Energy expenditure was significantly increased during a 12 h light/dark cycle after CLE and LU treatment when compared with the HFD group. Considering the suppressed hepatic lipogenesis and enhanced energy expenditure by CLE and LU treatment [17], it was evident that CLE and LU have a potential to attenuate obesity in mice.

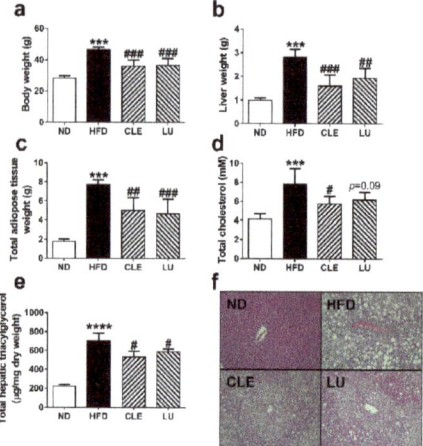

Figure 2. Effect of *Chrysanthemum morifolium* Ramat leaf extracts (CLE; 1.5%) and luteolin (LU; 0.003%) on body weight (**a**), liver weight (**b**), total adipose tissue weight (**c**), total cholesterol level (**d**), total hepatic triacylglycerol contents (**e**), and hepatic morphology (original magnification × 100) (**f**) in C57BL/6J mice fed a high-fat diet (HFD). The data are shown as mean ± standard deviation (SD) (*n* = 6). *, # different letters indicate significant difference compared with normal diet (ND) group (*) and HFD group (#), as determined by Tukey's multiple comparisons test. (*** $p < 0.001$, **** $p < 0.0001$, # $p < 0.05$, ## $p < 0.01$, ### $p < 0.001$).

3.2. Multivariate Statistical Analysis of Mice Plasma Lipid Levels

Representative pooled mice plasma samples were used to identify lipids therein. Approximately 140 individual lipid molecular species covering 9 lipid classes, comprising 16 LPC, 27 PC, 6 LPE, 11 PE, 41 TAG, 5 DAG, 14 SM, 14 CE, and 6 CER, were identified from pooled plasma samples of the mice [26]. The lipid profiles thus obtained from the ND, HFD, CLE, and LU groups were analyzed by multivariate statistical analysis to identify the extent of differences among the four groups. In the PCA score plot (Figure 3a), QC samples (NIST SRM1950 standard blood plasma, [40]) were tightly clustered, suggesting that the mass spectrometric analysis data has excellent stability and reproducibility. Performance of the constructed principal component analysis (PCA) and partial least-squares discriminant analysis (PLS-DA) model was assessed by fitness (R^2) and predictability (Q^2), and the performance levels of the good models are higher than 50%. The significance of the PLS-DA model was evaluated using cross-validated analysis of variance (CV-ANOVA) [41]. Each group showed a clear distinction in the PCA ($R^2X = 95\%$, $Q^2 = 85\%$) and PLS-DA ($R^2X = 93\%$, $Q^2 = 37\%$, $p = 0.038$) score plots with a good model quality. Clusters of lipid species from the CLE and LU groups were observed as separate clusters from those of the HFD group (Figure 3b,c).

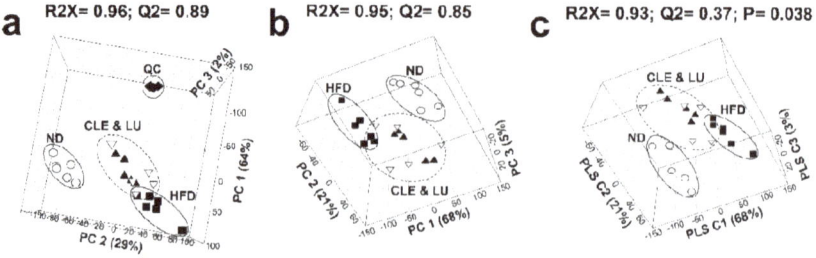

Figure 3. Principal component analysis (PCA) three-dimensional (3D) score plots (**a**), PCA 3D score

plots excluding quality control (QC) (**b**), and partial least-squares discriminant analysis (PLS-DA) 3D score plots (**c**) based on the serum lipidomic profiling among four groups. (Circle (○): normal diet (ND); Box (■): high-fat diet (HFD); Inverted triangle (▽): HFD plus *Chrysanthemum morifolium* Ramat leaf extract 1.5% diet (CLE); Triangle (▲): HFD plus luteolin 0.003% diet (LU); Diamond (♦): Quality control (QC)).

3.3. Effect of a High-Fat Diet on Mice

The sum (total) levels of the lipid species quantified in the plasma samples of mice were significantly elevated by HFD, and the lipid species contributing to these changes were LPC, PC, CE, SM, and CER. In contrast, the levels of LPE, PE, TAG, and DAG did not differ between the groups (Figure 4). The levels of 13 of 14 CE species, 12 of 27 PC species, 12 of 16 LPC species, all SM species, and 5 of 6 CER species were significantly increased by HFD, as shown in Supplementary Table S1. Similar to our results, accumulation of CE, PC, LPC, and sphingolipids (CER and SM) in plasma of HFD-induced obese and dyslipidemic mice has been reported [23,24,26,42–44]. The PC/PE ratio is a well-known marker associated with health and disease and regulates a variety of cellular processes [45]. Recently, an increase in these indicators has also been observed in the plasma of dyslipidemic and diabetic mice [24] and WAT macrophages in leptin-deficient (*ob/ob*) mice [46]. Consistent with this result, our results also showed a significant elevation in the levels of PC and PC/PE ratio in the HFD group compared with those in the ND group (Figure 4).

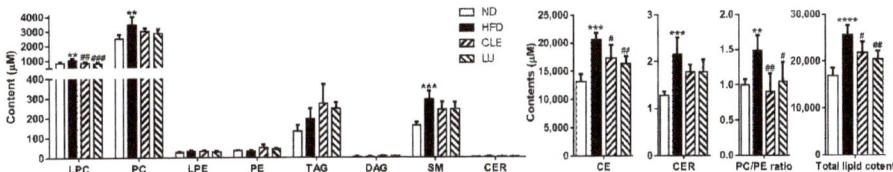

Figure 4. Overview of the effects of *Chrysanthemum morifolium* Ramat leaf extracts and luteolin on the serum lipidome in obese mice. The total lipid contents are expressed as the sum of contents of all identified lipids in mice plasma. Lipid classes are indicated on the *x*-axis: LPC, lysophosphatidylcholine; PC, phosphatidylcholine; LPE, lysophosphatidylethanolamine; PE, phosphatidylethanolamine; TAG, triacylglycerol; DAG, diacylglycerol; SM, sphingomyelin; CER, ceramide; CE, cholesteryl ester. The data are shown as mean ± standard deviation (SD) ($n = 6$). *, # different letters indicate significant difference compared with the normal diet (ND) group (*) and high-fat diet (HFD) group (#), as determined by Tukey's multiple comparisons test. CLE: HFD plus *Chrysanthemum morifolium* Ramat leaf extract 1.5% diet; LU: HFD plus luteolin 0.003% diet (** $p < 0.01$, *** $p < 0.001$, **** $p < 0.0001$, # $p < 0.05$, ## $p < 0.01$, ### $p < 0.001$).

3.4. Effect of Chrysanthemum morifolium Ramat leaf Extract (CLE) and Luteolin (LU) in Mice

We found that the sum (total) levels of LPC, PC, CE, SM, and CER were elevated in the HFD group compared to those in the ND group. Compared with the HFD group, CLE or LU treatment significantly reduced the sum total of the LPC and CE ($p < 0.05$), and also showed a tendency to decrease the SM and CER ($p = 0.08$) (Figure 4). However, even though CLE or LU had little effect on altering the sum total of the PC, the PC/PE ratio completely recovered to that of the ND group (Figure 4). The level of PC can be modulated by converting PE to PC by phosphatidylethanolamine *N*-methyltransferase (PEMT) as well as the Kennedy pathway that comprises Chpt1 and Cept1. The depletion of PC content by knockout of PEMT led to an increase in energy expenditure, weight loss, and insulin sensitivity, thereby preventing HFD-induced obesity and atherosclerosis [47–49]. Importantly, significantly higher hepatic expression of Chpt1 was observed in HFD-induced obese mice, however, CLE treatment significantly suppressed both the levels of Chpt1 and Cept1, while LU treatment significantly reduced only Cept1 (Figure 5a).

In contrast, no statistically significant change in the hepatic expression of PEMT was noted between the groups (data not shown). Thus, CLE or LU treatment appears to have an inhibitory effect on the Kennedy pathway rather than through the PEMT pathway.

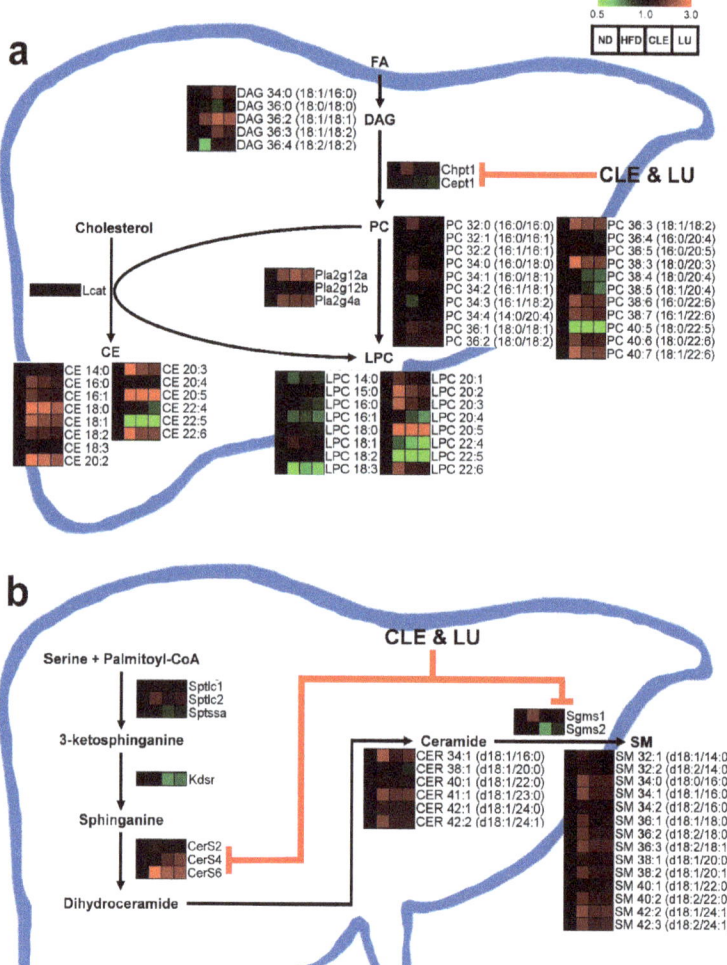

Figure 5. Scheme of the phospholipid synthesis (**a**) and sphingolipid synthesis (**b**) by which *Chrysanthemum morifolium* Ramat leaf extracts and luteolin regulates serum lipids and related hepatic gene-expression. The features of these compared to the ND group are color-coded by row, with red indicating high levels and green indicating low levels. ND: normal diet; HFD: high-fat diet; CLE: HFD plus *Chrysanthemum morifolium* Ramat leaf extract 1.5% diet; LU: HFD plus luteolin 0.003% diet; FA: fatty acid; DAG: diacylglycerol; PC: phosphatidylcholine; LPC: lysophosphatidylcholine; CE: cholesteryl ester; CER: ceramide; SM: sphingomyelin.

LPC is generated from the PC either via deacylation by phospholipase A_2 (PLA_2) isozymes or conversion by lecithin-cholesterol acyltransferase (LCAT) and is well known to be one of the major lipotoxic intermediates that promotes metabolic diseases through specific cell signaling, such as endoplasmic reticulum (ER) stress, chronic inflammation, apoptosis, and necrosis [50–52]. Consistent with our results, many previous studies have reported that the levels of most LPCs, including LPC 18:0, LPC 18:1, LPC 20:3, and LPC 22:6, were significantly increased in plasma of obese mice [26,42,44]. In addition to LPC, high plasma levels of CE are strongly recognized as a key marker to assess the risk and prediction of CVD [53,54]. Several studies have demonstrated that accumulation of high levels of CEs in plasma was observed in HFD-streptozotocin-induced diabetic (db/db) mice and HFD-induced obese mice, which are consistent with our findings [23,24,26,42]. In our study, one of the interesting findings was that significantly reduced levels of most LPC and CE were observed after CLE or LU treatment. However, no significant changes in the hepatic gene expressions, including LCAT, PLA_2 isozymes, and lysophosphatidylcholine acyltransferase (LPCAT) isozymes that are involved in synthesis of these lipids, were observed between all the groups ($p > 0.05$; data not shown). Therefore, CLE or LU treatment might have a potential therapeutic effect through reduced levels of lipotoxic intermediates (LPC and CE).

Among the 63 lipid metabolites increased by the HFD, we identified 22 potential markers associated with anti-obesity effects of CLE or LU in the plasma of mice using Tukey's multiple comparison test. In particular, the levels of 6 CE (20:2, 20:3, 20:4, 20:5, 22:4, and 22:6), 7 LPC (16:0, 18:0, 18:1, 20:2, 20:3, 20:4, and 22:6), 5 PC (34:0 (16:0/18:0), 38:4 (18:0/20:4), 38:5 (18:1/20:4), 40:6 (18:0/22:6), and 40:7 (18:1/22:6)), and 4 sphingolipid (CER 34:1 (d18:1/16:0), SM 34:1 (d18:1/16:0), SM 36:1 (d18:1/18:0), and SM 36:2 (d18:2/18:0)) were significantly lowered in the HFD group treated with CLE or LU (Supplementary Table S1).

CER, a precursor and major molecule of sphingolipids, and SM, which may act as a pool for the generation of CER, are the most abundant sphingolipids in lipoproteins and constitute about 3% and 87% of plasma sphingolipids, respectively [55]. Similar to our study, several studies have reported that CER and SM levels were significantly increased in plasma and liver of animal models caused by a HFD or leptin deficiency [56–59]. In addition, upregulation of genes involved in sphingolipid biosynthesis has been frequently observed in obesity and dyslipidemia. The synthesis of sphingolipids is initiated by serine palmitoyl-coenzyme A (CoA) transferase (SPT) using serine and palmitoyl-CoA as substrates, and CER is generated through a two-step process by ceramide synthase (CerS) and dihydroceramide desaturase (DES1), which is then converted to SM by a transfer of the head group of PC via the action of sphingomyelin synthase (Sgms) [60]. The gene expression of the SPT isozymes, 3-ketodihydrosphingosine reductase (kdsr), CerS isozymes, and Sgms isozymes, which are involved in regulating the de novo sphingolipid biosynthetic pathway and the levels of pro-ceramide gene expression, including sptlc2, CerS6, and sgms1, were significantly increased in the HFD group compared to those in the ND group ($p < 0.05$). Similar to our results, a previous study has reported that sptlc2, which is responsible for the initial steps in sphingolipid biosynthesis, was significantly elevated in HFD-induced insulin-resistant mice relative to a low-fat diet group [61]. In addition, upregulated expression levels of ceramide synthases (CerS1, CerS2, CerS4, and CerS6) have been observed in HFD-induced insulin resistance [61–63].

In the present study, CLE or LU treatment markedly decreased the levels of sphingolipids (CER and SM) in plasma (Figure 5b). As a result, the hepatic mRNA expression levels of CerS4, CerS6, Sgms1, and Sgms2 were significantly reduced after CLE or LU treatment ($p < 0.05$) (Figure 5b). CER 34:1 (d18:1/16:0) synthesized by CerS6 is specifically distinguished as a key CER compared to other CERs in obesity-related diseases, which worsens the overall health status through disruption of insulin signaling, induction of apoptosis, and suppression of energy expenditure or fatty acid oxidation [63–66]. Similar to our study (Figure 6), Raichur et al. also showed that treatment with antisense oligonucleotides as a selective CerS6 inhibitor prevented the development of obesity and T2D through improved insulin sensitivity and reduced body weight gain, together with approximately a 50% reduction of CER 34:1 (d18:1/16:0) levels in both the plasma and liver [64]. In addition, sgms1 gene knockout mice showed dramatic attenuation of SM levels in plasma and liver with suppression of inflammatory cytokines [67]. Additionally, some studies reported that Sgms2 knockout could prevent the development of liver steatosis [68,69]. These results indicated that CLE or LU treatment ameliorated HFD-induced dyslipidemia in mice by lowering the lipotoxic intermediates (CER and SM) in the liver and plasma through inhibition of de novo synthesis of sphingolipids.

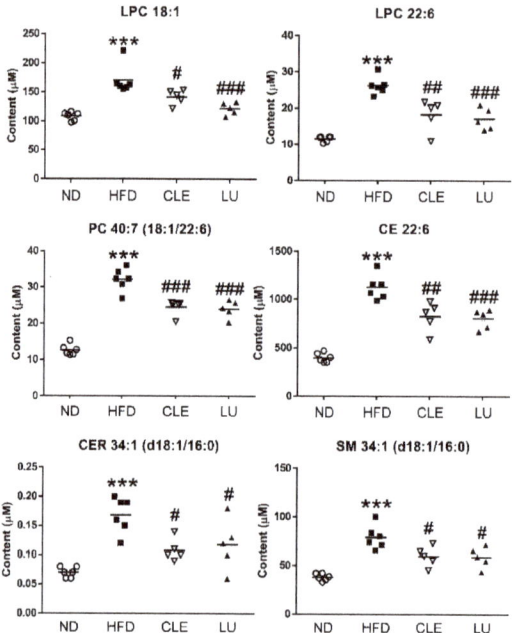

Figure 6. Scatter plot showing significant differences in the levels of the lipid biomarkers with the same lipid compositions among the normal diet (ND), high-fat diet (HFD), HFD plus *Chrysanthemum morifolium* Ramat leaf extract 1.5% diet (HFD + CLE), and HFD plus luteolin 0.003% diet (HFD + LU) groups. Each symbol represents an individual mouse (Circle (○): ND; Box (■): HFD; Inverted triangle (▽): CLE; Triangle (▲): LU; Diamond (◆): Quality control (QC)). *, # different letters indicate significant difference compared with the normal diet (ND) group (*) and the HFD group (#), as determined by Tukey's multiple comparisons test. (*** $p < 0.001$, # $p < 0.05$, ## $p < 0.01$, ### $p < 0.001$). LPC: lysophosphatidylcholine; PC: phosphatidylcholine; CE: cholesteryl ester; CER: ceramide; SM: sphingomyelin.

Taken together, our study demonstrated that treatment with CLE significantly reduced lipotoxic intermediates, such as PC, LPC, CER, SM, and CE, in the plasma of HFD-induced obesity and dyslipidemia model. Especially, six metabolites, LPC 18:1, LPC 22:6, PC 40:7, CE 22:6, CER 34:1, and SM 34:1, might be used as biomarker candidates which could explain the pharmacological effects of CLE or LU on dyslipidemic mice (Figure 6). Elevated hepatic expression levels of genes involved in the Kennedy pathway and sphingolipid metabolism related to synthesis of lipotoxic intermediates in the group of HFD-induced obese mice were dramatically recovered to the levels of the ND group after CLE or LU treatment. Consequently, the supplementation of CLE and LU was shown to ameliorate HFD-induced dyslipidemia and these lipid biomarkers can be used to better understand obesity-related metabolic disorders and to investigate their beneficial effects associated with such disorders.

Supplementary Materials: The following are available online at http://www.mdpi.com/2072-6643/12/10/2973/s1, Figure S1: Effect of *Chrysanthemum morifolium* Ramat leaf extracts (CLE) and Luteolin (LU) supplements for 16 weeks on individual TAG species in the liver. *, # different letters indicate significant difference compared with normal diet (ND) group (*) and HFD groups (#), as determined by Tukey's multiple comparisons test (*** $p < 0.001$, # $p < 0.05$, ## $p < 0.01$, ### $p < 0.001$). Table S1: Identified potential lipid biomarkers in plasma indicating statistically significant difference among sampling groups.

Author Contributions: Conceptualization, K.-H.L.; Project administration, K.-H.L. and M.-S.C.; Funding acquisition, K.-H.L. and M.-S.C.; Supervision, K.-H.L. and M.-S.C.; Methodology, J.C.S. and W.C.K.; Formal analysis, J.C.S. and R.R.; Software, J.C.S. and Z.W.; Investigation, J.C.S. and R.R.; Writing—Original Draft, J.C.S.; Writing—Review and Editing, J.-S.S. and Z.W. All authors have read and agreed to the published version of the manuscript.

Funding: This research was funded by the Bio-Synergy Research Project (NRF-2014M3A9C4066462 and NRF-2014M3A9C4066459) of the Ministry of Science and ICT through the National Research Foundation (NRF).

Conflicts of Interest: The authors declare no conflict of interest.

Abbreviations

Abbreviations	Definition
BHT	butylhydroxytoluene
CE	cholesteryl ester
Cept	ethanolamine phosphotransferase
CER	ceramide
CerS	ceramide synthase
Chpt	choline phosphotransferase
CLE	*Chrysanthemum morifolium* Ramat leaf extracts
CM	*Chrysanthemum morifolium* Ramat
CVD	cardiovascular disease
DAG	diacylglycerol
DES1	dihydroceramide desaturase
HFD	high-fat diet
HPLC	high-performance liquid chromatography
IS	internal standard
kdsr	3-ketodihydrosphingosine reductase
LCAT	lecithin-cholesterol acyltransferase
LC-MS/MS	liquid chromatography coupled with tandem mass spectrometry
LDL	low-density lipoprotein
LPC	lysophosphatidylcholine
LPE	lysophosphatidylethanolamine
LU	HFD plus luteolin 0.003% diet
MTBE	methyl-*tert*-butyl ether
ND	normal diet
PC	phosphatidylcholine
PCA	principal component analysis
PE	phosphatidylethanolamine
PEMT	Phosphatidylethanolamine *N*-methyltransferase
PLA$_2$	phospholipase A$_2$
PLS-DA	partial least squares-discriminant analysis
PPAR	peroxisome proliferator-activated receptor
QC	quality control
Sgms	sphingomyelin synthase
SM	sphingomyelin

SPT	serine palmitoyltransferase
SRM	selected reaction monitoring
TAG	triacylglycerol
TNF	tumor necrosis factor
T2DM	type 2 diabetes mellitus
WAT	white adipose tissue

References

1. Cheng, H.; Xu, N.; Zhao, W.; Su, J.; Liang, M.; Xie, Z.; Wu, X.; Li, Q. (-)-Epicatechin regulates blood lipids and attenuates hepatic steatosis in rats fed high-fat diet. *Mol. Nutr. Food Res.* **2017**, *61*. [CrossRef] [PubMed]
2. Collaborators, G.B.D.O.; Afshin, A.; Forouzanfar, M.H.; Reitsma, M.B.; Sur, P.; Estep, K.; Lee, A.; Marczak, L.; Mokdad, A.H.; Moradi-Lakeh, M.; et al. Health Effects of Overweight and Obesity in 195 Countries over 25 Years. *N. Engl. J. Med.* **2017**, *377*, 13–27. [CrossRef]
3. Gadde, K.M.; Martin, C.K.; Berthoud, H.R.; Heymsfield, S.B. Obesity: Pathophysiology and Management. *J. Am. Coll. Cardiol.* **2018**, *71*, 69–84. [CrossRef] [PubMed]
4. Wong, S.K.; Chin, K.Y.; Suhaimi, F.H.; Fairus, A.; Ima-Nirwana, S. Animal models of metabolic syndrome: A review. *Nutr. Metab. Lond.* **2016**, *13*, 65. [CrossRef] [PubMed]
5. Wang, C.Y.; Liao, J.K. A mouse model of diet-induced obesity and insulin resistance. *Methods Mol. Biol.* **2012**, *821*, 421–433. [CrossRef] [PubMed]
6. Buettner, R.; Scholmerich, J.; Bollheimer, L.C. High-fat diets: Modeling the metabolic disorders of human obesity in rodents. *Obesity* **2007**, *15*, 798–808. [CrossRef]
7. Han, A.R.; Kim, H.Y.; So, Y.; Nam, B.; Lee, I.S.; Nam, J.W.; Jo, Y.D.; Kim, S.H.; Kim, J.B.; Kang, S.Y.; et al. Quantification of Antioxidant Phenolic Compounds in a New Chrysanthemum Cultivar by High-Performance Liquid Chromatography with Diode Array Detection and Electrospray Ionization Mass Spectrometry. *Int. J. Anal. Chem.* **2017**, *2017*, 1254721. [CrossRef]
8. Kim, H.J.; Lee, Y.S. Identification of new dicaffeoylquinic acids from Chrysanthemum morifolium and their antioxidant activities. *Planta Med.* **2005**, *71*, 871–876. [CrossRef]
9. Li, Y.; Yang, P.; Luo, Y.; Gao, B.; Sun, J.; Lu, W.; Liu, J.; Chen, P.; Zhang, Y.; Yu, L.L. Chemical compositions of chrysanthemum teas and their anti-inflammatory and antioxidant properties. *Food Chem.* **2019**, *286*, 8–16. [CrossRef]
10. Ukiya, M.; Akihisa, T.; Tokuda, H.; Suzuki, H.; Mukainaka, T.; Ichiishi, E.; Yasukawa, K.; Kasahara, Y.; Nishino, H. Constituents of Compositae plants III. Anti-tumor promoting effects and cytotoxic activity against human cancer cell lines of triterpene diols and triols from edible chrysanthemum flowers. *Cancer Lett.* **2002**, *177*, 7–12. [CrossRef]
11. Gao, T.; Zhu, Z.Y.; Zhou, X.; Xie, M.L. Chrysanthemum morifolium extract improves hypertension-induced cardiac hypertrophy in rats by reduction of blood pressure and inhibition of myocardial hypoxia inducible factor-1alpha expression. *Pharm. Biol.* **2016**, *54*, 2895–2900. [CrossRef] [PubMed]
12. Cui, Y.; Wang, X.; Xue, J.; Liu, J.; Xie, M. Chrysanthemum morifolium extract attenuates high-fat milk-induced fatty liver through peroxisome proliferator-activated receptor alpha-mediated mechanism in mice. *Nutr. Res.* **2014**, *34*, 268–275. [CrossRef] [PubMed]
13. Nepali, S.; Cha, J.Y.; Ki, H.H.; Lee, H.Y.; Kim, Y.H.; Kim, D.K.; Song, B.J.; Lee, Y.M. Chrysanthemum indicum Inhibits Adipogenesis and Activates the AMPK Pathway in High-Fat-Diet-Induced Obese Mice. *Am. J. Chin. Med.* **2018**, *46*, 119–136. [CrossRef] [PubMed]
14. Shang, X.; Zhu, Z.-Y.; Wang, F.; Liu, J.-C.; Liu, J.-Y.; Xie, M.-L. Hypoglycemic effect of Chrysanthemum morifolium extract on alloxan-induced diabetic mice is associated with peroxisome proliferator-activated receptor α/γ-mediated hepatic glycogen synthesis. *J. Appl. Biomed.* **2017**, *15*, 81–86. [CrossRef]
15. Lai, J.P.; Lim, Y.H.; Su, J.; Shen, H.M.; Ong, C.N. Identification and characterization of major flavonoids and caffeoylquinic acids in three Compositae plants by LC/DAD-APCI/MS. *J. Chromatogr. B Anal. Technol. Biomed Life Sci.* **2007**, *848*, 215–225. [CrossRef]
16. Wang, T.; Shen, X.G.; Guo, Q.S.; Zhou, J.S.; Mao, P.F.; Shen, Z.G. Comparison of major bioactive components from leaves of Chrysanthemum morifolium. *China J. Chin. Mater. Med.* **2015**, *40*, 1670–1675.

17. Ryu, R.; Kwon, E.Y.; Choi, J.Y.; Shon, J.C.; Liu, K.H.; Choi, M.S. Chrysanthemum Leaf Ethanol Extract Prevents Obesity and Metabolic Disease in Diet-Induced Obese Mice via Lipid Mobilization in White Adipose Tissue. *Nutrients* **2019**, *11*. [CrossRef]
18. Huynh, K.; Barlow, C.K.; Jayawardana, K.S.; Weir, J.M.; Mellett, N.A.; Cinel, M.; Magliano, D.J.; Shaw, J.E.; Drew, B.G.; Meikle, P.J. High-Throughput Plasma Lipidomics: Detailed Mapping of the Associations with Cardiometabolic Risk Factors. *Cell Chem. Biol.* **2019**, *26*, 71–84. [CrossRef]
19. Kaddurah-Daouk, R.; Baillie, R.A.; Zhu, H.; Zeng, Z.B.; Wiest, M.M.; Nguyen, U.T.; Watkins, S.M.; Krauss, R.M. Lipidomic analysis of variation in response to simvastatin in the Cholesterol and Pharmacogenetics Study. *Metabolomics* **2010**, *6*, 191–201. [CrossRef]
20. Zhang, Z.H.; Vaziri, N.D.; Wei, F.; Cheng, X.L.; Bai, X.; Zhao, Y.Y. An integrated lipidomics and metabolomics reveal nephroprotective effect and biochemical mechanism of Rheum officinale in chronic renal failure. *Sci. Rep.* **2016**, *6*, 22151. [CrossRef]
21. Ramakrishanan, N.; Denna, T.; Devaraj, S.; Adams-Huet, B.; Jialal, I. Exploratory lipidomics in patients with nascent Metabolic Syndrome. *J. Diabetes Complicat.* **2018**, *32*, 791–794. [CrossRef] [PubMed]
22. Shah, C.; Yang, G.; Lee, I.; Bielawski, J.; Hannun, Y.A.; Samad, F. Protection from high fat diet-induced increase in ceramide in mice lacking plasminogen activator inhibitor 1. *J. Biol. Chem.* **2008**, *283*, 13538–13548. [CrossRef] [PubMed]
23. Eisinger, K.; Liebisch, G.; Schmitz, G.; Aslanidis, C.; Krautbauer, S.; Buechler, C. Lipidomic analysis of serum from high fat diet induced obese mice. *Int. J. Mol. Sci.* **2014**, *15*, 2991–3002. [CrossRef] [PubMed]
24. Zhai, L.; Ning, Z.W.; Huang, T.; Wen, B.; Liao, C.H.; Lin, C.Y.; Zhao, L.; Xiao, H.T.; Bian, Z.X. Cyclocarya paliurus Leaves Tea Improves Dyslipidemia in Diabetic Mice: A Lipidomics-Based Network Pharmacology Study. *Front. Pharmacol.* **2018**, *9*, 973. [CrossRef] [PubMed]
25. Nam, M.; Choi, M.S.; Choi, J.Y.; Kim, N.; Kim, M.S.; Jung, S.; Kim, J.; Ryu, D.H.; Hwang, G.S. Effect of green tea on hepatic lipid metabolism in mice fed a high-fat diet. *J. Nutr. Biochem.* **2018**, *51*, 1–7. [CrossRef]
26. Shon, J.C.; Shin, H.S.; Seo, Y.K.; Yoon, Y.R.; Shin, H.; Liu, K.H. Direct infusion MS-based lipid profiling reveals the pharmacological effects of compound K-reinforced ginsenosides in high-fat diet induced obese mice. *J. Agric. Food Chem.* **2015**, *63*, 2919–2929. [CrossRef] [PubMed]
27. Ye, Q.; Liang, Y.; Lu, J. Effect of different extracting methods on quality of Chrysanthemum Morifolium Ramat. Infusion. *Asia Pac. J. Clin. Nutr.* **2007**, *16 (Suppl. 1)*, 183–187.
28. Duan, K.; Yuan, Z.; Guo, W.; Meng, Y.; Cui, Y.; Kong, D.; Zhang, L.; Wang, N. LC-MS/MS determination and pharmacokinetic study of five flavone components after solvent extraction/acid hydrolysis in rat plasma after oral administration of Verbena officinalis L. extract. *J. Ethnopharmacol.* **2011**, *135*, 201–208. [CrossRef]
29. Lin, L.-Z.; Harnly, J.M. Identification of the phenolic components of chrysanthemum flower (Chrysanthemum morifolium Ramat). *Food Chem.* **2010**, *120*, 319–326. [CrossRef]
30. Tsimogiannis, D.; Samiotaki, M.; Panayotou, G.; Oreopoulou, V. Characterization of flavonoid subgroups and hydroxy substitution by HPLC-MS/MS. *Molecules* **2007**, *12*, 593–606. [CrossRef]
31. Matyash, V.; Liebisch, G.; Kurzchalia, T.V.; Shevchenko, A.; Schwudke, D. Lipid extraction by methyl-tert-butyl ether for high-throughput lipidomics. *J. Lipid Res.* **2008**, *49*, 1137–1146. [CrossRef] [PubMed]
32. Shon, J.C.; Noh, Y.J.; Kwon, Y.S.; Kim, J.H.; Wu, Z.; Seo, J.S. The impact of phenanthrene on membrane phospholipids and its biodegradation by Sphingopyxis soli. *Ecotoxicol. Environ. Saf.* **2020**, *192*, 110254. [CrossRef] [PubMed]
33. Im, S.S.; Park, H.Y.; Shon, J.C.; Chung, I.S.; Cho, H.C.; Liu, K.H.; Song, D.K. Plasma sphingomyelins increase in pre-diabetic Korean men with abdominal obesity. *PLoS ONE* **2019**, *14*, e0213285. [CrossRef]
34. Cajka, T.; Fiehn, O. Comprehensive analysis of lipids in biological systems by liquid chromatography-mass spectrometry. *Trends Anal. Chem.* **2014**, *61*, 192–206. [CrossRef] [PubMed]
35. Cajka, T.; Smilowitz, J.T.; Fiehn, O. Validating Quantitative Untargeted Lipidomics Across Nine Liquid Chromatography-High-Resolution Mass Spectrometry Platforms. *Anal. Chem.* **2017**, *89*, 12360–12368. [CrossRef] [PubMed]
36. Karsai, G.; Kraft, F.; Haag, N.; Korenke, G.C.; Hanisch, B.; Othman, A.; Suriyanarayanan, S.; Steiner, R.; Knopp, C.; Mull, M.; et al. DEGS1-associated aberrant sphingolipid metabolism impairs nervous system function in humans. *J. Clin. Investig.* **2019**, *129*, 1229–1239. [CrossRef] [PubMed]

37. Trapnell, C.; Roberts, A.; Goff, L.; Pertea, G.; Kim, D.; Kelley, D.R.; Pimentel, H.; Salzberg, S.L.; Rinn, J.L.; Pachter, L. Differential gene and transcript expression analysis of RNA-seq experiments with TopHat and Cufflinks. *Nat. Protoc.* **2012**, *7*, 562–578. [CrossRef]
38. Want, E.J.; Wilson, I.D.; Gika, H.; Theodoridis, G.; Plumb, R.S.; Shockcor, J.; Holmes, E.; Nicholson, J.K. Global metabolic profiling procedures for urine using UPLC-MS. *Nat. Protoc.* **2010**, *5*, 1005–1018. [CrossRef]
39. Burla, B.; Arita, M.; Arita, M.; Bendt, A.K.; Cazenave-Gassiot, A.; Dennis, E.A.; Ekroos, K.; Han, X.; Ikeda, K.; Liebisch, G.; et al. MS-based lipidomics of human blood plasma: A community-initiated position paper to develop accepted guidelines. *J. Lipid Res.* **2018**, *59*, 2001–2017. [CrossRef]
40. Lange, M.; Fedorova, M. Evaluation of lipid quantification accuracy using HILIC and RPLC MS on the example of NIST(R) SRM(R) 1950 metabolites in human plasma. *Anal. Bioanal. Chem.* **2020**, *412*, 3573–3584. [CrossRef]
41. Eriksson, L.; Trygg, J.; Wold, S. CV-ANOVA for significance testing of PLS and OPLS® models. *J. Chemom.* **2008**, *22*, 594–600. [CrossRef]
42. Zacek, P.; Bukowski, M.; Mehus, A.; Johnson, L.; Zeng, H.; Raatz, S.; Idso, J.P.; Picklo, M. Dietary saturated fatty acid type impacts obesity-induced metabolic dysfunction and plasma lipidomic signatures in mice. *J. Nutr. Biochem.* **2019**, *64*, 32–44. [CrossRef] [PubMed]
43. Kim, J.; Choi, J.N.; Choi, J.H.; Cha, Y.S.; Muthaiya, M.J.; Lee, C.H. Effect of fermented soybean product (Cheonggukjang) intake on metabolic parameters in mice fed a high-fat diet. *Mol. Nutr. Food Res.* **2013**, *57*, 1886–1891. [CrossRef] [PubMed]
44. Kim, H.J.; Kim, J.H.; Noh, S.; Hur, H.J.; Sung, M.J.; Hwang, J.T.; Park, J.H.; Yang, H.J.; Kim, M.S.; Kwon, D.Y.; et al. Metabolomic analysis of livers and serum from high-fat diet induced obese mice. *J. Proteome Res.* **2011**, *10*, 722–731. [CrossRef] [PubMed]
45. Van der Veen, J.N.; Kennelly, J.P.; Wan, S.; Vance, J.E.; Vance, D.E.; Jacobs, R.L. The critical role of phosphatidylcholine and phosphatidylethanolamine metabolism in health and disease. *Biochim. Biophys. Acta Biomembr.* **2017**, *1859*, 1558–1572. [CrossRef]
46. Petkevicius, K.; Virtue, S.; Bidault, G.; Jenkins, B.; Cubuk, C.; Morgantini, C.; Aouadi, M.; Dopazo, J.; Serlie, M.J.; Koulman, A.; et al. Accelerated phosphatidylcholine turnover in macrophages promotes adipose tissue inflammation in obesity. *Elife* **2019**, *8*. [CrossRef]
47. Jacobs, R.L.; Zhao, Y.; Koonen, D.P.; Sletten, T.; Su, B.; Lingrell, S.; Cao, G.; Peake, D.A.; Kuo, M.S.; Proctor, S.D.; et al. Impaired de novo choline synthesis explains why phosphatidylethanolamine N-methyltransferase-deficient mice are protected from diet-induced obesity. *J. Biol. Chem.* **2010**, *285*, 22403–22413. [CrossRef]
48. Zhao, Y.; Su, B.; Jacobs, R.L.; Kennedy, B.; Francis, G.A.; Waddington, E.; Brosnan, J.T.; Vance, J.E.; Vance, D.E. Lack of phosphatidylethanolamine N-methyltransferase alters plasma VLDL phospholipids and attenuates atherosclerosis in mice. *Arter. Thromb. Vasc. Biol.* **2009**, *29*, 1349–1355. [CrossRef]
49. Funai, K.; Lodhi, I.J.; Spears, L.D.; Yin, L.; Song, H.; Klein, S.; Semenkovich, C.F. Skeletal Muscle Phospholipid Metabolism Regulates Insulin Sensitivity and Contractile Function. *Diabetes* **2016**, *65*, 358–370. [CrossRef]
50. Neuschwander-Tetri, B.A. Hepatic lipotoxicity and the pathogenesis of nonalcoholic steatohepatitis: The central role of nontriglyceride fatty acid metabolites. *Hepatology* **2010**, *52*, 774–788. [CrossRef]
51. Schmitz, G.; Ruebsaamen, K. Metabolism and atherogenic disease association of lysophosphatidylcholine. *Atherosclerosis* **2010**, *208*, 10–18. [CrossRef] [PubMed]
52. Law, S.H.; Chan, M.L.; Marathe, G.K.; Parveen, F.; Chen, C.H.; Ke, L.Y. An Updated Review of Lysophosphatidylcholine Metabolism in Human Diseases. *Int. J. Mol. Sci.* **2019**, *20*. [CrossRef] [PubMed]
53. Stegemann, C.; Pechlaner, R.; Willeit, P.; Langley, S.R.; Mangino, M.; Mayr, U.; Menni, C.; Moayyeri, A.; Santer, P.; Rungger, G.; et al. Lipidomics profiling and risk of cardiovascular disease in the prospective population-based Bruneck study. *Circulation* **2014**, *129*, 1821–1831. [CrossRef] [PubMed]
54. Alshehry, Z.H.; Mundra, P.A.; Barlow, C.K.; Mellett, N.A.; Wong, G.; McConville, M.J.; Simes, J.; Tonkin, A.M.; Sullivan, D.R.; Barnes, E.H.; et al. Plasma Lipidomic Profiles Improve on Traditional Risk Factors for the Prediction of Cardiovascular Events in Type 2 Diabetes Mellitus. *Circulation* **2016**, *134*, 1637–1650. [CrossRef] [PubMed]
55. Hammad, S.M.; Pierce, J.S.; Soodavar, F.; Smith, K.J.; Al Gadban, M.M.; Rembiesa, B.; Klein, R.L.; Hannun, Y.A.; Bielawski, J.; Bielawska, A. Blood sphingolipidomics in healthy humans: Impact of sample collection methodology. *J. Lipid Res.* **2010**, *51*, 3074–3087. [CrossRef]

56. Samad, F.; Hester, K.D.; Yang, G.; Hannun, Y.A.; Bielawski, J. Altered adipose and plasma sphingolipid metabolism in obesity: A potential mechanism for cardiovascular and metabolic risk. *Diabetes* **2006**, *55*, 2579–2587. [CrossRef]
57. Yang, G.; Badeanlou, L.; Bielawski, J.; Roberts, A.J.; Hannun, Y.A.; Samad, F. Central role of ceramide biosynthesis in body weight regulation, energy metabolism, and the metabolic syndrome. *Am. J. Physiol. Endocrinol. Metab.* **2009**, *297*, E211–E224. [CrossRef]
58. Kasumov, T.; Li, L.; Li, M.; Gulshan, K.; Kirwan, J.P.; Liu, X.; Previs, S.; Willard, B.; Smith, J.D.; McCullough, A. Ceramide as a mediator of non-alcoholic Fatty liver disease and associated atherosclerosis. *PLoS ONE* **2015**, *10*, e0126910. [CrossRef]
59. Adams, J.M., 2nd; Pratipanawatr, T.; Berria, R.; Wang, E.; DeFronzo, R.A.; Sullards, M.C.; Mandarino, L.J. Ceramide content is increased in skeletal muscle from obese insulin-resistant humans. *Diabetes* **2004**, *53*, 25–31. [CrossRef]
60. Cowart, L.A. *Sphingolipids and Metabolic Disease*; Springer Science & Business Media: Berlin, Germany, 2011; Volume 721.
61. Longato, L.; Tong, M.; Wands, J.R.; de la Monte, S.M. High fat diet induced hepatic steatosis and insulin resistance: Role of dysregulated ceramide metabolism. *Hepatol. Res.* **2012**, *42*, 412–427. [CrossRef]
62. Cinar, R.; Godlewski, G.; Liu, J.; Tam, J.; Jourdan, T.; Mukhopadhyay, B.; Harvey-White, J.; Kunos, G. Hepatic cannabinoid-1 receptors mediate diet-induced insulin resistance by increasing de novo synthesis of long-chain ceramides. *Hepatology* **2014**, *59*, 143–153. [CrossRef] [PubMed]
63. Turpin, S.M.; Nicholls, H.T.; Willmes, D.M.; Mourier, A.; Brodesser, S.; Wunderlich, C.M.; Mauer, J.; Xu, E.; Hammerschmidt, P.; Bronneke, H.S.; et al. Obesity-induced CerS6-dependent C16:0 ceramide production promotes weight gain and glucose intolerance. *Cell Metab.* **2014**, *20*, 678–686. [CrossRef]
64. Raichur, S.; Brunner, B.; Bielohuby, M.; Hansen, G.; Pfenninger, A.; Wang, B.; Bruning, J.C.; Larsen, P.J.; Tennagels, N. The role of C16:0 ceramide in the development of obesity and type 2 diabetes: CerS6 inhibition as a novel therapeutic approach. *Mol. Metab.* **2019**, *21*, 36–50. [CrossRef]
65. Raichur, S.; Wang, S.T.; Chan, P.W.; Li, Y.; Ching, J.; Chaurasia, B.; Dogra, S.; Ohman, M.K.; Takeda, K.; Sugii, S.; et al. CerS2 haploinsufficiency inhibits beta-oxidation and confers susceptibility to diet-induced steatohepatitis and insulin resistance. *Cell Metab.* **2014**, *20*, 687–695. [CrossRef]
66. Fucho, R.; Casals, N.; Serra, D.; Herrero, L. Ceramides and mitochondrial fatty acid oxidation in obesity. *FASEB J.* **2017**, *31*, 1263–1272. [CrossRef] [PubMed]
67. Li, Z.; Fan, Y.; Liu, J.; Li, Y.; Huan, C.; Bui, H.H.; Kuo, M.S.; Park, T.S.; Cao, G.; Jiang, X.C. Impact of sphingomyelin synthase 1 deficiency on sphingolipid metabolism and atherosclerosis in mice. *Arter. Thromb. Vasc. Biol.* **2012**, *32*, 1577–1584. [CrossRef] [PubMed]
68. Mitsutake, S.; Zama, K.; Yokota, H.; Yoshida, T.; Tanaka, M.; Mitsui, M.; Ikawa, M.; Okabe, M.; Tanaka, Y.; Yamashita, T.; et al. Dynamic modification of sphingomyelin in lipid microdomains controls development of obesity, fatty liver, and type 2 diabetes. *J. Biol. Chem.* **2011**, *286*, 28544–28555. [CrossRef] [PubMed]
69. Li, Y.; Dong, J.; Ding, T.; Kuo, M.S.; Cao, G.; Jiang, X.C.; Li, Z. Sphingomyelin synthase 2 activity and liver steatosis: An effect of ceramide-mediated peroxisome proliferator-activated receptor gamma2 suppression. *Arter. Thromb. Vasc. Biol.* **2013**, *33*, 1513–1520. [CrossRef] [PubMed]

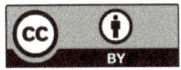

© 2020 by the authors. Licensee MDPI, Basel, Switzerland. This article is an open access article distributed under the terms and conditions of the Creative Commons Attribution (CC BY) license (http://creativecommons.org/licenses/by/4.0/).

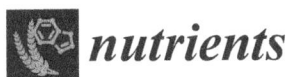

Article

Red Propolis and Its Dyslipidemic Regulator Formononetin: Evaluation of Antioxidant Activity and Gastroprotective Effects in Rat Model of Gastric Ulcer

Marcio A. A. de Mendonça [1], Ana R. S. Ribeiro [2], Adriana K. de Lima [1], Gislaine B. Bezerra [1], Malone S. Pinheiro [1], Ricardo L. C. de Albuquerque-Júnior [1,3], Margarete Z. Gomes [1,3], Francine F. Padilha [1,3], Sara M. Thomazzi [2], Ettore Novellino [4], Antonello Santini [4,*], Patricia Severino [1,3,5], Eliana B. Souto [6,7,*] and Juliana C. Cardoso [1,3,*]

1. University of Tiradentes, Av. Murilo Dantas, 300, Aracaju CEP 49032-490, Sergipe, Brazil; andrade.mendonca@oi.com.br (M.A.A.d.M.); adrianaklima@live.com (A.K.d.L.); gislaine.proativa@yahoo.com.br (G.B.B.); malonepinheiro@hotmail.com (M.S.P.); ricardo.patologia@uol.com.br (R.L.C.d.A.-J.); guetezanardo@yahoo.com.br (M.Z.G.); fpadilha@yahoo.com (F.F.P.); pattypharma@gmail.com (P.S.)
2. Departament of Physiology, Federal University of Sergipe, Av. Marechal Rondon, Cidade Universitária, São Cristóvão CEP 49100-000, Sergipe, Brazil; ana_farmaunit@hotmail.com (A.R.S.R.); sthomazzi@gmail.com (S.M.T.)
3. Institute of Technology and Research (ITP), Av. Murilo Dantas, 300, Aracaju CEP 49032-490, Sergipe, Brazil
4. Department of Pharmacy, University of Napoli Federico II, Via D. Montesano 49, 80131 Napoli, Italy; ettore.novellino@unina.it
5. Tiradentes Institute, 150 Mt Vernon St, Dorchester, MA 02125, USA
6. Department of Pharmaceutical Technology, Faculty of Pharmacy, University of Coimbra, Pólo das Ciências da Saúde, Azinhaga de Santa Comba, 3000-548 Coimbra, Portugal
7. CEB—Centre of Biological Engineering, University of Minho, Campus de Gualtar, 4710-057 Braga, Portugal
* Correspondence: asantini@unina.it (A.S.); ebsouto@ff.uc.pt (E.B.S.); juaracaju@yahoo.com.br (J.C.C.); Tel.: +39-81-253-9317 (A.S.); +351-239-488-400 (E.B.S.); +55-79-3218-2190 (J.C.C.)

Received: 31 August 2020; Accepted: 24 September 2020; Published: 26 September 2020

Abstract: Propolis has various pharmacological properties of clinical interest, and is also considered a functional food. In particular, hydroalcoholic extracts of red propolis (HERP), together with its isoflavonoid formononetin, have recognized antioxidant and anti-inflammatory properties, with known added value against dyslipidemia. In this study, we report the gastroprotective effects of HERP (50–500 mg/kg, p.o.) and formononetin (10 mg/kg, p.o.) in ethanol and non-steroidal anti-inflammatory drug-induced models of rat ulcer. The volume, pH, and total acidity were the evaluated gastric secretion parameters using the pylorus ligature model, together with the assessment of gastric mucus contents. The anti-*Helicobacter pylori* activities of HERP were evaluated using the agar-well diffusion method. In our experiments, HERP (250 and 500 mg/kg) and formononetin (10 mg/kg) reduced ($p < 0.001$) total lesion areas in the ethanol-induced rat ulcer model, and reduced ($p < 0.05$) ulcer indices in the indomethacin-induced rat ulcer model. Administration of HERP and formononetin to pylorus ligature models significantly decreased ($p < 0.01$) gastric secretion volumes and increased ($p < 0.05$) mucus production. We have also shown the antioxidant and anti-*Helicobacter pylori* activities of HERP. The obtained results indicate that HERP and formononetin are gastroprotective in acute ulcer models, suggesting a prominent role of formononetin in the effects of HERP.

Keywords: propolis; formononetin; dyslipidemia; gastric ulcer; rats

1. Introduction

Dyslipidaemia is a condition defined either by the high levels of total or low-density lipoprotein (LDL) cholesterol, and/or by the low levels of high-density lipoprotein (HDL). Such lipid metabolic dysfunction, resulting from, e.g., lipid peroxidation or oxidative stress, plays an important role in the pathogenesis of atherosclerosis and other chronic diseases [1]. Changes in lifestyle (e.g., adoption of a heart-healthy diet and exercise) and the use of drugs (e.g., fibrates to reduce triacylglycerols, statins to reduce bad cholesterol (LDL), and niacin to increase the overall (HDL) cholesterol) are commonly implemented to ameliorate these metabolic diseases. Atherogenesis results from the imbalance between the antioxidant capacity and the activity of oxidative species (reactive oxygen, nitrogen, and halogen). The oxidizing cellular protein, lipid, and DNA directly injure cells or these can even die from disturbances in signaling pathways. Reactive oxygen species (ROS) participate as signaling molecules in fundamental cellular functions in ambient conditions. Oxidative stress, and activation of ROS, is triggered when a cell is depleted in small molecule antioxidants or when antioxidase systems are overloaded or not operating at all.

The interest in natural products as sources of new drugs and therapeutic strategies for chronic diseases is increasingly growing. Among those sources, natural antioxidants from different plants (e.g., *Dirmophandra mollis* Benth, *Ruta graveolens* L., *Ginkgo biloba* L., *Vitis vinifera* L, *Thymus zygis*, *Croton argyrophyllus* Kunth, *Hordeum vulgare*, *Dalbergia ecastophyllum*, *Origanum vulgare* L.) are receiving particular attention [2–7].

Propolis (or bee glue) is a complex mixture of molecules obtained from several resinous secretions (e.g., resins, mucilage, gums, lattices, leaf buds) collected by worker-bees from different plant species [8]. Its composition is thus strongly influenced by the diversity of local flora, harvesting place and season, and by the genetics of the bees [9]. Briefly, these plant resinous secretions are mixed with salivary and enzymatic secretions of honey bees, producing a cementing material, used to close open cracks occurring in beehives. Propolis is used for sealing the spaces in beehives and to smooth their internal walls, providing antiseptic activity, as it protects the bees' larvae and comb from microbial invasions [8].

Among several species, red propolis obtained from *Dalbergia ecastophyllum* (L.) Taub. (Fabaceae, [10]) shows various pharmacological properties of clinical interest, also being considered a functional food [11–13]. In particular, and due to its significant antioxidant activity [14–16], Brazilian red propolis has been proposed for dermal healing [17,18], and for the treatment of cancer cells [14,15,19,20], as an antimicrobial [16], antiproliferative [21,22], antihypertensive [23], and as a neuroprotective [11]. Several compounds have been identified in this resin, including the isoflavonoids formononetin, biochanin A, medicarpin, and pinocembrin [24,25]. Reported biological activities of these isolated compounds include the anti-inflammatory activities of biochanin A [26], pinocembrin [27], neovestitol, and vestitol [28], the antioxidant activities of formononetin [29], biochanin A [30], pinocembrin [31], the gastroprotective properties of biochanin A [32], the antifungal and dyslipidemic activities of formononetin [33,34], and the antimicrobial actions of neovestitol and vestitol [28].

Inhibitors of the HMG-CoA (3-hydroxy-3-methyl-glutaryl-coenzyme A) reductase play an active role in the treatment of hypercholesterolemia and have been found to play a protective role in several bacteria-associated diseases such as *Helicobacter pylori*-induced gastric ulcer. Association between *Helicobacter pylori* infection and dyslipidemia has been reported significantly [35]. Gastric ulcer is a chronic disease of high worldwide prevalence, associated to unexpected complications such as bleeding, perforation, and stenosis [36]. The imbalances of gastric mucosal defense mechanisms (prostaglandins, mucus, mucosal blood flow, bicarbonate, nitric oxide, and sulfhydryl compounds, and ATP sensitive K^+ channels) against exposure to endogenous and exogenous factors (e.g., non-steroidal anti-inflammatory drugs (NSAIDs), pepsin, bile acids, alcohol, stress, and trauma, *Helicobacter pylori* infection, hemorrhagic shock, sepsis, and burns) promote the development of gastric ulcers [36,37].

It is also known that a long-term use of NSAID, and/or the presence of *Helicobacter pylori* infection, are the main causes of incidence and recurrence of gastric ulcers [38–40]. Furthermore, excessive alcohol consumption is an independent risk factor for the set-up of gastric ulcer, being thus a serious public health concern [41,42].

Using a rat model of inflammatory and neurogenic pain, without emotional or motor side effects, we have already demonstrated that hydroalcoholic extracts of red propolis (HERP) have significant anti-inflammatory and antinociceptive activities [43]. We have also described the anti-inflammatory activity of the dyslipidemic isoflavonoid formononetin [11,43]. In the present work, we proposed the in vivo characterization of the gastroprotective effects of HERP and formononetin, using an experimental rat model of gastric ulcer, as a suitable approach for phytomedical uses.

2. Materials and Methods

2.1. Drugs and Reagents

Alcian blue (Cas. No: 33864-99-2), carbenoxolone (Cas. No: 5697-56-3), cimetidine (Cas. No: 51481-61-9), formononetin (Cas. No: 485-72-3), indomethacin (Cas. No: 53-86-1), and omeprazole (Cas. No: 73590-58-6) were obtained from Sigma Chemical Co. (St. Louis, MO, USA). All other used reagents were of analytical grade. Test substances were dissolved in 0.9% NaCl solution containing 2% Tween 80 (polysorbate 80), while indomethacin was dissolved in 2% sodium bicarbonate, all from Sigma-Aldrich (Darmstadt, Germany). HERP and formononetin doses were based on our preliminary experiments [5].

2.2. Red Propolis Collection, Hydroalcoholic Extracts Preparation and Characterization

Red propolis was collected from species of Brejo Grande, Sergipe, Brazil (10°28′25″ S, 36°26′12″ W). The material was labeled, and stored in sterile and refrigerated containers. For the extraction, a volume of 12.5 mL of ethanol (70%) was used to extract 1 g of propolis samples using an ultrasound bath for 1 h, at room temperature as described by Pinheiro et al. [22]. After extraction, the obtained mixture was centrifuged, and the obtained supernatant evaporated under low pressure resulting in HERP, which was stored at refrigerated temperature until further use. The obtained extraction yield was 34% (w/w). Analysis of hydroalcoholic extracts of red propolis (HERP) was performed using HPLC as described by Cavendish et al. [43], and formononetin (ca. 2%) was confirmed as the major component.

2.3. Antioxidant Activity

The antioxidant activity of HERP was determined as the capacity of the antioxidants present in the sample to scavenge the stable radical 2 2-diphenyl-1-picrylhydrazyl (DPPH·), applying a previously described methodology [44,45]. A volume of 3 mL of extract, at concentrations between 2.5 and 15.0 mg/mL, was homogenized with 750 μL of DPPH solution (200 mM). After 15 min at room temperature, the spectrophotometric reading was done at 517 nm. Ethanol 70% was used as control and subject to the same procedure. Experiments were done in triplicate. To determine the % of free radical inhibition (%I), the following equation was used:

$$\%I = 100 - (A_C/A_A) \times 100$$

where A_C is the absorbance of the control and A_A is the absorbance of the sample. The mean inhibition index (IC50) was obtained from the %I values at each tested concentration by non-linear regression by computing the data in Prism GraphPad software (San Diego, CA, USA).

2.4. Microorganism

Helicobacter pylori strain ATCC 43504 was obtained from the Instituto Nacional de Controle de Qualidade em Saúde (INCQS—Fundação Oswaldo Cruz—Fiocruz/RJ, Brazil). The stock cultures were kept in Brucella broth at −20 °C until further use.

2.5. Animals

Wistar rats of both sexes, of 280–320 g mean weight, were received from the animal facilities of the Tiradentes University biotherium (Aracaju, Brazil). Animals were housed at 21 ± 2 °C in plastic cages, with free access to food (Purina®) and water ad libitum, under a 12-h light/12-h dark cycle. Twenty-four hours prior to the experiments, rats were provided with water ad libitum. All experiments and protocols were approved by the Institutional Ethics Committee (250608) of the Tiradentes University (Aracaju, Brazil) and were performed according to the EEC Directive of 1986, following the principles for laboratory animal use and care.

2.6. Antiulcerogenic Activity

2.6.1. Ethanol-Induced Ulcers

These experiments were conducted according to the method described by Robert et al. [46]. Briefly, rats ($n = 6$/group) were fasted for 24 h and were then pre-treated orally with 50, 250, or 500 mg/kg HERP, 10 mg/kg formononetin, 100 mg/kg omeprazole, or vehicle (2% Tween 80, 10 mL/kg). Thirty minutes after treatment, all rats received 1 mL of absolute ethanol to induce gastric ulcers and were anaesthetized (3% halothane) and one hour later were euthanized by cervical dislocation.

The stomachs of the animals were then removed and opened along the greater curvature. To remove gastric contents and blood clots, the stomachs were gently rinsed with water. Tissues images were recorded as described by Pinto et al. [47], and total lesion areas were measured (mm^2). Stomach samples from 50, 250, and 500 mg/kg HERP, formononetin, omeprazole, and vehicle treated animals were cut into serial 5 μm thick sections and were stained with hematoxylin-eosin (HE) according to laboratorial techniques.

Microscopic scores were determined for the interstitial edema and for the disruption of superficial regions of the gastric gland with epithelial cell loss Intensities of epithelial cell loss and interstitial edema were categorized as follows: absence (0); focal limited to the upper third (1); focal beyond the upper third (2); and diffuse in the upper third (3). Three histological sections for each animal ($n = 6$/group) were randomly analyzed (without previous knowledge of the treatments).

2.6.2. Non-Steroidal Anti-Inflammatory Drug (NSAID)-Induced Ulcers

These experiments were adopted from the method described by Djahanguiri, with a few modifications [48]. Briefly, rats ($n = 6$/group) were pre-treated orally with HERP (50, 250, or 500 mg/kg), formononetin (10 mg/kg), cimetidine (100 mg/kg), or vehicle (2% Tween 80) for 30 min, and were then treated with indomethacin (100 mg/kg, p.o.) to induce gastric ulcers. Animals were euthanized by cervical dislocation six hours later after anesthesia with 3% halothane. Stomachs were then removed and opened for the scoring of ulcer index as follows: (i) score 1, standing for loss of mucosal folding, mucosal discoloration, edema, or hemorrhage; (ii) score 2, standing for less than 10 petechiae; and (iii) score 3, standing for more than 10 petechiae [49].

2.7. Determination of Gastric Juice Parameters Following Pyloric Ligature

For the determination of the gastric juice parameters, the methods described by Shay et al. were followed with some modifications [50]. Animals were anaesthetized with ketamine/xylazine (60 and 10 mg/kg, respectively, i.p.) after 24 h of fasting, followed by laparotomy and pylorus ligation. Rats ($n = 6$/group) were then treated intraduodenally with HERP (50, 250, or 500 mg/kg), formononetin (10 mg/kg), cimetidine (100 mg/kg), or vehicle (2% Tween 80). Four hours later, animals were anesthetized with halothane (3%) and euthanized by cervical dislocation. Abdomens were then opened, stomachs removed, and gastric contents collected and centrifuged for 10 min at 8000× g (25 °C). The pH and volume of the gastric juice values were measured and total acid secretions in total gastric juice supernatants determined by titration with 0.01 N NaOH solution using phenolphthalein as indicator.

2.8. Determination of Gastric Mucus Contents

For the determination of the mucus contents the methods described by Sun et al. were followed, with some modifications [51]. Animals were anaesthetized with ketamine/xylazine (60 and 10 mg/kg, respectively, i.p.) after 24 h of fasting, followed by laparotomy and pylorus ligation. Rats ($n = 6$/group) were immediately treated intraduodenally with HERP (50, 250, or 500 mg/kg), formononetin (10 mg/kg), carbenoxolone (200 mg/kg), or vehicle (2% Tween 80). Four hours later, animals were anesthetized with halothane (3%) followed euthanasia by cervical dislocation. The removed stomach contents were immersed in 10 mL of solution containing 0.16-M sucrose, 0.02% Alcian blue, and 0.05-M sodium acetate (pH 5.8), and were kept at room temperature for 24 h. Alcian blue binding extracts were then centrifuged at $3000 \times g$ for 10 min and absorbances of supernatants were measured using spectrophotometry at 620 nm. Free gastric mucus contents were calculated from quantities of bound Alcian blue (mg/g tissue).

2.9. Agar-Well Diffusion Assays

Antibacterial activity was investigated using a modified agar-well diffusion method [52]. Wells of 8 mm in diameter were sub-cultured with blood agar (Mueller-Hinton agar with 10% sheep blood) plates and inoculated with *Helicobacter pylori* suspensions of 6×10^8 CFU/mL (McFarland turbidity standard 0.5). Wells were then filled with 80 µL of 100 mg/mL HERP and tetracycline (0.03 mg/mL) was used as a standard compound. Plates were stored for 30 min at room temperature and then incubated for another 48 h at 37 °C under microaerophilic conditions. Subsequently, growth inhibition halos were measured using a digital pachymeter. The size of the inhibitory zones (diameter) was measured in triplicate and mean values of ≥08 mm considered active.

2.10. Statistical Analysis

Data are presented as the mean ± standard error of the mean (SEM) of n animals per group. Differences between the treated groups were identified using the one-way analysis of variance (ANOVA) and Bonferroni's test. Changes in microscopy parameters of indomethacin-induced ulcers (scores) were analyzed using Kruskal–Wallis test followed by Dunn's test. Differences were considered significant when $p < 0.05$.

3. Results

From the in vitro antioxidant activity test against free radical DPPH, an IC50 of 294 µg/mL was recorded for HERP. This result demonstrates the antioxidant potential of the variety of propolis used in this study. The antioxidant activity of the extract may be related to its ability to inhibit ethanol damage on the gastric mucosa. Ethanol is metabolized in the body, releasing superoxide anion and hydroperoxides. Such free radicals are known to be involved in the mechanism of acute and chronic ulceration. The sequestration of these chemical entities plays an important role in the healing process of gastric injury [53].

Free radicals are chemical entities capable of causing irreversible damage to the cell [4,54]. The antioxidant process includes the scavenging of these radicals (preventing their propagation), enzymatic hydrolysis of the ester linkage to remove peroxidized fatty acids from lipids, scavenging of transition metal ions, and reduction of peroxide catalyst enzymes. The pathogenesis of peptic ulcer is associated with endogenous and exogenous factors. Ethanol causes oxidative stress, which can happen by decreasing the release of nitric oxide, which has an important role in the metabolism of free radicals [55].

Following the induction of ulcers using ethanol, pre-treatments with the HERP at different doses (50, 250, or 500 mg/kg) inhibited the total lesion areas in a dose dependently fashion, when compared to the group treated with Tween 80 (2%) solution ($p < 0.001$; Figure 1). Formononetin (FOR, 10 mg/kg) and omeprazole (OMEP, 100 mg/kg) also reduced the areas of the total lesions significantly ($p < 0.001$)

(Figure 1). Table 1 depicts the quantification effects of HERP and formononetin on ethanol-induced damage of gastric mucosa. Histopathological analyses of gastric mucosa after the administration of absolute ethanol are shown in Figure 2.

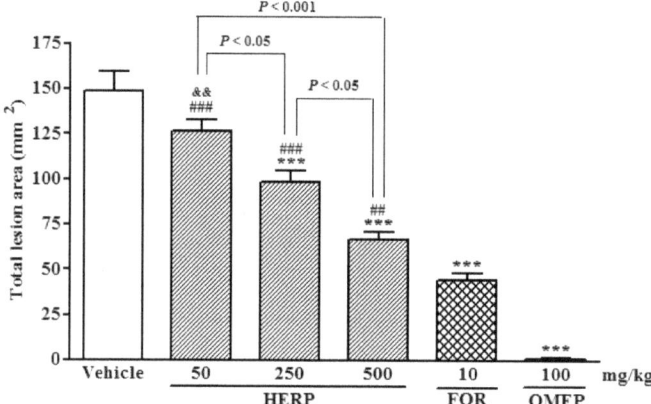

Figure 1. Effects of hydroalcoholic extracts of red propolis (HERP) and formononetin (FOR) on the ethanol-induced gastric damage; rats were pre-treated with a solution of 2% Tween 80 (vehicle), HERP (50–500 mg/kg), formononetin (10 mg/kg), or omeprazole (OMEP, 100 mg/kg) for 30 min prior to one hour treatment with absolute ethanol (1 mL). Total lesion areas were then determined and are presented as the means ± standard errors of the mean (SEM; $n = 6$/group); ANOVA followed by Bonferroni's test; *** $p < 0.001$ vs. vehicle group; ## $p < 0.01$ and ### $p < 0.001$ vs. OMEP group; && $p < 0.01$ vs. FOR group.

Table 1. Effects of HERP and formononetin on ethanol-induced microscopic damage in gastric mucosa.

Treatment (p.o.)	Dose (mg/kg)	Epithelial Cell Loss (Score 0–3)	Edema (Score 0–3)
Vehicle	-	3.0 (2.0–3.0)	3.0 (2.0–3.0)
HERP	50	3.0 (2.0–3.0) ###	0.0 (0.0–2.0) ***
	250	1.0 (0.0–2.0) ***	0.0 (0.0–1.0) ***
	500	1.0 (0.0–2.0) ***	0.0 (0.0–1.0) ***
Formononetin	10	0.0 (0.0–1.0) ***	0.0 (0.0–1.0) ***
Omeprazole	100	0.0 (0.0–1.0) ***	0.0 (0.0–1.0) ***

Data are presented as medians with minimum and maximal scores in brackets; differences were identified using Kruskal–Wallis followed by Dunn's test; *** $p < 0.001$ vs. vehicle group; and ### $p < 0.001$ vs. HERP groups at 250 and 500 mg/kg; three histological sections from each animal, $n = 6$/group.

The oral administration of absolute ethanol administration (vehicle-treated group) promoted microscopic damage, with a pronounced edema of the submucosa and a consistent epithelial cell loss, and presence of inflammatory cells. Ethanol-induced gastric ulcer resulted from the disruption of the vascular endothelium, increase of vascular permeability, formation of edema, and promotion of epithelial lifting. The gastric tissue of the animals treated with HERP (250 and 500 mg/kg, p.o.) showed less mucosal damage than those that were treated with the vehicle. The total lesion area was reduced in a concentration dependent manner, i.e., the increase of the HERP dose promoted a significant reduction of the total lesion area. Pre-treatment with formononetin and omeprazole also inhibited the formation of ethanol-induced lesions (vehicle group). Omeprazole is a proton-pump inhibitor thus it reduces the acid produced in the stomach. It is commonly used to promote the healing of erosive esophagitis and for the treatment of other gastrointestinal conditions (e.g., gastroesophageal reflux disease, peptic ulcer). Omeprazole treatment (OMEP, 100 mg/kg) for 30 min resulted in a total lesion area close to zero (mm^2).

The macroscopic effects of HERP shown in Figure 2 clearly demonstrate a significant tissue recovery in the animals treated with HERP (250 and 500 mg/kg, $p < 0.05$) and formononetin (10 mg/kg, $p < 0.001$), against the positive control (vehicle). Pre-treatments with HERP doses (250 and 500 mg/kg, $p < 0.05$) and formononetin (10 mg/kg, $p < 0.001$) significantly reduced ulcer indices of indomethacin-induced ulcers in comparison with the those of the vehicle-treated group (Table 2). Cimetidine (100 mg/kg) also significantly reduced ulcer indices ($p < 0.01$, Table 2). Indomethacin is an indol derivative that is the first-choice approach for gastric-ulcer induction in laboratory. Cimetidine belongs to the histamine H2 receptor antagonists and acts by inhibiting the production of acid in the stomach. It is commonly used to treat and prevent certain types of stomach ulcer.

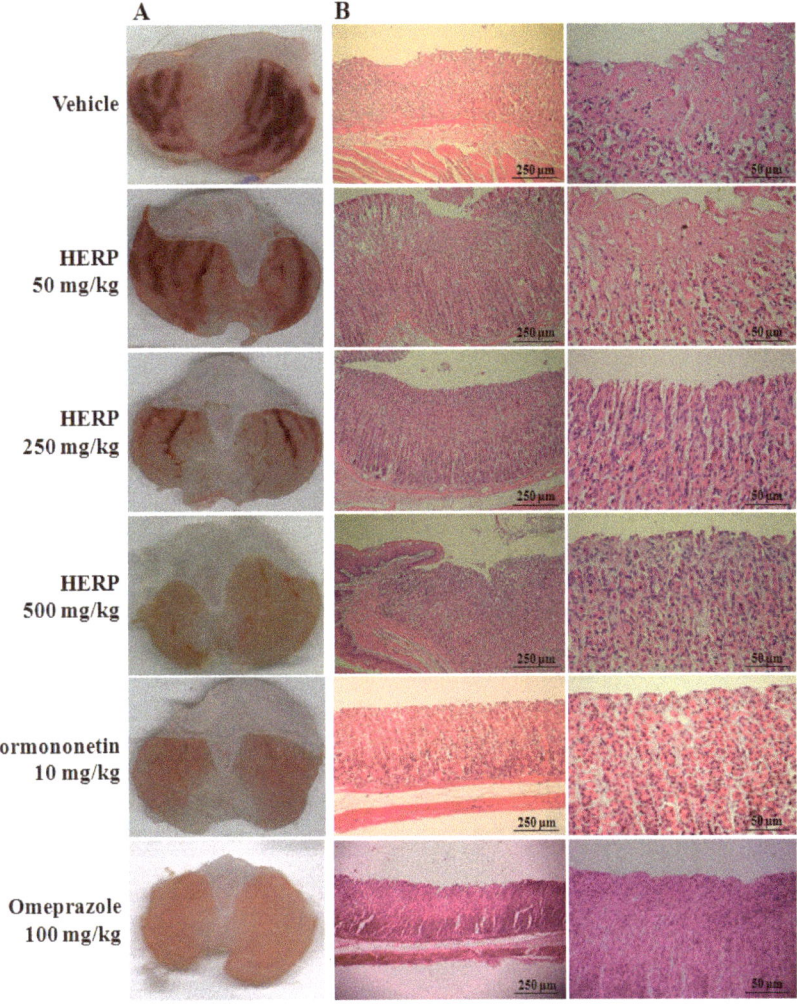

Figure 2. (**A**) Macroscopic effects of HERP, formononetin, and omeprazole in ethanol-induced gastric ulcers; (**B**) hematoxylin/eosin-stained histological sections of gastric mucosa specimens from ethanol treated rats; representative photomicrographs were generated from the same areas and were quantified (Table 1).

Table 2. Effects of HERP and formononetin on indomethacin-induced ulcers in rats.

Treatment (p.o.)	Dose (mg/kg)	Ulcer Index	Inhibition (%)
Vehicle	-	2.29 ± 0.18	-
HERP	50	1.86 ± 0.14 ##	18.78
	250	0.29 ± 0.18 *	87.34
	500	0.00 ± 0.00 ***	100.00
Formononetin	10	0.00 ± 0.00 ***&&	100.00
Cimetidine	100	0.29 ± 0.29 **&	87.34

Results are presented as means ± SEM (n = 6/group). Differences were identified using Kruskal–Wallis test followed by Dunn's test; * $p < 0.05$, ** $p < 0.01$, and *** $p < 0.001$ vs. vehicle group; ## $p < 0.01$ vs. 500-mg/kg HERP group; & $p < 0.05$ and && $p < 0.01$ vs. 50-mg/kg HERP group.

The treatment with 50 and 250 mg/kg HERP in the pylorus ligature model of gastric secretion significantly reduced secretion volumes ($p < 0.01$) and increased H^+ concentrations (50 mg/kg, $p < 0.01$) (Table 3). Similarly, treatments with formononetin (10 mg/kg) significantly reduced secretion volumes ($p < 0.01$). However, HERP and formononetin treatments both did not succeed in significantly increasing the pH values compared to those in the group treated with the vehicle. In contrast, cimetidine affected all gastric juice parameters significantly ($p < 0.01$).

Table 3. Effects of intraduodenal treatments with HERP and formononetin on the biochemical parameters of gastric juice collected from the pylorus ligature rats.

Treatment	Dose (mg/kg)	Volume (mL)	pH	$[H^+]$mEq/L/4 h
Vehicle	-	1.20 ± 0.04	3.36 ± 0.05	46.8 ± 2.85
HERP	50	0.70 ± 0.08 ***#	3.40 ± 0.12	65.9 ± 2.69 **###
	250	0.80 ± 0.08 **	3.40 ± 0.12	56.0 ± 3.35 ##
	500	1.00 ± 0.08	3.30 ± 0.00	36.3 ± 3.55
Formononetin	10	0.82 ± 0.05 **	3.14 ± 0.14	42.7 ± 3.78
Cimetidine	100	0.80 ± 0.04 **	6.10 ± 0.45 ***	27.5 ± 3.14 **

Results are presented as means ± SEM (n = 6/group) and differences between treatment groups were identified using ANOVA followed by Bonferroni's test; ** $p < 0.01$ and *** $p < 0.001$ vs. vehicle group; # $p < 0.05$, ## $p < 0.01$, and ### $p < 0.001$ vs. 500-mg/kg HERP group.

Compared to the vehicle treated controls (Table 4), the production of mucus was significantly increased with HERP (500 mg/kg) treatment ($p < 0.05$). Treatments with formononetin (FOR, 10 mg/kg) and carbenoxolone (200 mg/kg) also increased the production of mucus ($p < 0.05$ and $p < 0.001$, respectively, when compared to the control).

Table 4. Effects of intraduodenal treatments with HERP and formononetin on Alcian blue binding to free gastric mucus from pylorus ligatures in rats.

Treatment	Dose (mg/kg)	Alcian Blue Bound (mg/g Tissue)
Vehicle	-	1.14 ± 0.03
HERP	50	1.21 ± 0.02
	250	1.25 ± 0.02
	500	1.30 ± 0.02 *
Formononetin	10	1.34 ± 0.07 *
Carbenoxolone	200	1.53 ± 0.03 ***

Results are presented as means ± SEM (n = 6/group) and differences were identified using ANOVA followed by the Bonferroni's test; * $p < 0.05$ and *** $p < 0.001$ vs. vehicle group.

In assessments of anti-*H. Pylori* activity, HERP treatments reduced the diameter of the inhibitory zone to 13.0 ± 2.0 mm at 100 mg/mL, whereas inhibition halos were 35.0 ± 0.5 mm in the presence of the standard tetracycline (0.03 mg/mL).

4. Discussion

Propolis is a product obtained from honey bee hives, characterized chiefly by a beeswax and a resin (obtained from apical buds, young leaves and exudates) [56]. Red propolis is ranked as the second most produced type of Brazilian propolis. Its characteristics (e.g., texture, odor, color) vary according to the source and type, but also harvesting season. The interest in Brazilian red propolis is attributed to its several beneficial effects for a range of health conditions, due to the presence of phytoestrogens. Phytoestrogens are naturally occurring compounds with a chemical structure similar to 17-β-estradiol, the mammalian estrogen. These compounds show the capacity to bind to estrogen receptors, either as agonists or antagonist, to promote, respectively, estrogenic or antiestrogenic activity [57]. They have been recommended for the treatment of estrogen-related diseases, as happens with dyslipidemia resulting from the high levels of estrogen in post-menopause women. On the other hand, during physiologic menstrual cycle bicarbonate secretion increases with estrogenic levels, which may contribute to reduce the risk of gastric ulcer.

In our study, two rat ulcer models were used (ethanol-induced and indomethacin-induced ulcers) and tested for the potential of hydroalcoholic extracts of red propolis (HERP), and its isoflavonoid formononetin, for gastric protection. The phytoestrogen formononetin is an O-methylated isoflavone (Figure 3) that was found to be present in hydroalcoholic extract of Brazilian red propolis.

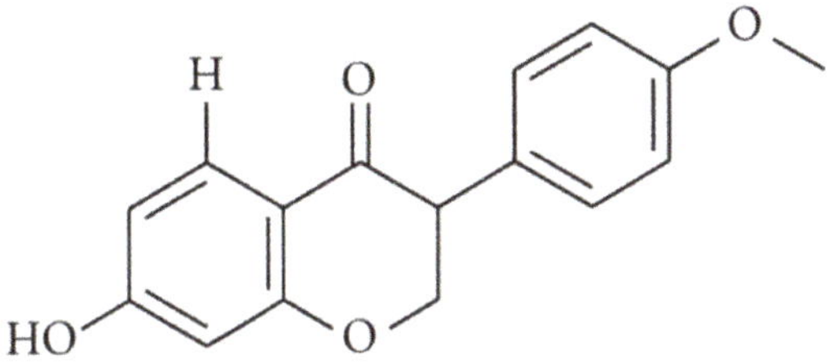

Figure 3. Chemical structure of formononetin (C16H12O4, molecular weight 268.26 g/mol).

Our results demonstrate that HERP in the tested concentrations of 50, 250, and 500 mg/kg exhibited acute gastroprotective effects against ethanol- and indomethacin-induced ulcers, in a concentration dependent manner, with the highest dose increasing the mucus production significantly (Table 4). HERP and its major isoflavonoid formononetin (10 mg/kg) decreased gastric secretion volumes and increased mucus production in the present pylorus ligature model, while HERP depicted anti-*H. Pylori* activity. Oral administration of HERP decreased the total lesion areas (Figure 1) induced by absolute ethanol in a dose dependent fashion, and reduced the associated macroscopic and microscopic damage to mucosa (Figure 2), at doses which were considered safe, according to the toxicological study described by Silva et al. [58]. Similar reductions were also observed after formononetin treatment when compared to the vehicle-treated animals, which showed severe ulceration of gastric mucosa (vehicle group).

Ethanol has been previously used to induce ulcers in rodents, leading to gastric mucosal injury through the direct and indirect effects of reactive oxygen species (ROS) and cytokines [34]. Moreover, this process is reportedly mediated by activated neutrophils, and is associated with cellular lipid and protein peroxidation [59]. However, several studies have shown that natural products with antioxidant activity protect gastric mucosa against damage [60–63]. The advantages of HERP for human use have been extensively discussed in the literature, relying on the many identified beneficial effects, mostly attributed to its antioxidant properties [5,64–67]. Various phenolic antioxidants, such as flavonoids, coumarins, tannins, procyanidins, and xanthenes, act as radical scavengers, neutralizing ROS, inhibiting lipid peroxidation and other free radical-mediated pathologies, in a dose-dependent fashion. Plants enriched with antioxidants, such as isoflavonoid, may thus be considered as an alternative approach for the management and treatment of the chronic diseases related to oxidative stress. Among flavonoids present in HERP, biochanin A has demonstrated gastroprotective effects by a strong induction of superoxide dismutase (SOD) and nitric oxide enzymes, and reduced release of malondialdehyde [32]. Asif et al. have reported a strong correlation between the antioxidant and antiglycation activities of biochanin A present in organic fractions of *Hordeum vulgare* [6].

The therapeutic potential of biochanin-A against myocardial infarction has also been proposed, and attributed to its capacity in compromising lipid peroxidation. Male Wistar rats were first subjected to isoproterenol-induced myocardial infarction [68], resulting in a significant increase of creatine kinase-MB and cardiac troponin, serum glutamic oxaloacetic transaminase, serum glutamic pyruvic transaminase, and lactate dehydrogenase, and reduction of the activity of antioxidant enzymes (i.e., SOD, catalase, glutathione peroxidase, glutathione-S-transferase, and glutathione reductase) in the heart. Such antioxidant enzymes catalyze reactions to counterbalance free radicals and ROS, thus forming endogenous defense mechanisms. The authors reported the cardioprotective effects of biochanin-A by modulation of lipid peroxidation, through enhancing antioxidants and detoxifying enzyme systems [68]. The effect of biochanin-A on a high-fat diet-induced hyperlipidemia in mice has been studied by Xue et al. [69]. The authors have demonstrated the capacity of biochanin A in decreasing the LDL-cholesterol in about 85% and total cholesterol ca. 39% in a moderate dose, increasing the activity of lipoprotein lipase in 96% and of hepatic triglyceride lipase in 78%. The results also showed the increase of fecal lipid levels and decrease of epididymal fat index in hyperlipidemic mice in comparison to the control mice. Jia et al. demonstrated that formononetin attenuates hydrogen peroxide-induced apoptosis and nuclear factor-kappa B (NF-κB) activation in retinal ganglion cells, exposed to oxidative stress over a period of 24 h [70].

The abovementioned beneficial effects of flavonoids (biochanin-A, formononetin) identified in HERP, substantiate the rationale for exploiting additional biological activities related to their antioxidant properties. Fukai et al. anticipated the potential use of these compounds as chemopreventive agents for peptic ulcer or gastric cancer in *Helicobacter pylori*-infected individuals [71].

Helicobacter pylori infections are associated with dyslipidemia. Epidemiologic and clinical data suggest that such an infection can be a contributing factor in the progression of atherosclerosis [35]. In 2010, Satoh et al. reported that *Helicobacter pylori* infection was significantly associated with high LDL-cholesteremia and low HDL-cholesteremia in Japanese male subjects [72]. The association of this infection with metabolic syndrome in the Japanese population, has also been reported in the past [73]. Thus, treating *Helicobacter pylori* infections and protecting gastric mucosa from ulceration may have a synergistic effect in prophylaxis of dyslipidemia as well.

From our results, the histological analyses obtained from ethanol-induced ulcers show that HERP and formononetin attenuate lymphocytic infiltration, suggesting immunomodulatory effects on the release of cytokines (Figure 2). Furthermore, bioactive fractions of geopropolis that were collected from the same region reportedly decreased neutrophil migration and reduced NO-related inflammatory interactions between leukocytes and endothelial cells [74].

Numerous studies have demonstrated enhanced immune responses in the presence of propolis [75–78]. Moreover, the isoflavonoid biochanin A inhibited lipopolysaccharide (LPS)-induced activation of microglia, and production of tumor necrosis factor (TNF)-α, NO, and SOD in mesencephalic neuron-glia cultures and microglia-enriched cultures [79]. Formononetin also inhibited TNF-α and interleukin (IL)-6 expression, and improved SOD activity in traumatic brain injury [29] and LPS-induced acute lung injury models [80]. These studies suggest that the gastroprotective properties of HERP are mediated, at least partially, by formononetin.

NSAIDs are the most commonly used treatment for inflammatory diseases, but are proven to cause gastric and duodenal ulcers in rats and humans [81]. The potent NSAID indomethacin causes gastric legions by inhibiting cyclo-oxygenase (COX), resulting in decreased prostaglandin synthesis [82]. The ensuing injury is characterized by reduced bicarbonate and mucus secretion and blood flow, increased acid back-diffusion, and inhibition of repair. In the present study, HERP and its flavonoid formononetin inhibited the formation of indomethacin-induced gastric lesions. Flavonoids were previously shown to inhibit COX-1 and COX-2 enzymes [83], and the isoflavonoids genistein and daidzein significantly reduced COX activity [84]. Hence, the present observations of increased mucus production in the presence of HERP or formononetin were attributed to COX inhibition.

Flavonoid treatments reportedly increased the production of mucus and bicarbonate, and affected proton pump activities in parietal cells [85]. Hence, the present effects of HERP likely reflect formononetin contents. Hajrezaie et al. showed that biochanin A increases mucus secretion in ethanol-induced ulcer models [32], and De Barros et al. showed that quercitrin and afzelin increase the secretion of mucus and reduce H^+- and K^+-ATPase activity in vitro [86].

In further experiments, HERP and formononetin decreased gastric secretion volumes after pylorus ligature. As HERP and formononetin treatments were administered via a intraduodenal route, systemic effects are likely not to be related to the local neutralization of gastric acid or physical barriers. Moreover, physiological gastric acid secretion by parietal cells is activated by several stimuli. These include acetylcholine, which acts directly via M_3 receptors and indirectly by M_2 and M_4 receptors, and is associated with the inhibition of somatostatin secretion, histamine, which acts directly via H_2 receptors, and gastrin, which predominantly acts indirectly via cholecystokinin-2 (CCK-2) receptors on enterochromaffin-like cells and is associated with histamine release [87]. Flavonoids have been shown to induce the expression of acetylcholinesterase, which hydrolyzes acetylcholine in cultured osteoblast synapses [88]. Additionally, flavonoids reportedly increase mucosal prostaglandin levels and reduce histamine production by mast cells by inhibiting histidine decarboxylase [89].

Herein, we showed increased H^+ concentrations following treatments with HERP, likely reflecting the presence of acid phenolic compounds [16]. However, no significant changes in pH were observed under these conditions, whereas cimetidine treatment modified all biochemical parameters of gastric mucosa, suggesting distinct mechanisms of action. Similarly, formononetin treatments reduced gastric secretion volumes, but had no significant effects on pH or total acid secretion, indicating that changes in gastric acid secretions do not play an important role in the gastroprotective mechanisms of this compound. H. Pylori is associated with various gastric diseases and is a frequently encountered human pathogen [90]. In our study, we demonstrated that HERP treatment (100 mg/mL) inhibited the growth of H. Pylori in vitro, highlighted by the identification of an inhibitory zone of 13.0 ± 2.0 mm, in comparison to the 35.0 ± 0.5 mm inhibition halos in the presence of standard tetracycline (0.03 mg/mL). The anti-H. Pylori effect has been demonstrated for several propolis varieties. Using the same agar-well diffusion method, Boyanova et al. (2003) reported the increase of mean diameters of H. Pylori growth inhibition from 17.8, 21.2, 28.2 mm when treated, respectively, by 30, 60, and 90 mL of ethanolic propolis extract (30%), whereas the treatment with of ethanol alone (30 mL) resulted in a mean diameter of 8.5 mm [91]. More recently, Baltas et al. (2016) reported inhibition diameters ranging from 31.0 to 47.0 mm from 15 different ethanolic propolis extracts tested at 75 µg/mL [92]. The authors found a significant positive correlation between the reported anti-H. Pylori activity of the extracts and the total phenolic content.

5. Conclusions

In this work, we reported the gastroprotective effect of HERP, and its predominant isoflavonoid formononetin, known for its hypolipidemia effects. Our results demonstrated that treating animals with HERP resulted in the reduction of mucosal damage, in particular with doses as high as 200 and 500 mg/kg (p.o.), with a significant reduction in the loss of epithelial cells and on edema. The macroscopic effects of sample-treated rats corroborate these results. The treatment with HERP increased H^+ concentration, as well as the mucus production, both contributing to enhance the protection of gastrointestinal mucosa, and to reducing the aggressive effects in gastric mucosa, thus reducing the risk of ulcers. The antioxidant activity of HERP was also shown, reporting a IC50 of 294 µg/mL. Together with the prophylactic role in reducing the lipid accumulation, formononetin was shown to have a prominent role in increased mucus production. HERP can be further exploited as an alternative phytomedicine for the treatment of ulcers with hypolipidemic profile. HERP and formononetin have recognized gastroprotective properties, as they significantly inhibit the development of acute ulcers in the presence of ethanol and indomethacin, ameliorated inflammatory cell infiltration and edema, reducing gastric secretion volumes, and increasing gastric mucus contents.

Author Contributions: M.A.A.d.M., A.R.S.R., A.K.d.L., G.B.B., M.S.P., R.L.C.d.A.-J. and M.Z.G. contributed to the methodology, formal analysis, investigation, resources, and data curation; red propolis collection, preparation of the hydroalcoholic extracts, and sample characterization have been carried out by F.F.P., S.M.T., A.S. and P.S.; in vivo experiments have been performed by R.L.C.d.A.-J., M.Z.G., F.F.P., S.M.T., P.S. and J.C.C.; quantification analyses and antibacterial activities have been run by E.B.S., L.K.H.; writing of the original manuscript was the contribution of M.A.A.d.M., E.B.S., A.S., and P.S.; conceptualization, review, and editing of the manuscript, as well as project administration, supervision, and funding acquisition was contributed to by A.S., P.S., E.B.S., E.N. and J.C.C. All authors have made a substantial contribution to the work and have approved its publication. All authors have read and agreed to the published version of the manuscript.

Funding: This work has been funded by the Fundação de Apoio à Pesquisa e à Inovação Tecnológica do Estado de Sergipe (FAPITEC/SE), by the Conselho Nacional de Desenvolvimento Científico e Tecnológico (CNPq). R.L.C.d.A.-J., S.M.T., and J.C.C. received CNPq productivity grants. E.B.S. acknowledges the sponsorship of the project UIDB/04469/2020 (strategic fund), from the Portuguese Science and Technology Foundation, Ministry of Science and Education (FCT/MEC) through national funds, and was co-financed by FEDER, under the Partnership Agreement PT2020. E.N. and A.S. acknowledge the support of the research project: Nutraceutica come supporto nutrizionale nel paziente oncologico, CUP: B83D18000140007.

Conflicts of Interest: The authors declare no conflict of interest.

References

1. Ito, F.; Sono, Y.; Ito, T. Measurement and Clinical Significance of Lipid Peroxidation as a Biomarker of Oxidative Stress: Oxidative Stress in Diabetes, Atherosclerosis, and Chronic Inflammation. *Antioxidants* **2019**, *8*, 72. [CrossRef] [PubMed]
2. Carbone, C.; Martins-Gomes, C.; Caddeo, C.; Silva, A.M.; Musumeci, T.; Pignatello, R.; Puglisi, G.; Souto, E.B. Mediterranean essential oils as precious matrix components and active ingredients of lipid nanoparticles. *Int. J. Pharm.* **2018**, *548*, 217–226. [CrossRef] [PubMed]
3. Cefali, L.C.; Ataide, J.; Fernandes, A.R.; Sanchez-Lopez, E.; Sousa, I.; Figueiredo, M.C.; Ruiz, A.; Foglio, M.; Mazzola, P.G.; Souto, E.B. Evaluation of In Vitro Solar Protection Factor (SPF), Antioxidant Activity, and Cell Viability of Mixed Vegetable Extracts from Dirmophandra mollis Benth, *Ginkgo biloba* L., *Ruta graveolens* L., and *Vitis vinifera* L. *Plants* **2019**, *8*, 453. [CrossRef] [PubMed]
4. Silva, A.M.; Martins-Gomes, C.; Souto, E.B.; Schäfer, J.; Dos Santos, J.A.; Bunzel, M.; Nunes, F.M. Thymus zygis subsp. zygis an Endemic Portuguese Plant: Phytochemical Profiling, Antioxidant, Anti-Proliferative and Anti-Inflammatory Activities. *Antioxidants* **2020**, *9*, 482. [CrossRef]
5. Carvalho, F.M.D.A.D.; Schneider, J.K.; De Jesus, C.V.F.; Andrade, L.; Amaral, R.G.; David, J.M.; Krause, L.C.; Severino, P.; Soares, C.; Caramão, E.B.; et al. Brazilian Red Propolis: Extracts Production, Physicochemical Characterization, and Cytotoxicity Profile for Antitumor Activity. *Biomolecules* **2020**, *10*, 726. [CrossRef]
6. Asif, A.; Zeeshan, N.; Mehmood, S. Antioxidant and antiglycation activities of traditional plants and identification of bioactive compounds from extracts of Hordeum vulgare by LC–MS and GC–MS. *J. Food Biochem.* **2020**, 13381. [CrossRef]
7. Souto, E.B.; Severino, P.; Marques, C.; Andrade, L.N.; Durazzo, A.; Lucarini, M.; Atanasov, A.G.; El Maimouni, S.; Novellino, E.; Santini, A. *Croton argyrophyllus* Kunth Essential Oil-Loaded Solid Lipid Nanoparticles: Evaluation of Release Profile, Antioxidant Activity and Cytotoxicity in a Neuroblastoma Cell Line. *Sustainability* **2020**, *12*, 7697. [CrossRef]
8. Anjum, S.I.; Ullah, A.; Khan, K.A.; Attaullah, M.; Khan, H.; Ali, H.; Bashir, M.A.; Tahir, M.; Ansari, M.J.; Ghramh, H.A.; et al. Composition and functional properties of propolis (bee glue): A review. *Saudi J. Boil. Sci.* **2019**, *26*, 1695–1703. [CrossRef]
9. Santos, L.M.; Da Fonseca, M.S.; Sokolonski, A.R.; Deegan, K.R.; Araújo, R.P.C.; Umsza-Guez, M.A.; Barbosa, J.D.V.; Portela, R.D.; Machado, B.A.S. Propolis: Types, composition, biological activities, and veterinary product patent prospecting. *J. Sci. Food Agric.* **2019**, *100*, 1369–1382. [CrossRef]
10. Daugsch, A.; Moraes, C.S.; Fort, P.; Park, Y.K. Brazilian Red Propolis—Chemical Composition and Botanical Origin. *Evid. Based Complement. Altern. Med.* **2008**, *5*, 435–441. [CrossRef]

11. Barbosa, R.A.; Nunes, T.L.G.M.; Nunes, T.L.G.M.; Da Paixão, A.O.; Neto, R.B.; Moura, S.; Júnior, R.L.C.A.; Cândido, E.A.F.; Padilha, F.F.; Quintans, J.S.; et al. Hydroalcoholic extract of red propolis promotes functional recovery and axon repair after sciatic nerve injury in rats. *Pharm. Boil.* **2015**, *54*, 993–1004. [CrossRef] [PubMed]
12. Batista, C.; Alves, A.; Queiroz, L.; Lima, B.; Filho, R.; Araújo, A.; Júnior, R.D.A.; Cardoso, J. The photoprotective and anti-inflammatory activity of red propolis extract in rats. *J. Photochem. Photobiol. B Boil.* **2018**, *180*, 198–207. [CrossRef] [PubMed]
13. Cavalcante, D.R.R.; De Oliveira, P.S.; Góis, S.M.; Soares, A.F.; Cardoso, J.C.; Padilha, F.F.; Júnior, R.L.C.D.A. Effect of green propolis on oral epithelial dysplasia in rats. *Braz. J. Otorhinolaryngol.* **2011**, *77*, 278–284. [CrossRef] [PubMed]
14. Frozza, C.O.D.S.; Garcia, C.S.C.; Gambato, G.; De Souza, M.D.O.; Salvador, M.; Moura, S.; Padilha, F.F.; Seixas, F.K.; Collares, T.; Borsuk, S.; et al. Chemical characterization, antioxidant and cytotoxic activities of Brazilian red propolis. *Food Chem. Toxicol.* **2013**, *52*, 137–142. [CrossRef]
15. De Mendonça, I.C.G.; Porto, I.C.C.D.M.; Nascimento, T.G.D.; De Souza, N.S.; Oliveira, J.M.D.S.; Arruda, R.E.D.S.; Mousinho, K.C.; Santos, A.F.; Júnior, I.D.B.; Parolia, A.; et al. Brazilian red propolis: Phytochemical screening, antioxidant activity and effect against cancer cells. *BMC Complement. Altern. Med.* **2015**, *15*, 357. [CrossRef]
16. Righi, A.A.; Alves, T.R.; Negri, G.; Marques, L.M.; Breyer, H.; Salatino, A. Brazilian red propolis: Unreported substances, antioxidant and antimicrobial activities. *J. Sci. Food Agric.* **2011**, *91*, 2363–2370. [CrossRef]
17. Júnior, R.L.A.; Barreto, A.L.S.; Pires, J.A.; Reis, F.P.; Lima, S.O.; Ribeiro, M.; Cardoso, J.C. Effect of Bovine Type-I Collagen-Based Films Containing Red Propolis on Dermal Wound Healing in Rodent Model. *Int. J. Morphol.* **2009**, *27*, 1105–1110. [CrossRef]
18. De Almeida, E.B.; Cardoso, J.C.; De Lima, A.K.; De Oliveira, N.L.; De Pontes-Filho, N.T.; Lima, S.O.; Souza, I.C.L.; De Albuquerque-Júnior, R.L.C. The incorporation of Brazilian propolis into collagen-based dressing films improves dermal burn healing. *J. Ethnopharmacol.* **2013**, *147*, 419–425. [CrossRef]
19. Awale, S.; Li, F.; Onozuka, H.; Esumi, H.; Tezuka, Y.; Kadota, S. Constituents of Brazilian red propolis and their preferential cytotoxic activity against human pancreatic PANC-1 cancer cell line in nutrient-deprived condition. *Bioorg. Med. Chem.* **2008**, *16*, 181–189. [CrossRef]
20. Ribeiro, D.R.; Ângela, V.F.A.; Dos Santos, E.P.; Padilha, F.F.; Gomes, M.Z.; Rabelo, A.S.; Cardoso, J.C.; Massarioli, A.P.; De Alencar, S.M.; De Albuquerque-Júnior, R.L.C.; et al. Inhibition of DMBA-induced Oral Squamous Cells Carcinoma Growth by Brazilian Red Propolis in Rodent Model. *Basic Clin. Pharmacol. Toxicol.* **2015**, *117*, 85–95. [CrossRef]
21. Frozza, C.O.D.S.; Ribeiro, T.D.S.; Gambato, G.; Menti, C.; Moura, S.; Pinto, P.M.; Staats, C.C.; Padilha, F.F.; Begnini, K.R.; De Leon, P.M.M.; et al. Proteomic analysis identifies differentially expressed proteins after red propolis treatment in Hep-2 cells. *Food Chem. Toxicol.* **2014**, *63*, 195–204. [CrossRef] [PubMed]
22. Pinheiro, K.S.; Ribeiro, D.R.; Alves, A.V.F.; Pereira-Filho, R.N.; De Oliveira, C.R.; Cardoso, J.C.; Lima, S.O.; Reis, F.P.; Júnior, R.L.A. Modulatory activity of brazilian red propolis on chemically induced dermal carcinogenesis. *Acta Cir. Bras.* **2014**, *29*, 111–117. [CrossRef] [PubMed]
23. Teles, F.; Da Silva, T.M.; Júnior, F.P.D.C.; Honorato, V.H.; Costa, H.D.O.; Barbosa, A.P.F.; De Oliveira, S.G.; Porfírio, Z.; Libório, A.B.; Borges, R.L.; et al. Brazilian Red Propolis Attenuates Hypertension and Renal Damage in 5/6 Renal Ablation Model. *PLoS ONE* **2015**, *10*, e0116535. [CrossRef] [PubMed]
24. López, B.G.-C.; Schmidt, E.M.; Eberlin, M.N.; Sawaya, A.C.H.F. Phytochemical markers of different types of red propolis. *Food Chem.* **2014**, *146*, 174–180. [CrossRef] [PubMed]
25. Trusheva, B.; Popova, M.; Bankova, V.; Simova, S.; Marcucci, M.C.; Miorin, P.L.; Pasin, F.D.R.; Tsvetkova, I. Bioactive Constituents of Brazilian Red Propolis. *Evid. Based Complement. Altern. Med.* **2006**, *3*, 249–254. [CrossRef] [PubMed]
26. Wang, W.; Tang, L.; Li, Y.; Wang, Y. Biochanin A protects against focal cerebral ischemia/reperfusion in rats via inhibition of p38-mediated inflammatory responses. *J. Neurol. Sci.* **2015**, *348*, 121–125. [CrossRef] [PubMed]
27. Zhou, L.-T.; Wang, K.-J.; Li, L.; Li, H.; Geng, M. Pinocembrin inhibits lipopolysaccharide-induced inflammatory mediators production in BV2 microglial cells through suppression of PI3K/Akt/NF-κB pathway. *Eur. J. Pharmacol.* **2015**, *761*, 211–216. [CrossRef] [PubMed]

28. Bueno-Silva, B.; De Alencar, S.M.; Koo, H.; Ikegaki, M.; Da Silva, G.V.J.; Napimoga, M.H.; Rosalen, P.L. Anti-Inflammatory and Antimicrobial Evaluation of Neovestitol and Vestitol Isolated from Brazilian Red Propolis. *J. Agric. Food Chem.* **2013**, *61*, 4546–4550. [CrossRef]
29. Li, Z.; Dong, X.; Zhang, J.; Zeng, G.; Zhao, H.; Liu, Y.; Qiu, R.; Mo, L.; Ye, Y. Formononetin protects TBI rats against neurological lesions and the underlying mechanism. *J. Neurol. Sci.* **2014**, *338*, 112–117. [CrossRef]
30. Wang, J.; He, C.; Wu, W.-Y.; Chen, F.; Wu, Y.-Y.; Li, W.; Chen, H.-Q.; Yin, Y.-Y. Biochanin A protects dopaminergic neurons against lipopolysaccharide-induced damage and oxidative stress in a rat model of Parkinson's disease. *Pharmacol. Biochem. Behav.* **2015**, *138*, 96–103. [CrossRef]
31. Saad, M.A.; Abdelsalam, R.M.; Kenawy, S.A.; Attia, A.S. Pinocembrin attenuates hippocampal inflammation, oxidative perturbations and apoptosis in a rat model of global cerebral ischemia reperfusion. *Pharmacol. Rep.* **2015**, *67*, 115–122. [CrossRef] [PubMed]
32. Hajrezaie, M.; Salehen, N.; Karimian, H.; Zahedifard, M.; Shams, K.; Al Batran, R.; Majid, N.A.; Khalifa, S.A.M.; Ali, H.M.; El-Seedi, H.; et al. Biochanin A Gastroprotective Effects in Ethanol-Induced Gastric Mucosal Ulceration in Rats. *PLoS ONE* **2015**, *10*, e0121529. [CrossRef] [PubMed]
33. Das Neves, M.V.M.; Da Silva, T.M.S.; Lima, E.D.O.; Da Cunha, E.V.L.; Oliveira, E.J. Isoflavone formononetin from red propolis acts as a fungicide against Candida sp. *Braz. J. Microbiol.* **2016**, *47*, 159–166. [CrossRef]
34. Abdel-Salam, O.M.E.; Czimmer, J.; Debreceni, A.; Szolcsányi, J.; Mózsik, G. Gastric mucosal integrity: Gastric mucosal blood flow and microcirculation. An overview. *J. Physiol.* **2001**, *95*, 105–127. [CrossRef]
35. Kim, T.J.; Lee, H.; Kang, M.; Kim, J.E.; Choi, Y.-H.; Min, Y.W.; Min, B.-H.; Lee, J.H.; Son, H.J.; Rhee, P.-L.; et al. Helicobacter pylori is associated with dyslipidemia but not with other risk factors of cardiovascular disease. *Sci. Rep.* **2016**, *6*, 38015. [CrossRef]
36. Gao, H.; Li, L.; Zhang, C.; Tu, J.; Geng, X.; Wang, J.; Zhou, X.; Jing, J.; Pan, W. Comparison of efficacy of pharmacological therapies for gastric endoscopic submucosal dissection-induced ulcers: A systematic review and network meta-analysis. *Expert Rev. Gastroenterol. Hepatol.* **2020**, 1–13. [CrossRef]
37. Milivojevic, V.; Milosavljevic, T. Burden of Gastroduodenal Diseases from the Global Perspective. *Curr. Treat. Options Gastroenterol.* **2020**, *18*, 148–157. [CrossRef]
38. Takahashi, M.; Katayama, Y.; Takada, H.; Kuwayama, H.; Terano, A. The effect of NSAIDs and a COX-2 specific inhibitor on Helicobacter pylori-induced PGE2 and HGF in human gastric fibroblasts. *Aliment. Pharmacol. Ther.* **2000**, *14*, 44–49. [CrossRef]
39. Tytgat, G.N. Etiopathogenetic Principles and Peptic Ulcer Disease Classification. *Dig. Dis.* **2011**, *29*, 454–458. [CrossRef]
40. Venerito, M.; Goni, E.; Malfertheiner, P. Helicobacter pyloriscreening: Options and challenges. *Expert Rev. Gastroenterol. Hepatol.* **2016**, *10*, 497–503. [CrossRef]
41. Kaufman, D.W.; Kelly, J.P.; Wiholm, B.-E.; Laszlo, A.; Sheehan, J.E.; Koff, R.S.; Shapiro, S. The Risk of Acute Major Upper Gastrointestinal Bleeding Among Users of Aspirin and Ibuprofen at Various Levels of Alcohol Consumption. *Am. J. Gastroenterol.* **1999**, *94*, 3189–3196. [CrossRef] [PubMed]
42. Li, T.-K. Quantifying the risk for alcohol-use and alcohol-attributable health disorders: Present findings and future research needs. *J. Gastroenterol. Hepatol.* **2008**, *23*, S2–S8. [CrossRef] [PubMed]
43. Cavendish, R.L.; Santos, J.D.S.; Neto, R.B.; Paixão, A.O.; Oliveira, J.V.; Araújo, E.D.; E Silva, A.A.B.; Thomazzi, S.M.; Cardoso, J.C.; Gomes, M.Z. Antinociceptive and anti-inflammatory effects of Brazilian red propolis extract and formononetin in rodents. *J. Ethnopharmacol.* **2015**, *173*, 127–133. [CrossRef] [PubMed]
44. Souto, E.; Souto, S.B.; Zielińska, A.; Durazzo, A.; Lucarini, M.; Santini, A.; Horbańczuk, O.K.; Atanasov, A.; Marques, C.; Andrade, L.; et al. Perillaldehyde 1,2-epoxide Loaded SLN-Tailored mAb: Production, Physicochemical Characterization and In Vitro Cytotoxicity Profile in MCF-7 Cell Lines. *Pharmaceutics* **2020**, *12*, 161. [CrossRef] [PubMed]
45. Souto, E.; Zielińska, A.; Souto, S.B.; Durazzo, A.; Lucarini, M.; Santini, A.; Silva, A.M.; Atanasov, A.; Marques, C.; Andrade, L.; et al. (+)-Limonene 1,2-Epoxide-Loaded SLNs: Evaluation of Drug Release, Antioxidant Activity, and Cytotoxicity in an HaCaT Cell Line. *Int. J. Mol. Sci.* **2020**, *21*, 1449. [CrossRef]
46. Robert, A.; Nezamis, J.E.; Lancaster, C.; Hanchar, A.J. Cytoprotection by prostaglandins in rats. *Gastroenterology* **1979**, *77*, 433–443. [CrossRef]
47. Pinto, L.A.; Cordeiro, K.W.; Carrasco, V.; Carollo, C.A.; Cardoso, C.A.L.; Argadoña, E.J.S.; Freitas, K.D.C. Antiulcerogenic activity of Carica papaya seed in rats. *Naunyn Schmiedeberg's Arch. Pharmacol.* **2014**, *388*, 305–317. [CrossRef]

48. Djahanguiri, B. The production of acute gastric ulceration by indomethacin in the rat. *Scand. J. Gastroenterol* **1969**, *4*, 265–267.
49. Gamberini, M.T.; Skorupa, L.A.; Souccar, C.; Lapa, A.J. Inhibition of gastric secretion by a water extract from Baccharis triptera. *Mem. Inst. Oswaldo Cruz* **1991**, *86*, 137–139. [CrossRef]
50. Shay, H. A simple method for the uniform production of gastric ulceration in the rat. *Gastroenterology* **1945**, *5*, 43–61.
51. Sun, X.-B.; Matsumoto, T.; Yamada, H. Effects of a Polysaccharide Fraction from the Roots of Bupleurum falcatum L. on Experimental Gastric Ulcer Models in Rats and Mice. *J. Pharm. Pharmacol.* **1991**, *43*, 699–704. [CrossRef] [PubMed]
52. Okunji, C.; Okeke, C.N.; Gugnani, H.C.; Iwu, M.M. An Antifungal Spirostanol Saponin from Fruit Pulp of Dracaena mannii. *Int. J. Crude Drug Res.* **1990**, *28*, 193–199. [CrossRef]
53. Lobo, V.; Patil, A.; Phatak, A.; Chandra, N. Free radicals, antioxidants and functional foods: Impact on human health. *Pharmacogn. Rev.* **2010**, *4*, 118–126. [CrossRef] [PubMed]
54. Silva, A.M.; Martins-Gomes, C.; Fangueiro, J.F.; Andreani, T.; Souto, E.B. Comparison of antiproliferative effect of epigallocatechin gallate when loaded into cationic solid lipid nanoparticles against different cell lines. *Pharm. Dev. Technol.* **2019**, *24*, 1243–1249. [CrossRef] [PubMed]
55. Bhattacharyya, A.; Chattopadhyay, R.; Mitra, S.; Crowe, S.E. Oxidative stress: An essential factor in the pathogenesis of gastrointestinal mucosal diseases. *Physiol. Rev.* **2014**, *94*, 329–354. [CrossRef] [PubMed]
56. Salatino, A. Brazilian Red Propolis: Legitimate Name of the Plant Resin Source. *MOJ Food Process. Technol.* **2018**, *6*, 1–2. [CrossRef]
57. Raheja, S.; Girdhar, A.; Lather, V.; Pandita, D. Biochanin A: A phytoestrogen with therapeutic potential. *Trends Food Sci. Technol.* **2018**, *79*, 55–66. [CrossRef]
58. Da Silva, R.O.; Andrade, V.M.; Rêgo, E.S.B.; Dória, G.A.A.; Lima, B.D.S.; Da Silva, F.A.; Araújo, A.A.D.S.; Júnior, R.L.C.D.A.; Cardoso, J.C.; Gomes, M.Z. Acute and sub-acute oral toxicity of Brazilian red propolis in rats. *J. Ethnopharmacol.* **2015**, *170*, 66–71. [CrossRef]
59. Rocha, N.F.M.; De Oliveira, G.V.; De Araújo, F.Y.R.; Rios, E.R.V.; Carvalho, A.M.R.; De Vasconcelos, S.M.M.; Macedo, D.; Soares, P.M.G.; De Sousa, D.P.; De Sousa, F.C.F. (−)-α-Bisabolol-induced gastroprotection is associated with reduction in lipid peroxidation, superoxide dismutase activity and neutrophil migration. *Eur. J. Pharm. Sci.* **2011**, *44*, 455–461. [CrossRef]
60. Lucarini, M.; Durazzo, A.; Kiefer, J.; Santini, A.; Lombardi-Boccia, G.; Souto, E.B.; Romani, A.; Lampe, A.; Nicoli, S.F.; Gabrielli, P.; et al. Grape Seeds: Chromatographic Profile of Fatty Acids and Phenolic Compounds and Qualitative Analysis by FTIR-ATR Spectroscopy. *Foods* **2019**, *9*, 10. [CrossRef]
61. Ribeiro, A.R.S.; Diniz, P.B.; Estevam, C.S.; Pinheiro, M.S.; Albuquerque-Júnior, R.L.; Thomazzi, S.M. Gastroprotective activity of the ethanol extract from the inner bark of Caesalpinia pyramidalis in rats. *J. Ethnopharmacol.* **2013**, *147*, 383–388. [CrossRef] [PubMed]
62. Salehi, B.; Venditti, A.; Sharifi-Rad, J.; Kregiel, D.; Sharifi-Rad, J.; Durazzo, A.; Lucarini, M.; Santini, A.; Souto, E.B.; Novellino, E.; et al. The Therapeutic Potential of Apigenin. *Int. J. Mol. Sci.* **2019**, *20*, 1305. [CrossRef] [PubMed]
63. Sánchez-Mendoza, M.E.; Rodríguez-Silverio, J.; Rivero-Cruz, J.F.; Rocha-González, H.I.; Pineda-Farías, J.B.; Arrieta, J. Antinociceptive effect and gastroprotective mechanisms of 3,5-diprenyl-4-hydroxyacetophenone from Ageratina pichinchensis. *Fitoterapia* **2013**, *87*, 11–19. [CrossRef] [PubMed]
64. Hotta, S.; Uchiyama, S.; Ichihara, K. Brazilian red propolis extract enhances expression of antioxidant enzyme genes in vitro and in vivo. *Biosci. Biotechnol. Biochem.* **2020**, *84*, 1–11. [CrossRef] [PubMed]
65. Osés, S.; Marcos, P.; Azofra, P.; De Pablo, A.; Fernández-Muíño, M.Á.; Sancho, M.T. Phenolic Profile, Antioxidant Capacities and Enzymatic Inhibitory Activities of Propolis from Different Geographical Areas: Needs for Analytical Harmonization. *Antioxidants* **2020**, *9*, 75. [CrossRef]
66. Rivero-Cruz, J.F.; Granados-Pineda, J.; Pedraza-Chaverri, J.; Rojas, J.M.P.; Passari, A.K.; Díaz-Ruiz, G.; Rivero-Cruz, B.E. Phytochemical Constituents, Antioxidant, Cytotoxic, and Antimicrobial Activities of the Ethanolic Extract of Mexican Brown Propolis. *Antioxidants* **2020**, *9*, 70. [CrossRef]
67. Svečnjak, L.; Marijanović, Z.; Okińczyc, P.; Kuś, P.M.; Jerković, I. Mediterranean Propolis from the Adriatic Sea Islands as a Source of Natural Antioxidants: Comprehensive Chemical Biodiversity Determined by GC-MS, FTIR-ATR, UHPLC-DAD-QqTOF-MS, DPPH and FRAP Assay. *Antioxidants* **2020**, *9*, 337. [CrossRef]

68. Govindasami, S.; Uddandrao, V.V.S.; Raveendran, N.; Sasikumar, V. Therapeutic Potential of Biochanin-A Against Isoproterenol-Induced Myocardial Infarction in Rats. *Cardiovasc. Hematol. Agents Med. Chem.* **2020**, *18*, 31–36. [CrossRef]
69. Xue, Z.; Zhang, Q.; Yu, W.; Wen, H.; Hou, X.; Li, D.; Kou, X. Potential Lipid-Lowering Mechanisms of Biochanin A. *J. Agric. Food Chem.* **2017**, *65*, 3842–3850. [CrossRef]
70. Jia, W.C.; Liu, G.; Zhang, C.D.; Zhang, S.P. Formononetin attenuates hydrogen peroxide (H_2O_2)-induced apoptosis and NF-κB activation in RGC-5 cells. *Eur. Rev. Med. Pharm. Sci.* **2014**, *18*, 2191–2197.
71. Fukai, T.; Marumo, A.; Kaitou, K.; Kanda, T.; Terada, S.; Nomura, T. Anti-Helicobacter pylori flavonoids from licorice extract. *Life Sci.* **2002**, *71*, 1449–1463. [CrossRef]
72. Satoh, H.; Saijo, Y.; Yoshioka, E.; Tsutsui, H. Helicobacter Pylori Infection is a Significant Risk for Modified Lipid Profile in Japanese Male Subjects. *J. Atheroscler. Thromb.* **2010**, *17*, 1041–1048. [CrossRef] [PubMed]
73. Gunji, T.; Matsuhashi, N.; Sato, H.; Fujibayashi, K.; Okumura, M.; Sasabe, N.; Urabe, A. Helicobacter PyloriInfection Is Significantly Associated with Metabolic Syndrome in the Japanese Population. *Am. J. Gastroenterol.* **2008**, *103*, 3005–3010. [CrossRef] [PubMed]
74. Franchin, M.; Da Cunha, M.G.; Denny, C.; Napimoga, M.H.; Cunha, F.Q.; Bueno-Silva, B.; De Alencar, S.M.; Ikegaki, M.; Rosalen, P.L. Bioactive Fraction of Geopropolis fromMelipona scutellarisDecreases Neutrophils Migration in the Inflammatory Process: Involvement of Nitric Oxide Pathway. *Evid. Based Complement. Altern. Med.* **2013**, *2013*, 1–9. [CrossRef] [PubMed]
75. Kalil, M.A.; Santos, L.M.; Barral, T.D.; Rodrigues, D.M.; Pereira, N.P.; Sá, M.D.C.A.; Umsza-Guez, M.A.; Machado, B.A.S.; Meyer, R.; Portela, R.D. Brazilian Green Propolis as a Therapeutic Agent for the Post-surgical Treatment of Caseous Lymphadenitis in Sheep. *Front. Vet. Sci.* **2019**, *6*, 399. [CrossRef] [PubMed]
76. Pineros, A.; De Lima, M.; Rodrigues, T.S.; Gembre, A.F.; Bertolini, T.B.; Fonseca, M.D.; Berretta, A.A.; Ramalho, L.N.Z.; Cunha, F.Q.; Hori, J.I.; et al. Green propolis increases myeloid suppressor cells and CD4+Foxp3+ cells and reduces Th2 inflammation in the lungs after allergen exposure. *J. Ethnopharmacol.* **2020**, *252*, 112496. [CrossRef]
77. Shedeed, H.A.; Farrag, B.; Elwakeel, E.A.; El-Hamid, I.S.A.; El-Rayes, M.A.H. Propolis supplementation improved productivity, oxidative status, and immune response of Barki ewes and lambs. *Vet. World* **2019**, *12*, 834–843. [CrossRef]
78. Usman, A.N.; Abdullah, A.Z.; Raya, I.; Budiaman, B.; Bukhari, A. Glucocorticoid and cortisol hormone in response to honey and honey propolis supplementation in mild stress women. *Enferm. Clín.* **2020**, *30*, 1–4. [CrossRef]
79. Chen, H.-Q.; Jin, Z.; Li, G.-H. Biochanin A protects dopaminergic neurons against lipopolysaccharide-induced damage through inhibition of microglia activation and proinflammatory factors generation. *Neurosci. Lett.* **2007**, *417*, 112–117. [CrossRef]
80. Ma, Z.; Ji, W.; Fu, Q.; Ma, S. Formononetin Inhibited the Inflammation of LPS-Induced Acute Lung Injury in Mice Associated with Induction of PPAR Gamma Expression. *Inflammation* **2013**, *36*, 1560–1566. [CrossRef]
81. Konturek, P.C.; Konturek, S.J.; Cześnikiewicz, M.; Płonka, M.; Bielański, W. Interaction of Helicobacter pylori (Hp) and nonsteroidal anti-inflammatory drugs (NSAID) on gastric mucosa and risk of ulcerations. *Med. Sci. Monit.* **2002**, *8*, 197–209.
82. Wallace, J.L.; McKnight, W.; Reuter, B.K.; Vergnolle, N. NSAID-induced gastric damage in rats: Requirement for inhibition of both cyclooxygenase 1 and 2. *Gastroenterology* **2000**, *119*, 706–714. [CrossRef] [PubMed]
83. Ribeiro, D.; Freitas, M.; Tomé, S.M.; Silva, A.M.S.; Laufer, S.; Lima, J.L.F.C.; Fernandes, E. Flavonoids Inhibit COX-1 and COX-2 Enzymes and Cytokine/Chemokine Production in Human Whole Blood. *Inflammation* **2014**, *38*, 858–870. [CrossRef] [PubMed]
84. Yu, J.; Bi, X.; Yu, B.; Chen, D. Isoflavones: Anti-Inflammatory Benefit and Possible Caveats. *Nutrients* **2016**, *8*, 361. [CrossRef]
85. Gracioso, J.D.S.; Vilegas, W.; Lima, C.A.H.; Brito, A.R.M.S. Effects of tea from Turnera ulmifolia L. on mouse gastric mucosa support the Turneraceae as a new source of antiulcerogenic drugs. *Boil. Pharm. Bull.* **2002**, *25*, 487–491. [CrossRef]
86. De Barros, M.; Da Silva, L.M.; Boeing, T.; Somensi, L.B.; Cury, B.J.; Burci, L.D.M.; Santin, J.R.; De Andrade, S.F.; Monache, F.D.; Cechinel-Filho, V. Pharmacological reports about gastroprotective effects of methanolic extract from leaves of Solidago chilensis (Brazilian arnica) and its components quercitrin and afzelin in rodents. *Naunyn Schmiedeberg's Arch. Pharmacol.* **2016**, *389*, 403–417. [CrossRef]

87. Hou, W.; Schubert, M.L. Gastric secretion. *Curr. Opin. Gastroenterol.* **2006**, *22*, 593–598. [CrossRef]
88. Xu, M.L.; Bi, C.W.; Kong, A.Y.; Dong, T.T.; Wong, Y.H.; Tsim, K.W. Flavonoids induce the expression of acetylcholinesterase in cultured osteoblasts. *Chem. Interact.* **2016**, *259*, 295–300. [CrossRef]
89. Borrelli, F.; Izzo, A.A. The plant kingdom as a source of anti-ulcer remedies. *Phytother. Res.* **2000**, *14*, 581–591. [CrossRef]
90. Atherton, J.C. The Pathogenesis Ofhelicobacter Pylori–Induced Gastro–Duodenal Diseases. *Annu. Rev. Pathol. Mech. Dis.* **2006**, *1*, 63–96. [CrossRef]
91. Boyanova, L.; Derejian, S.; Koumanova, R.; Katsarov, N.; Gergova, G.; Mitov, I.; Nikolov, R.; Krastev, Z. Inhibition of Helicobacter pylori growth in vitro by Bulgarian propolis: Preliminary report. *J. Med. Microbiol.* **2003**, *52*, 417–419. [CrossRef] [PubMed]
92. Baltas, N.; Karaoglu, S.A.; Tarakci, C.; Kolayli, S. Effect of propolis in gastric disorders: Inhibition studies on the growth of Helicobacter pylori and production of its urease. *J. Enzym. Inhib. Med. Chem.* **2016**, *31*, 1–5. [CrossRef] [PubMed]

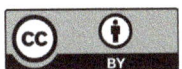

© 2020 by the authors. Licensee MDPI, Basel, Switzerland. This article is an open access article distributed under the terms and conditions of the Creative Commons Attribution (CC BY) license (http://creativecommons.org/licenses/by/4.0/).

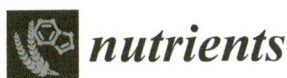

Article

Protective Effects of Black Raspberry (*Rubus occidentalis*) Extract against Hypercholesterolemia and Hepatic Inflammation in Rats Fed High-Fat and High-Choline Diets

Taehwan Lim, Juhee Ryu, Kiuk Lee, Sun Young Park and Keum Taek Hwang *

Department of Food and Nutrition, and Research Institute of Human Ecology, Seoul National University, Seoul 08826, Korea; imtae86@snu.ac.kr (T.L.); issue221@snu.ac.kr (J.R.); leku@snu.ac.kr (K.L.); sunyoung.park@snu.ac.kr (S.Y.P.)
* Correspondence: keum@snu.ac.kr; Tel.: +82-2-880-2531; Fax: +82-2-884-0305

Received: 24 July 2020; Accepted: 12 August 2020; Published: 14 August 2020

Abstract: Choline is converted to trimethylamine by gut microbiota and further oxidized to trimethylamine-*N*-oxide (TMAO) by hepatic flavin monooxygenases. Positive correlation between TMAO and chronic diseases has been reported. Polyphenols in black raspberry (BR), especially anthocyanins, possess various biological activities. The objective of this study was to determine the effects of BR extract on the level of choline-derived metabolites, serum lipid profile, and inflammation markers in rats fed high-fat and high-choline diets. Forty female Sprague-Dawley (SD) rats were randomly divided into four groups and fed for 8 weeks as follows: CON (AIN-93G diet), HF (high-fat diet), HFC (HF + 1.5% choline water), and HFCB (HFC + 0.6% BR extract). Serum levels of TMAO, total cholesterol, and low-density lipoprotein (LDL)-cholesterol and cecal trimethylamine (TMA) level were significantly higher in the HFC than in the HFCB. BR extract decreased mRNA expression of pro-inflammatory genes including nuclear factor-κB (NF-κB), interleukin (IL)-1β, IL-6, and cyclooxygenase-2 (COX-2), and protein expression of NF-κB and COX-2 in liver tissue. These results suggest that consistent intake of BR extract might alleviate hypercholesterolemia and hepatic inflammation induced by excessive choline with a high-fat diet via lowering elevated levels of cecal TMA and serum TMAO in rats.

Keywords: black raspberry; excessive choline; TMAO; hypercholesterolemia; hepatic inflammation

1. Introduction

Choline, one of the components of phospholipids in cell membrane and neurotransmitter, is regarded as an essential nutrient [1]. However, choline is also a precursor of trimethylamine-*N*-oxide (TMAO), which has been reported to act as a putative promoter of chronic diseases in human [2–6]. A part of excessive dietary choline is metabolized by gut microbiota to produce trimethylamine (TMA). Once TMA is absorbed from intestine, it is transported to liver via portal circulation and further oxidized to TMAO by hepatic flavin monooxygenases [2].

Since various epidemiological studies revealed connection between TMAO and cardiovascular diseases (CVD) [5,7,8], studies on TMAO and its precursors, such as choline, lecithin, and L-carnitine, have focused on vascular inflammation, endothelial dysfunction, and cholesterol homeostasis [3–5,9–12]. In addition, the effects of TMAO and its precursors on glucose intolerance [6] and hepatotoxicity [9,12] have been investigated. Taken together, it would likely be possible that TMAO can act in various organs throughout the body. More recently, TMAO has been demonstrated to induce expressions of cytokines and adhesion molecules in primary human aortic endothelial cells and vascular smooth muscle cells [3]. These inflammatory responses were also reported to be mediated via activation of nuclear factor-κB (NF-κB) signaling pathway, which is pivotal in inflammation, immunity, and cell death of various cell types [3].

Both epidemiological and experimental studies have revealed positive correlation between TMAO and chronic diseases such as CVD, renal disease, and diabetes [5–8,13–16]. Besides, evidences that TMAO might be able to cause hepatotoxicity or inflammation in adipose tissue have been provided [6,9,12]. However, consumption of fruits and vegetables has been widely known to be able to prevent incidence of chronic diseases. Phytochemicals, bioactive compounds in plants, contribute to reduce risks of those diseases mostly by their anti-oxidant activity [17].

Black raspberry (*Rubus occidentalis*; BR) is relatively high in anthocyanins among *Rubus* fruits [18]. It has been found that the major bioactive compounds in BR were anthocyanins, mainly cyanidin-3-rutinoside (C3R), cyanidin-3-glucoside (C3G), and cyanidin-3-xylosylrutinoside (C3XR) [19,20]. BR has been known to possess anti-oxidative, anti-inflammatory, and anti-cancer activities [21]. Especially, C3R and C3G were demonstrated to have anti-inflammatory activity through down-regulating NF-κB expression and inhibiting inhibitory κB (I-κB) degradation in lipopolysaccharide (LPS)-treated murine macrophages [19]. However, to the best of our knowledge, protective effects of polyphenols in BR on inflammation induced by excessive choline intake have not been reported.

The aims of this study were to investigate the effect of excessive choline intake on serum lipid profile and inflammation in rats fed high-fat diet and to evaluate the effect of polyphenols including anthocyanins in BR on choline-induced inflammation of the rats.

2. Materials and Methods

2.1. Materials and Chemicals

BR (*Rubus occidentalis*) fruits harvested in 2017 were purchased from Gochang, Korea. C3G, C3R, TMA, TMAO, and Folin-Ciocalteu reagent were the products of Sigma-Aldrich Chemical Co. (St. Louis, MO, USA). Choline chloride was obtained from Jinan Pengbo Biotechnology Co., Ltd. (Jinan, China). Trizol reagent was purchased from Invitrogen (Carlsbad, CA, USA). Radioimmune precipitation assay (RIPA) buffer and protease inhibitor cocktail (PIC) #6 were purchased from Biosesang Inc. (Seongnam, Korea). Anti-I-κB, anti-NF-κB, and horseradish peroxidase (HRP)-linked anti-rabbit immunoglobulin G (IgG) were purchased from Cell Signaling Technology (Danvers, MA, USA); anti-COX-2 from Novus Biologicals (Littleton, CO, USA); and anti-β-actin from Abcam (Cambridge, England). Enhanced chemiluminescence (ECL) solution was obtained from GenDEPOT (Katy, TX, USA).

2.2. Preparation of BR Extract

BR fruits (60 g) were crushed by hand and mixed with 80% (*v/v*) ethanol solution (300 mL) for 1 h by an overhead stirrer (WiseStir HS-30D, Daihan Scientific, Wonju, Korea). The extract was filtered with Whatman No. 2 filter paper (Whatman International Ltd., Maidstone, UK). The filtrate was concentrated using a vacuum rotary evaporator (A-10005, Eyela Co., Tokyo, Japan). The concentrate was freeze-dried using a freeze dryer (FDI06-85, Soritech, Hwaseong, Korea) to obtain powder form of the extract and stored at −20 °C for further studies.

2.3. Determination of Total Phenolic Content (TPC)

TPC in the BR extract was determined according to the method of Singleton et al. with a slight modification [22]. The BR extract (10 mg) was dissolved in 1 mL water followed by addition of 100 μL Folin-Ciocalteu reagent. After 3 min, 300 μL 20% (*w/v*) sodium bicarbonate solution was added to the mixture. The mixture was incubated at 40 °C for 30 min and then absorbance was measured at 765 nm by a spectrophotometer (Spectramax190, Molecular Devices, San Jose, CA, USA). TPC was presented as gallic acid equivalent (GAE).

2.4. HPLC-UV Analysis of Anthocyanins in BR Extract

The BR extract powder (100 mg) was dissolved in 10 mL methanol containing 0.01% (*v/v*) hydrochloric acid. To separate anthocyanin fraction, 3 mL of the dissolved BR extract was injected into a Sep-Pak Plus C-18 cartridge (Waters Co., Milford, MA, USA), and the eluate was filtered using a 0.22 µm syringe filter (Pall Co., Port Washington, NY, USA). Composition and content of anthocyanins in the fraction were analyzed using a reversed-phase HPLC (Waters 2996 Separation Module, Waters Co., Milford, MA, USA) equipped with an XBridge C18 column (4.6 × 250 mm, 5 µm, Waters Co., Milford, MA, USA). Mobile phase was 5% (*v/v*) formic acid aqueous solution (A) and acetonitrile (B) with a gradient as follows: 0–1 min, 2% B; 1–2 min, 2–10% B; 2–15.5 min, 10–12.5% B; 15.5–21 min, 12.5–60% B; 21–26 min, 60–2% B; and 26–30 min, 2% B. Flow rate and column temperature were 1 mL min^{-1} and 30 °C. Anthocyanins were identified and quantified matching retention times of C3R and C3G standards at 520 nm.

2.5. Animals and Diets

Forty female Sprague-Dawley (SD) rats (5 weeks old) were purchased from Koatech (Pyeongtaek, Korea). Female rats were selected since hepatic activity of flavin monooxygenase 3 is relatively higher in females than in males; therefore, they are prone to accumulation of TMAO in blood [5,23]. The rats were acclimatized to laboratory environment for 1 week under controlled temperature (23 ± 3 °C), humidity (50 ± 10%), and 12/12 h light-dark cycle. All the rats had free access to autoclaved tap water and normal chow diet during acclimation period of 1 week. After acclimated, they were randomly divided into 4 groups. Compositions of control AIN (American Institute of Nutrition)-93G diet and high-fat diet were shown in Table S1. High-fat diet supplemented with 0.6% BR extract was customized by Raonbio (Yongin, Korea). Treated groups were as follows: CON (AIN-93G diet (16% calories from fat)), HF (high-fat diet (45% calories from fat)), HFC (high-fat diet with 1.5% (*w/w*) choline water), and HFCB (high-fat diet with 1.5% (*w/w*) choline water and 0.6% BR extract). The CON and HF groups were given autoclaved tap water. All the animals were allowed free access to diet and water for 8 weeks and the water was replaced every two days. All protocols for animal experiment used in this study were conducted in accordance with institutional policies for animal health and well-being and approved by the Institutional Animal Care and Use Committee of Seoul National University (Approval No.: SNU-171103-1-5).

2.6. Blood and Tissue Collection

At the end of the experiment, all the rats were fasted for 6 h but allowed free access to water. All the animals were euthanized by asphyxiation with CO_2. Blood was collected by cardiac puncture and centrifuged to get serum at 3000× *g* at 4 °C for 20 min after coagulation. Liver and adipose tissue were isolated and washed with saline. All the tissues were immediately stored at −80 °C until analysis.

2.7. Quantification of Choline, TMA, and TMAO

To determine the effect of choline intake on the production of choline-derived metabolites, cecal choline, TMA, and TMAO and serum TMAO were measured. To analyze the levels of choline-derived metabolites in cecum, cecal content was mixed with 80% (*v/v*) ice-cold methanol solution, vortexed for 5 min, and then centrifuged at 12,000× *g* for 5 min at 4 °C. The supernatant was filtered using a 0.22 µm syringe filter (Pall Co.) and the filtrate was concentrated by centrifugation (15,000× *g*, 25 min, 4 °C) in a Vivaspin centrifugal concentrator (Vivaspin 500, MWCO 3000, VS0192; Sartorius Stedim Lab, Stonehouse, UK). The concentrate was used for further analysis. Serum samples were mixed with 80% (*v/v*) ice-cold methanol solution, vortexed for 1 min, and then centrifuged at 12,000× *g* for 5 min at 4 °C. The supernatant was filtered using a 0.22 µm syringe filter (Pall Co.) and the filtrate was used for further analysis.

All the analytes were separated on an Acquity UPLC (Waters Co., Milford, MA, USA) equipped with Acquity UPLC BEH amide column (2.1 mm × 100 mm, 1.7 μm, Waters Co., Milford, MA, USA) heated at 50 °C. Mobile phase consisted of two eluents: (A) 0.5 mM ammonium formate (pH 8.1) in water and (B) acetonitrile. The gradient program was: 0–2.5 min, 95–5% B; 2.5–5 min, 5–95% B; 5–6 min, 95% B. Flow rate was 0.6 mL min^{-1}. The ion transitions (m/z 104.08 → 60.08 for choline; m/z 60.08 → 44.05 for TMA; and m/z 76.07 → 59.07 for TMAO) were used for quantitation. Samples were analyzed by SYNAPT G2-Si mass spectrometer (Waters Co., Milford, MA, USA) in positive ion electrospray mode. Capillary voltage and sampling cone voltage were set at 0.5 kV and 15 V, respectively. Flow rates of desolvation gas and cone gas were 650 L/h and 250 L/h, respectively. Desolvation temperature was 150 °C. Data acquisition and quantitation were carried out using MassLynx software 4.1 (Waters Co., Milford, MA, USA).

2.8. Serum Lipid Profile

Serum triglyceride (TG), total cholesterol (TC), and high-density lipoprotein-cholesterol (HDL-C) concentrations were determined with commercially available kits (Asan Pharmaceutical Co., Ltd., Seoul, Korea) according to the manufacturer's instructions which are based on enzymatic colorimetric methods. Absorbance was measured by a spectrophotometer (Spectramax190, Molecular Devices). Serum low-density lipoprotein-cholesterol (LDL-C) level was calculated from Friedewald formula [24].

2.9. Total RNA Extraction, cDNA Synthesis, and Real-Time Quantitative Polymerase Chain Reaction (qPCR)

Total RNA were extracted from liver and adipose tissue using Trizol reagent according to the manufacturer's instruction. Purity and quantity of RNA were evaluated by a NanoDrop spectrophotometer (NANO-200, Allsheng, Hangzhou, China). The RNA samples were reverse-transcribed using a GoScript Reverse Transcription kit (Promega, Madison, WI, USA) with random primers. qPCR was carried out with SYBR Green PCR Master mix (Applied Biosystems, Foster City, CA, USA) using Applied Biosystems StepOne Real-Time PCR system (Applied Biosystems, Foster City, CA, USA) under following conditions: 2 min at 95 °C for initiation, 15 s at 95 °C for denaturation, and 60 s at 60 °C for annealing up to 40 cycles. All qPCR primer sequences used in this study are listed in Table 1. All the relative expressions of genes were normalized to glyceraldehyde-3-phosphate dehydrogenase (GAPDH) expression and quantified using $2^{-\Delta\Delta Ct}$ method [25].

Table 1. Primer sequences used in real-time quantitative PCR.

Gene	Sequence
GAPDH	Forward (5'-3'): ACCACAGTCCATGCCATCAC Reverse (5'-3'): TCCACCACCCTGTTGCTGTA
NF-κB	Forward (5'-3'): TGGACGATCTGTTTCCCCTC Reverse (5'-3'): CCCTCGCACTTGTAACGGAA
TNF-α	Forward (5'-3'): GTAGCCCACGTCGTAGCAAAC Reverse (5'-3'): ACCACCAGTTGGTTGTCTTTGA
IL-6	Forward (5'-3'): TCCTACCCCAACTTCCAATGCTC Reverse (5'-3'): TTGGATGGTCTTGGTCCTTAGCC
IL-1β	Forward (5'-3'): GACTTCACCATGGAACCCGT Reverse (5'-3'): CAGGGAGGGAAACACACGTT
IL-10	Forward (5'-3'): GCTAACGGGAGCAACTCCTT Reverse (5'-3'): ATGTCCCCTATGGAAACAGCTT
COX-2	Forward (5'–3'): TGTATGCTACCATCTGGCTTCGG Reverse (5'-3'): GTTTGGAACAGTCGCTCGTCATC
iNOS	Forward (5'-3'): GCCATCCCGCTGCTCTAATA Reverse (5'-3'): GTTGGGAGTGGACGAAGGTA

GAPDH (glyceraldehyde-3-phosphate dehydrogenase), NF-κB (nuclear factor-κB), TNF-α (tumor necrosis factor-α), IL (interleukin), COX-2 (cyclooxygenase-2), and iNOS (inducible nitric oxide synthase).

2.10. Western Blot Analysis

Liver tissue (100 mg) was homogenized with the mixture of RIPA buffer and PIC #6 at a ratio of 100:1 (1 mL) using a Tissuelyser (DE/85220, Qiazen, Hilden, Germany). The homogenized sample was agitated at 4 °C for 1 h and centrifuged at 12,000× g at 4 °C for 30 min (Smart R17, Hanil Scientific Inc., Gimpo, Korea). The supernatant was used to determine protein concentration using a modified Lowry protein assay kit (Thermo Fisher Scientific Inc., Waltham, MA, USA) according to the manufacturer's instruction. The protein samples were loaded at 10 μL per well into 10% sodium dodecyl sulfate polyacrylamide gel and separated out at 60 V for 20 min and then at 120 V for 80 min. After the electrophoresis, proteins were transferred to nitrocellulose membrane (Bio-Rad Laboratories Inc., Hercules, CA, USA) at 370 mA for 100 min. Membranes were washed with Tris-buffered saline containing 0.1% (v/v) Tween 20 (TBST) and then blocked in blocking buffer (TBST containing 5% skim milk) for 1 h.

Each of primary antibodies, anti-NF-κB, anti-COX-2, and anti-β-actin, was diluted to 1:500 in blocking buffer. Anti-I-κB was diluted to 1:250 in blocking buffer. Secondary antibody, HRP-linked anti-rabbit IgG, was diluted to 1:1000 in blocking buffer. After blocking, the membranes were incubated with primary antibodies on a shaker for 2 h. In turn, the membranes were washed 4 times for 5 min each using TBST and incubated with secondary antibody for 1 h. The membranes were then washed 4 times for 5 min each with TBST. Protein bands were visualized by ECL followed by densitometric analysis using Chemidoc XRS+ (Bio-Rad Laboratories Inc., Hercules, CA, USA).

2.11. Statistical Analysis

Results were expressed as means ± standard deviations. All statistical analyses were performed using SPSS program (version 23.0, SPSS, Chicago, IL, USA). Data were evaluated for normal distribution by means of Shapiro-Wilk test. Thereafter, either one-way analysis of variance (ANOVA) with Duncan's multiple range test or Kruskal-Wallis test with Mann-Whitney U test was performed where applicable for analysis of differences among mean values at $p < 0.05$.

3. Results and Discussion

3.1. Chemical Properties of the BR Extract

A previous study reported that the major component of the BR extract using ethanol solution was carbohydrates (approximately 70% of the BR extract, wet basis) and small amounts of soluble proteins, ash, and anthocyanins [26]. Since biological properties of BR and its extract have been largely related to their phenolic-type phytochemicals [27,28], bioactive compounds in the BR extract used in this study would most likely be polyphenols.

In the present study, TPC in the BR extract was 42.7 ± 6.9 mg GAE g^{-1}. Since C3XR standard was not commercially available, it was identified by comparison with chromatograms from Jung et al. [19] and presented as C3R equivalent (C3RE). The contents of C3XR, C3G, and C3R in the anthocyanin fraction were 0.83 ± 0.02 mg C3RE g^{-1}, 0.50 ± 0.01 mg g^{-1}, and 2.08 ± 0.08 mg g^{-1} (dry basis), respectively. C3R was the major anthocyanin accounting for 60% of total anthocyanins, which agrees with a previous study [19].

3.2. Body Weights and Food and Water Intakes

At the end of the experimental period, body weight and daily food intake were significantly higher in the CON and HF groups than in the HFC and HFCB (Table 2). This result might be due to the difference in food intake. Although notable difference was not observed between the body weights of the CON and HF, the HF group showed a significant increase in food efficiency ratio. In addition, no matter which became obese or not, hyperlipidemia, oxidative stress, and inflammation could be induced in high-fat diet-fed SD rats [29,30]. Meanwhile, supplementation of black raspberry resulted in a significant reduction in food efficiency ratio.

Table 2. Body weights, weight gain, food and water intakes, and food efficiency ratio (FER) of rats.

	Group			
	CON	HF	HFC	HFCB
Initial body weight (g)	135.3 ± 8.9	137.1 ± 6.1	137.5 ± 7.5	137.0 ± 7.9
Final body weight (g)	249.2 ± 25.5 [a]	255.5 ± 19.3 [a]	214.0 ± 22.1 [b]	207.6 ± 22.7 [b]
Weight gain (g·d^{-1})	2.0 ± 0.3 [a]	2.1 ± 0.3 [a]	1.4 ± 0.4 [b]	1.3 ± 0.4 [b]
Food intake (g·d^{-1}) *	26.5 ± 2.3 [a]	24.7 ± 4.3 [a]	18.3 ± 2.3 [b]	17.6 ± 2.7 [b]
Water intake (mL·d^{-1}) *	40.2 ± 4.3	41.7 ± 4.0	43.4 ± 1.9	39.3 ± 8.3
FER *	0.15 ± 0.01 [a,b]	0.17 ± 0.01 [a]	0.15 ± 0.01 [a,b]	0.14 ± 0.02 [b]

FER = weight gain (g·d^{-1})/food intake (g·d^{-1}). Values represent means and standard deviations (n = 10). * n = 5. Values with different superscripts within each row are significantly different among the groups (p < 0.05; one-way ANOVA and Duncan's multiple range test). CON (AIN-93G diet), HF (45% high-fat diet), HFC (HF + 1.5% choline water), and HFCB (HFC + 0.6% black raspberry extract).

3.3. Serum TMAO Level and Cecal Choline, TMA, and TMAO Levels

The groups fed choline water showed significant higher level of choline in cecal content of the rats compared to the group fed autoclaved tap water (Figure 1A). The HFC group showed the highest level of TMA in cecum and supplementation of BR extract decreased the choline-induced elevated cecal TMA level. Likewise, serum TMAO level was significantly higher in the HFC group, while lower in the HFCB (Figure 1B). However, cecal TMAO levels were not significantly different when compared between the HFC and HFCB (Figure 1A). Dietary choline can be transformed into TMA by gut bacteria having TMA lyase (CutC) activity [31]. TMA produced once in the gut is absorbed from intestine and further oxidized to TMAO in liver. Therefore, it is necessary to reduce cecal TMA level for reduction of circulating plasma TMAO level. Some researchers reported that polyphenols, such as resveratrol, and probiotics, such as *Lactobacillus plantarum*, *Bifidobacterium animalis*, and *Enterobacter aerogenes* could be good sources to reduce elevated level of TMAO in blood by reduction of microbial TMA production [4,32–34]. There are also several studies showing that polyphenol-rich extract from various natural sources could have a prebiotic-like activity [35,36]. Therefore, the result suggests that BR extract rich in polyphenols, especially anthocyanins, might have potent to reduce cecal TMA level via modulation of gut bacteria.

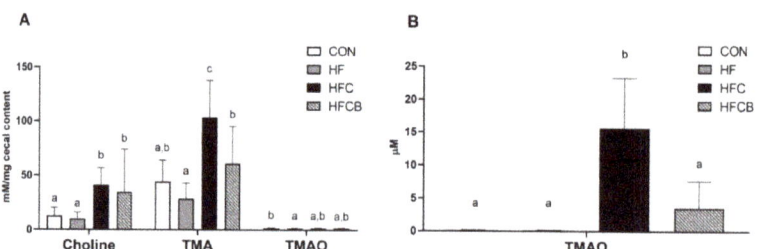

Figure 1. Effect of excessive choline intake on choline-derived metabolites in Sprague-Dawley rats. (**A**) Choline, trimethylamine (TMA), and trimethylamine-*N*-oxide (TMAO) in cecal content of the rats. (**B**) Serum TMAO level in the rats. All data represent the means and standard deviations (n = 8). Within the same metabolite, different small letters above bars indicate significant differences among the groups (p < 0.05; one-way ANOVA and Duncan's multiple range test). CON (AIN-93G diet), HF (45% high-fat diet), HFC (HF + 1.5% choline water), and HFCB (HFC + 0.6% black raspberry extract).

3.4. Serum Lipid Profile

Serum TG level of the HFC group was 27.9% and 16.1% higher than those of the CON and HF, respectively, with no significant difference (Figure 2A). Serum TG level of the HFCB group was 21.6%

and 34.3% lower than those of the HF and HFC, respectively, with no significant difference. It has been reported that intake of 3% choline water could elevate serum TG level in male Kunming mice [9,12]. However, in female LDL-receptor$^{-/-}$ C57BL/6J mice, intake of 1.3% choline water did not change plasma TG level compared to control group [3]. It remains unclear whether and how excessive choline or TMAO intake affect blood TG level.

Serum levels of TC and LDL-C in the HFC group were higher than those in the CON, HF, and HFCB ($p < 0.05$), while these three groups had no significant difference (Figure 2B,D). There was no significant difference in serum HDL-C level among the groups (Figure 2C). The elevated serum TC level in the HFC group is in agreement with the results of Chen et al. [4] and Ren et al. [12], who reported that diet containing 1% choline and water containing 3% choline could raise serum TC in apolipoprotein E (ApoE)$^{-/-}$ mice and healthy mice, respectively. It was suggested that the choline-induced elevation of serum TC might be because TMAO down-regulates expression of hepatic cholesterol 7 alpha-hydroxylase (CYP7A1), which is a key enzyme in bile acid synthesis from cholesterol [4].

In the present study, when the rats were fed both excessive choline and BR extract, serum TC level was significantly lower than the ones fed excessive choline alone. It was demonstrated that C3G intake could lower serum TC via up-regulating hepatic CYP7A1 expression in ApoE$^{-/-}$ mice [37]. Therefore, BR extract rich in anthocyanins might lower choline-induced elevation of serum TC.

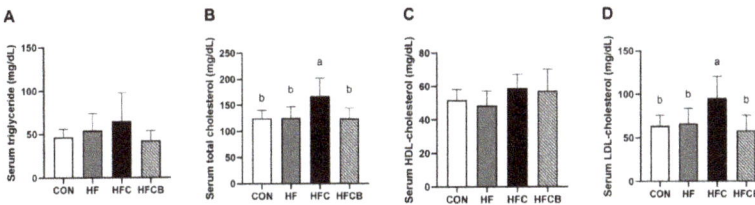

Figure 2. Serum triglycerides (**A**), total cholesterol (**B**), high-density lipoprotein (HDL)-cholesterol (**C**), and low-density lipoprotein (LDL)-cholesterol (**D**) in Sprague-Dawley rats. All data represent the means and standard deviations ($n = 7$–8). Different small letters above bars indicate significant differences among the groups ($p < 0.05$; one-way ANOVA and Duncan's multiple range test). CON (AIN-93G diet), HF (45% high-fat diet), HFC (HF + 1.5% choline water), and HFCB (HFC + 0.6% black raspberry extract).

3.5. Relative mRNA Expression of Genes Involved in Inflammatory Response in the Liver and Adipose Tissue

The mRNA expressions of NF-κB, interleukin (IL)-1β, IL-6, IL-10, tumor necrosis factor (TNF)-α, cyclooxygenase (COX)-2, and inducible nitric oxide synthase (iNOS) in liver and adipose tissue were determined by qPCR. NF-κB plays an important role in an inflammation response via regulating the expression of pro-inflammatory genes of cytokines, chemokines, and adhesion molecules [38]. In this study, the HFC group showed higher hepatic mRNA expression of NF-κB than the CON and HF ($p > 0.05$) (Figure 3). Although precise mechanism regarding effects of TMAO on NF-κB signaling pathway has not been clarified, trace amine-associated receptor (TAAR) 5, which is activated by TMA, has been suggested to be a possible mediator of TMAO activation due to the structural similarity between TMA and TMAO [3]. Also, another possible molecular mechanism has been suggested that uptake of TMAO into cells would mediate activation of NF-κB through collaborating with protein kinase C activator [11]. Despite these hypotheses, the exact mechanism of TMAO activity is still unclear. However, it might be able to regulate NF-κB expression in some ways. In the present study, NF-κB mRNA expression of the HFCB group was significantly lower than that of the HFC. Similar to this result, it was reported that anthocyanins from mulberry and sweet cherry (mainly C3G and C3R, respectively) down-regulate hepatic mRNA expression of NF-κB in diet-induced obese mice [39].

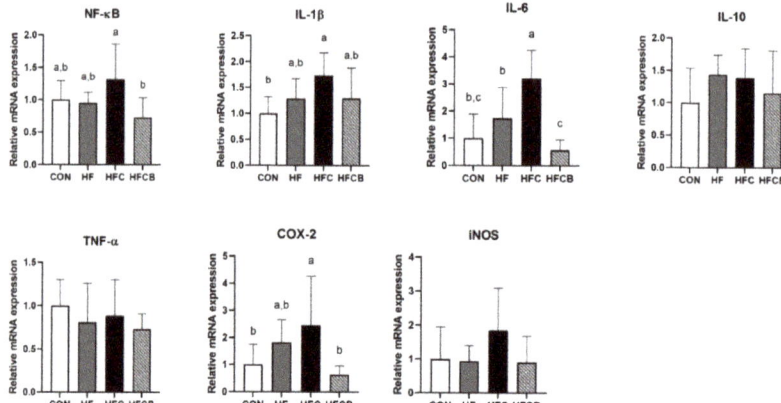

Figure 3. Relative mRNA level of genes involved in pro- and anti-inflammation in the liver of Sprague-Dawley rats. All the relative expressions of genes were normalized to glyceraldehyde-3-phosphate dehydrogenase expression. All data represent the means and standard deviations (n = 7–8). Different small letters above bars indicate significant differences among the groups ($p < 0.05$; one-way ANOVA and Duncan's multiple range test). CON (AIN-93G diet), HF (45% high-fat diet), HFC (HF + 1.5% choline water), and HFCB (HFC + 0.6% black raspberry extract).

Once NF-κB is activated, it starts to induce inflammatory cytokines that can regulate immune response, such as IL-1β, IL-6, and TNF-α [38]. In the present study, hepatic mRNA expressions of IL-1β and IL-6 in the HF group were higher than in the CON ($p > 0.05$) and those in the HFC group were even higher than in the HF ($p > 0.05$) (Figure 3). Gao et al. [6] reported that mice fed high-fat diet containing 0.2% TMAO had higher mRNA expressions of those genes in epididymal adipose tissue than mice fed high-fat diet alone. In the present study, mRNA expressions of IL-1β and IL-6 in the HFCB group were markedly suppressed compared to the HFC. Likewise, intake of C3G-rich jaboticaba peel powder was able to suppress the expressions of IL-1β and IL-6 genes via decreasing phosphorylation of I-κB in liver of high-fat diet-fed mice [40]. IL-10 is known to be an anti-inflammatory cytokine inhibiting synthesis of pro-inflammatory cytokines such as IL-1, TNF-α, and interferon-γ secreted from macrophages and monocytes [41]. The mRNA expression level of IL-10 did not differ among all the groups in this study. In contrast to this result, intake of high-fat diet containing 0.2% TMAO decreased IL-10 mRNA expression in the epididymal adipose tissue of mice [6]. In the present study, there was no significant difference in mRNA level of TNF-α among all the groups. Effect of choline or TMAO intake on TNF-α mRNA expression has been reported to vary from organ to organ [3,6,10].

COX-2 and iNOS are highly inducible enzymes in specific circumstances associated with pro-oxidant and pro-inflammatory responses under regulation of NF-κB [42]. iNOS is regarded as a biomarker of inflammatory response because it can induce overexpression of nitric oxide, which can react with superoxide and further cause cytotoxicity [43]. In the present study, mRNA expression of COX-2 in the HFC group was higher than that in the HF ($p > 0.05$) and HFCB ($p < 0.05$) (Figure 3). However, there was no significant difference in mRNA expression of iNOS among all the groups. According to Seldin et al. [3], chronic intake of choline could up-regulate mRNA expression of COX-2 in aorta of atherosclerosis-prone LDLR$^{-/-}$ mice.

In the adipose tissue, mRNA expressions of IL-6 and COX-2 in the HFC group tended to be higher than in the CON and HF, and those in the HFCB group tended to be lower than those of the HFC ($p > 0.05$) (Figure 4). The mRNA levels of NF-κB, IL-1β, IL-10, TNF-α, and iNOS did not significantly differ among the groups. It was reported that the mRNA expressions of inflammatory cytokines such as IL-6 and IL-1β in epididymal adipose tissue were upregulated when the mice were fed high-fat diet containing 0.2% TMAO for 12 weeks [6]. Thus, previous studies have reported that inflammatory responses of macrophages in adipose tissue only occurred in prolonged (≥8 weeks) high-fat feeding in the rat [44–46]. Accordingly, long-term (≥8 weeks) experiment should be needed to evaluate the effect of excessive choline and BR extract on adipose tissue of rats fed high-fat diet.

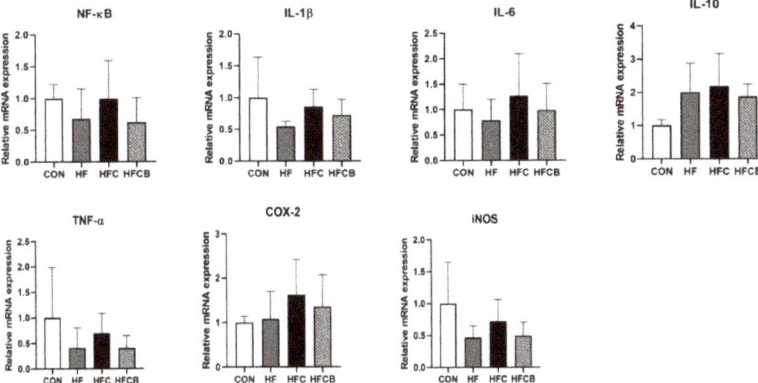

Figure 4. Relative mRNA levels involved in pro- and anti-inflammation in the adipose tissue of Sprague-Dawley rats. All the relative expressions of genes were normalized to glyceraldehyde-3-phosphate dehydrogenase expression. All data represent the means and standard deviations (n = 4–6). CON (AIN-93G diet), HF (45% high-fat diet), HFC (HF + 1.5% choline water), and HFCB (HFC + 0.6% black raspberry extract).

Collectively, excessive dietary choline might exacerbate hepatic inflammation in rats fed high-fat diet via up-regulating mRNA expressions of NF-κB, IL-6, IL-1β, and COX-2. BR extract could ameliorate choline-induced inflammation via down-regulating those genes. However, eight weeks of experiment might not be enough to change the expressions of genes related to inflammatory response in adipose tissue of the rats fed high-fat diet with or without BR extract and choline.

3.6. Protein Expression of NF-κB, I-κB, and COX-2 in the Liver

NF-κB dimer exists in the cytoplasm as an inactivated complex combined with I-κB. When cells are stimulated by specific stimuli such as antigen receptors, cytokines, reactive oxygen, and LPS, phosphorylation of I-κB occurs and then phosphorylated I-κB is degraded by protesome, releasing NF-κB dimer. NF-κB dimer then translocates into nucleus and binds to κB site of target genes [47]. In the present study, protein expression of NF-κB and COX-2 were significantly higher in the HFC group than in the CON, HF, and HFCB (Figure 5A–C,E). Similarly, it was reported that intake of C3R-rich black currant extract suppressed the hepatic protein expressions of NF-κB and COX-2 in diethylnitrosamine-initiated hepatocarcinogenesis of SD rats, as C3G-rich riceberry bran extract also did in gentamicin-induced liver damage [48,49]. Meanwhile, there was no effect of excessive choline or BR extract intake on the hepatic protein expression of I-κB (Figure 5A,D). In contrast to Jung et al. [19], who reported anthocyanins of BR could protect I-κB from LPS-induced degradation in macrophages, neither excessive choline nor BR extract affects protein expression of I-κB in this study.

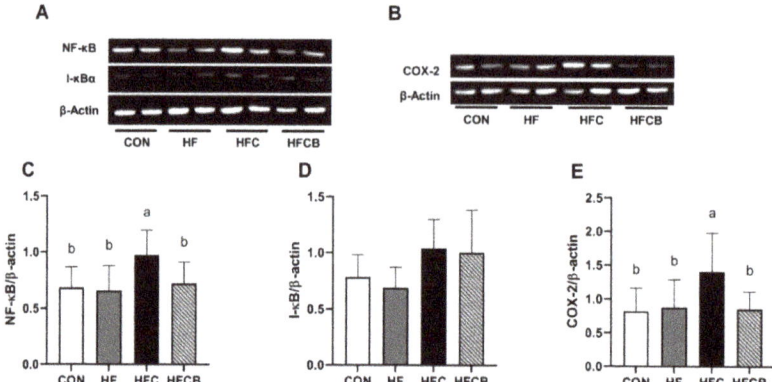

Figure 5. Protein expressions of NF-κB (**A,C**), I-κB (**A,D**), and COX-2 (**B,E**) in the liver of Sprague-Dawley rats. All data represent the means and standard deviations (n = 6–8). Different small letters above bars indicate significant differences among the groups ($p < 0.05$; one-way ANOVA and Duncan's multiple range test). CON (AIN-93G diet), HF (45% high-fat diet), HFC (HF + 1.5% choline water), and HFCB (HFC + 0.6% black raspberry extract).

4. Conclusions

Excessive choline can cause hypercholesterolemia and induce hepatic inflammation via, in part, NF-κB signaling pathway in rats fed high-fat diet. It might be due to elevated levels of cecal TMA and serum TMAO. Consistent intake of BR extract could lower the levels of cecal TMA and serum TMAO, which might result in the improvement of serum lipid profile in diet-induced hypercholesterolemia in rats. The result that BR could alter cecal TMA level suggests that BR polyphenols may act as a prebiotic in human gut as well. It could also alleviate hepatic inflammation via down-regulating the mRNA and protein expressions of genes related to inflammation. Further study, such as microbiome analysis, may be needed to elucidate the role of BR polyphenols, which seem to have a potent activity in reduction of cecal TMA level via modulation of gut bacteria.

Supplementary Materials: The following are available online at http://www.mdpi.com/2072-6643/12/8/2448/s1, Table S1: Composition of experimental diets.

Author Contributions: Conceptualization, T.L.; Funding acquisition, T.L. and K.T.H.; Investigation, T.L., J.R., K.L. and S.Y.P.; Methodology, T.L., K.L. and S.Y.P.; Supervision, K.T.H.; Visualization, T.L. and J.R.; Writing—original draft, J.R.; Writing—review & editing, T.L., J.R., K.L., S.Y.P. and K.T.H. All authors have read and agreed to the published version of the manuscript.

Funding: This research has been supported by Basic Science Research Program through the National Research Foundation of Korea (NRF) funded by the Ministry of Education (NRF-2017R1D1A1B03028407).

Conflicts of Interest: The authors declare no conflict of interest.

References

1. Zeisel, S.H.; Da Costa, K.A. Choline: An essential nutrient for public health. *Nutr. Rev.* **2009**, *67*, 615–623. [CrossRef]
2. Zeisel, S.H.; Warrier, M. Trimethylamine N-oxide, the microbiome, and heart and kidney disease. *Annu. Rev. Nutr.* **2017**, *37*, 157–181. [CrossRef] [PubMed]
3. Seldin, M.M.; Meng, Y.; Qi, H.; Zhu, W.; Wang, Z.; Hazen, S.L.; Lusis, A.J.; Shih, D.M. Trimethylamine N-oxide promotes vascular inflammation through signaling of mitogen-activated protein kinase and nuclear factor-κB. *J. Am. Heart Assoc.* **2016**, *5*, e002767. [CrossRef]
4. Chen, M.L.; Yi, L.; Zhang, Y.; Zhou, X.; Ran, L.; Yang, J.; Zhu, J.D.; Zhang, Q.Y.; Mi, M.T. Resveratrol attenuates trimethylamine-N-oxide (TMAO)-induced atherosclerosis by regulating TMAO synthesis and bile acid metabolism via remodeling of the gut microbiota. *MBio* **2016**, *7*, e02210–e02215. [CrossRef] [PubMed]

5. Wang, Z.; Klipfell, E.; Bennett, B.J.; Koeth, R.; Levison, B.S.; Dugar, B.; Feldstein, A.E.; Britt, E.B.; Fu, X.; Chung, Y.M.; et al. Gut flora metabolism of phosphatidylcholine promotes cardiovascular disease. *Nature* **2011**, *472*, 57–63. [CrossRef] [PubMed]
6. Gao, X.; Xu, J.; Jiang, C.; Zhang, Y.; Xue, Y.; Li, Z.; Wang, J.; Xue, C.; Wang, Y. Fish oil ameliorates trimethylamine N-oxide-exacerbated glucose intolerance in high-fat diet-fed mice. *Food Funct.* **2015**, *6*, 1117–1125. [CrossRef]
7. Wang, Z.; Tang, W.H.; Buffa, J.A.; Fu, X.; Britt, E.B.; Koeth, R.A.; Levison, B.S.; Fan, Y.; Wu, Y.; Hazen, S.L. Prognostic value of choline and betaine depends on intestinal microbiota-generated metabolite trimethylamine-N-oxide. *Eur. Heart J.* **2014**, *35*, 904–910. [CrossRef]
8. Tang, W.H.; Wang, Z.; Levison, B.S.; Koeth, R.A.; Britt, E.B.; Fu, X.; Wu, Y.; Hazen, S.L. Intestinal microbial metabolism of phosphatidylcholine and cardiovascular risk. *N. Engl. J. Med.* **2013**, *368*, 1575–1584. [CrossRef]
9. Jia, M.; Ren, D.; Nie, Y.; Yang, X. Beneficial effects of apple peel polyphenols on vascular endothelial dysfunction and liver injury in high choline-fed mice. *Food Funct.* **2017**, *8*, 1282–1292. [CrossRef]
10. He, Z.; Lei, L.; Kwek, E.; Zhao, Y.; Liu, J.; Hao, W.; Zhu, H.; Liang, N.; Ma, K.Y.; Ho, H.M.; et al. Ginger attenuates trimethylamine-N-oxide (TMAO)-exacerbated disturbance in cholesterol metabolism and vascular inflammation. *J. Funct. Foods* **2019**, *52*, 25–33. [CrossRef]
11. Ma, G.; Pan, B.; Chen, Y.; Guo, C.; Zhao, M.; Zheng, L.; Chen, B. Trimethylamine N-oxide in atherogenesis: Impairing endothelial self-repair capacity and enhancing monocyte adhesion. *Biosci. Rep.* **2017**, *37*, BSR20160244. [CrossRef] [PubMed]
12. Ren, D.; Liu, Y.; Zhao, Y.; Yang, X. Hepatotoxicity and endothelial dysfunction induced by high choline diet and the protective effects of phloretin in mice. *Food Chem. Toxicol.* **2016**, *94*, 203–212. [CrossRef] [PubMed]
13. Organ, C.L.; Otsuka, H.; Bhushan, S.; Wang, Z.; Bradley, J.; Trivedi, R.; Polhemus, D.J.; Tang, W.H.; Wu, Y.; Hazen, S.L.; et al. Choline diet and its gut microbe–derived metabolite, trimethylamine N-oxide, exacerbate pressure overload–induced heart failure. *Circ. Heart Fail.* **2016**, *9*, e002314. [CrossRef] [PubMed]
14. Tang, W.H.; Wang, Z.; Kennedy, D.J.; Wu, Y.; Buffa, J.A.; Agatisa-Boyle, B.; Li, X.S.; Levison, B.S.; Hazen, S.L. Gut microbiota-dependent trimethylamine N-oxide (TMAO) pathway contributes to both development of renal insufficiency and mortality risk in chronic kidney disease. *Circ. Res.* **2015**, *116*, 448–455. [CrossRef] [PubMed]
15. Missailidis, C.; Hällqvist, J.; Qureshi, A.R.; Barany, P.; Heimbürger, O.; Lindholm, B.; Stenvinkel, P.; Bergman, P. Serum trimethylamine-N-oxide is strongly related to renal function and predicts outcome in chronic kidney disease. *PLoS ONE* **2016**, *11*, e0141738. [CrossRef] [PubMed]
16. Koeth, R.A.; Wang, Z.; Levison, B.S.; Buffa, J.A.; Org, E.; Sheehy, B.T.; Britt, E.B.; Fu, X.; Wu, Y.; Li, L.; et al. Intestinal microbiota metabolism of L-carnitine, a nutrient in red meat, promotes atherosclerosis. *Nat. Med.* **2013**, *19*, 576. [CrossRef]
17. Liu, R.H. Health benefits of fruit and vegetables are from additive and synergistic combinations of phytochemicals. *Am. J. Clin. Nutr.* **2003**, *78*, 517S–520S. [CrossRef]
18. Torre, L.C.; Barritt, B.H. Quantitative evaluation of *Rubus* fruit anthocyanin pigments. *J. Food Sci.* **1977**, *42*, 488–490. [CrossRef]
19. Jung, H.; Kwak, H.K.; Hwang, K.T. Antioxidant and antiinflammatory activities of cyanidin-3-glucoside and cyanidin-3-rutinoside in hydrogen peroxide and lipopolysaccharide-treated RAW264.7 cells. *Food Sci. Biotechnol.* **2014**, *23*, 2053–2062. [CrossRef]
20. Paudel, L.; Wyzgoski, F.J.; Scheerens, J.C.; Chanon, A.M.; Reese, R.N.; Smiljanic, D.; Wesdemiotis, C.; Blakeslee, J.J.; Riedl, K.M.; Rinaldi, P. Nonanthocyanin secondary metabolites of black raspberry (*Rubus occidentalis* L.) fruits: Identification by HPLC-DAD, NMR, HPLC-ESI-MS, and ESI-MS/MS analyses. *J. Agric. Food Chem.* **2013**, *61*, 12032–12043. [CrossRef]
21. Kula, M.; Krauze-Baranowska, M. *Rubus occidentalis*: The black raspberry—Its potential in the prevention of cancer. *Nutr. Cancer* **2016**, *68*, 18–28. [CrossRef] [PubMed]
22. Singleton, V.L.; Orthofer, R.; Lamuela-Raventós, R.M. Analysis of total phenols and other oxidation substrates and antioxidants by means of folin-ciocalteu reagent. *Meth. Enzymol.* **1999**, *299*, 152–178.
23. Bennett, B.J.; de Aguiar Vallim, T.Q.; Wang, Z.; Shih, D.M.; Meng, Y.; Gregory, J.; Allayee, H.; Lee, R.; Graham, M.; Crooke, R.; et al. Trimethylamine-N-oxide, a metabolite associated with atherosclerosis, exhibits complex genetic and dietary regulation. *Cell Metab.* **2013**, *17*, 49–60. [CrossRef] [PubMed]

24. Friedewald, W.T.; Levy, R.I.; Fredrickson, D.S. Estimation of the concentration of low-density lipoprotein cholesterol in plasma, without use of the preparative ultracentrifuge. *Clin. Chem.* **1972**, *18*, 499–502. [CrossRef] [PubMed]
25. Livak, K.J.; Schmittgen, T.D. Analysis of relative gene expression data using real-time quantitative PCR and the 2−$^{\Delta\Delta CT}$ method. *Methods* **2001**, *25*, 402–408. [CrossRef] [PubMed]
26. Shaddel, R.; Hesari, J.; Azadmard-Damirchi, S.; Hamishehkar, H.; Fathi-Achachlouei, B.; Huang, Q. Double emulsion followed by complex coacervation as a promising method for protection of black raspberry anthocyanins. *Food Hydrocoll.* **2018**, *77*, 803–816. [CrossRef]
27. Jeong, J.H.; Jung, H.; Lee, S.R.; Lee, H.J.; Hwang, K.T.; Kim, T.Y. Anti-oxidant, anti-proliferative and anti-inflammatory activities of the extracts from black raspberry fruits and wine. *Food Chem.* **2010**, *123*, 338–344. [CrossRef]
28. Seeram, N.P. Berry fruits: Compositional elements, biochemical activities, and the impact of their intake on human health, performance, and disease. *J. Agric. Food Chem.* **2008**, *56*, 627–629. [CrossRef]
29. Wu, Q.; Li, S.; Li, X.; Sui, Y.; Yang, Y.; Dong, L.; Xie, B.; Sun, Z. Inhibition of advanced glycation endproduct formation by lotus seedpod oligomeric procyanidins through RAGE–MAPK signaling and NF-κB activation in high-fat-diet rats. *J. Agric. Food Chem.* **2015**, *63*, 6989–6998. [CrossRef]
30. Xu, Z.J.; Fan, J.G.; Ding, X.D.; Qiao, L.; Wang, G.L. Characterization of high-fat, diet-induced, non-alcoholic steatohepatitis with fibrosis in rats. *Dig. Dis. Sci.* **2010**, *55*, 931–940. [CrossRef]
31. Smaranda, C.; Emily, P.B. Microbial conversion of choline to trimethylamine requires a glycyl radical enzyme. *Proc. Natl. Acad. Sci. USA* **2012**, *109*, 21307–21312.
32. Liang, X.; Zhang, Z.; Lv, Y.; Tong, L.; Liu, T.; Yi, H.; Zhou, X.; Yu, Z.; Tian, X.; Cui, Q.; et al. Reduction of intestinal trimethylamine by probiotics ameliorated lipid metabolic disorders associated with atherosclerosis. *Nutrition* **2020**, 110941. [CrossRef]
33. Qiu, L.; Yang, D.; Tao, X.; Yu, J.; Xiong, H.; Wei, H. *Enterobacter aerogenes* ZDY01 attenuates choline-induced trimethylamine *N*-oxide levels by remodeling gut microbiota in mice. *J. Microbiol. Biotechnol.* **2017**, *27*, 1491–1499. [CrossRef] [PubMed]
34. Qiu, L.; Tao, X.; Xiong, H.; Yu, J.; Wei, H. *Lactobacillus plantarum* ZDY04 exhibits a strain-specific property of lowering TMAO via the modulation of gut microbiota in mice. *Food Funct.* **2018**, *9*, 4299–4309. [CrossRef] [PubMed]
35. Yang, Q.; Liang, Q.; Balakrishnan, B.; Belobrajdic, D.P.; Feng, Q.-J.; Zhang, W. Role of Dietary Nutrients in the Modulation of Gut Microbiota: A Narrative Review. *Nutrients* **2020**, *12*, 381. [CrossRef] [PubMed]
36. Loo, Y.T.; Howell, K.; Chan, M.; Zhang, P.; Ng, K. Modulation of the human gut microbiota by phenolics and phenolic fiber-rich foods. *Compr. Rev. Food Sci. Food Saf.* **2020**, 1–31. [CrossRef]
37. Wang, D.; Xia, M.; Gao, S.; Li, D.; Zhang, Y.; Jin, T.; Ling, W. Cyanidin-3-O-β-glucoside upregulates hepatic cholesterol 7α-hydroxylase expression and reduces hypercholesterolemia in mice. *Mol. Nutr. Food Res.* **2012**, *56*, 610–621. [CrossRef]
38. Tornatore, L.; Thotakura, A.K.; Bennett, J.; Moretti, M.; Franzoso, G. The nuclear factor kappa B signaling pathway: Integrating metabolism with inflammation. *Trends Cell Biol.* **2012**, *22*, 557–566. [CrossRef]
39. Wu, T.; Yin, J.; Zhang, G.; Long, H.; Zheng, X. Mulberry and cherry anthocyanin consumption prevents oxidative stress and inflammation in diet-induced obese mice. *Mol. Nutr. Food Res.* **2016**, *60*, 687–694. [CrossRef]
40. Dragano, N.R.; Cintra, D.E.; Solon, C.; Morari, J.; Leite-Legatti, A.V.; Velloso, L.A.; Maróstica-Júnior, M.R. Freeze-dried jaboticaba peel powder improves insulin sensitivity in high-fat-fed mice. *Br. J. Nutr.* **2013**, *110*, 447–455. [CrossRef]
41. Hasko, G.; Szabó, C.; Németh, Z.H.; Kvetan, V.; Pastores, S.M.; Vizi, E.S. Adenosine receptor agonists differentially regulate IL-10, TNF-alpha, and nitric oxide production in RAW 264.7 macrophages and in endotoxemic mice. *J. Immunol.* **1996**, *157*, 4634–4640. [PubMed]
42. Liu, D.; Ji, L.; Wang, Y.; Zheng, L. Cyclooxygenase-2 expression, prostacyclin production and endothelial protection of high-density lipoprotein. *Cardiovasc. Haematol. Disord. Drug Targets* **2012**, *12*, 98–105. [CrossRef] [PubMed]
43. Aktan, F. iNOS-mediated nitric oxide production and its regulation. *Life Sci.* **2004**, *75*, 639–653. [CrossRef] [PubMed]

44. Turner, N.; Kowalski, G.M.; Leslie, S.J.; Risis, S.; Yang, C.; Lee-Young, R.S.; Babb, J.R.; Meikle, P.J.; Lancaster, G.I.; Henstridge, D.C.; et al. Distinct patterns of tissue-specific lipid accumulation during the induction of insulin resistance in mice by high-fat feeding. *Diabetologia* **2013**, *56*, 1638–1648. [CrossRef] [PubMed]
45. Weisberg, S.P.; McCann, D.; Desai, M.; Rosenbaum, M.; Leibel, R.L.; Ferrante, A.W. Obesity is associated with macrophage accumulation in adipose tissue. *J. Clin. Investig.* **2003**, *112*, 1796–1808. [CrossRef]
46. Xu, H.; Barnes, G.T.; Yang, Q.; Tan, G.; Yang, D.; Chou, C.J.; Sole, J.; Nichols, A.; Ross, J.S.; Tartaglia, L.A.; et al. Chronic inflammation in fat plays a crucial role in the development of obesity-related insulin resistance. *J. Clin. Investig.* **2003**, *112*, 1821–1830. [CrossRef]
47. Luedde, T.; Schwabe, R.F. NF-κB in the liver—linking injury, fibrosis and hepatocellular carcinoma. *Nat. Rev. Gastroenterol. Hepatol.* **2011**, *8*, 108. [CrossRef]
48. Bishayee, A.; Thoppil, R.J.; Mandal, A.; Darvesh, A.S.; Ohanyan, V.; Meszaros, J.G.; Háznagy-Radnai, E.; Hohmann, J.; Bhatia, D. Black currant phytoconstituents exert chemoprevention of diethylnitrosamine-initiated hepatocarcinogenesis by suppression of the inflammatory response. *Mol. Carcinog.* **2013**, *52*, 304–317. [CrossRef]
49. Arjinajarn, P.; Chueakula, N.; Pongchaidecha, A.; Jaikumkao, K.; Chatsudthipong, V.; Mahatheeranont, S.; Norkaew, O.; Chattipakorn, N.; Lungkaphin, A. Anthocyanin-rich riceberry bran extract attenuates gentamicin-induced hepatotoxicity by reducing oxidative stress, inflammation and apoptosis in rats. *Biomed. Pharmacother.* **2017**, *92*, 412–420. [CrossRef]

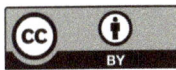
© 2020 by the authors. Licensee MDPI, Basel, Switzerland. This article is an open access article distributed under the terms and conditions of the Creative Commons Attribution (CC BY) license (http://creativecommons.org/licenses/by/4.0/).

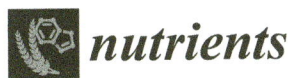

Article

Blackcurrant (*Ribes nigrum*) Extract Prevents Dyslipidemia and Hepatic Steatosis in Ovariectomized Rats

Naoki Nanashima [1,*,†], Kayo Horie [1,†], Kanako Yamanouchi [1], Toshiko Tomisawa [2], Maiko Kitajima [2], Indrawati Oey [3,4] and Hayato Maeda [5]

- [1] Department of Bioscience and Laboratory Medicine, Hirosaki University Graduate School of Health Sciences, 66-1 Hon-cho, Hirosaki, Aomori 036-8564, Japan; k-horie@hirosaki-u.ac.jp (K.H.); kanako.8@hirosaki-u.ac.jp (K.Y.)
- [2] Department of Nursing Sciences, Hirosaki University Graduate School of Health Sciences, 66-1 Hon-cho, Hirosaki, Aomori 036-8564, Japan; tmtott@hirosaki-u.ac.jp (T.T.); kitajima@hirosaki-u.ac.jp (M.K.)
- [3] Department of Food Science, University of Otago, PO Box 56, Dunedin 9054, New Zealand; indrawati.oey@otago.ac.nz
- [4] Riddet Institute, Private Bag 11 222, Palmerston North 4442, New Zealand
- [5] Faculty of Agriculture and Life Science, Hirosaki University, 3 Bunkyo-cho, Hirosaki 036-8561, Japan; hayatosp@hirosaki-u.ac.jp
- * Correspondence: nnaoki@hirosaki-u.ac.jp; Tel.: +81-172-5968
- † These authors contributed equally to this manuscript.

Received: 23 April 2020; Accepted: 21 May 2020; Published: 25 May 2020

Abstract: Estrogen is involved in lipid metabolism. Menopausal women with low estrogen secretion usually gain weight and develop steatosis associated with abnormal lipid metabolism. A previous study showed that blackcurrant (*Ribes nigrum* L.) extract (BCE) had phytoestrogen activity. In this study, we examined whether BCE improved lipid metabolism abnormalities and reduced liver steatosis in ovariectomized rats, as a menopausal animal model. Twelve-week-old ovariectomized (OVX) rats were fed a regular diet (Ctrl) or a 3% BCE supplemented diet while sham rats were fed a regular diet for three months. Body weight, visceral fat weight, levels of serum triglycerides, total cholesterol, and LDL cholesterol decreased in the BCE-treated OVX and sham rats, but not in OVX Ctrl rats. The results of hematoxylin and eosin staining revealed that BCE decreased the diameters of adipocytes and the nonalcoholic fatty liver disease activity score. Furthermore, quantitative RT-PCR indicated a decreased expression of hepatitis-related genes, such as tumor necrosis factor-α, IL-6, and IL-1β in OVX rats after BCE treatment. This is the first study that reported improvement of lipid metabolism abnormalities in OVX rats by BCE administration. These results suggest that the intake of BCE alleviated dyslipidemia and prevented nonalcoholic steatohepatitis during menopause in this animal model.

Keywords: blackcurrant; dyslipidemia; liver steatosis; ovariectomized; phytoestrogen

1. Introduction

Estrogen is directly related to lipid metabolism. After menopause, estrogen levels suddenly decrease. Previous studies found that menopausal women and mice with decreased estrogen secretion experience an increase in weight and symptoms of menopause, such as abnormal lipid metabolism and hepatic steatosis [1–3]. In postmenopausal women, total cholesterol (TC), LDL cholesterol (LDL-C), and triglyceride (TG) contents are increased [4], and these changes promote arteriosclerosis and adversely affect the heart and blood vessels [5,6]. Furthermore, dyslipidemia or hepatic steatosis induces nonalcoholic fatty liver disease (NAFLD) or nonalcoholic steatohepatitis (NASH) [7], leading to diseases that are major threats to public health, such as cirrhosis and hepatocellular carcinoma [8]. Estrogen plays an important role in liver lipid metabolism, and its deficiency increases the risk of NAFLD and NASH with menopausal dyslipidemia [2,9]. Thus, decreased estrogen secretion adversely affects menopausal women.

Phytoestrogens are a chemically diverse group of plant compounds with estrogenic effects in animals. Phytoestrogens, which include isoflavones, lignans, coumestans, flavonoids, and resveratrol, are present in several foods [10–13]. More importantly, some reports indicated that daily intake of phytoestrogen reduced climacteric symptoms [14]. Recently, we reported that blackcurrant (Ribes nigrum L.) extract (BCE) had phytoestrogen activity by signaling through both estrogen receptors α and β [15,16].

Blackcurrant contains high levels of polyphenols, especially four anthocyanins, cyanidin-3-glucoside, cyanidin-3-rutinoside, delphinidin-3-glucoside, and delphinidin-3-rutinoside [17]. These compounds elicited health beneficial effects, such as blood flow improvement and cancer suppression effects. Furthermore, previous studies showed that BCE had a cosmetic effect on the skin [18], alleviated hair loss [19], and improved vascular endothelium function in menopausal model rats [20]. A few studies have reported the effectiveness of BCE in alleviating dyslipidemia and NASH caused by the consumption of a high-fat diet [21,22]. However, there are no reports on whether BCE affects dyslipidemia in menopausal women or animals. Therefore, this study aimed to investigate whether BCE reduced dyslipidemia. Ovariectomized (OVX) rats were used as the menopausal animal model to examine whether BCE was effective in reducing dyslipidemia and associated hepatic steatosis during menopause. This is the first study that reports the effects of BCE treatment on lipid metabolism abnormalities in OVX rats.

2. Materials and Methods

2.1. Animals and Diets

OVX female Sprague-Dawley and sham surgery rats (12 weeks of age; weight 249.7 ± 10.2 g) were purchased from CLEA Japan Inc. (Tokyo, Japan). The rats were housed in air-conditioned rooms, with a 12 h light/dark cycle and with free access to water and food, at the Institute for Animal Experiments of Hirosaki University Graduate School of Medicine.

The BCE powder, CaNZac-35, was purchased from Koyo Mercantile Co. (Tokyo, Japan). BCE contains high concentrations of polyphenols (37.6 g/100 g BCE) and anthocyanins (38 g/100 g BCE) [16]. Since our previous studies showed that 3% BCE elicited phytoestrogen effects in the skin and vascular endothelium of rats [18–20], all rats in this study received an AIN-93M diet, with or without 3% BCE, and were assigned into three groups (n = 9–10 rats/group): 1) OVX rats treated with 3% BCE for 3 months (OVX BCE group), 2) OVX control rats without BCE treatment (OVX Ctrl group), and 3) sham surgery rats without BCE treatment (sham group). Blood, uterus, visceral fat, and liver tissues were collected from euthanized animals after 3 months, and the body, uterus, and liver weights were measured. This experiment was approved by the Animal Research Committee of Hirosaki University (permission number: G16004) and was conducted in accordance with the rules for Animal Experimentation of Hirosaki University.

2.2. Biochemical Analysis of Serum

Serum TG, glucose, AST (aspartate transaminase), ALT (alanine transaminase), and γ-GT (γ-glutamyl transferase) levels were examined using SPOTCHEM EZ SP-4430 (ARKRAY, Inc., Kyoto, Japan), while TC, HDL-C, and LDL-C contents were measured using the EnzyChrom HDL and LDL/VLDL Assay Kit (BioAssay Systems, CA, USA). Adiponectin and leptin concentrations were determined using CircuLex Rat Adiponectin ELISA Kit (Circulex, CycLex Co. Ltd., Nagano, Japan) and Rat Leptin ELISA Kit (Yanaihara Institute Co. Ltd., Shizuoka, Japan), respectively.

2.3. Histological Analysis of Liver and Adipose Tissues

Each tissue was fixed in 10% formaldehyde and embedded in paraffin for histological examination. Liver and adipose tissue sections (4 μm thick) were mounted onto silane-coated slides. The sections were deparaffinized by passing through xylene and a graded alcohol series before staining with hematoxylin and eosin. Digital images were acquired using a fluorescence microscope (FSX100; Olympus, Tokyo, Japan). Adipocyte diameters were measured, and liver steatosis grades were estimated using NAFLD activity score: steatosis (0–3), lobular inflammation foci (0–2), and hepatocellular ballooning (0–2), quantified according to the criteria proposed by Kleiner et al. [23]

2.4. RT-qPCR Analysis

Total RNA was prepared using an RNeasy mini kit (Qiagen, Valencia, CA, USA) according to the manufacturer's instructions. RNA was reverse-transcribed into cDNA using PrimeScript RT Master Mix (TaKaRa, Tokyo, Japan). Levels of *TNF-α*, *IL-6*, and *IL-1β* mRNAs were quantified by qPCR using TB Green Premix Ex Taq II (Tli RNaseH Plus; TaKaRa). The PCR amplification protocol consisted of 30 s at 94 °C, 30 s at 58 °C, and 30 s at 72 °C for 40 cycles. Transcript levels were normalized to those of glyceraldehyde 3-phosphate dehydrogenase (GAPDH) cDNA. The primer sequences were as follows (5′→3′) [24]: *TNF-α*, forward ACCACGCTCTTCTGTCTACTG and reverse CTTGGTGGTTTGCTACGAC; *IL-6*, forward TCTCTCCGCAAGAGACTTCCA and reverse ATACTGGTCTGTTGTGGGTGG; *IL-1β*, forward GCAATGGTCGGGACATAGTT and reverse AGACCTGACTTGGCAGAGGA; and *GAPDH*, forward TGAGAACGGGAAGTCTGTCA and reverse TCTCCATGGTGGTGAAGACG. PCR specificity was checked using a melting curve analysis. All samples were analyzed in duplicates, and relative gene expression was calculated according to the $2^{-\Delta\Delta Ct}$ method [25].

2.5. Statistical Analysis

Results are expressed as the mean ± standard deviation. Graphs were generated using the Graph Pad Prism 7.0 ver. 7.03 software (Graph Pad Prism, San Diego, CA, USA). Statistically significant differences were determined using Kruskal–Wallis analysis with the Steel post hoc test using the bell curve for Excel ver. 3.2 software (Social Survey Research Information Co., Ltd., Tokyo, Japan). Results with *p*-values <0.05 were considered statistically significant.

3. Results and Discussion

3.1. Weight of Body, Visceral Fat, Uterine and Volume of Food Intake

Before the experiment, the rats were grown up to 12 weeks old, and there was no significant difference in body weight (data not shown) among the rats. After three months, rats in the OVX Ctrl group increased in body weight compared to those in the sham group. However, BCE intake alleviated weight gain in OVX rats by 14%, comparable to sham rats (15%) (Figure 1A). By examining the food intake, it was 18.9 ± 1.0 g/rat/day in the OVX control group compared to the sham group, but decreased to 15.4 ± 1.2 g/rat/day in the sham group. However, the food intake in the OVX BCE group was 18.9 ± 2.9 g/rat/day, which was not different from that in the OVX control group (Figure 1B). Therefore, in this study, the food intake was the same between OVX control rats and OVX BCE rats. It is known that food intake increases with reduced estrogen levels, but in this research, the food intake of OVX BCE rats was not decreased [26]. Therefore, we concluded that phytoestrogen did not have the same strength as estrogen. It was also suggested that the decrease in the body weights of OVX BCE rats was not due to a decrease in food intake. The amount of BCE employed in the present animal study is equivalent to a daily dose of 1.9 g polyphenols [27], for a 60 kg human. This phenolic intake is considered realistic, and it could be provided by 5.1 g of BCE.

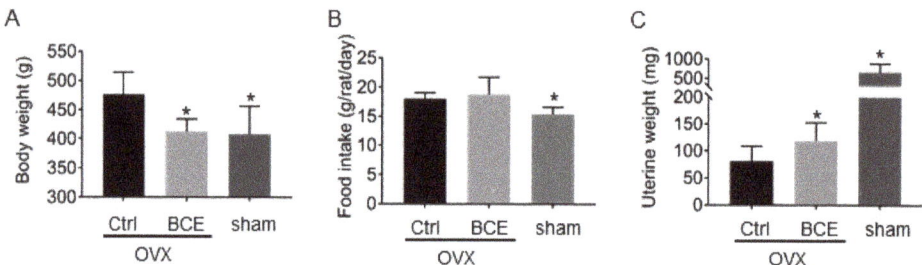

Figure 1. Effect of blackcurrant (*Ribes nigrum* L.) extract (BCE) on (**A**) body weight, (**B**) food intake, and (**C**) uterine weight of rats. Ovariectomized (OVX) rats treated with 3% BCE for 3 months (OVX BCE, n = 9), OVX rats without BCE treatment (OVX Ctrl, n = 10), and sham surgery rats without BCE treatment (sham, n = 9). Data represent the means ± SD. * $p < 0.05$ vs. Ctrl.

In addition, uterine weight increased with BCE intake (Figure 1C). Estrogens and phytoestrogens enlarge the uterus and promote the thickening of the endometrium. In our previous study, oral administration of 1000 mg/kg BCE to four-week-old young rats for three days without estrogen secretion did not increase the weight of the uterus, but the endometrium was partially thickened. In this study, as BCE was administered for three months, the weight of the uterus may have been affected. Thus, this result confirmed that BCE functioned as a phytoestrogen.

3.2. Visceral Adipose Tissue Mass and Adipocyte Sizes

OVX rats had a greater visceral adipose tissue mass (34.3 ± 10.9 g) than did sham (17.3 ± 8.8 g) rats ($p = 0.023$). However, OVX BCE rats did not increase in adipose tissue mass (24.3 ± 18.8 g) as much as did OVX Ctrl rats. (Figure 2A). As shown in Figure 2B,C, the average adipocyte diameter also increased in OVX Ctrl rats (172.3 ± 23.1 μm) compared to sham rats (117.2 ± 29.4 μm, $p < 0.001$). However, BCE treatment reduced adipocyte diameters to the levels observed in OVX Ctrl rats (136 ± 24 μm, $p < 0.001$).

Estrogens are known to play an important role in energy control and lipid metabolism, and menopausal women are at an increased risk of lifestyle-related diseases due to their decreased metabolism [28]. Several phytoestrogens have been previously reported to be effective in reducing these risks in OVX rats, but BCE has been shown to have similar effects [29,30].

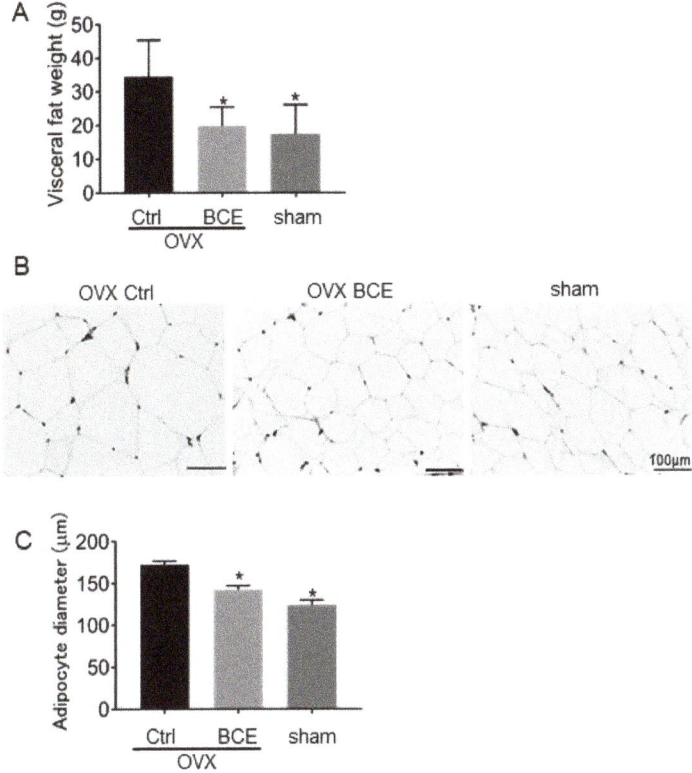

Figure 2. Effect of BCE on visceral adipose tissue mass and size. (**A**) Visceral fat mass, (**B**) images of paraffin-embedded adipocyte hematoxylin and eosin-stained sections of OVX rats treated with 3% BCE for 3 months (OVX BCE, n = 9), OVX rats without BCE treatment (OVX Ctrl, n = 10), and sham surgery rats without BCE treatment (sham, n = 9). Scale bar = 100 µm. (**C**) Average adipocyte diameters were measured in each of the three fields. Data represent the means ± SD. * $p < 0.05$ vs. Ctrl.

3.3. Serum Lipid Profiles

We investigated whether BCE intake affected serum lipids. TG, TC, and LDL-C levels increased in OVX Ctrl rats compared to sham rats. However, BCE intake reduced these serum lipids. There was no difference in HDL-C (Table 1). These results suggested that abnormal lipid metabolism occurred in OVX Ctrl rats. Serum lipid abnormalities frequently occur in menopausal women and OVX rodents [31,32]. Therefore, our results suggested that BCE alleviated menopausal lipid metabolism abnormality. TG, TC, and LDL-C are risk factors of dyslipidemia, arteriosclerosis, and cardiovascular disease. Moreover, it is known that serum glucose level rises due to a decrease in estrogen levels, causing diabetes and insulin resistance in menopausal women and OVX animals [33,34]. In this study, the serum glucose levels in OVX Ctrl rats were higher than those of sham rats, but BCE intake slightly decreased them; however, there was no significant difference between them (Supplementary Table S1).

Table 1. Serum lipid profile in OVX Ctrl (OVX Ctrl) and sham (sham) rats fed with regular diet and OVX rats treated with BCE diet (OVX BCE) after 3 months.

	OVX Ctrl	OVX BCE	Sham
TG (mg/dL)	269.8 ± 57	151.4 ± 64.6 *	212.3 ± 40.2 *
TC (mg/dL)	213.4 ± 98.8	140.5 ± 12.6 *	98.2 ± 53.3 *
LDL-C (mg/dL)	43 ± 5.8	31.7 ± 7.7 *	26.2 ± 14.8 *
HDL-C (mg/dL)	66.2 ± 28	53.1 ± 26.9	65.7 ± 15.5

Data represent the means ± SD of 9–10 animals. * $p < 0.05$ vs. Ctrl.

3.4. Serum Leptin and Adiponectin Levels

Adipocytokine is a general term for cytokines, such as adiponectin and leptin, secreted from adipose tissues. Levels of these adipocytokines increased in OVX rats more than in sham rats, but decreased with BCE intake (Table 2). Adiponectin can prevent arteriosclerosis, enhance the action of insulin, and lower blood pressure, while leptin reduces the appetite; these adipocytokines are effective in treating lifestyle-related diseases [35,36]. Adiponectin and leptin concentrations increase due to late postmenopause in women and estrogen deficiency in animals, such as OVX mice [37–39]. The results of this study were consistent with these previous reports, suggesting that this is a compensatory effect due to weight gain and adipocyte growth.

Table 2. Serum adipocytokine levels in OVX Ctrl (OVX Ctrl) and sham (sham) rats, and OVX rats treated with BCE diet (OVX BCE) after 3 months.

	OVX Ctrl	OVX BCE	sham
Adiponectin (µg/mL)	21.2 ± 4.3	16.1 ± 3.4 **	12.0 ± 4.9 **
Leptin (ng/mL)	1.96 ± 0.56	1.29 ± 0.37 *	1.23 ± 0.41 *

Data represent the means ± SD of 9–10 animals. * $p < 0.05$ and ** $p < 0.01$ vs. Ctrl.

3.5. Evaluation of Hepatic Steatosis and Inflammation

Menopausal women and OVX animals may develop NAFLD from dyslipidemia. In this study, we examined whether BCE was effective in preventing NAFLD onset by analyzing the liver of OVX rats. Hematoxylin and eosin staining revealed no steatosis in sham rats, but marked steatosis in OVX Ctrl rats; ingestion of BCE decreased the degree of steatosis (Figure 3A). Inflammatory foci and balloons in the liver were not observed, but mild inflammation such as lymphocyte infiltration was detected in OVX Ctrl rats (Figure 3B, black arrow). In contrast, no inflammation was observed in the OVX BCE or sham groups. The NAFLD activity score in the sham group was 0.3 ± 0.5, and it increased to 2.6 ± 0.9 ($p = 0.0016$) in the OVX Ctrl group. However, it decreased to 1.3 ± 0.5 ($p = 0.006$, Figure 3C) in the OVX BCE group. Furthermore, in the livers of OVX Ctrl rats, the expression of hepatic inflammatory marker genes such as *TNF-α*, *IL-6*, and *IL-1β* was higher than that in sham rats, but their levels decreased after BCE intake (Figure 3D).

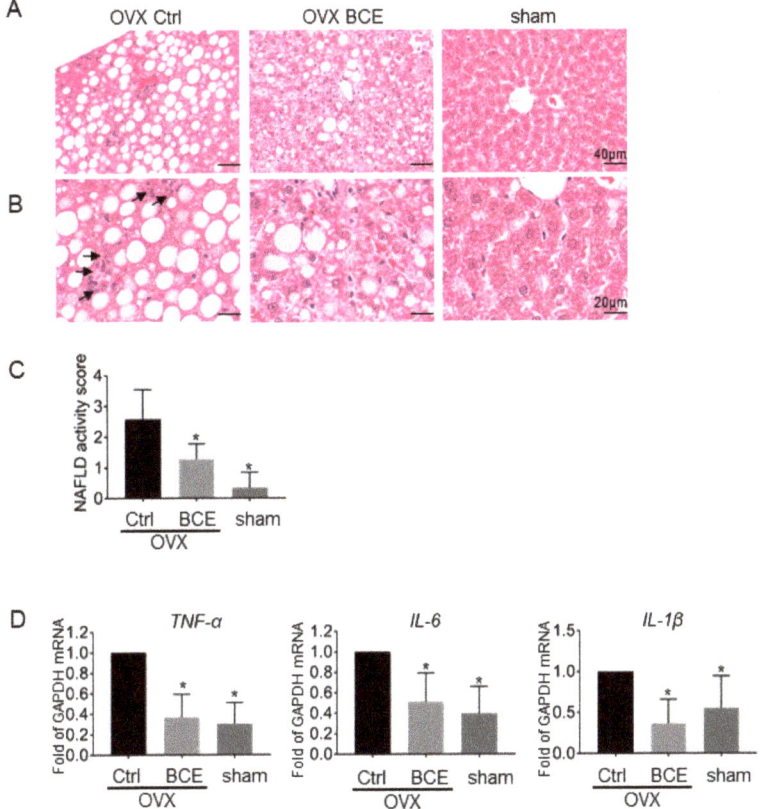

Figure 3. Effects of BCE on liver steatosis. Images of paraffin-embedded hematoxylin and eosin-stained liver sections of OVX rats treated with 3% BCE for 3 months (OVX BCE, n = 9), OVX rats without BCE treatment (OVX Ctrl, n = 10), and sham surgery rats without BCE treatment (sham, n = 9). Magnifications of the upper and lower images are (**A**) 200× and (**C**) 400×, respectively, and scale bars are 40 μm and 20 μm, respectively. (**B**) Nonalcoholic fatty liver disease (NAFLD) activity scores in the liver were estimated in each of the three fields. Data represent the means ± SD. * $p < 0.05$ vs. Ctrl. (**D**) Effects of BCE on mRNA levels of liver inflammatory marker genes. Total mRNA levels in liver tissues from rats of each treatment group were quantified by RT-qPCR. Relative expression of *TNF-α*, *IL-6*, and *IL-1β* was normalized with that of *GAPDH*. Data represent the means ± SD of the means from three rats. * $p < 0.05$ vs. Ctrl.

Feeding OVX mice with a high-fat diet causes liver damage, indicated by an increase in the level of liver damage markers such as serum AST and ALT [30]. In this study, the serum AST and ALT levels increased in the OVX Ctrl rats compared to sham rats and decreased after BCE intake; however, the differences were not significant. Furthermore, there was no change in the serum level of the liver damage marker γ-GT (Supplementary Table S1).

Fat accumulation is known to cause liver fibrosis and weight increase, and blackcurrant was effective in preventing obesity-induced NASH caused by high-fat diet consumption in a previous study [21]. However, severe fibrosis progression (Figure 3A,C) and an increase in liver weight (Supplementary Figure S1) in the OVX Ctrl rats was not observed in this study. Only mild liver inflammation was observed because no high-fat diet was fed. However, BCE intake alleviated liver steatosis progression and the expression of inflammatory genes such as *TNF-α*, *IL-6*, and *IL-1β* in the

OVX rats, speculating that daily intake of BCE was effective in preventing NAFLD and NASH in this non-high-fat diet menopausal model rat.

This study used OVX rats as a menopausal dyslipidemia model, and BCE reduced this dyslipidemia. Since we have previously found that BCE has an effect of phytoestrogens [15,16,18–20], it is speculated that BCE may alleviate menopausal dyslipidemia via estrogen signaling. On the other hand, the ingestion of a high-fat food promotes oxidative stress [40,41] and induces dyslipidemia, and it is known that anthocyanins [42,43] and polyphenols [44] have antioxidant potentials and have an effect of reducing dyslipidemia. Polyphenols, such as flavanone [45] and resveratrol [46], as activators of the nuclear receptor, peroxisome proliferator-activated receptor γ, are known to promote adipocyte differentiation. Anthocyanins are also known to bind to some nuclear receptors [47]. Therefore, BCE may function in this menopausal dyslipidemia in addition to its effect as a phytoestrogen, and it is necessary to study this further.

4. Conclusions

So far, it has been known that BCE has a phytoestrogen effect, but it is unknown whether it has an effect on menopausal lipid abnormalities. In this study, increased body weights, fat weights, and adipocyte diameters in OVX rats were reduced by the ingestion of BCE. In addition, serum lipids, such as triglyceride and cholesterol, were also reduced. Furthermore, hepatic steatosis and levels of TNF-α, IL-6, IL-1β inflammatory genes increased in OVX rats, but were reduced after BCE intake. This is the first report to show that BCE intake is effective in preventing lipid metabolism abnormality and liver steatosis in menopausal model rats. The results of this study suggest that daily BCE intake is effective in preventing lipid metabolism abnormalities in rats with low estrogen secretion; however, these results should be confirmed in studies with menopausal women to warrant its future use in clinical settings.

Supplementary Materials: The following are available online at http://www.mdpi.com/2072-6643/12/5/1541/s1, Table S1: Serum glucose and liver injury marker levels of OVX Ctrl and sham (sham) rats fed with regular diet and OVX rats treated with BCE diet (OVX BCE) for 3 months. Figure S1: Effect of BCE on rat liver weight.

Author Contributions: N.N. and K.H. designed the study; N.N., K.H., T.T., and M.K. performed the experiments and analyzed the data; N.N., K.H., and H.M. acquired funding; N.N. and K.Y. cared for the animals; N.N. and K.H. wrote the manuscript; I.O. edited the manuscript. All authors reviewed and approved the manuscript.

Funding: This research was partially supported by the Japan Society for the Promotion of Science KAKENHI (grant number 16K00844, 20K02402), Hirosaki University Grant for Joint Researches Led by Women Researchers, and Interdisciplinary Collaborative Research Grant for Young Scientists, Hirosaki University.

Acknowledgments: We would like to thank Editage (www.editage.jp) for English language editing.

Conflicts of Interest: The authors declare no conflict of interest.

References

1. Quinn, M.A.; Xu, X.; Ronfani, M.; Cidlowski, J.A. Estrogen Deficiency Promotes Hepatic Steatosis via a Glucocorticoid Receptor-Dependent Mechanism in Mice. *Cell Rep.* **2018**, *22*, 2690–2701. [CrossRef]
2. Chen, K.L.; Madak-Erdogan, Z. Estrogens and female liver health. *Steroids* **2018**, *133*, 38–43. [CrossRef]
3. Lobo, R.A. Metabolic syndrome after menopause and the role of hormones. *Maturitas* **2008**, *60*, 10–18. [CrossRef]
4. Barton, M. Cholesterol and atherosclerosis: Modulation by oestrogen. *Curr. Opin. Lipidol.* **2013**, *24*, 214–220. [CrossRef] [PubMed]
5. Cifkova, R.; Krajcoviechova, A. Dyslipidemia and cardiovascular disease in women. *Curr. Cardiol. Rep.* **2015**, *17*, 609. [CrossRef] [PubMed]
6. Barrett-Connor, E. Menopause, atherosclerosis, and coronary artery disease. *Curr. Opin. Pharmacol.* **2013**, *13*, 186–191. [CrossRef] [PubMed]
7. Cohen, D.E.; Fisher, E.A. Lipoprotein metabolism, dyslipidemia, and nonalcoholic fatty liver disease. *Semin. Liver Dis.* **2013**, *33*, 380–388.

8. Anstee, Q.M.; Reeves, H.L.; Kotsiliti, E.; Govaere, O.; Heikenwalder, M. From NASH to HCC: Current concepts and future challenges. *Nat. Rev. Gastroenterol Hepatol.* **2019**, *16*, 411–428. [CrossRef]
9. Palmisano, B.T.; Zhu, L.; Stafford, J.M. Role of Estrogens in the Regulation of Liver Lipid Metabolism. *Adv. Exp. Med Biol.* **2017**, *1043*, 227–256.
10. Mahmoud, A.M.; Yang, W.; Bosland, M.C. Soy isoflavones and prostate cancer: A review of molecular mechanisms. *J. Steroid Biochem. Mol. Biol.* **2014**, *140*, 116–132. [CrossRef]
11. Lee, Y.M.; Kim, J.B.; Bae, J.H.; Lee, J.S.; Kim, P.S.; Jang, H.H.; Kim, H.R. Estrogen-like activity of aqueous extract from Agrimonia pilosa Ledeb. in MCF-7 cells. *BMC Complement. Altern. Med.* **2012**, *12*, 260. [CrossRef] [PubMed]
12. Guo, D.; Wang, J.; Wang, X.; Luo, H.; Zhang, H.; Cao, D.; Chen, L.; Huang, N. Double directional adjusting estrogenic effect of naringin from Rhizoma drynariae (Gusuibu). *J. Ethnopharmacol.* **2011**, *138*, 451–457. [CrossRef] [PubMed]
13. Limer, J.L.; Speirs, V. Phyto-oestrogens and breast cancer chemoprevention. *Breast Cancer Res.* **2004**, *6*, 119–127. [CrossRef] [PubMed]
14. Knight, D.C.; Eden, J.A. Phytoestrogens—A short review. *Maturitas* **1995**, *22*, 167–175. [CrossRef]
15. Nanashima, N.; Horie, K.; Maeda, H. Phytoestrogenic Activity of Blackcurrant Anthocyanins Is Partially Mediated through Estrogen Receptor Beta. *Molecules* **2017**, *23*, 74. [CrossRef]
16. Nanashima, N.; Horie, K.; Tomisawa, T.; Chiba, M.; Nakano, M.; Fujita, T.; Maeda, H.; Kitajima, M.; Takamagi, S.; Uchiyama, D.; et al. Phytoestrogenic activity of blackcurrant (Ribes nigrum) anthocyanins is mediated through estrogen receptor alpha. *Mol. Nutr. Food Res.* **2015**, *59*, 2419–2431. [CrossRef]
17. Gopalan, A.; Reuben, S.C.; Ahmed, S.; Darvesh, A.S.; Hohmann, J.; Bishayee, A. The health benefits of blackcurrants. *Food Funct.* **2012**, *3*, 795–809. [CrossRef]
18. Nanashima, N.; Horie, K.; Maeda, H.; Tomisawa, T.; Kitajima, M.; Nakamura, T. Blackcurrant Anthocyanins Increase the Levels of Collagen, Elastin, and Hyaluronic Acid in Human Skin Fibroblasts and Ovariectomized Rats. *Nutrients* **2018**, *10*, 495. [CrossRef]
19. Nanashima, N.; Horie, K. Blackcurrant Extract with Phytoestrogen Activity Alleviates Hair Loss in Ovariectomized Rats. *Molecules* **2019**, *24*, 1272. [CrossRef]
20. Horie, K.; Nanashima, N.; Maeda, H. Phytoestrogenic Effects of Blackcurrant Anthocyanins Increased Endothelial Nitric Oxide Synthase (eNOS) Expression in Human Endothelial Cells and Ovariectomized Rats. *Molecules* **2019**, *24*, 1259. [CrossRef]
21. Lee, Y.; Pham, T.X.; Bae, M.; Hu, S.; O'Neill, E.; Chun, O.K.; Han, M.J.; Koo, S.I.; Park, Y.K.; Lee, J.Y. Blackcurrant (*Ribes nigrum*) Prevents Obesity-Induced Nonalcoholic Steatohepatitis in Mice. *Obesity* **2019**, *27*, 112–120. [CrossRef] [PubMed]
22. Benn, T.; Kim, B.; Park, Y.K.; Yang, Y.; Pham, T.X.; Ku, C.S.; Farruggia, C.; Harness, E.; Smyth, J.A.; Lee, J.Y. Polyphenol-rich blackcurrant extract exerts hypocholesterolaemic and hypoglycaemic effects in mice fed a diet containing high fat and cholesterol. *Br. J. Nutr.* **2015**, *113*, 1697–1703. [CrossRef] [PubMed]
23. Kleiner, D.E.; Brunt, E.M.; Van Natta, M.; Behling, C.; Contos, M.J.; Cummings, O.W.; Ferrell, L.D.; Liu, Y.C.; Torbenson, M.S.; Unalp-Arida, A.; et al. Nonalcoholic Steatohepatitis Clinical Research, N. Design and validation of a histological scoring system for nonalcoholic fatty liver disease. *Hepatology* **2005**, *41*, 1313–1321. [CrossRef]
24. Li, H.B.; Qin, D.N.; Cheng, K.; Su, Q.; Miao, Y.W.; Guo, J.; Zhang, M.; Zhu, G.Q.; Kang, Y.M. Central blockade of salusin beta attenuates hypertension and hypothalamic inflammation in spontaneously hypertensive rats. *Sci. Rep.* **2015**, *5*, 11162. [CrossRef] [PubMed]
25. Livak, K.J.; Schmittgen, T.D. Analysis of relative gene expression data using real-time quantitative PCR and the 2(-Delta Delta C(T)) Method. *Methods* **2001**, *25*, 402–408. [CrossRef] [PubMed]
26. Hirschberg, A.L. Sex hormones, appetite and eating behaviour in women. *Maturitas* **2012**, *71*, 248–256. [CrossRef] [PubMed]
27. Nair, A.B.; Jacob, S. A simple practice guide for dose conversion between animals and human. *J. Basic Clin. Pharm.* **2016**, *7*, 27–31. [CrossRef]
28. D'Eon, T.M.; Souza, S.C.; Aronovitz, M.; Obin, M.S.; Fried, S.K.; Greenberg, A.S. Estrogen regulation of adiposity and fuel partitioning. Evidence of genomic and non-genomic regulation of lipogenic and oxidative pathways. *J. Biol. Chem.* **2005**, *280*, 35983–35991. [CrossRef]

29. Sutjarit, N.; Sueajai, J.; Boonmuen, N.; Sornkaew, N.; Suksamrarn, A.; Tuchinda, P.; Zhu, W.; Weerachayaphorn, J.; Piyachaturawat, P. Curcuma comosa reduces visceral adipose tissue and improves dyslipidemia in ovariectomized rats. *J. Ethnopharmacol.* **2018**, *215*, 167–175. [CrossRef]
30. Kim, J.; Lee, H.; Lim, J.; Lee, H.; Yoon, S.; Shin, S.S.; Yoon, M. The lemon balm extract ALS-L1023 inhibits obesity and nonalcoholic fatty liver disease in female ovariectomized mice. *Food Chem. Toxicol.* **2017**, *106*, 292–305. [CrossRef]
31. Ambikairajah, A.; Walsh, E.; Cherbuin, N. Lipid profile differences during menopause: A review with meta-analysis. *Menopause* **2019**, *26*, 1327–1333. [CrossRef] [PubMed]
32. Jeong, Y.H.; Hur, H.J.; Jeon, E.J.; Park, S.J.; Hwang, J.T.; Lee, A.S.; Lee, K.W.; Sung, M.J. Honokiol Improves Liver Steatosis in Ovariectomized Mice. *Molecules* **2018**, *23*, 194. [CrossRef] [PubMed]
33. Min, W.; Fang, P.; Huang, G.; Shi, M.; Zhang, Z. The decline of whole-body glucose metabolism in ovariectomized rats. *Exp. Gerontol.* **2018**, *113*, 106–112. [CrossRef] [PubMed]
34. Wellons, M.F.; Matthews, J.J.; Kim, C. Ovarian aging in women with diabetes: An overview. *Maturitas* **2017**, *96*, 109–113. [CrossRef]
35. Yanai, H.; Yoshida, H. Beneficial Effects of Adiponectin on Glucose and Lipid Metabolism and Atherosclerotic Progression: Mechanisms and Perspectives. *Int. J. Mol. Sci.* **2019**, *20*, 1190. [CrossRef]
36. Landecho, M.F.; Tuero, C.; Valenti, V.; Bilbao, I.; de la Higuera, M.; Fruhbeck, G. Relevance of Leptin and Other Adipokines in Obesity-Associated Cardiovascular Risk. *Nutrients* **2019**, *11*, 2664. [CrossRef]
37. Nag, S.; Khan, M.A.; Samuel, P.; Ali, Q.; Hussain, T. Chronic angiotensin AT2R activation prevents high-fat diet-induced adiposity and obesity in female mice independent of estrogen. *Metabolism* **2015**, *64*, 814–825. [CrossRef]
38. Moorthy, K.; Yadav, U.C.; Mantha, A.K.; Cowsik, S.M.; Sharma, D.; Basir, S.F.; Baquer, N.Z. Estradiol and progesterone treatments change the lipid profile in naturally menopausal rats from different age groups. *Biogerontology* **2004**, *5*, 411–419. [CrossRef]
39. Combs, T.P.; Berg, A.H.; Rajala, M.W.; Klebanov, S.; Iyengar, P.; Jimenez-Chillaron, J.C.; Patti, M.E.; Klein, S.L.; Weinstein, R.S.; Scherer, P.E. Sexual differentiation, pregnancy, calorie restriction, and aging affect the adipocyte-specific secretory protein adiponectin. *Diabetes* **2003**, *52*, 268–276. [CrossRef]
40. Wang, J.P.; Cui, R.Y.; Zhang, K.Y.; Ding, X.M.; Luo, Y.H.; Bai, S.P.; Zeng, Q.F.; Xuan, Y.; Su, Z.W. High-Fat Diet Increased Renal and Hepatic Oxidative Stress Induced by Vanadium of Wistar Rat. *Biol. Trace Elem. Res.* **2016**, *170*, 415–423. [CrossRef]
41. Tan, B.L.; Norhaizan, M.E. Effect of High-Fat Diets on Oxidative Stress, Cellular Inflammatory Response and Cognitive Function. *Nutrients* **2019**, *11*, 2579. [CrossRef] [PubMed]
42. Liu, C.; Sun, J.; Lu, Y.; Bo, Y. Effects of Anthocyanin on Serum Lipids in Dyslipidemia Patients: A Systematic Review and Meta-Analysis. *PLoS ONE* **2016**, *11*, e0162089. [CrossRef] [PubMed]
43. Song, H.; Wu, T.; Xu, D.; Chu, Q.; Lin, D.; Zheng, X. Dietary sweet cherry anthocyanins attenuates diet-induced hepatic steatosis by improving hepatic lipid metabolism in mice. *Nutrition* **2016**, *32*, 827–833. [CrossRef] [PubMed]
44. Musolino, V.; Gliozzi, M.; Scarano, F.; Bosco, F.; Scicchitano, M.; Nucera, S.; Carresi, C.; Ruga, S.; Zito, M.C.; Maiuolo, J.; et al. Bergamot Polyphenols Improve Dyslipidemia and Pathophysiological Features in a Mouse Model of Non-Alcoholic Fatty Liver Disease. *Sci. Rep.* **2020**, *10*, 2565. [CrossRef]
45. Saito, T.; Abe, D.; Sekiya, K. Flavanone exhibits PPARgamma ligand activity and enhances differentiation of 3T3-L1 adipocytes. *Biochem. Biophys. Res. Commun.* **2009**, *380*, 281–285. [CrossRef]
46. Hall, J.M.; Powell, H.A.; Rajic, L.; Korach, K.S. The Role of Dietary Phytoestrogens and the Nuclear Receptor PPARgamma in Adipogenesis: An in Vitro Study. *Environ. Health Perspect.* **2019**, *127*, 37007. [CrossRef]
47. Avior, Y.; Bomze, D.; Ramon, O.; Nahmias, Y. Flavonoids as dietary regulators of nuclear receptor activity. *Food Funct.* **2013**, *4*, 831–844. [CrossRef]

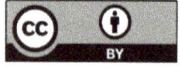

© 2020 by the authors. Licensee MDPI, Basel, Switzerland. This article is an open access article distributed under the terms and conditions of the Creative Commons Attribution (CC BY) license (http://creativecommons.org/licenses/by/4.0/).

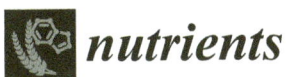

Review

Naturally Occurring PCSK9 Inhibitors

Maria Pia Adorni [1], Francesca Zimetti [2], Maria Giovanna Lupo [3], Massimiliano Ruscica [4] and Nicola Ferri [3,*]

1. Department of Medicine and Surgery-Unit of Neurosciences, University of Parma, 43125 Parma, Italy; mariapia.adorni@unipr.it
2. Dipartimento di Scienze degli Alimenti e del Farmaco, Università di Parma, 43124 Parma, Italy; francesca.zimetti@unipr.it
3. Dipartimento di Scienze del Farmaco, Università degli Studi di Padova, 35121 Padova, Italy; mariagiovanna.lupo@phd.unipd.it
4. Dipartimento di Scienze Farmacologiche e Biomolecolari, Università degli Studi di Milano, 20122 Milan, Italy; massimiliano.ruscica@unimi.it
* Correspondence: nicola.ferri@unipd.it; Tel.: +39-049-827-5080

Received: 20 April 2020; Accepted: 13 May 2020; Published: 16 May 2020

Abstract: Genetic, epidemiological and pharmacological data have led to the conclusion that antagonizing or inhibiting Proprotein convertase subtilisin/kexin type 9 (PCSK9) reduces cardiovascular events. This clinical outcome is mainly related to the pivotal role of PCSK9 in controlling low-density lipoprotein (LDL) cholesterol levels. The absence of oral and affordable anti-PCSK9 medications has limited the beneficial effects of this new therapeutic option. A possible breakthrough in this field may come from the discovery of new naturally occurring PCSK9 inhibitors as a starting point for the development of oral, small molecules, to be used in combination with statins in order to increase the percentage of patients reaching their LDL-cholesterol target levels. In the present review, we have summarized the current knowledge on natural compounds or extracts that have shown an inhibitory effect on PCSK9, either in experimental or clinical settings. When available, the pharmacodynamic and pharmacokinetic profiles of the listed compounds are described.

Keywords: nutraceuticals; PCSK9; SREBP; HNF1α; berberine; cholesterol

---

1. Introduction

Proprotein convertase subtilisin/kexin type 9 (PCSK9) is a pivotal regulator of low-density lipoprotein (LDL) receptor, and thus of LDL-cholesterol levels [1]. PCSK9 is mainly synthesized by the hepatocytes, where it undergoes an autocatalytic cleavage in the endoplasmic reticulum (ER) that allows the release of the mature PCSK9 from the endoplasmic reticulum (ER) to the Golgi [2–5]. PCSK9 is one of the 33 genes regulated by the sterol regulatory element (SRE) binding protein (SREBP) family of transcription factors [6]. When cell cholesterol depletion or inhibition of intracellular synthesis occurs, PCSK9 promoter activity is raised, leading to an increased transcription [7]. A second transcription factor involved in regulation of PCSK9 is the hepatocyte nuclear factor 1α (HNF1α) [8,9]. Once secreted, PCSK9 binds the epidermal growth factor-like repeat homology domain A (EGFA-like) of the LDL receptor (LDLR) through its catalytic domain. This phenomenon fosters the degradation of LDLR in lysosomes, instead of allowing it to recycle on the cell surface. This degrading activity reduces the number of LDLR on hepatocytes, and thus the uptake of circulating LDL particles by the liver. For this reason, PCSK9 genetic gain-of-function (GOF) mutations are associated to hypercholesterolemic conditions, and its pharmacological inhibition has been considered as a new line of intervention for preventing cardiovascular diseases [10–12].

At least two strategies have been developed to reduce PCSK9 plasma levels or to inhibit its binding to the LDLR, i.e., monoclonal antibodies and antisense oligonucleotides [5]. However, an optimal pharmacological strategy to inhibit PCSK9 may involve the identification and development of orally absorbed small molecules with anti-PCSK9 activity. The history of pharmacology has provided compelling evidence of the importance of identifying naturally occurring chemical entities with potential therapeutic activities. For this reason, in the present review, we summarized the current knowledge on natural compounds or extracts that have shown significant PCSK9 inhibitory activity.

2. Berberine

Plants belonging to the genus *Berberis* (Family: *Berberidaceae*) are widely distributed worldwide, with nearly 550 species. Several studies have reported traditional uses *Berberis* for the treatment of metabolic diseases (e.g., diabetes and hyperlipidemia). Various bioactive compounds, such as alkaloids, polyphenols, flavonoids, anthocyanins, etc., have been found in *Berberis* species.

Berberine, originally isolated from *Huanglian* (*Coptis chinensis*, Franch. *ranunculaceae*), is a quaternary ammonium salt belonging to a group of benzylisoquinoline alkaloids (Table 1). The chemical name of berberine is 5,6-dihydro-9,10-dimethoxybenzo[g]-1,3-benzodioxolo[5,6-α]quinolizinium. *Berberine* is the most active compound reported from *Berberis* species, and it is considered to be highly effective against diabetes and other metabolic diseases [13–15]. Berberine is present in roots, rhizomes, and stem bark of *Berberis*, and in other species of flowering plants *like Coptis rhizomes* and *Hydrastis Canadensis* [16].

The mechanism of action of the lipid-lowering effect of berberine was identified by screening 700 Chinese herbs with potential induction effect on LDLR expression [17]. Among different compounds tested, berberine showed the highest activity in increasing LDLR expression, suggesting a mechanism similar to hydroxymethylglutaryl-coenzyme A (HMG-CoA) reductase inhibitors, statins. However, berberine increases messenger ribonucleic acid (mRNA) and protein, as well as the function of hepatic LDLR, independently from the intracellular cholesterol levels. Thus, the upregulation of the LDLR, that is mediated by the activation of the transcription factor sterol regulatory element binding proteins (SREBPs) [18], is not involved in the action of berberine. Further investigation of the biological action of berberine led to the discovery that this natural compound prolongs the mRNA stability of LDLR approximately threefold (from 64 to 198 min).

After the discovery of the role of PCSK9 on LDLR, experimental studies were carried out in order to investigate if PCSK9 was involved in the mechanism of action of berberine. As previously described, the gene transcription of PCSK9 is mainly regulated by SREBP. However, key SRE motifs are usually adjacent to Sp1 (specific protein 1) or NF-Y (nuclear transcription factor Y) binding sites, and SREBPs work in concert with these coactivators to induce full transactivation. In this regard, the PCSK9 promoter has a unique sequence, with an HNF1 binding site, adjacent to SRE, as a critical regulatory sequence motif. HNF1α is, indeed, the predominant working partner for SREBP2 in the regulation of PCSK9 gene.

Starting from these relevant structural differences between the promoters of LDLR and PCSK9, berberine was shown to strongly reduce the PCSK9 mRNA levels in a time- and concentration-dependent manner [19]. This inhibitory effect is also independent from the SREBP pathway but related to HNF1α [9]. More interestingly, berberine inhibits PCSK9 protein expression and counteracts the inducing effect of various statins [9]. Indeed, berberine significantly reduced the expression of HNF1α (−60%), and only slightly of SREBP2 [9]. This effect is sufficient to block PCSK9 transcription without affecting LDLR expression. The synergy between SREBP2 and HNF1α is beneficial for LDLR expression, because SREBP2 is absolutely required for LDLR transcription. The fact that berberine increases LDLR protein level, both in vitro and in vivo [17,20,21], suggests that the balanced effects are in favor of LDLR mRNA stability. A more detailed study was conducted to investigate the mechanism underlying the inhibitory effect of berberine on HNF1α-mediated PCSK9 transcription. By using the proteasome inhibitor bortezomib, Dong et al. demonstrated that berberine accelerates the degradation of HNF1α by proteasome pathway. Thus, by blocking proteasome, the effect of berberine is antagonized, determining an increase of PCSK9 levels and a reduction of LDLR expression [22].

Finally, results from hamster experiments suggest that the effect of berberine on LDLR and plasma cholesterol is mainly derived from a systemic action, rather than an inhibition of gastrointestinal cholesterol absorption. These conclusions derive from the observation that intraperitoneal administration of berberine (20 mg/kg) has a stronger lipid-lowering effect than oral administration (100 mg/kg), and that oral berberine did not increase fecal lipids [21]. These results are particularly important considering that oral bioavailability of berberine is estimated to be around 0.37% [23]. In humans, the maximum concentration (Cmax) of berberine in plasma was measured at 0.4 ng/mL, after a single oral dose of 400 mg [24]. Intestinal first-pass elimination of berberine is considered the major barrier of its oral bioavailability, and that its high extraction and distribution in the liver could be other important factors that lead to its low plasma levels in rats. After intragastric dosing, berberine is widely distributed into various tissues, including liver, heart, kidney, spleen, lung, and even brain, with the liver being the most predominant organ, in which the mean level of berberine was approximately 70-fold greater than that in plasma [23].

Beyond the unfavorable physicochemical properties, a second factor that may negatively impact on the oral bioavailability of berberine is the fact that this compound is a substrate of some membrane transporters, including the P-glycoprotein (P-gp) and multidrug resistance protein 1 (MRP1) [25]. These transporters may limit berberine absorption by extruding it from the enterocytes.

At least four metabolites of berberine have been identified. Berberine phase I metabolites M1 via demethylation, M2 via demethylenation, and M3 (jatrorrhizine), from which derive phase II metabolites that are the corresponding glucuronide conjugates of M1, M2, and M3, respectively [23]. The unconjugated metabolites are the major forms present in tissues, including liver, heart, and kidney; however, glucuronides of phase I metabolites of berberine were the major forms in plasma after oral intake.

2.1. In Vitro Studies

The in vitro model utilized to predict the hypocholesterolemic action of nutraceuticals mainly involve the use of hepatoma cell line HepG2 or Huh7. The first report showing the effect of berberine on PCSK9 demonstrated that berberine, at concentration of 15 μg/mL (44 μM), reduced the amount of PCSK9 mRNA by 77%. Time course experiments demonstrated that berberine reduced PCSK9 mRNA within 8 h of incubation and reached a significant reduction at 12 h and 24 h (65% and 61%, respectively). The amount of PCSK9 secreted into the media of HepG2 cells treated with 15 μg/mL was reduced by 87% [19]. Under the same experimental condition, berberine increased the LDLR mRNA expression after 12 h and 24 h 1.9-fold and 2.1-fold, respectively [19]. Very similar results were observed by Li et al., with a significant reduction of PCSK9 levels at 12 h (−30%) in berberine-treated cells down to 23% after 48 h at the concentration of 20 μM (6.7 μg/mL) [9]. These studies also confirmed the antagonist effect of berberine on statin-induced PCSK9 mRNA levels [19].

When the analysis was extended to other genes involved in cholesterol homeostasis, berberine was shown to reduce the level of HMG-CoA reductase mRNA by 39%, without any significant effect on farnesyl-diphosphate synthase (FDPS) and 7-dehydrocholesterol reductase (DHCR7) mRNA, two enzymes involved in the synthesis of cholesterol. The same analysis conducted on non-SRE containing genes involved in lipid metabolism demonstrated that berberine increased the amounts of peroxisome proliferator-activated receptors alpha (PPARα) mRNA by 39% ($p < 0.05$), and SREBP2 mRNA by 74% ($p < 0.05$). These data demonstrated that there are no consistent effects of berberine on mRNA expression of genes with or without an SRE. Thus, berberine-mediated reduction in PCSK9 mRNA level does not involve the SREBP pathway. In addition, by using actinomycin D, berberine was shown to not alter the mRNA stability of PCSK9 while reducing its promoter activity [19].

Berberine metabolites can exert an extracellular signal-regulated kinase (ERK)-dependent PCSK9-lowering action, with berberrubine (M1) and its analogs being the most powerful [26].

2.2. In Vivo Studies

The first in vivo evidence of a lipid-lowering effect by berberine was reported in 2004 in hamsters fed high-fat and high-cholesterol diet (10% lard, 10% egg yolk powder and 1% cholesterol) [17]. This animal model was chosen since the kinetics of hepatic LDLR-mediated LDL clearance have been well characterized [27]. Treatment of these hyperlipidemic animals with berberine determined a time and dose-dependent reduction of total and LDL-cholesterol levels. According to the LDL kinetics, the effect on LDL-cholesterol was observed after 7 days of treatment, and at day 10 berberine reduced LDL-cholesterol by 26% and 42%, at a dose of 50 and 100 mg/kg/d, respectively. This effect was associated with increased LDLR mRNA (3.5-fold) and protein (2.6-fold) expressions in the liver [17]. However, the first in vivo report on the effect of berberine on PCSK9 derives from the analysis conducted in dyslipidemic C57BL/6 mice, in response to LPS-induced inflammation [28]. Berberine was given by oral gavage at the dose of 10 or 30 mg/kg per day and showed a significant and dose-dependent reduction of PCSK9 mRNA levels, induced by LPS, in the liver. This effect was associated with a significant increase of the LDLR mRNA [28]. Thus, although the animal model utilized cannot be consider optimal for studying the lipid-lowering properties of new agents, the data confirmed the in vitro analysis and reinforced the concept that berberine reduces PCSK9 transcription.

In contrast, different results were reported in a second study conducted in rats fed a high-fat diet (47% calories from fat, 20% calories from protein, 33% calories from carbohydrate) for 6 weeks [29]. 400 mg/kg/day of oral berberine significantly reduced LDL-cholesterol (−45%) and increased high-density lipoprotein (HDL) cholesterol (+45%), resulting in unchanged total cholesterol (TC) levels. Surprisingly, in response to high-fat diet, a significant increase of plasma levels of PCSK9 was observed, values that were further augmented in response to berberine (almost twofold higher) [29]. Similar trend was observed with simvastatin, utilized as control treated group.

To further investigate the effect of berberine on PCSK9, a third study was conducted in a similar model of hypercholesterolemic rats [30]. Rats were fed a high-fat diet (20% lard, 5% egg yolk powder, 2% cholesterol, 0.3% bile salts, and 0.2% Prothiucil) for 4 weeks, and then treated with berberine, at the dose of 156 mg/kg/day, by oral gavage once a day for 8 weeks. Berberine reduced TC, triglycerides (TG) and LDL-cholesterol by 68%, 66% and 83%, respectively. Interestingly, a berberine derivative, 8-hydroxydihydroberberine, considered to have a higher bioavailability than berberine, produced the same lipid-lowering effect when used at one fourth of the dose of berberine [30]. In this experimental model, a significant reduction of PCSK9 in the liver was found in berberine-treated animals compared to hypercholesterolemic controls [30].

Thus, it is possible to conclude that the animal models utilized had contrasting results, and are potentially not predictive of the human situation, where substantial differences on lipid metabolism are recognized.

2.3. Cilinical Studies

The first study that evaluated the effect of berberine in a Chinese population of hypercholesterolemic patients reported a significant cholesterol-lowering effect, with a 25% reduction of LDL-cholesterol and 35% of TG [17]; these effects were more evident in subjects that were not under therapy with other lipid-lowering drugs. The lipid-lowering effect of berberine was then evaluated in at least three meta-analyses [13,14,31]. The dose of berberine utilized in these studies was between 0.5 g and 1.5 g/day. The results clearly demonstrated that berberine reduces the LDL-cholesterol by approximately 25 mg/deciliter (dL) in patients with hypercholesterolemia and/or type 2 diabetes mellitus (T2DM). This variation was accompanied by a significant reduction in TG levels and a modest increase, albeit significant, of HDL-cholesterol levels [13,14,31].

Clinical evidence of the effect of berberine on circulating PCSK9 levels derives exclusively from studies conducted with combinations of nutraceuticals. For instance, the treatment of dyslipidemic subjects for 4 weeks with a nutraceutical formulation containing red yeast rice (monacolin K 3.3 mg), berberine 531.25 mg and leaf extract of *Morus alba* 200 mg, did not modify PCSK9 plasma levels [32].

The authors speculated that monacolin K, the statin produced by *Monascus purpureus* present in this combination, should increase plasma PCSK9 [33], and this effect may have been counteracted by the presence of berberine, a well-known negative modulator of PCSK9, as well as potentially by leaf extract of *Morus alba* [34]. Very similar results were observed in a double blind, randomized, placebo-controlled study that investigated the lipid-lowering effect of 12 weeks treatment with a nutraceutical containing chitosan, red yeast rice, and berberine, in individuals with hypercholesterolemia [35]. As expected, the treatment significantly reduced non-HDL-cholesterol and LDL-cholesterol compared to the placebo, while no changes were observed in PCSK9 plasma levels [35], further supporting the counteracting effect of berberine on monacolin K. On the contrary, the treatment of hypercholesterolemic patients with a nutraceutical combination of monacolin K, berberine, and silymarin determined a significant increase of PCSK9 plasma levels after 8 weeks [36]. This effect is likely due to the use of a different ratio of the monacolin and berberine doses, resulting in the increasing effect on PCSK9.

In an additional study, conducted in genotype-confirmed heterozygous familial hypercholesterolemic (HeFH) patients treated with statins or statins/ezetimibe combination, the supplementation with a nutraceutical containing berberine induced a further 10.5% reduction of plasma LDL-cholesterol level [37]. The mechanisms underlying this effect might consist of: (*i*) an increased expression of LDLR, encoded by the wild-type allele, coupled with their prolonged half-life; and/or (*ii*) a reduced expression of PCSK9. Unfortunately, in this study the levels of PCSK9 were not measured. However, the authors observed an inverse correlation between the reduction of LDL-cholesterol levels obtained with statins or statins/ezetimibe and the additional decrease induced by berberine [37]. Interestingly, a direct relationship between the hypolipidemic effect of statins and increased levels of PCSK9 has been observed [38,39], and the above-mentioned inverse correlation might be explained by the berberine-mediated inhibition of PCSK9.

Although berberine is usually very well tolerated at doses up to 1 mg per day, among its possible side effects are constipation, diarrhea, abdominal distension, and bitter taste. However, these effects were observed mainly in trials conducted with the highest doses [31]. It is also important to know that long-term administration of berberine was shown to reduce the activity of CYP2D6, CYP2D9 and CYP3A4 in healthy subjects [40], effects potentially associated with drug—drug interactions.

Another aspect needing further investigation is related to the bioavailability of different berberine preparations. Although it seems clear that berberine supplementation produces favorable effects on lipid metabolism, it is equally true that absorption of intestinal berberine is often minor and has a wide inter-individual variability [23,24]. This aspect could determine a high variability of the efficacy of the nutraceutical.

In this regard, several attempts have been pursued in order to improve the bioavailability of berberine, including the synthesis of non-natural derivatives [30,41], as well as drug delivery nanotechnology [42,43]. For instance, the synthetic derivative 8-hydroxy-dihydroberberine can produce similar lipid-lowering effects to berberine when only a quarter of the original dosage of berberine is administered, thus suggesting a better pharmacokinetic profile [30]. A second approach was based on the synthesis of a new series of indole-containing tetrahydroprotoberberine [41]. This study led to the identification of a new compound with potent inhibitory PCSK9 activity, that promoted LDL-cholesterol uptake in HepG2 cells and had an oral bioavailability of 21.9% [41]. This compound also showed a significant in vivo hypolipidemic potency in hamsters fed a high fat diet (0.5% cholesterol), when administered at the daily dose of 30 mg/kg [41].

To improve berberine bioavailability, Ochin and Garelnabi developed a new formulation consisting of the encapsulation of the compound within PLGA-PEG nanoparticles to negatively modulate PCSK9 [42]. Although this formulation was shown to be active in reducing PCSK9 expression in vitro, a direct comparison to berberine with in vivo evidence of a better oral bioavailability is still missing. Moreover, in vivo evidence of improved activity of berberine was recently reported with rational designed micelle (CTA-Mic) developed for an effective liver deposition of berberine. This new formulation has excellent in vivo lipid-lowering activity, although the authors did not provide data on PCSK9 levels [43].

3. Sterol/Stanols and Vegetable Proteins

Among available dietary supplements/substituents for cholesterol reduction, plant sterols/stanols have one of the widest uses [44]. There are, however, no clear data on these compounds, essentially showing no activity on PCSK9 levels and, in any case, they are not conclusive. Two groups have investigated the involvement of PCSK9 in the LDL-C lowering effect of plant stanols intake [45]. Simonen et al., in a randomized controlled double-blind trial in normal and hypercholesterolemic subjects, evaluated the effect of a 6 months consumption of vegetable-oil spread (20 g/day), enriched (plant stanol group) or not (control group) with plant stanols (3 g/day) as ester. The long-term intake of plant stanol esters reduced LDL-C by 7–10%, without affecting either PCSK9 plasma concentrations or the hepatic LDLR levels, indicating that plant stanol esters can lower LDL-C through inhibition of cholesterol absorption, without interfering with PCSK9 metabolism [46]. De Smet et al. showed that an acute intake of plant stanol esters (0.25 mg cholesterol + 50 mg plant stanol esters dissolved in olive oil) in mice up-regulated mRNA expression of intestinal PCSK9 and LDLR, and their main transcription factor SREBP-2, whereas hepatic expression of these genes was down-regulated after 15 min following oral intake. In parallel, reduced intestinal cholesterol absorption and decreased plasma LDL-C levels occurred [47].

Several food peptides from vegetable sources exert instead a cholesterol-lowering activity by a physical interaction with bile acid micelles [48]. These again show, however, no activity on PCSK9. A more interesting case is instead that of food peptides lowering LDL-cholesterol by statin-like mechanisms. This is the case of both soy and lupin peptide mixtures, achieving inhibition of HMG-CoA reductase activity of > 50% at 0.5 mg/mL levels [49]. A similar mechanism has been reported for soy β-conglycinin [50]. In addition, hempseed peptides (from *Cannabis sativa* L. Cannabaceae) appear to exert a hypocholesterolemic activity by a statin-like mechanism [51]. The mechanism of the HMG-CoA reductase inhibition was postulated for some peptides (TPMASD, HFKW and PMAS), based on molecular docking studies and enzyme assays, consistent with 3-dimensional similarity to statins [52]; the inhibitory activity was however far lower than the nanomolar IC_{50} values of known statins.

3.1. Lupin

Lupin is a protein-rich grain legume, is commonly represented by four domestic species, i.e., *Lupinus albus* (white lupin), *L. luteus* (yellow lupin), *L. mutabilis* (pearl lupin) and *L. angustifolius* (sweet leaf lupin; Fabaceae). Lupin proteins have been studied for a number of years mainly for their activity on plasma cholesterol reduction, attributable in large part to an LDLR-activating mechanism [53]. In animal models, lupin proteins have displayed hypolipidemic and a remarkable antiatherosclerotic effect [54]. Clinically, lupin proteins have been tested predominantly in hypercholesterolemic patients, with a positive effect on LDL-cholesterol and on the LDL:HDL cholesterol ratio shown in two studies, one with supplementation [55] and the other with diet enrichment [56]. Conversely, lupin protein combinations with cellulose led to a remarkable hypocholesterolemic effect [57], with a concomitant reduction of PCSK9 plasma levels (−8.5% vs. control) [58]. This trend was further confirmed in another randomized trial, on metabolic syndrome patients, in whom the dietary intervention with lupin proteins led to an 8% drop in LDL-cholesterol, with a decrease of 12.7% (vs. baseline) of PCSK9 levels [59]. Very recently, a mechanism has been hypothesized, i.e., in HepG2 cells, lupin proteins decrease both PCSK9 and HNF1α protein levels (Figure 1) [60]. In addition, lupin protein-derived peptides were found to inhibit the interaction between PCSK9 and LDLR, with the peptide LILPKHSDAD generated from lupin β-2 conglutin being the best candidate (Figure 1 and Table 1). This peptide dose-dependently inhibits PCSK9-LDLR binding, thus increasing LDL-uptake in HepG2 cells [61]. Besides inhibiting this interaction, these peptides have been found to lower the expression level of PCSK9 protein, thus reducing circulating enzyme levels. Thus, two main hypotheses could explain the activity of lupin proteins on PCSK9: (*i*) inhibition of protein–protein interaction between PCSK9 and the LDLR [61]; and (*ii*) reduced protein expression of HNF1α [58], at least in HepG2 cells (Figure 1).

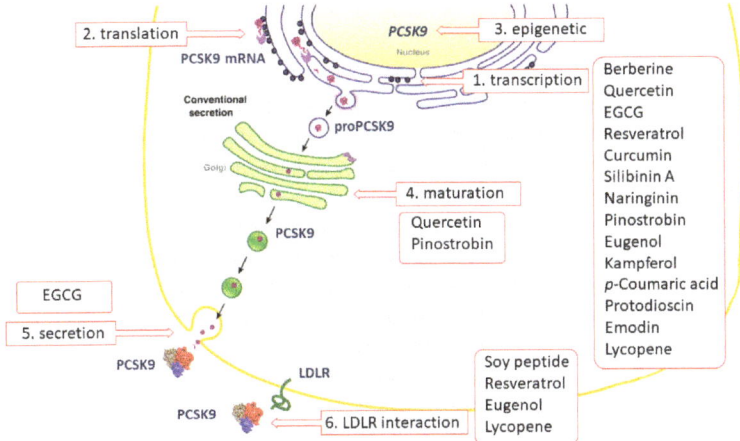

Figure 1. Schematic representation of the to-date-known mechanism of action of natural Proprotein convertase subtilisin/kexin type 9 (PCSK9) inhibitors.

This novel inhibitory pathway of functional foods, related to both the LDLR upregulation and possible PCSK9 antagonism, are of major interest these days, and may lead to new approaches to cardiovascular prevention.

3.2. Soy Proteins

Soy proteins are the most widely evaluated dietary proteins for metabolic control [62]. Proteins from *Glycine max* are the prototype plant proteins and, as such, have reached the attention, as reported in a recent position paper [63], on the effects of plant vs. animal protein sources on cholesterol reduction. The intake of active daily soy doses, in a range of 30 g, leads to an LDL-cholesterol reduction between 3% and 10%, an effect not associated with changes in PCSK9 circulating levels [64].

4. Polyphenols

Polyphenols are plant-derived secondary metabolites found in fruits, vegetables, nuts, seeds, herbs, spices, stems and flowers, as well as in tea and red wine. This class includes a huge number of different molecules such as flavonoids, lignans, stilbenes, and condensed (flavan-3-ol polymers known as proanthocyanidins) or hydrolyzable (such as tannic acid) phenolic polymers [65]. Several epidemiological studies, as well as clinical trials, have reported many cardiovascular benefits of polyphenols, occurring through multiple mechanisms of action, including plasma LDL-cholesterol-lowering activity [66–68]. From the mechanistic side, most of these molecules act by upregulating the LDLR at the hepatic surface, as described for berberine in the above section. This evidence led researchers to investigate the potential influence of polyphenols on PSCK9.

Although some data is available on the effect of polyphenols on PCSK9, it must be remembered that the main problem related to research on polyphenols in vitro is that concentrations of tested compounds are often higher than those detected in vivo, limiting the physiological relevance of these observations. In addition, the extensive metabolism that polyphenols undergo by intestinal microbiota in vivo may generate bioactive compounds, making it very hard to traverse the in vitro findings to the in vivo situation. We critically discussed these aspects that have been deeply reviewed elsewhere [69,70].

4.1. Quercetin

Quercetin [2-(3,4-dihydroxyphenyl)-3,5,7-trihydroxy-4H-chromen-4-one] is a flavonoid ubiquitous in fruit and vegetables (Table 1). Quercetin strongly upregulates the LDLR gene expression in hepatic cells, resulting in increased LDL uptake. This effect seems to be mediated by the activation of the transcription factor SREBP2 [71].

In vitro studies revealed that quercetin in its glicosidated form, incubated with HepG-2 cells at a concentration range from 1 to 10 μM, reduced PCSK9 mRNA levels by 20–30%. In addition, authors observed a 20–90% increase in intracellular PCSK9 levels and a 30–35% reduction in PCSK9 secretion in the culture medium [72]. The latter effect occurred through a negative modulation of sortilin, a protein inducing the cellular secretion of PCSK9 from the trans-Golgi network to the plasma membrane (Figure 1) [73]. Interestingly, quercetin 20 μM affects the expression of PCSK9 not only in hepatic cells, but also in a foam cell macrophages model [74]. This may unravel a direct antiatherogenic and LDL-cholesterol-independent effect of quercetin, since PCSK9 negatively modulates cholesterol metabolism and inflammation in macrophages [75,76]. Differently from hepatic cells and macrophages, quercetin 3-glucoside increased both PCSK9 and LDLR expression in mouse pancreatic cells. However, this was interpreted as a beneficial effect. In fact, the greater increase of PCSK9 relative to LDLR induced by quercetin may prevent cholesterol uptake, thus avoiding cholesterol-dependent dysfunction in these cells [77].

It should be noted that the high concentration of quercetin, and the use of its glicosidated form instead of the free aglycone, the active component, strongly limits the relevance of the above in vitro works. However, similar effects on PCSK9 were also observed in vivo, in which the enzymatic cleavage by the microbiota releases aglycon, which could undergo absorption. In fact, the supplementation with quercetin-3-gucoside (0.05 and 0.1% w/w) in high-cholesterol diet-fed mice reduced PCSK9 circulating levels, leading to increased LDLR expression at the hepatocyte surface. As observed in vitro, the supplementation significantly increased the amount of pancreatic PCSK9 [77]. A reduction of PCSK9 expression, both in liver and aorta, has also been observed after supplementation for 12 weeks with 12.5 mg/kg of quercetin, in apoE$^{-/-}$ mice fed with a high-fat diet, suggesting a anti-atherogenic effect occurring at multiple levels (Figure 1 and Table 1) [78].

Specific clinical evidence of the effect of quercetin on circulating PCSK9 levels is still missing. However, several studies in humans undoubtedly highlighted the cholesterol-lowering properties of this flavonoid. As example, quercetin supplementation has shown to reduce by approximately 12% LDL-C levels, as emerged from a recent meta-analysis of randomized controlled trials [79].

From the pharmacokinetic side, like the most of polyphenols, quercetin is characterized by a poor solubility and low oral absorption, leading to physiological plasma concentrations lower than micromolar levels [80]. Moreover, quercetin is known to be a substrate and inhibitor of the P-gp and of breast cancer resistance protein (BCRP), and this further reduces its bioavailability (Table 1) [81–84]. Quercetin glycosides, the major form present in nature, undergo deglycosylation in the intestine, generating the quercetin-free form that successively is a substrate of liver enzymes [85], responsible for the production of the metabolites quercetin-3-sulfate, quercetin-3'-sulfate, and quercetin-3-glucuronide [86]. Quercetin is also metabolized by gut microbiota into 3,4-dihydroxyphenylacetic acid, 3-(3-hydroxyphenyl) propionic acid, 3,4-dihydroxybenzoic acid and 4-hydroxybenzoic acid [85].

Several formulations have been made to improve polyphenol bioavailability, by enhancing their solubility or preventing their degradation or metabolism [87]. Among them, a novel lecithin-based formulation of quercetin has been tested in healthy volunteers, showing a significant improvement in solubility, and consequently bioavailability [88].

4.2. Epigallocatechin Gallate

Epigallocatechin gallate (EGCG), the most active catechin found in green tea, has shown hypocholesterolemic activity occurring by an increase of LDLR mRNA levels and protein expression in human hepatoma cells line, in an ERK-signaling pathway-dependent manner. Moreover, EGCG reduced the production of apolipoprotein B (apoB), the main protein component of LDL [89]. This effect was shown to be independent of the 67 kDa laminin receptor, the main receptor described for EGCG [90]. Other evidence of the mechanism of action of EGCG is provided by Li and colleagues, who demonstrated EGCG's capacity to inhibit the endogenous cholesterol synthesis via the suppression of SREBP2 with a sirtuin 1/forkhead box protein O1 (SIRT1/FOXO1) signaling pathway-dependent mechanism [91].

A marked reduced secretion of PCSK9 was observed in hepatic cells treated with 25 µM EGCG, with a maximum effect already evident after 3 h of incubation. In the same study, EGCG was able to counteract the inducing effect of lovastatin on PCSK9 secretion (Table 1). These effects were not accompanied by changes in PCSK9 mRNA, or in the intracellular precursor/mature protein level (Figure 1) [92].

Direct evidence of EGCG's effect on circulating PCSK9 in humans is not yet available. However, several studies found a significant association between green tea drinking and lower plasma levels of total and LDL-cholesterol. For instance, the isolated EGCG has shown hypocholesterolemic effects (LDL-cholesterol −9.29%) in healthy subjects [93]. Similarly, the administration for 6 weeks of green tea extract lowered, by about 5%, LDL-cholesterol in overweight and obese women [94].

As discussed for quercetin, the oral bioavailability of EGCG is also low in humans (Table 1) [95]. The administration of 300 mg/day for 4 days, followed by an extra 150 mg the fifth day, led to a mean Cmax of 275.4 µg/mL, with more than sixfold variability among individuals. The reason for such variability is the high rate of metabolism: ECGC is mainly biotransformed in the liver and in the small intestine, leading to methylated, sulfated and glucuronidated metabolites, as well as phenylvalerolactones and phenylvaleric acids, that successively undergo glucuronidation [85,96,97]. The bioavailability of EGCG is also influenced by polymorphism in genes coding for multidrug resistance-associated protein 2 (MRP2) and organic anion transporter polypeptide 1 B1 (OATP1B1), transporters involved in the excretion and uptake of these molecules [98].

4.3. Resveratrol

Resveratrol (3,5,4'-trihydroxy-trans-stilbene) is a non-flavonoid polyphenol first isolated and identified from the roots of *Veratrum grandiflorum (Maxim. ex Miq), O. Loes (Melanthiaceae)*, and it is found in red wine, grapes, and peanuts (Table 1). It was previously demonstrated that red wine polyphenols upregulated LDLR expression and activity, and suppressed the secretion of apolipoprotein B-100 from human HepG2 cells. After this discovery, researchers specifically focused on the mechanism of action of resveratrol, the main bioactive polyphenol, finding a remarkable effect in inducing the transcription of the *LDLR* gene in hepatic cells, specifically occurring through the processing of SREBP, but independently of the adenosine monophosphate-activated protein (AMP) kinase (AMPK)-mediated signaling pathway [99]. Resveratrol also induced LDLR mRNA levels and protein expression in steatotic hepatic cells, by acting on the PCSK9 promoter with a mechanism involving SREBP1c [100]. In the same cells, 20 µM resveratrol reduced the expression of PCSK9 and promoted LDL uptake, with important implications for the pathogenesis of non-alcoholic fatty liver disease (NAFLD), the leading cause of liver damage [100]. The upregulating action on LDLR has been also seen for polydatin (piceid), the resveratrol natural precursor [101]. Indeed, polydatin has shown a potential interfering action on the PCSK9/LDLR interaction, as suggested by an in vitro screening work (Figure 1) [102]. The direct binding of polydatin to the active pocket of PCSK9 has been further highlighted, demonstrating that this interaction occurs through several hydrogen bonds. In the same study, authors found that the treatment with 20 µM of polydatin abrogated the inducing effect of palmitic acid on PCSK9 protein levels in an insulin-resistant hepatic cell model, suggesting a potential beneficial effect of polydatin on T2DM [101]. As discussed for quercetin, a strong limitation of these studies relates to the use of glucosides instead of free aglycone.

The beneficial effect of polydatin in the context of glucose intolerance and diabetes emerged also from in vivo studies: gene and protein expression of PCSK9 was found reduced in the liver and serum of diabetes (db/db) C57BL/6 mice treated with polydatin 100 mg/Kg, 6 d/week for 4 weeks. This effect was accompanied by an improvement in glucose metabolism, by a PCSK9-dependent upregulation of glucokinase (GCK) [101].

Concerning humans, no data are available so far on the effect of resveratrol on PCSK9, and even its efficacy on the lipid profile itself is still debated. The results of a recent metanalysis of 20 studies did not find an association between the administration of resveratrol and the LDL-cholesterol plasma levels, suggesting that the described cardioprotective effects of resveratrol may occur through an influence on other factors beyond lipids [103]. On the other hand, the results of another metanalysis concluded that longer resveratrol intervention trials (≥3 months) led to a significant reduction of plasma LDL-cholesterol [104]. Based on these available data, wider and longer studies are still needed to unequivocally determine the hypocholesterolemic effects of resveratrol.

Resveratrol demonstrates photosensitivity, poor solubility, and rapid metabolism, with negative consequences on bioavailability and bioactivity. The administration of an oral dose of 25 mg of resveratrol in humans resulted in plasma concentration from 1 to 5 nanograms (ng)/mL [105]. Due to its lipophilic nature, resveratrol may accumulate in several tissues and organs such as the brain, liver, and the intestine. About 20 resveratrol-derived metabolites have been reported in human plasma, urine, and human tissues. Among these, resveratrol-3-O-sulfate is reported as the most abundant liver-derived circulating metabolite [106]. Resveratrol and its metabolites may also be biotransformed in the colon by the gut microbiota, leading to generation of dihydroresveratrol [107].

4.4. Other Polyphenols

Few other polyphenolic compounds have demonstrated an influence on PCSK9 from preliminary data obtained in vivo or in vitro. However, data are too scarce and further investigations are needed to better characterize the bioactivity of these compounds with respect to PCSK9. For instance, silibinin A, a flavonolignan, has emerged as a repressor of PCSK9 promoter activity from the results of a drug-screening assay (Figure 1 and Table 1) [108]. In HepG2, increasing concentrations of silibinin A, from 10 to 100 µM, reduced PCSK9 mRNA levels and protein expression in a dose-dependent manner. This activity was dependent on the suppression of the p38 mitogen-activated protein kinase (MAPK) pathway. Importantly, silibinin A was able to attenuate the atorvastatin-induced PCSK9, with a complete counteracting effect observed at 50 µM, suggesting silibinin A as promising agent to abrogate the negative effect of statin on PCSK9 [108,109]. Silibin can be metabolized by both the liver, generating sulfate and glucuronide derivatives [109], and by the gut microbiota, leading to demethylated compounds, as highlighted by an ex vivo study [110].

Naringin, a flavanone-7-O-glycoside (naringenin 7-O-neohesperidoside), isolated from grapefruit and other citrus (Rutaceae), administered at doses of 25, 50 or 100 mg/kg/day for 8 weeks, reduced the hepatic expression of PCSK9, SREBP1 and SREBP2 in obese mice, and the LDLR was consequently induced (Figure 1 and Table 1). Plasma levels of PCSK9 and LDL-cholesterol were also measured and they have been found to both be dose-dependently reduced by naringenin [111]. When orally administered, naringin is hydrolyzed to its aglycon naringenin by hydrolase and intestinal microflora [112]. Naringenin is partly absorbed and then engaged in both phase I and phase II metabolism. Meanwhile, unabsorbed naringenin and the metabolites excreted by the enterohepatic circulation are further degraded into phenolic catabolites by intestinal microbiota [112].

Finally, pinostrobin, a flavanone found in honey and in other plants [*Pinus strobus* L. Pinaceae, *Cajanus cajan* (L.) Millsp., Fabaceae, *Boesenbergia rotunda* (L.) Mansf., and *Boesenbergia pandurata* (Roxb.) Schltr., Zingiberaceae], was studied with respect of its potential influence on PCSK9. The treatment of HepG2 with 20 and 40 µM of pinostrobin led to a dose-dependent reduction of mRNA and protein expression of PCSK9, and a reduction of its catalytic activity, resulting in increased LDLR expression and LDL uptake by the cells [113]. Stereospecific differences in the pharmacokinetic profile of pinostrobin have been observed in rats after iv and oral administrations (Figure 1 and Table 1) [114].

4.5. Eugenol

Eugenol (4-allyl-2-methoxyphenol), a major component of the essential oil of clove [*Syzygium aromaticum* (L.)], is a phenolic nutraceutical with known hypocholesterolemic activities (Table 1). It has been considered as a safe nutrient, with the acceptable daily intake of up to 2.5 mg/kg body weight in humans. Animal studies have shown that eugenol lowers serum cholesterol levels and inhibits lipogenesis in the liver, thus suggesting a protective effect on atherosclerosis and fatty liver disease [115,116]. More recently, a molecular docking analysis revealed hydrophobic interactions between ligand eugenol and PCSK9 (Figure 1) [117]. In addition, eugenol was found to reduce the expression of PCSK9 in Jurkat cells [117]. This effect can be the result of a physical interaction between the two molecules, or an indirect inhibitory effect of eugenol on the SREBP pathway (Figure 1) [115]. The pharmacokinetic profile of eugenol has only been investigated in experimental models (Table 1) [118].

5. Nutrients

5.1. Curcumin

Curcumin [1,7-bis(4-hydroxy-3-methoxyphenyl)-1,6-heptadiene-3,5-dione] is one of the main bioactive polyphenolic components of the spice turmeric, prepared from the rhizome of *Curcuma longa* L. (Zingiberaceae) (Table 1).

Curcumin increased the expression of the LDLR and LDL uptake in HepG2 in a dose- and time-dependent manner. This activity occurred through the activation of the SREBP pathway [119], although this result was not confirmed in other studies [120,121]. More recently, the stimulating effect of curcumin on LDLR expression and activity was further observed, but this increase was not accompanied by changes in *LDLR* transcription and mRNA stability, suggesting a regulation at the transcriptional level [122]. Indeed curcumin 10 and 20 µM for 24 h markedly reduced PCSK9 mRNA and protein expression in hepatic cells. In this work, the transcription factor HNF1α, but not SREBP, was involved in the curcumin-mediated effect on PCSK9. Interestingly, curcumin almost completely abrogated the PCSK9-inducing effect of lovastatin, suggesting that curcumin could counteract the effect of statin on circulating PCSK9 [123] and opening new perspectives on novel nutraceutical cholesterol-lowering combination approaches (Figure 1). However, the higher concentrations of curcumin, although widely used in cell culture system, are higher than what can be achieved in vivo, reducing the relevance of these findings.

The only evidence of curcumin influence on PCSK9 in vivo was reported in 2017. The authors suggest an anti-endotoxemic action of curcumin, that would be able to improve LPS detoxification via the LDLR. In detail, authors observed that treatment of cirrhotic rats with curcumin 200 mg/kg/day for 12 weeks, despite no change in mRNA, induced an increase in LDLR protein expression in their liver. This occurred because of a curcumin-inhibition effect on PCSK9 mRNA and protein level [124].

Although no report is so far available on the influence of curcumin on PCSK9 in humans, several studies have examined the effect on LDL-cholesterol levels. Results of these investigations are controversial [125], reporting weak effect or no change, as suggested by the results of a metanalysis of randomized controlled trials [126]. The reason for this discrepancy may be related to the population studied, to the length of treatment and the type of formulation that can lead to different bioavailability.

Indeed, low poor aqueous solubility, bioavailability, and an unfavorable pharmacokinetic profile, limits curcumin's therapeutic use. In particular, curcumin presents a poor stability under physiological conditions, with a $t_{1/2}$ of less than 10 min [127]. Curcumin and its hepatic-derived metabolites, mainly conjugated with glucuronide, sulfate and glutathione, are further transformed by the gut microbiota, generating more than 10 different molecules, including tetrahydrocurcumin, demethylcurcumin, bisdemethylcurcumin, etc. [128,129]. To overcame curcumin pharmacokinetic issues, several formulation approaches have been proposed, that will need to be tested in appropriate pharmacological studies [130].

5.2. Welsh Onion

Welsh onion (*Allium fistulosum* L., Amaryllidaceae) is a perennial plant that is widely cultivated throughout the world, especially in Asia. The ethanol extract of welsh onion contains 0.5 g/100 g of total fat, and is rich in vitamins B2 (riboflavin, 1.3 mg/100 g), B3 (niacin, 284.3 mg/100 g), B6 (pyridoxine, 5.4 mg/100 g), and B9 (folic acid, 2.2 mg/100 g), and mineral iron (20.8 mg/100 g). In addition, welsh onion contains 0.53 ± 0.02 mg/g of ferulic acid and 0.61 ± 0.01 mg/g of quercetin [131]. A second study confirmed that ferulic acid is the most abundant phenolic compound present in welsh onion extract (0.16 ± 0.01 mg/g of extract), followed by *p*-coumaric acid and kaempferol (0.11 ± 0.01 and 0.10 ± 0.01 mg/g of extract, respectively) [132]. Quercetin was also found in the extract, but the amount was negligible (0.04 ± 0.01 mg/g extract).

In HepG2 cells, welsh onion ethanol extract was shown to control the induction of different genes involved in lipid and cholesterol metabolism in response to lipid-deprived serum [132]. The extract was active at 50 μg/mL up to 200 μg/mL concentration, and effectively controlled LDLR protein expression. Importantly, at the same concentrations, a significant reduction of PCSK9 mRNA levels were also observed [132], suggesting a negative impact on gene transcription. In accordance with this hypothesis, the authors observed a strong reduction of both SREBP2 and HNF1α [132]. Welsh onion ethanol extract also reduced PCSK9 protein expression, determined by western blot analysis of total protein extracts, without any significant changes in the LDLR levels. These data suggest that, despite a significant inhibitory effect on PCSK9, welsh onion did not increase LDLR expression [132].

The ethanol extract was also shown to counteract the induction of PCSK9 by statins, further supporting a negative effect on SREBP or HNF1α-dependent regulation of PCSK9 transcription [132].

Among the active components identified in the extract, kaempferol, quercetin, and *p*-coumaric acid significantly reduced the PCSK9 level under lipid depletion conditions in HepG2 cells, albeit this effect was observed at considerably high in vitro concentrations (40 μM). On the contrary, ferulic acid did not show any significant effect (Figure 1 and Table 1) [132].

The hypolipidemic effect of welsh onion ethanol extract was investigated in C57BL6/J mice fed a high-fat diet (60% of energy as fat, 20% as protein and 20% as carbohydrates) [133]. Welsh onion extract was dissolved in normal saline and was orally administered to the mice at a dose of 400 mg/kg/day for 6.5 weeks. This supplementation lead to a significant reduction of body weight and food intake, with a significant reduction of TG (−46%), TC (−11%) and LDL-cholesterol (−24%) [133]. Interestingly, the authors also observed a reduction in the expression of SREBP1c in the liver, confirming the data obtained in vitro [133] and suggesting a possible effect on PCSK9, although this analysis has not been performed [132].

5.3. Cashew Nuts (Anacardium Occidentale L., Anacardiaceae)

The last guidelines of European Atherosclerosis Society (EAS) and European Society of Cardiology (ESC) clearly state that higher consumption of fruit, non-starchy vegetables, nuts, legumes, fish, vegetable oils, yoghurt and wholegrains, along with a lower intake of red and processed meats, foods higher in refined carbohydrates, and salt, is associated with a lower incidence of cardiovascular (CV) events [134]. These data indicate that the replacement of animal fats with vegetable sources of fats and polyunsaturated fatty acids (PUFAs) may decrease the risk of CV disease (CVD). However, clinical trials relating cashew nuts to cardiovascular disease risk factors, including LDL-cholesterol, are limited to four conflicting studies [135–138]. In one controlled-feeding study conducted on a total of 42 adults as a randomized crossover trial, the addition of 42 g of cashews/day was associated with a significant reduction of PCSK9 plasma levels (270.8 ng/mL vs. 252.6 ng/mL) [135]. This effect was not associated to any significant change of the LDL-cholesterol, and the active component responsible for the inhibition of PCSK9 is still unknown.

5.4. Kenaf

Kenaf (*Hibiscus cannabinus* L., Malvaceae) and defatted kenaf seed meal (DKSM) is a low-cost agricultural waste, but potentially a value-added functional food ingredient with hypocholesterolemic properties [139]. Phenolics and saponins are two major bioactive classes in DKSM that confer superior antioxidant properties compared to common edible flours, i.e., wheat, rice and sweet potato flours [139]. The hypocholesterolemic effect of DKSM was recently tested in rats fed high-fat and cholesterol-containing atherogenic diet, containing either 15% or 30% DKSM. Alternatively, rats were fed with the same diet but supplemented with 2.3% or 4.6% of phenolic-saponin rich extract (PSRE) of DKSM. The main active components detected in DKSM or PSRE were *p*-coumaric acid, caffeic acid, (+)-catechin and gallic acid [139].

Supplementation with DKSM, and the equivalent levels of PSRE, in hypercholesteremic rats for 10 weeks, exhibited substantial atherogenic risk reduction, with reduced levels of total and LDL-cholesterol and increased HDL-cholesterol [139]. DKSM and PSRE reduced HMG-CoA reductase in the liver, and more importantly serum PCSK9 levels. These effects are probably to be attributed to phenolic and saponin components. *p*-Coumaric acid, caffeic acid, (+)-catechin and gallic acid have been reported to exhibit anti-hypercholesterolemic properties in different animal models [140–142]. In particular, saponins appear to interfere with SREBP transcription factor, and are the most likely components that affected PCSK9 expression (Figure 1 and Table 1) [143].

5.5. Vitamin MK7

Vitamin K occurs in two dietary forms, i.e., vitamin K1 (phylloquinone) and vitamin K2 (menaquinones, MK). Vitamin K2 is mainly found in fermented foods such as cheese and "natto", a Japanese soybean product [144]. More than 12 different types of MK-n have been identified, from MK-4 to MK-15, where "n" indicates the number of unsaturated isoprenoid residues linked to the menaquinone (Table 1). MK-7 is produced mainly by submerged fermentation using *Bacillus subtilis* and shows a more favorable pharmacokinetic profile compared to MK-4, including a longer half-life time and higher bioavailability [145]. After its intestinal absorption, vitamin K is solubilized by bile salts and pancreatic juice and packaged into chylomicrons [146]. European experts suggested that the Recommended Daily Intake (RDI) of vitamin K, preferably in the form of vitamin K2, is 200–500 µg/day (200 µg/day for MK7), which is required for optimal carboxylation of extrahepatic γ-carboxyglutamic acid (GLA)-proteins.

The hypocholesterolemic action of vitamin K derives from an old study conducted on chronic renal failure patients treated with continuous ambulatory peritoneal dialysis. Vitamin K2 was administered at very high dose (45 mg daily) for several months, and the biochemical analysis showed that TC concentrations at 3 months were significantly higher than those at 7 months or later. Similar effects were observed on LDL-cholesterol [147].

More recently, we have observed a reduction of TC levels in uremic rats after the administration of a nutraceutical combination named RenaTris®, containing MK-7, magnesium carbonate, and Sucrosomial® Iron [148]. By in vitro experiments conducted in hepatoma cells, it was found that MK7 alone reduces the cholesterol biosynthesis, by potentially affecting an enzymatic step of the mevalonate pathway upstream of the squalene synthase [148]. In response to the inhibition of cholesterol synthesis, MK7 induces LDLR, similarly to statins, and this effect was prevented by the co-incubation with squalene [148]. However, differently from statin, which induces PCSK9 expression, MK7 was shown to suppress PCSK9 synthesis and secretion by hepatoma cells [148]. This is thus very similar to what is observed with berberine, although the mechanism of action of MK7 is still unknown (Table 1).

5.6. Lycopene

Lycopene belongs to the family of the lipid-soluble antioxidants called carotenoids, which are found in fruits and vegetables [149,150] but mainly present in tomatoes, or tomato-containing products, which account for about 80% of total lycopene ingestion (Table 1). Growing evidence points to several beneficial effects of lycopene in the maintenance of CV function and health. Among the carotenoids, lycopene exhibits the highest potent antioxidant activity, but it seems to exert additional cardioprotective functions, such as anti-inflammatory properties, platelet aggregation inhibition and endothelial protection [151]. In a recent in vivo study, it was shown for the first time that lycopene administration in hypertriglyceridemic rats (5, 10 and 50 mg/kg body weigth/day) suppressed the hepatic PCSK9 mRNA expression two- and threefold through the ubiquitin-induced proteasomal degradation of HNF1α [152]. This effect partly explains the reduced plasma levels of atherogenic lipoproteins in lycopene-treated rats, as treatment with lycopene significantly decreased the level of plasma LDL-cholesterol and very low-density lipoprotein (VLDL)-cholesterol, as well as TG, with the maximum effect reached at the highest dose (−85.3%, −55.5% and 55.5%, respectively). In light of the reported reciprocal regulation between PCSK9 and inflammatory cytokines [153], the authors [152] hypothesized that the lycopene-induced inhibition of PCSK9 expression in hypercholesterolemic rats might be related to the suppression of inflammatory markers mediated by lycopene, as treatment induced a significant decrease, of 45, 39.3%, 29.8% and 47.8%, respectively, in the concentrations of circulating interleukin (IL)-1β, IL-6, tumor necrosis factor (TNF)-α and C-reactive protein (CRP), with maximum effect at the highest dose of lycopene. Finally, from in-silico molecular modelling studies, the authors demonstrated that lycopene reduces the affinity of PCSK9 with the complex EGFA (epidimal growth factor-A) of LDLR (Figure 1). In another study, the same group also showed that lycopene, through inhibition of HNF1α expression and possibly through the upregulation of farnesoid X receptor (FXR) and/or PPARα, reduces twofold the LPS-induced hepatic upregulation of PCSK9 in rats [154]. Again, the observed restoration of the inflammatory cascades in LPS-treated mice by lycopene treatment (−64.1%, −25.7%, 20% and −27.4% on circulating TNF-α, IL-1β, IL-6 and CRP, respectively, when compared to the LPS control group) is likely related to the suppression of PCSK9 expression (Figure 1).

The main problem is related to lycopene's low bioavailability; in the human organism only 10–30% of the lycopene in trans-isomeric form is absorbed from the alimentary sources [155]. Its bioavailability depends on several factors, such as the different lycopene biochemical isoforms, the lycopene sources, doses, food co-ingestion, and genetic factors. Indeed, lycopene bioavailability and metabolism is strongly influenced by genetic variability, being described as at least 28 single nucleotide polymorphisms in 16 genes, among which are those coding for the cholesterol membrane transporter scavenger receptor class B, member 1 (SCARB1), the molecular guidance cue slit homolog 3 gene (SLIT3), and the steroid-breakdown enzyme dehydrogenase/reductase (SDR family) member 2 (DHRS2). New technologies to overcome bioavailability problems have been recently investigated, by testing nanodrugs in a nano-emulsion composed of lycopene as anti-inflammatory agent in an animal model of rheumatoid arthritis [156]. With respect to lycopene metabolites, it has been reported that the enzyme b,b-carotene 9',10'-dioxygenase (BCO2) may catalyze the eccentric cleavage of both provitamin and non–provitamin A carotenoids to form apo-10'-carotenoids, including apo-10'-lycopenoids from lycopene [157], which have been demonstrated to mediate some of the biological activities of lycopene [158].

5.7. Omega 3

Omega-3 (ω-3 or n-3) polyunsaturated fatty acids (PUFA) are characterized by having the last double bond between carbon numbers 3 and 4 in the hydrocarbon (acyl) chain, counting the terminal methyl carbon as number one. Longer chain n-3 fatty acids include eicosapentaenoic acid (EPA; 20:5n-3), docosapentaenoic acid (DPA; 22:5n-3) and docosahexaenoic acid (DHA; 22:6n-3), found in significant amounts in fatty fish, fish oil and in other seafood. These exert a number of cardioprotective effects by favorably modulating several risk factors for CVD, such as blood lipids, blood pressure, heart rate and heart rate variability, platelet aggregation, endothelial function and inflammation [159]. With respect to cholesterol metabolism, EPA and DHA have been shown to reduce production, and may induce a faster clearance of triglyceride-rich lipoproteins (TGRL), with a paralleled more rapid clearance of LDL particles and slower production of VLDL particles [160]. These effects seem to be mediated by the inhibition of the SREBP1 mediated pathways, including the activation of the nuclear transcription factors, hepatocyte nuclear factor-4 alpha (HNF4), FXR, liver X receptor (LXR), and PPARs [161,162]. Studies conducted in animal models showed that long term intake of n-3 PUFA-enriched fish oil (10% in diet) reduces hepatic PCSK9 expression, with a consequent significant 84% reduction of LDL-cholesterol plasma levels [163], and that an omega-3 fatty acid-rich diet reduced PCSK9 plasma levels in association with 40% less plasma VLDL- and LDL-cholesterol [164]. Consistently, in subjects with at least one of the metabolic syndrome risk factors, a diet supplemented with canola oil enriched with DHA (by 6%) lowered circulating PCSK9 and TG levels compared to canola and canola oleic diets. In the same study, circulating PCSK9 levels were found to be significantly and positively associated with LDL-cholesterol, TG and apoB levels [165]. Moreover, daily consumption of marine n-3 PUFAs (containing 38.5% EPA, 25.9% DHA and 6.0% DPA) decreased circulating PCSK9 levels by 11.4% and 9.8% in premenopausal and postmenopausal women, respectively, without affecting plasma LDL-cholesterol levels [166].

Despite the several beneficial effects of long-chain omega-3 PUFA supplementation, DHA and EPA have been shown to also increase LDL-cholesterol levels [167], with DHA being more potent than EPA [168]. Consistently, in a recent study in men and women at high risk of cardiovascular disease, it has been observed that, compared with EPA, supplementation with DHA increased LDL-cholesterol concentrations (+3.3%; $p = 0.038$) and the mean LDL particle size, and reduced the proportion of small LDL (23.2%; $p = 0.01$) [169]. Despite the increase in LDL-cholesterol, compared to control both DHA and EPA reduced PCSK9 concentrations in a similar manner (DHA, −225.0 ng/mL; EPA, −218.2 ng/mL). Moreover, changes in PCSK9 correlated positively with changes in the LDL apoB-100 concentrations, and negatively with changes in LDL apoB-100 fractional catabolic rate, after DHA but not after EPA, suggesting a partial role of PCSK9 in the differential effects of DHA and EPA supplementation on LDL metabolism. Allaire et al. also observed that the responders to DHA or to EPA, in terms of TG reduction, had greater serum PCSK9 concentration at baseline than non-responders, suggesting a modulatory role of this protein in the n-3 PUFA-mediated effects [170]. With respect to the mechanism underlying the relationship between omega-3 and PCSK9, it has been hypothesized to be a modulation of SREBP2-mediated pathways [171]. In the context of the reciprocal regulating relation between long chain n-3 PUFAs and PCSK9, there has recently observed a significant interaction between the common *PCSK9* variant rs11206510 located in the promoter region of the *PCSK9* gene, identified for early onset myocardial infarction (MI) through a genome-wide association study (GWAS) [172], and long chain n-3 PUFA intake in Costa Rican Hispanics. Carriers of this variant reported a lower risk of nonfatal MI as compared to non–carriers [173].

Several omega-3 formulations naturally concentrated or purified from fish oil have been approved by the US Food and Drug Administration (FDA) for the treatment of severe hypertriglyceridemia. Some of these formulations provide EPA and/or DHA in either ethyl ester (EE), that requires digestion with carboxyl ester lipase (bile salt-dependent lipase). Therefore, the bioavailability of EPA and DHA from n-3 EE products is strictly dependent on their consumption with a fat meal to stimulate the release of bile salts. In this regard, technologies have been developed to enhance EPA and DHA absorption and to facilitate bioavailability [174]. A very recent study in humans showed that pre-digested omega-3-sn-1(3)-monoacylglycerol lipid structure (OM3-MAG) has a significantly greater absorption at high therapeutic doses (2.9 g/day) than the most common omega-3-EE (3.1 g/day) forms used in hypertriglyceridemia, suggesting the use of the pre-digested OM3-MAG as a more efficacious therapy in severe CV conditions, where high doses of omega-3 are required and a low-fat diet is indicated [175].

6. Other Inhibitors

6.1. Probiotics

Gut microbiota has a relevant impact on cholesterol metabolism, and thus on the pathogenesis of atherosclerosis [176]. For this reason, the use of selected probiotics with specific biological properties has been proposed as a new therapeutic approach for controlling hypercholesterolemia. Within this context, only one study reported data on PCSK9 levels [177]. This clinical trial evaluated the efficacy and safety of a nutraceutical combination containing *Bifidobacterium longum* BB536, red yeast rice extract, niacin and coenzyme Q10, on the improvement of LDL-cholesterol level, as well as the efficacy and safety of a set of clinical and experimental markers of cardiovascular risk. The results of this randomized, double-blind, placebo-controlled study demonstrated that 12 week-treatment significantly reduced TC (−16.7%), LDL-cholesterol (−25.7%) and apoB (−17%), without any changes in PCSK9 plasma levels. From the analysis of the circulating levels of lathosterol, markers of cholesterol synthesis, and campesterol, markers of intestinal cholesterol absorption, it was concluded that *Bifidobacterium longum* BB536 may counteract increased cholesterol absorption potentially induced by monacolin K present in the red yeast rice. On the same line, *Bifidobacterium longum* BB536 might dampen the induction of PCSK9 plasma levels observed in statin-treated patients. However, how *Bifidobacterium longum* BB536 may regulate PCSK9 expression is not known.

6.2. Dioscorea

The aqueous extracts from the root of the *Dioscorea zingiberensis* C.H. Wright, and from rhizome of *Dioscorea nipponica* Makino (Dioscoreaceae), have been used in the prevention and treatment of atherosclerotic CVD for nearly 30 years in China. In 2012, these products were also approved in the Netherlands. Several clinical reports have shown that *Dioscorea nipponica* can decrease the levels of TC, LDL-cholesterol and TG [178,179]. More recently, in a classical mouse model of atherosclerosis, involving apoE$^{-/-}$ mice fed a high-fat diet for 18 weeks, dioscorea showed potent lipid-lowering and anti-atherosclerotic effects [179]. More importantly, dioscorea downregulated hepatic PCSK9 mRNA and reduced circulating PCSK9. The analysis of the composition of the extract of *Dioscorea nipponica* rhizome revealed the presence of protodioscin, pseudoprodioscin and dioscin. These steroidal saponins are considered the main active components. However, some dioscin terpenoids are conjugated with a polysaccharide and cannot be absorbed at gastrointestinal level, while their respective aglycones may be bioavailable. Interestingly, protodioscin, pseudoprotodioscin and methylprotodioscin have been shown to suppress PCSK9 expression (Figure 1 and Table 1) [180]. This effect was associated with the inhibition of SREBP transcription factors and was responsible of the induction of the LDLR protein in HepG2 cells [180]. It is still unclear whether the aglycone of protodioscin and pseudoprotodioscin is released under in vitro conditions, and thus the active component on PCSK9 is unknown. Indeed, HepG2 cells are known to show extremely low activity of numerous xenobiotic metabolizing enzymes, which could provide misleading results in pharmacological tests with compounds that require biotransformation [181–183]. This is particularly true for natural compounds that need to be activated by enzymes of gut microbiota that are not present in cultured cells.

6.3. Emodin

Emodin (6-methyl-1,3,8-trihydroxyanthraquinone) is one of the active anthraquinone derivatives from *Rheum palmatum* L. (Polygonaceae) and some other Chinese herbs (Table 1) [184]. In C57BL6/J mice fed high-fat diets for 12 weeks, emodin supplementation at the dose of 40 and 80 mg/kg/day showed an improvement of lipid levels associated with a reduction of SREBP expression [185]. In addition, in rats fed high-fat diets, emodin was shown to prevent hypercholesterolemic status through the bile acids-CYP7A1 pathway. Emodin binds and reduces the reabsorption of bile acids, leading to cholesterol being shunted into bile acid production, which determines its lipid-lowering effects [186]. More recently, 100 mg/kg per day of aloe, which also contains emodin, was shown to reduce TC and

LDL-cholesterol levels in diet-induced hypercholesterolemic rats. Interestingly, aloe ameliorates the liver fat content, and in vitro studies on HepG2 cells show a negative effect on SREBP and HNF1α. As expected, the inhibition of both transcription factors determined a downregulation of PCSK9, associated with increased expression of LDLR and LDL uptake (Figure 1) [187].

Table 1. Pharmacokinetic and pharmacodinamic characteristics of natural compounds affecting PCSK9.

Natural Compound	Chemical Structure	Bioavail.	Tmax (h)	Half-Life Time (h)	Metabolism	Mechanism of Action	Transport.	Level of Evidence on PCSK9	Counteracts Statins	Ref.
Berberine		0.37%	9.8	28.6	Demethylation and glucuronide	Inhibits SREBP; HNF1α	P-gp and MRP1	In vitro, in vivo and clinical	Yes	[23,24,28,30,33,35–37,188]
Sterol/Stanols and Vegetable Proteins										
Lupin peptide	LILPKHSDAD	Poor (predicted)	Not known	Not known	Proteases	Inhibits interaction PCSK9-LDLR; Reduces HNF1α	No (predicted)	In vitro. Clinic (negative)	Not known	[61,64]
Polyphenols										
Quercetin		0.31%	2.5 ÷ 3	2.1	Liver: Sulfate and methyl glucuronide; Gut microbiota: free aglycone; 3,4-dihydroxyphenylacetic acid, 3-(3-hydroxyphenyl) propionic acid, 3,4-dihydroxybenzoic acid and 4-hydroxybenzoic acid	Inhibits secretion (sortilin) and SREBP	P-gp sand BCRP	In vitro and in vivo	Not known	[72,73] [78,80,81]
Epigallocatechin gallate		0.1%	1 ÷ 2	3.4	Liver: Methyl, sulfate, and glucuronide; Gut microbiota: phenylvalerolactones and phenylvaleric acids	Inhibits secretion and SREBP	MRP2 and OATP1B1	In vitro	Yes	[85,91,92,95–98]
Resveratrol		<1%	3	9.2	Liver: Sulfate and glucuronide; Gut microbiota: dihydroresveratrol	Inhibits SREBP1c and interaction PCSK9-LDLR	Not known	In vivo and in vivo	Not known	[100–102,105–107]
Curcumin		<1%	Not known	Not known	Liver: reduction and glucuronide, sulfate, and glutathione; Gut microbiota: tetrahydrocurcumin, demethylcurcumin, bisdemethylcurcumin etc.	Inhibits; HNF1α	Not known	In vivo and in vivo	Yes	[122–124,127–129]
Silibinin A		<1%	1.4	Not known	Sulfate and glucuronide	Inhibits transcription	P-gp inhibitor	In vitro	Yes	[108–110]

Table 1. Cont.

Natural Compound	Chemical Structure	Bioavail.	Tmax (h)	Half-Life Time (h)	Metabolism	Mechanism of Action	Transport.	Level of Evidence on PCSK9	Counteracts Statins	Ref.
Naringin		<1%	0.5	9.5	Liver: Hydrolysis and then glucuronide, sulfate, methylation; Gut microbiota: Phenolic derivatives	Inhibits SREBP	P-gp and OATP1A5 inhibitor	In vivo	Not known	[111,112]
Pinostrobin		1.8% (S); 13.8% (R)	6.0	38.1	Glucuronide	Inhibits transcription and catalytic activity	Not known	In vitro	Not known	[113,114]
Eugenol		<1%	2.1	14.0	Phenol, glucuronide and sulphate	Direct interaction with PCSK9 and inhibits SREBP	Not known	In vitro	Not known	[115,117,118]
Nutrients										
Kaempferol		2.5%	Not known	Not known	Glucuronide and sulphate	Inhibits transcription	Not known	In vitro	Yes	[86,132]
p-Coumaric acid		24%	0.17	0.25	Glucuronide and sulphate	Inhibits transcription	Not known	In vitro	Yes	[132]
Vitamin K7		2%	6.0	60	Not known	Not known	Not known	In vitro and in vivo	Not known	[145,148,189]
Lycopene		33.9%	24	235	Phase I, oxidation	Inhibits transcription and interaction PCSK9-LDLR	Not Known	In vitro and in vivo	Not Known	[151,152,154,190]
Other Inhibitors										
Protodioscin		0.2%	20	20	Oxidation, deglycosylation and glucuronide	Inhibits transcription	Not known	In vitro and in vivo	Not known	[179,180]
Emodin		low	0.13	8.6	Glucuronide and sulphate	Inhibits SREBP; HNF1α	Not known	In vitro	Not known	[191,192]

Most of the individualized compounds have been shown to inhibit PCSK9 transcription factors, such as SREBP and HNF1α. However, there is evidence that compounds with different mechanisms of PCSK9 inhibition also exist, including: Epigallocatechin gallate (EGCG), which affects PCSK9 secretion; soy peptides, resveratrol, eugenol and lycopene, which inhibit the interaction of PCSK9 with the LDL receptor (LDLR); and finally, quercetin and pinostrobin, which impair the autocatalytic processing and maturation of PCSK9 in the endoplasmic reticulum. Today there is no evidence of natural compounds affecting PCSK9 at the translational level and by epigenetic mechanisms.

7. Conclusions

The relevance of PCSK9 as a new molecular target for treating hypercholesterolemia and associated cardiovascular diseases is demonstrated by the clinical efficacy of two FDA/EMA-approved monoclonal antibodies: alirocumab and evolocumab [5]. However, these monoclonal antibodies, the only currently available anti-PCSK9 therapies, have several drawbacks: (*i*) very high costs; (*ii*) subcutaneous administration (poor compliance and convenience); (*iii*) potential immunogenicity with long term treatment. A more recent alternative to anti-PCSK9 antibodies is represented by Inclisiran, a short interfering RNA (siRNA) designed to target hepatic PCSK9 mRNA. However, this approach still has some drawbacks, such as the long pharmacokinetic profile, parenteral administration, and an as yet undefined safety profile [193]. Thus, cheaper, orally administrable, small-molecule drugs are greatly needed. The response to this issue can potentially come from the identification of natural compounds with lipid-lowering activity associated with anti-PCSK9 inhibitory action. In the present review, we identified many compounds with effective anti-PCSK9 inhibitory activity, mainly by acting at the transcriptional levels, and only few examples of the autocatalytic secretion step or PCSK9 interaction with the LDL receptor. A critical aspect of all these potentially valid PCSK9 inhibitors is represented by their limited oral bioavailability, and the restricted evidence of their efficacy only in in vivo experimental models. Nevertheless, a number of drug delivery approaches and chemical derivatives of natural compounds, aiming to improve the oral bioavailability, are emerging. In addition, it must be recognized that, as elsewhere reviewed [194], when assessing the efficacy of a nutraceutical, the following key aspects are worth of consideration: (*i*) to identify differences in purity and origin between products on the market [195]; (*ii*) to find evidence of clinical efficacy evaluated via placebo-controlled, double-blind studies [196]; (*iii*) to evaluate the effects of combining active ingredients. Finally, evidence has to be grounded on the mechanisms of action of active ingredients in vitro, followed by pre-clinical studies in experimental animals, to finally explore safety and efficacy in humans [194]. All these aspects have not always been provided for the natural compounds described in the present review. Thus, the selected molecules can only be considered as starting points for the eventual development of oral PCSK9 inhibitors.

Author Contributions: Writing—Original draft preparation, N.F.; F.Z.; M.P.A.; M.R.; Writing—Review and editing, M.G.L. All authors have read and agreed to the published version of the manuscript.

Funding: This research was funded by Italian MIUR (PRIN 2017).

Conflicts of Interest: F.Z.; M.P.A.; M.G.L. and M.R. declare no conflict of interest. N.F. has received a financial grant from PharmaNutra S.P.A.

References

1. Ferri, N.; Ruscica, M. Proprotein convertase subtilisin/kexin type 9 (PCSK9) and metabolic syndrome: Insights on insulin resistance, inflammation, and atherogenic dyslipidemia. *Endocrinology* **2016**, *54*, 588–601. [CrossRef]
2. Seidah, N.G.; Benjannet, S.; Wickham, L.; Marcinkiewicz, J.; Jasmin, S.B.; Stifani, S.; Basak, A.; Prat, A.; Chrétien, M. The secretory proprotein convertase neural apoptosis-regulated convertase 1 (NARC-1): Liver regeneration and neuronal differentiation. *Proc. Natl. Acad. Sci. USA* **2003**, *100*, 928–933. [CrossRef]
3. Tavori, H.; Christian, D.C.; Minnier, J.; Plubell, D.; Shapiro, M.D.; Yeang, C.; Giunzioni, I.; Croyal, M.; Duell, P.B.; Lambert, G.; et al. PCSK9 Association with Lipoprotein(a). *Circ. Res.* **2016**. [CrossRef]

4. Ruscica, M.; Simonelli, S.; Botta, M.; Ossoli, A.; Lupo, M.G.; Magni, P.; Corsini, A.; Arca, M.; Pisciotta, L.; Veglia, F.; et al. Plasma PCSK9 levels and lipoprotein distribution are preserved in carriers of genetic HDL disorders. *Biochim. Biophys. Acta (BBA) Mol. Cell Boil. Lipids* **2018**, *1863*, 991–997. [CrossRef] [PubMed]
5. Macchi, C.; Banach, M.; Corsini, A.; Sirtori, C.R.; Ferri, N.; Ruscica, M. Changes in circulating pro-protein convertase subtilisin/kexin type 9 levels—Experimental and clinical approaches with lipid-lowering agents. *Eur. J. Prev. Cardiol.* **2019**, *26*, 930–949. [CrossRef] [PubMed]
6. Horton, J.D.; Shah, N.A.; Warrington, J.A.; Anderson, N.N.; Park, S.W.; Brown, M.S.; Goldstein, J.L. Combined analysis of oligonucleotide microarray data from transgenic and knockout mice identifies direct SREBP target genes. *Proc. Natl. Acad. Sci. USA* **2003**, *100*, 12027–12032. [CrossRef] [PubMed]
7. Dubuc, G.; Chamberland, A.; Wassef, H.; Davignon, J.; Seidah, N.G.; Bernier, L.; Prat, A. Statins UpregulatePCSK9, the Gene Encoding the Proprotein Convertase Neural Apoptosis-Regulated Convertase-1 Implicated in Familial Hypercholesterolemia. *Arter. Thromb. Vasc. Boil.* **2004**, *24*, 1454–1459. [CrossRef] [PubMed]
8. Ruscica, M.; Ricci, C.; Macchi, C.; Magni, P.; Cristofani, R.; Liu, J.; Corsini, A.; Ferri, N. Suppressor of Cytokine Signaling-3 (SOCS-3) Induces Proprotein Convertase Subtilisin Kexin Type 9 (PCSK9) Expression in Hepatic HepG2 Cell Line*. *J. Boil. Chem.* **2015**, *291*, 3508–3519. [CrossRef]
9. Li, H.; Dong, B.; Park, S.W.; Lee, H.-S.; Chen, W.; Liu, J. Hepatocyte Nuclear Factor 1α Plays a Critical Role in PCSK9 Gene Transcription and Regulation by the Natural Hypocholesterolemic Compound Berberine*. *J. Boil. Chem.* **2009**, *284*, 28885–28895. [CrossRef]
10. Cohen, J.; Pertsemlidis, A.; Kotowski, I.K.; Graham, R.; Garcia, C.K.; Hobbs, H.H. Low LDL cholesterol in individuals of African descent resulting from frequent nonsense mutations in PCSK9. *Nat. Genet.* **2005**, *37*, 161–165. [CrossRef]
11. Abifadel, M.; Varret, M.; Rabès, J.-P.; Allard, D.; Ouguerram, K.; Devillers, M.; Cruaud, C.; Benjannet, S.; Wickham, L.; Erlich, D.; et al. Mutations in PCSK9 cause autosomal dominant hypercholesterolemia. *Nat. Genet.* **2003**, *34*, 154–156. [CrossRef] [PubMed]
12. Ferri, N.; Corsini, A.; Macchi, C.; Magni, P.; Ruscica, M. Proprotein convertase subtilisin kexin type 9 and high-density lipoprotein metabolism: Experimental animal models and clinical evidence. *Transl. Res.* **2016**, *173*, 19–29. [CrossRef] [PubMed]
13. Dong, H.; Wang, N.; Zhao, L.; Lu, F. Berberine in the Treatment of Type 2 Diabetes Mellitus: A Systemic Review and Meta-Analysis. *Evid. Based Complement. Altern. Med.* **2012**, *2012*, 1–12. [CrossRef] [PubMed]
14. Lan, J.; Zhao, Y.; Dong, F.; Yan, Z.; Zheng, W.; Fan, J.; Sun, G. Meta-analysis of the effect and safety of berberine in the treatment of type 2 diabetes mellitus, hyperlipemia and hypertension. *J. Ethnopharmacol.* **2015**, *161*, 69–81. [CrossRef] [PubMed]
15. Wang, L.; Ye, X.; Hua, Y.; Song, Y. Berberine alleviates adipose tissue fibrosis by inducing AMP-activated kinase signaling in high-fat diet-induced obese mice. *Biomed. Pharmacother.* **2018**, *105*, 121–129. [CrossRef]
16. Andola, H.C.; Gaira, K.S.; Rawal, R.S.; Rawat, M.S.; Bhatt, I.D. Habitat-dependent variations in berberine content of Berberis asiatica Roxb. ex. DC. in Kumaon, Western Himalaya. *Chem. Biodivers.* **2010**, *7*, 415–420. [CrossRef]
17. Kong, W.; Wei, J.; Abidi, P.; Lin, M.; Inaba, S.; Li, C.; Wang, Y.; Wang, Z.; Si, S.; Pan, H.; et al. Berberine is a novel cholesterol-lowering drug working through a unique mechanism distinct from statins. *Nat. Med.* **2004**, *10*, 1344–1351. [CrossRef]
18. Horton, J.D.; Goldstein, J.L.; Brown, M.S. SREBPs: Activators of the complete program of cholesterol and fatty acid synthesis in the liver. *J. Clin. Investig.* **2002**, *109*, 1125–1131. [CrossRef]
19. Cameron, J.; Ranheim, T.; Kulseth, M.A.; Leren, T.P.; Berge, K.E. Berberine decreases PCSK9 expression in HepG2 cells. *Atherosclerosis* **2008**, *201*, 266–273. [CrossRef]
20. Abidi, P.; Chen, W.; Kraemer, F.B.; Li, H.; Liu, J. The medicinal plant goldenseal is a natural LDL-lowering agent with multiple bioactive components and new action mechanisms. *J. Lipid Res.* **2006**, *47*, 2134–2147. [CrossRef]
21. Kong, W.-J.; Zhang, H.; Song, D.-Q.; Xue, R.; Zhao, W.; Wei, J.; Wang, Y.-M.; Shan, N.; Zhou, Z.-X.; Yang, P.; et al. Berberine reduces insulin resistance through protein kinase C–dependent up-regulation of insulin receptor expression. *Metabolism* **2009**, *58*, 109–119. [CrossRef] [PubMed]

22. Dong, B.; Li, H.; Singh, A.B.; Cao, A.; Liu, J. Inhibition ofPCSK9Transcription by Berberine Involves Down-regulation of Hepatic HNF1α Protein Expression through the Ubiquitin-Proteasome Degradation Pathway. *J. Boil. Chem.* **2014**, *290*, 4047–4058. [CrossRef] [PubMed]
23. Liu, Y.; Hao, H.; Xie, H.-G.; Lai, L.; Wang, Q.; Liu, C.; Wang, G. Extensive Intestinal First-Pass Elimination and Predominant Hepatic Distribution of Berberine Explain Its Low Plasma Levels in Rats. *Drug Metab. Dispos.* **2010**, *38*, 1779–1784. [CrossRef] [PubMed]
24. Hua, W.; Ding, L.; Chen, Y.; Gong, B.; He, J.; Xu, G. Determination of berberine in human plasma by liquid chromatography–electrospray ionization–mass spectrometry. *J. Pharm. Biomed. Anal.* **2007**, *44*, 931–937. [CrossRef]
25. Shitan, N.; Tanaka, M.; Terai, K.; Ueda, K.; Yazaki, K. Human MDR1 and MRP1 Recognize Berberine as Their Transport Substrate. *Biosci. Biotechnol. Biochem.* **2007**, *71*, 242–245. [CrossRef]
26. Cao, S.; Xu, P.; Yan, J.; Liu, H.; Liu, L.; Cheng, L.; Qiu, F.; Kang, N. Berberrubine and its analog, hydroxypropyl-berberrubine, regulate LDLR and PCSK9 expression via the ERK signal pathway to exert cholesterol-lowering effects in human hepatoma HepG2 cells. *J. Cell. Biochem.* **2018**, *120*, 1340–1349. [CrossRef]
27. Horton, J.D.; A Cuthbert, J.; Spady, D.K. Dietary fatty acids regulate hepatic low density lipoprotein (LDL) transport by altering LDL receptor protein and mRNA levels. *J. Clin. Investig.* **1993**, *92*, 743–749. [CrossRef]
28. Xiao, H.-B.; Sun, Z.-L.; Zhang, H.-B.; Zhang, D.-S. Berberine inhibits dyslipidemia in C57BL/6 mice with lipopolysaccharide induced inflammation. *Pharmacol. Rep.* **2012**, *64*, 889–895. [CrossRef]
29. Jia, Y.-J.; Xu, R.-X.; Sun, J.; Tang, Y.; Li, J.-J. Enhanced circulating PCSK9 concentration by berberine through SREBP-2 pathway in high fat diet-fed rats. *J. Transl. Med.* **2014**, *12*, 103. [CrossRef]
30. Liu, D.-L.; Xu, L.-J.; Dong, H.; Chen, G.; Huang, Z.-Y.; Zou, X.; Wang, K.-F.; Luo, Y.-H.; Lu, F. Inhibition of proprotein convertase subtilisin/kexin type 9: A novel mechanism of berberine and 8-hydroxy dihydroberberine against hyperlipidemia. *Chin. J. Integr. Med.* **2014**, *21*, 132–138. [CrossRef]
31. Dong, H.; Zhao, Y.; Zhao, L.; Lu, F. The Effects of Berberine on Blood Lipids: A Systemic Review and Meta-Analysis of Randomized Controlled Trials. *Planta Med.* **2013**, *79*, 437–446. [CrossRef] [PubMed]
32. Adorni, M.P.; Ferri, N.; Marchianò, S.; Trimarco, V.; Rozza, F.; Izzo, R.; Bernini, F.; Zimetti, F. Effect of a novel nutraceutical combination on serum lipoprotein functional profile and circulating PCSK9. *Ther. Clin. Risk Manag.* **2017**, *13*, 1555–1562. [CrossRef] [PubMed]
33. Sahebkar, A.; Simental-Mendía, L.E.; Guerrero-Romero, F.; Golledge, J.; Watts, G.F. Effect of statin therapy on plasma proprotein convertase subtilisin kexin 9 (PCSK9) concentrations: A systematic review and meta-analysis of clinical trials. *Diabetes Obes. Metab.* **2015**, *17*, 1042–1055. [CrossRef] [PubMed]
34. Lupo, M.G.; Macchi, C.; Marchianò, S.; Cristofani, R.; Greco, M.F.; Dall'Acqua, S.; Chen, H.; Sirtori, C.R.; Corsini, A.; Ruscica, M.; et al. Differential effects of red yeast rice, Berberis aristata and Morus alba extracts on PCSK9 and LDL uptake. *Nutr. Metab. Cardiovasc. Dis.* **2019**, *29*, 1245–1253. [CrossRef]
35. Spigoni, V.; Aldigeri, R.; Antonini, M.; Micheli, M.M.; Fantuzzi, F.; Fratter, A.; Pellizzato, M.; Derlindati, E.; Zavaroni, I.; Bonadonna, R.C.; et al. Effects of a New Nutraceutical Formulation (Berberine, Red Yeast Rice and Chitosan) on Non-HDL Cholesterol Levels in Individuals with Dyslipidemia: Results from a Randomized, Double Blind, Placebo-Controlled Study. *Int. J. Mol. Sci.* **2017**, *18*, 1498. [CrossRef]
36. Formisano, E.; Pasta, A.; Cremonini, A.L.; Favari, E.; Ronca, A.; Carbone, F.; Semino, T.; Di Pierro, F.; Sukkar, G.S.; Pisciotta, L. Efficacy of Nutraceutical Combination of Monacolin K, Berberine, and Silymarin on Lipid Profile and PCSK9 Plasma Level in a Cohort of Hypercholesterolemic Patients. *J. Med. Food* **2019**. [CrossRef]
37. Pisciotta, L.; Bellocchio, A.; Bertolini, S. Nutraceutical pill containing berberine versus ezetimibe on plasma lipid pattern in hypercholesterolemic subjects and its additive effect in patients with familial hypercholesterolemia on stable cholesterol-lowering treatment. *Lipids Heal. Dis.* **2012**, *11*, 123. [CrossRef]
38. Dubuc, G.; Tremblay, M.; Paré, G.; Jacques, H.; Hamelin, J.; Benjannet, S.; Boulet, L.; Genest, J.; Bernier, L.; Seidah, N.G.; et al. A new method for measurement of total plasma PCSK9: Clinical applications. *J. Lipid Res.* **2009**, *51*, 140–149. [CrossRef]
39. Awan, Z.; Seidah, N.G.; MacFadyen, J.G.; Benjannet, S.; I Chasman, D.; Ridker, P.M.; Genest, J. Rosuvastatin, Proprotein Convertase Subtilisin/Kexin Type 9 Concentrations, and LDL Cholesterol Response: The JUPITER Trial. *Clin. Chem.* **2012**, *58*, 183–189. [CrossRef]

40. Guo, Y.; Chen, Y.; Tan, Z.-R.; Klaassen, C.D.; Zhou, H.-H. Repeated administration of berberine inhibits cytochromes P450 in humans. *Eur. J. Clin. Pharmacol.* **2011**, *68*, 213–217. [CrossRef]
41. Wu, C.; Xi, C.; Tong, J.; Zhao, J.; Jiang, H.; Wang, J.; Wang, Y.; Liu, H. Design, synthesis, and biological evaluation of novel tetrahydroprotoberberine derivatives (THPBs) as proprotein convertase subtilisin/kexin type 9 (PCSK9) modulators for the treatment of hyperlipidemia. *Acta Pharm. Sin. B* **2019**, *9*, 1216–1230. [CrossRef] [PubMed]
42. Ochin, C.; Garelnabi, M. Berberine Encapsulated PLGA-PEG Nanoparticles Modulate PCSK-9 in HepG2 Cells. *Cardiovasc. Hematol. Disord. Targets* **2018**, *18*, 61–70. [CrossRef] [PubMed]
43. Guo, H.-H.; Feng, C.-L.; Zhang, W.-X.; Luo, Z.-G.; Zhang, H.-J.; Zhang, T.-T.; Ma, C.; Zhan, Y.; Li, R.; Wu, S.; et al. Liver-target nanotechnology facilitates berberine to ameliorate cardio-metabolic diseases. *Nat. Commun.* **2019**, *10*, 1981. [CrossRef] [PubMed]
44. Ras, R.T.; Geleijnse, J.M.; Trautwein, E.A. LDL-cholesterol-lowering effect of plant sterols and stanols across different dose ranges: A meta-analysis of randomised controlled studies. *Br. J. Nutr.* **2014**, *112*, 214–219. [CrossRef]
45. Momtazi-Borojeni, A.A.; Banach, M.; Pirro, M.; Katsiki, N.; Sahebkar, A. Regulation of PCSK9 by nutraceuticals. *Pharmacol. Res.* **2017**, *120*, 157–169. [CrossRef]
46. Simonen, P.; Stenman, U.-H.; Gylling, H. Serum proprotein convertase subtilisin/kexin type 9 concentration is not increased by plant stanol ester consumption in normo- to moderately hypercholesterolaemic non-obese subjects. The BLOOD FLOW intervention study. *Clin. Sci.* **2015**, *129*, 439–446. [CrossRef]
47. De Smet, E.; Mensink, R.P.; Konings, M.; Brufau, G.; Groen, A.K.; Havinga, R.; Schonewille, M.; Kerksiek, A.; Lütjohann, D.; Plat, J. Acute intake of plant stanol esters induces changes in lipid and lipoprotein metabolism-related gene expression in the liver and intestines of mice. *Lipids* **2015**, *50*, 529–541. [CrossRef]
48. Boachie, R.; Yao, S.; Udenigwe, C.C. Molecular mechanisms of cholesterol-lowering peptides derived from food proteins. *Curr. Opin. Food Sci.* **2018**, *20*, 58–63. [CrossRef]
49. Lammi, C.; Zanoni, C.; Scigliuolo, G.M.; D'Amato, A.; Arnoldi, A. Lupin Peptides Lower Low-Density Lipoprotein (LDL) Cholesterol through an Up-regulation of the LDL Receptor/Sterol Regulatory Element Binding Protein 2 (SREBP2) Pathway at HepG2 Cell Line. *J. Agric. Food Chem.* **2014**, *62*, 7151–7159. [CrossRef]
50. Lammi, C.; Zanoni, C.; Arnoldi, A.; Vistoli, G. Two Peptides from Soy beta-Conglycinin Induce a Hypocholesterolemic Effect in HepG2 Cells by a Statin-Like Mechanism: Comparative in Vitro and in Silico Modeling Studies. *J. Agric. Food Chem.* **2015**, *63*, 7945–7951. [CrossRef]
51. Zanoni, C.; Aiello, G.; Arnoldi, A.; Lammi, C. Hempseed Peptides Exert Hypocholesterolemic Effects with a Statin-Like Mechanism. *J. Agric. Food Chem.* **2017**, *65*, 8829–8838. [CrossRef]
52. Lin, S.-H.; Chang, D.-K.; Chou, M.-J.; Huang, K.-J.; Shiuan, D. Peptide inhibitors of human HMG-CoA reductase as potential hypocholesterolemia agents. *Biochem. Biophys. Res. Commun.* **2015**, *456*, 104–109. [CrossRef]
53. Sirtori, C.R.; Lovati, M.R.; Manzoni, C.; Castiglioni, S.; Duranti, M.; Magni, C.; Morandi, S.; D'Agostina, A.; Arnoldi, A. Proteins of White Lupin Seed, a Naturally Isoflavone-Poor Legume, Reduce Cholesterolemia in Rats and Increase LDL Receptor Activity in HepG2 Cells. *J. Nutr.* **2004**, *134*, 18–23. [CrossRef]
54. Marchesi, M.; Parolini, C.; Diani, E.; Rigamonti, E.; Cornelli, L.; Arnoldi, A.; Sirtori, C.R.; Chiesa, G. Hypolipidaemic and anti-atherosclerotic effects of lupin proteins in a rabbit model. *Br. J. Nutr.* **2008**, *100*, 707–710. [CrossRef]
55. Bähr, M.; Fechner, A.; Krämer, J.; Kiehntopf, M.; Jahreis, G. Lupin protein positively affects plasma LDL cholesterol and LDL:HDL cholesterol ratio in hypercholesterolemic adults after four weeks of supplementation: A randomized, controlled crossover study. *Nutr. J.* **2013**, *12*, 107. [CrossRef]
56. Bähr, M.; Fechner, A.; Kiehntopf, M.; Jahreis, G. Consuming a mixed diet enriched with lupin protein beneficially affects plasma lipids in hypercholesterolemic subjects: A randomized controlled trial. *Clin. Nutr.* **2015**, *34*, 7–14. [CrossRef]
57. Sirtori, C.R.; Triolo, M.; Bosisio, R.; Bondioli, A.; Calabresi, L.; De Vergori, V.; Gomaraschi, M.; Mombelli, G.; Pazzucconi, F.; Zacherl, C.; et al. Hypocholesterolaemic effects of lupin protein and pea protein/fibre combinations in moderately hypercholesterolaemic individuals. *Br. J. Nutr.* **2011**, *107*, 1176–1183. [CrossRef]
58. Lammi, C.; Zanoni, C.; Calabresi, L.; Arnoldi, A. Lupin protein exerts cholesterol-lowering effects targeting PCSK9: From clinical evidences to elucidation of the in vitro molecular mechanism using HepG2 cells. *J. Funct. Foods* **2016**, *23*, 230–240. [CrossRef]

59. Pavanello, C.; Lammi, C.; Ruscica, M.; Bosisio, R.; Mombelli, G.; Zanoni, C.; Calabresi, L.; Sirtori, C.R.; Magni, P.; Arnoldi, A. Effects of a lupin protein concentrate on lipids, blood pressure and insulin resistance in moderately dyslipidaemic patients: A randomised controlled trial. *J. Funct. Foods* **2017**, *37*, 8–15. [CrossRef]
60. Lammi, C.; Bollati, C.; Lecca, D.; Abbracchio, M.P.; Arnoldi, A. Lupin Peptide T9 (GQEQSHQDEGVIVR) Modulates the Mutant PCSK9D374Y Pathway: In vitro Characterization of its Dual Hypocholesterolemic Behavior. *Nutrients* **2019**, *11*, 1665. [CrossRef]
61. Lammi, C.; Zanoni, C.; Aiello, G.; Arnoldi, A.; Grazioso, G. Lupin Peptides Modulate the Protein-Protein Interaction of PCSK9 with the Low Density Lipoprotein Receptor in HepG2 Cells. *Sci. Rep.* **2016**, *6*, 29931. [CrossRef]
62. Sirtori, C.R.; Pavanello, C.; Calabresi, L.; Ruscica, M. Nutraceutical approaches to metabolic syndrome. *Ann. Med.* **2017**, *49*, 678–697. [CrossRef]
63. Banach, M.; Patti, A.M.; Giglio, R.V.; Cicero, A.F.G.; Atanasov, A.G.; Bajraktari, G.; Bruckert, É; Descamps, O.; Djuric, D.M.; Ezhov, M.; et al. The Role of Nutraceuticals in Statin Intolerant Patients. *J. Am. Coll. Cardiol.* **2018**, *72*, 96–118. [CrossRef]
64. Ruscica, M.; Pavanello, C.; Gandini, S.; Gomaraschi, M.; Vitali, C.; Macchi, C.; Morlotti, B.; Aiello, G.; Bosisio, R.; Calabresi, L.; et al. Effect of soy on metabolic syndrome and cardiovascular risk factors: A randomized controlled trial. *Eur. J. Nutr.* **2016**, *57*, 499–511. [CrossRef]
65. Durazzo, A.; Lucarini, M.; Souto, E.; Cicala, C.; Caiazzo, E.; Izzo, A.A.; Novellino, E.; Santini, A. Polyphenols: A concise overview on the chemistry, occurrence, and human health. *Phytother. Res.* **2019**, *33*, 2221–2243. [CrossRef]
66. Potì, F.; Santi, D.; Spaggiari, G.; Zimetti, F.; Zanotti, I. Polyphenol Health Effects on Cardiovascular and Neurodegenerative Disorders: A Review and Meta-Analysis. *Int. J. Mol. Sci.* **2019**, *20*, 351. [CrossRef]
67. Cicero, A.F.G.; Colletti, A. Polyphenols Effect on Circulating Lipids and Lipoproteins: From Biochemistry to Clinical Evidence. *Curr. Pharm. Des.* **2018**, *24*, 178–190. [CrossRef]
68. Chambers, K.F.; Day, P.E.; Aboufarrag, H.T.; Kroon, P.A. Polyphenol Effects on Cholesterol Metabolism via Bile Acid Biosynthesis, CYP7A1: A Review. *Nutrients* **2019**, *11*, 2588. [CrossRef]
69. Fraga, C.G.; Croft, K.D.; Kennedy, D.O.; Tomás-Barberán, F.A. The effects of polyphenols and other bioactives on human health. *Food Funct.* **2019**, *10*, 514–528. [CrossRef]
70. Del Rio, D.; Rodriguez-Mateos, A.; Spencer, J.P.; Tognolini, M.; Borges, G.; Crozier, A. Dietary (poly)phenolics in human health: Structures, bioavailability, and evidence of protective effects against chronic diseases. *Antioxid. Redox Signal.* **2012**, *18*, 1818–1892. [CrossRef]
71. Moon, J.; Lee, S.-M.; Do, H.J.; Cho, Y.; Chung, J.H.; Shin, M.-J. Quercetin Up-regulates LDL Receptor Expression in HepG2 Cells. *Phytother. Res.* **2012**, *26*, 1688–1694. [CrossRef]
72. Mbikay, M.; Sirois, F.; Simões, S.; Mayne, J.; Chrétien, M. Quercetin-3-glucoside increases low-density lipoprotein receptor (LDLR) expression, attenuates proprotein convertase subtilisin/kexin 9 (PCSK9) secretion, and stimulates LDL uptake by Huh7 human hepatocytes in culture. *FEBS Open Bio* **2014**, *4*, 755–762. [CrossRef]
73. Nishikido, T.; Ray, K.K. Non-antibody Approaches to Proprotein Convertase Subtilisin Kexin 9 Inhibition: siRNA, Antisense Oligonucleotides, Adnectins, Vaccination, and New Attempts at Small-Molecule Inhibitors Based on New Discoveries. *Front. Cardiovasc. Med.* **2019**, *5*. [CrossRef]
74. Li, S.; Cao, H.; Shen, D.; Jia, Q.; Chen, C.; Xing, S.L. Quercetin protects against ox-LDL-induced injury via regulation of ABCA1, LXR-α and PCSK9 in RAW264.7 macrophages. *Mol. Med. Rep.* **2018**, *18*, 799–806. [CrossRef]
75. Adorni, M.P.; Cipollari, E.; Favari, E.; Zanotti, I.; Zimetti, F.; Corsini, A.; Ricci, C.; Bernini, F.; Ferri, N. Inhibitory effect of PCSK9 on Abca1 protein expression and cholesterol efflux in macrophages. *Atherosclerosis* **2017**, *256*, 1–6. [CrossRef]
76. Ricci, C.; Ruscica, M.; Camera, M.; Rossetti, L.; Macchi, C.; Colciago, A.; Zanotti, I.; Lupo, M.G.; Adorni, M.P.; Cicero, A.F.G.; et al. PCSK9 induces a pro-inflammatory response in macrophages. *Sci. Rep.* **2018**, *8*, 2267. [CrossRef]
77. Mbikay, M.; Mayne, J.; Sirois, F.; Fedoryak, O.; Raymond, A.; Noad, J.; Chrétien, M. Mice Fed a High-Cholesterol Diet Supplemented with Quercetin-3-Glucoside Show Attenuated Hyperlipidemia and Hyperinsulinemia Associated with Differential Regulation of PCSK9 and LDLR in their Liver and Pancreas. *Mol. Nutr. Food Res.* **2018**, *62*, e1700729. [CrossRef]

78. Jia, Q.; Cao, H.; Shen, D.; Li, S.; Yan, L.; Chen, C.; Xing, S.; Dou, F. Quercetin protects against atherosclerosis by regulating the expression of PCSK9, CD36, PPARgamma, LXRalpha and ABCA1. *Int. J. Mol. Med.* **2019**, *44*, 893–902.
79. Tabrizi, R.; Tamtaji, O.R.; Mirhosseini, N.; Lankarani, K.B.; Akbari, M.; Heydari, S.T.; Dadgostar, E.; Asemi, Z. The effects of quercetin supplementation on lipid profiles and inflammatory markers among patients with metabolic syndrome and related disorders: A systematic review and meta-analysis of randomized controlled trials. *Crit. Rev. Food Sci. Nutr.* **2019**, 1–14. [CrossRef]
80. Terao, J. Factors modulating bioavailability of quercetin-related flavonoids and the consequences of their vascular function. *Biochem. Pharmacol.* **2017**, *139*, 15–23. [CrossRef]
81. Moon, Y.J.; Wang, L.; DiCenzo, R.; Morris, A.M.E. Quercetin pharmacokinetics in humans. *Biopharm. Drug Dispos.* **2008**, *29*, 205–217. [CrossRef]
82. Cooray, H.C.; Janvilisri, T.; Van Veen, H.W.; Hladky, S.B.; A Barrand, M. Interaction of the breast cancer resistance protein with plant polyphenols. *Biochem. Biophys. Res. Commun.* **2004**, *317*, 269–275. [CrossRef]
83. Hsiu, S.-L.; Hou, Y.-C.; Wang, Y.-H.; Tsao, C.-W.; Su, S.-F.; Chao, P.-D.L. Quercetin significantly decreased cyclosporin oral bioavailability in pigs and rats. *Life Sci.* **2002**, *72*, 227–235. [CrossRef]
84. Scambia, G.; Ranelletti, F.O.; Panici, P.B.; De Vincenzo, R.; Bonanno, G.; Ferrandina, G.; Piantelli, M.; Bussa, S.; Rumi, C.; Cianfriglia, M.; et al. Quercetin potentiates the effect of adriamycin in a multidrug-resistant MCF-7 human breast-cancer cell line: P-glycoprotein as a possible target. *Cancer Chemother. Pharmacol.* **1994**, *34*, 459–464. [CrossRef]
85. Santangelo, R.; Silvestrini, A.; Mancuso, C. Ginsenosides, catechins, quercetin and gut microbiota: Current evidence of challenging interactions. *Food Chem. Toxicol.* **2019**, *123*, 42–49. [CrossRef]
86. Dabeek, W.; Marra, M.V. Dietary Quercetin and Kaempferol: Bioavailability and Potential Cardiovascular-Related Bioactivity in Humans. *Nutrients* **2019**, *11*, 2288. [CrossRef]
87. Zhao, J.; Yang, J.; Xie, Y. Improvement strategies for the oral bioavailability of poorly water-soluble flavonoids: An overview. *Int. J. Pharm.* **2019**, *570*, 118642. [CrossRef]
88. Riva, A.; Ronchi, M.; Petrangolini, G.; Bosisio, S.; Allegrini, P. Improved Oral Absorption of Quercetin from Quercetin Phytosome(R), a New Delivery System Based on Food Grade Lecithin. *Eur. J. Drug Metab. Pharmacokinet.* **2019**, *44*, 169–177. [CrossRef]
89. Li, L.; Stillemark-Billton, P.; Beck, C.; Boström, P.; Andersson, L.; Rutberg, M.; Ericsson, J.; Magnusson, B.; Marchesan, D.; Ljungberg, A.; et al. Epigallocatechin gallate increases the formation of cytosolic lipid droplets and decreases the secretion of apoB-100 VLDL. *J. Lipid Res.* **2005**, *47*, 67–77. [CrossRef]
90. Zanka, K.; Kawaguchi, Y.; Okada, Y.; Nagaoka, S. Epigallocatechin Gallate Induces Upregulation of LDL Receptor via the 67 kDa Laminin Receptor-Independent Pathway in HepG2 Cells. *Mol. Nutr. Food Res.* **2020**, *64*, e1901036. [CrossRef]
91. Li, Y.; Wu, S. Epigallocatechin gallate suppresses hepatic cholesterol synthesis by targeting SREBP-2 through SIRT1/FOXO1 signaling pathway. *Mol. Cell Biochem.* **2018**, *448*, 175–185. [CrossRef]
92. Kitamura, K.; Okada, Y.; Okada, K.; Kawaguchi, Y.; Nagaoka, S. Epigallocatechin gallate induces an up-regulation of LDL receptor accompanied by a reduction of PCSK9 via the annexin A2-independent pathway in HepG2 cells. *Mol. Nutr. Food Res.* **2017**, *61*, 1600836. [CrossRef]
93. Momose, Y.; Maeda-Yamamoto, M.; Nabetani, H. Systematic review of green tea epigallocatechin gallate in reducing low-density lipoprotein cholesterol levels of humans. *Int. J. Food Sci. Nutr.* **2016**, *67*, 606–613. [CrossRef]
94. Huang, L.-H.; Liu, C.-Y.; Wang, L.-Y.; Huang, C.-J.; Hsu, C.-H. Effects of green tea extract on overweight and obese women with high levels of low density-lipoprotein-cholesterol (LDL-C): A randomised, double-blind, and cross-over placebo-controlled clinical trial. *BMC Complement. Altern. Med.* **2018**, *18*, 294. [CrossRef]
95. Lee, M.-J.; Maliakal, P.; Chen, L.; Meng, X.; Bondoc, F.Y.; Prabhu, S.; Lambert, G.; Mohr, S.; Yang, C.S. Pharmacokinetics of tea catechins after ingestion of green tea and (-)-epigallocatechin-3-gallate by humans: Formation of different metabolites and individual variability. *Cancer Epidemiol. Biomarkers Prev.* **2002**, *11*, 1025–1032.
96. Del Rio, D.; Calani, L.; Cordero, C.E.I.; Salvatore, S.; Pellegrini, N.; Brighenti, F. Bioavailability and catabolism of green tea flavan-3-ols in humans. *Nutrients* **2010**, *26*, 1110–1116. [CrossRef]
97. Sang, S.; Lambert, J.D.; Ho, C.-T.; Yang, C.S. The chemistry and biotransformation of tea constituents. *Pharmacol. Res.* **2011**, *64*, 87–99. [CrossRef]

98. Scholl, C.; Lepper, A.; Lehr, T.; Hanke, N.; Schneider, K.L.; Brockmöller, J.; Seufferlein, T.; Stingl, J. Population nutrikinetics of green tea extract. *PLoS ONE* **2018**, *13*, e0193074. [CrossRef]
99. Yashiro, T.; Nanmoku, M.; Shimizu, M.; Inoue, J.; Sato, R. Resveratrol increases the expression and activity of the low density lipoprotein receptor in hepatocytes by the proteolytic activation of the sterol regulatory element-binding proteins. *Atherosclerosis* **2012**, *220*, 369–374. [CrossRef]
100. Jing, Y.; Hu, T.; Lin, C.; Xiong, Q.; Liu, F.; Yuan, J.; Zhao, X.; Wang, R. Resveratrol downregulates PCSK9 expression and attenuates steatosis through estrogen receptor α-mediated pathway in L02 cells. *Eur. J. Pharmacol.* **2019**, *855*, 216–226. [CrossRef]
101. Wang, Y.; Ye, J.; Li, J.; Chen, C.; Huang, H.; Liu, P.-Q.; Huang, H. Polydatin ameliorates lipid and glucose metabolism in type 2 diabetes mellitus by downregulating proprotein convertase subtilisin/kexin type 9 (PCSK9). *Cardiovasc. Diabetol.* **2016**, *15*, 19. [CrossRef] [PubMed]
102. Li, L.; Shen, C.; Huang, Y.X.; Li, Y.N.; Liu, X.F.; Liu, X.M.; Liu, J.H. A New Strategy for Rapidly Screening Natural Inhibitors Targeting the PCSK9/LDLR Interaction In Vitro. *Molecules* **2018**, *23*, 2397. [CrossRef] [PubMed]
103. Haghighatdoost, F.; Hariri, M. Effect of resveratrol on lipid profile: An updated systematic review and meta-analysis on randomized clinical trials. *Pharmacol. Res.* **2018**, *129*, 141–150. [CrossRef] [PubMed]
104. Guo, X.-F.; Li, J.; Tang, J.; Li, D. Effects of resveratrol supplementation on risk factors of non-communicable diseases: A meta-analysis of randomized controlled trials. *Crit. Rev. Food Sci. Nutr.* **2017**, *58*, 3016–3029. [CrossRef]
105. Wang, P.; Sang, S. Metabolism and pharmacokinetics of resveratrol and pterostilbene. *BioFactors* **2018**, *44*, 16–25. [CrossRef]
106. Singh, A.P.; Singh, R.; Verma, S.S.; Rai, V.; Kaschula, C.H.; Maiti, P.; Gupta, S.C. Health benefits of resveratrol: Evidence from clinical studies. *Med. Res. Rev.* **2019**, *39*, 1851–1891. [CrossRef]
107. Springer, M.; Moco, S. Resveratrol and Its Human Metabolites—Effects on Metabolic Health and Obesity. *Nutrients* **2019**, *11*, 143. [CrossRef]
108. Dong, Z.; Zhang, W.; Chen, S.; Liu, C. Silibinin A decreases statin-induced PCSK9 expression in human hepatoblastoma HepG2 cells. *Mol. Med. Rep.* **2019**, *20*, 1383–1392. [CrossRef]
109. Barzaghi, N.; Crema, F.; Gatti, G.; Pifferi, G.; Perucca, E. Pharmacokinetic studies on IdB 1016, a silybin-phosphatidylcholine complex, in healthy human subjects. *Eur. J. Drug Metab. Pharmacokinet.* **1990**, *15*, 333–338. [CrossRef]
110. Valentová, K.; Havlik, J.; Kosina, P.; Papoušková, B.; Jaimes, J.D.; Káňová, K.; Petrásková, L.; Ulrichová, J.; Kren, V. Biotransformation of Silymarin Flavonolignans by Human Fecal Microbiota. *Metabolism* **2020**, *10*, 29. [CrossRef]
111. Sui, G.-G.; Xiao, H.-B.; Lu, X.-Y.; Sun, Z.-L. Naringin Activates AMPK Resulting in Altered Expression of SREBPs, PCSK9, and LDLR To Reduce Body Weight in Obese C57BL/6J Mice. *J. Agric. Food Chem.* **2018**, *66*, 8983–8990. [CrossRef] [PubMed]
112. Zeng, X.; Su, W.; Zheng, Y.; He, Y.; He, Y.; Rao, H.; Peng, W.; Yao, H. Pharmacokinetics, Tissue Distribution, Metabolism, and Excretion of Naringin in Aged Rats. *Front. Pharmacol.* **2019**, *10*, 34. [CrossRef] [PubMed]
113. Gao, W.-Y.; Chen, P.-Y.; Chen, S.-F.; Wu, M.-J.; Chang, H.-Y.; Yen, J.-H. Pinostrobin Inhibits Proprotein Convertase Subtilisin/Kexin-type 9 (PCSK9) Gene Expression through the Modulation of FoxO3a Protein in HepG2 Cells. *J. Agric. Food Chem.* **2018**, *66*, 6083–6093. [CrossRef] [PubMed]
114. Sayre, C.; Alrushaid, S.; Martinez, S.E.; Anderson, H.D.; Davies, N.M.; Sayre, C.L.; Alrushaid, S.; Martinez, S.E.; Anderson, H.D.; Pharmacy, N.M.D.O.; et al. Pre-Clinical Pharmacokinetic and Pharmacodynamic Characterization of Selected Chiral Flavonoids: Pinocembrin and Pinostrobin. *J. Pharm. Pharm. Sci.* **2015**, *18*, 368. [CrossRef] [PubMed]
115. Jo, H.K.; Kim, G.W.; Jeong, K.J.; Kim, D.Y.; Chung, S.H. Eugenol Ameliorates Hepatic Steatosis and Fibrosis by Down-Regulating SREBP1 Gene Expression via AMPK-mTOR-p70S6K Signaling Pathway. *Boil. Pharm. Bull.* **2014**, *37*, 1341–1351. [CrossRef]
116. Elbahy, D.A.; Madkour, H.I.; Abdel-Raheem, M.H. Evaluation of antihyperlipidemic activity of eugenol in triton induced hyperlipidemia in rats. *Int. J. Res. Stud. Biosci.* **2015**, *3*, 19–26.
117. Zia, S.; Batool, S.; Shahid, R. Could PCSK9 be a new therapeutic target of Eugenol? In vitro and in silico evaluation of hypothesis. *Med. Hypotheses* **2020**, *136*, 109513. [CrossRef]

118. Guénette, S.A.; Ross, A.; Marier, J.-F.; Beaudry, F.; Vachon, P. Pharmacokinetics of eugenol and its effects on thermal hypersensitivity in rats. *Eur. J. Pharmacol.* **2007**, *562*, 60–67. [CrossRef]
119. Dou, X.; Fan, C.; Wo, L.; Wo, X.; Yan, J.; Qian, Y. Curcumin Up-Regulates LDL Receptor Expression via the Sterol Regulatory Element Pathway in HepG2 Cells. *Planta Med.* **2008**, *74*, 1374–1379. [CrossRef]
120. Peschel, D.; Koerting, R.; Nass, N. Curcumin induces changes in expression of genes involved in cholesterol homeostasis. *J. Nutr. Biochem.* **2007**, *18*, 113–119. [CrossRef]
121. Kang, Q.; Chen, A. Curcumin inhibits srebp-2 expression in activated hepatic stellate cells in vitro by reducing the activity of specificity protein-1. *Endocrinology* **2009**, *150*, 5384–5394. [CrossRef]
122. Tai, M.-H.; Chen, P.-K.; Chen, P.-Y.; Wu, M.-J.; Ho, C.-T.; Yen, J.-H. Curcumin enhances cell-surface LDLR level and promotes LDL uptake through downregulation of PCSK9 gene expression in HepG2 cells. *Mol. Nutr. Food Res.* **2014**, *58*, 2133–2145. [CrossRef] [PubMed]
123. Nozue, T. Lipid Lowering Therapy and Circulating PCSK9 Concentration. *J. Atheroscler. Thromb.* **2017**, *24*, 895–907. [CrossRef] [PubMed]
124. Cai, Y.; Lu, D.; Zou, Y.; Zhou, C.; Liu, H.; Tu, C.; Li, F.; Zhang, S. Curcumin Protects Against Intestinal Origin Endotoxemia in Rat Liver Cirrhosis by Targeting PCSK9. *J. Food Sci.* **2017**, *82*, 772–780. [CrossRef] [PubMed]
125. Panahi, Y.; Ahmadi, Y.; Teymouri, M.; Johnston, T.P.; Sahebkar, A. Curcumin as a potential candidate for treating hyperlipidemia: A review of cellular and metabolic mechanisms. *J. Cell. Physiol.* **2017**, *233*, 141–152. [CrossRef] [PubMed]
126. Simental-Mendía, L.E.; Pirro, M.; Gotto, A.M.; Banach, M.; Atkin, S.L.; Majeed, M.; Sahebkar, A. Lipid-modifying activity of curcuminoids: A systematic review and meta-analysis of randomized controlled trials. *Crit. Rev. Food Sci. Nutr.* **2017**, *59*, 1178–1187. [CrossRef]
127. Nelson, K.M.; Dahlin, J.L.; Bisson, J.; Graham, J.; Pauli, G.F.; A Walters, M. The Essential Medicinal Chemistry of Curcumin. *J. Med. Chem.* **2017**, *60*, 1620–1637. [CrossRef]
128. Stohs, S.; Chen, O.; Ray, S.; Ji, J.; Bucci, L.; Preuss, H. Highly Bioavailable Forms of Curcumin and Promising Avenues for Curcumin-Based Research and Application: A Review. *Molecules* **2020**, *25*, 1397. [CrossRef]
129. Di Meo, F.; Margarucci, S.; Galderisi, U.; Crispi, S.; Peluso, G. Curcumin, Gut Microbiota, and Neuroprotection. *Nutrients* **2019**, *11*, 2426. [CrossRef]
130. Nasery, M.M.; Abadi, B.; Poormoghadam, D.; Zarrabi, A.; Keyhanvar, P.; Khanbabaei, H.; Ashrafizadeh, M.; Mohammadinejad, R.; Tavakol, S.; Sethi, G. Curcumin Delivery Mediated by Bio-Based Nanoparticles: A Review. *Molecules* **2020**, *25*, 689. [CrossRef]
131. Sung, Y.-Y.; Kim, S.H.; Kim, D.-S.; Park, S.H.; Yoo, B.W.; Kim, H.K. Nutritional composition and anti-obesity effects of cereal bar containing Allium fistulosum (welsh onion) extract. *J. Funct. Foods* **2014**, *6*, 428–437. [CrossRef]
132. Choi, H.-K.; Hwang, J.; Nam, T.G.; Kim, S.H.; Min, D.-K.; Park, S.W.; Chung, M.-Y. Welsh onion extract inhibits PCSK9 expression contributing to the maintenance of the LDLR level under lipid depletion conditions of HepG2 cells. *Food Funct.* **2017**, *8*, 4582–4591. [CrossRef] [PubMed]
133. Kim, H.K.; Sung, Y.-Y.; Yoon, T.; Kim, S.J.; Yang, W.-K. Anti-obesity activity of Allium fistulosum L. extract by down-regulation of the expression of lipogenic genes in high-fat diet-induced obese mice. *Mol. Med. Rep.* **2011**, *4*, 431–435. [CrossRef] [PubMed]
134. Mach, F.; Baigent, C.; Catapano, A.L.; Koskinas, K.C.; Casula, M.; Badimon, L.; Chapman, M.J.; De Backer, G.G.; Delgado, V.; A Ference, B.; et al. 2019 ESC/EAS Guidelines for the management of dyslipidaemias: Lipid modification to reduce cardiovascular risk. *Eur. Hear. J.* **2019**, *41*, 111–188. [CrossRef] [PubMed]
135. Baer, D.J.; A Novotny, J. Consumption of cashew nuts does not influence blood lipids or other markers of cardiovascular disease in humans: A randomized controlled trial. *Am. J. Clin. Nutr.* **2019**, *109*, 269–275. [CrossRef] [PubMed]
136. Mukuddem-Petersen, J.; (Oosthuizen), W.S.; Jerling, J.C.; Hanekom, S.M.; White, Z. Effects of a high walnut and high cashew nut diet on selected markers of the metabolic syndrome: A controlled feeding trial. *Br. J. Nutr.* **2007**, *97*, 1144–1153. [CrossRef]
137. Mah, E.; A Schulz, J.; Kaden, V.N.; Lawless, A.L.; Rotor, J.; Mantilla, L.B.; Liska, D.J. Cashew consumption reduces total and LDL cholesterol: A randomized, crossover, controlled-feeding trial. *Am. J. Clin. Nutr.* **2017**, *105*, 1070–1078. [CrossRef]
138. Mohan, V.; Gayathri, R.; Jaacks, L.M.; Lakshmipriya, N.; Anjana, R.M.; Spiegelman, D.; Jeevan, R.G.; Balasubramaniam, K.K.; Shobana, S.; Jayanthan, M.; et al. Cashew Nut Consumption Increases HDL

Cholesterol and Reduces Systolic Blood Pressure in Asian Indians with Type 2 Diabetes: A 12-Week Randomized Controlled Trial. *J. Nutr.* **2018**, *148*, 63–69. [CrossRef]
139. Chan, K.W.; Ismail, M.; Imam, M.U.; Ooi, D.J.; Khong, N.; Maznah, I.; Esa, N.M.; Der-Jiun, O. Dietary supplementation of defatted kenaf (Hibiscus cannabinus L.) seed meal and its phenolics–saponins rich extract effectively attenuates diet-induced hypercholesterolemia in rats. *Food Funct.* **2018**, *9*, 925–936. [CrossRef]
140. Yeh, Y.H.; Lee, Y.T.; Hsieh, H.S.; Hwang, D.F. Dietary caffeic acid, ferulic acid and coumaric acid supplements on cholesterol metabolism and antioxidant activity in rats. *J. Food Drug Anal.* **2009**, *17*, 123–132.
141. Hsu, C.-L.; Yen, G.-C. Effect of gallic acid on high fat diet-induced dyslipidaemia, hepatosteatosis and oxidative stress in rats. *Br. J. Nutr.* **2007**, *98*, 727–735. [CrossRef] [PubMed]
142. Kim, A.; Chiu, A.; Barone, M.K.; Avino, D.; Wang, F.; Coleman, C.I.; Phung, O.J. Green Tea Catechins Decrease Total and Low-Density Lipoprotein Cholesterol: A Systematic Review and Meta-Analysis. *J. Am. Diet. Assoc.* **2011**, *111*, 1720–1729. [CrossRef] [PubMed]
143. Zhao, D. Challenges associated with elucidating the mechanisms of the hypocholesterolaemic activity of saponins. *J. Funct. Foods* **2016**, *23*, 52–65. [CrossRef]
144. Van Ballegooijen, A.J.; Beulens, J.W. The Role of Vitamin K Status in Cardiovascular Health: Evidence from Observational and Clinical Studies. *Curr. Nutr. Rep.* **2017**, *6*, 197–205. [CrossRef] [PubMed]
145. Sato, T.; Schurgers, L.J.; Uenishi, K. Comparison of menaquinone-4 and menaquinone-7 bioavailability in healthy women. *Nutr. J.* **2012**, *11*, 93. [CrossRef] [PubMed]
146. Shearer, M.J.; Fu, X.; Booth, S.L. Vitamin K Nutrition, Metabolism, and Requirements: Current Concepts and Future Research12. *Adv. Nutr.* **2012**, *3*, 182–195. [CrossRef]
147. Nagasawa, Y.; Fujii, M.; Kajimoto, Y.; Imai, E.; Hori, M. Vitamin K2 and serum cholesterol in patients on continuous ambulatory peritoneal dialysis. *Lancet* **1998**, *351*, 724. [CrossRef]
148. Lupo, M.G.; Biancorosso, N.; Brilli, E.; Tarantino, G.; Adorni, M.P.; Vivian, G.; Salvalaio, M.; Dall'Acqua, S.; Sut, S.; Neutel, C.; et al. Cholesterol-Lowering Action of a Novel Nutraceutical Combination in Uremic Rats: Insights into the Molecular Mechanism in a Hepatoma Cell Line. *Nutrients* **2020**, *12*, 436. [CrossRef]
149. Tapiero, H.; Townsend, D.; Tew, K. The role of carotenoids in the prevention of human pathologies. *Biomed. Pharmacother.* **2004**, *58*, 100–110. [CrossRef]
150. El-Agamey, A.; Lowe, G.M.; McGarvey, D.J.; Mortensen, A.; Phillip, D.M.; Truscott, T.; Young, A. Carotenoid radical chemistry and antioxidant/pro-oxidant properties. *Arch. Biochem. Biophys.* **2004**, *430*, 37–48. [CrossRef]
151. Costa-Rodrigues, J.; Pinho, O.; Monteiro, P.R.R. Can lycopene be considered an effective protection against cardiovascular disease? *Food Chem.* **2018**, *245*, 1148–1153. [CrossRef]
152. Alvi, S.S.; Ansari, I.A.; Khan, I.; Iqbal, J.; Khan, M.S. Potential role of lycopene in targeting proprotein convertase subtilisin/kexin type-9 to combat hypercholesterolemia. *Free Radic. Boil. Med.* **2017**, *108*, 394–403. [CrossRef] [PubMed]
153. Tang, Z.; Jiang, L.; Peng, J.; Ren, Z.; Wei, D.; Wu, C.; Pan, L.; Jiang, Z.; Liu, L. PCSK9 siRNA suppresses the inflammatory response induced by oxLDL through inhibition of NF-kappaB activation in THP-1-derived macrophages. *Int. J. Mol. Med.* **2012**, *30*, 931–938. [CrossRef] [PubMed]
154. Alvi, S.S.; Ansari, I.A.; Ahmad, M.K.; Iqbal, J.; Khan, M.S. Lycopene amends LPS induced oxidative stress and hypertriglyceridemia via modulating PCSK-9 expression and Apo-CIII mediated lipoprotein lipase activity. *Biomed. Pharmacother.* **2017**, *96*, 1082–1093. [CrossRef] [PubMed]
155. Story, E.N.; Kopec, R.E.; Schwartz, S.J.; Harris, G.K. An update on the health effects of tomato lycopene. *Annu. Rev. Food Sci. Technol.* **2010**, *1*, 189–210. [CrossRef] [PubMed]
156. Moia, V.M.; Portilho, F.L.; Pádua, T.A.; Corrêa, L.B.; Ricci-Junior, E.; Rosas, E.C.; Alencar, L.M.R.; Sinfronio, F.S.M.; Sampson, A.; Iram, S.H.; et al. Lycopene used as Anti-inflammatory Nanodrug for the Treatment of Rheumathoid Arthritis: Animal assay, Pharmacokinetics, ABC Transporter and Tissue Deposition. *Coll. Surf. B Biointerf.* **2020**, *188*, 110814. [CrossRef]
157. Kiefer, C.; Hessel, S.; Lampert, J.M.; Vogt, K.; Lederer, M.O.; Breithaupt, D.E.; Von Lintig, J. Identification and Characterization of a Mammalian Enzyme Catalyzing the Asymmetric Oxidative Cleavage of Provitamin A. *J. Boil. Chem.* **2001**, *276*, 14110–14116. [CrossRef]
158. Wang, X.-D. Lycopene metabolism and its biological significance. *Am. J. Clin. Nutr.* **2012**, *96*, 1214S–1222S. [CrossRef]

159. Innes, J.; Calder, P.C. Marine Omega-3 (N-3) Fatty Acids for Cardiovascular Health: An Update for 2020. *Int. J. Mol. Sci.* **2020**, *21*, 1362. [CrossRef]
160. Mason, R.P.; Libby, P.; Bhatt, D.L. Emerging Mechanisms of Cardiovascular Protection for the Omega-3 Fatty Acid Eicosapentaenoic Acid. *Arter. Thromb. Vasc. Boil.* **2020**, *40*, 1135–1147. [CrossRef]
161. Scorletti, E.; Byrne, C.D. Omega-3 fatty acids and non-alcoholic fatty liver disease: Evidence of efficacy and mechanism of action. *Mol. Asp. Med.* **2018**, *64*, 135–146. [CrossRef]
162. Pizzini, A.; Lunger, L.; Demetz, E.; Hilbe, R.; Weiss, G.; Ebenbichler, C.; Tancevski, I. The Role of Omega-3 Fatty Acids in Reverse Cholesterol Transport: A Review. *Nutrients* **2017**, *9*, 1099. [CrossRef]
163. Yuan, F.; Wang, H.; Tian, Y.; Li, Q.; He, L.; Li, N.; Liu, Z. Fish oil alleviated high-fat diet–induced non-alcoholic fatty liver disease via regulating hepatic lipids metabolism and metaflammation: A transcriptomic study. *Lipids Heal. Dis.* **2016**, *15*, 20. [CrossRef]
164. Sorokin, A.V.; Yang, Z.-H.; Vaisman, B.; Thacker, S.; Yu, Z.-X.; Sampson, M.; Serhan, C.N.; Remaley, A.T. Addition of aspirin to a fish oil-rich diet decreases inflammation and atherosclerosis in ApoE-null mice. *J. Nutr. Biochem.* **2016**, *35*, 58–65. [CrossRef]
165. Pu, S.; Rodriguez-Perez, C.; Ramprasath, V.R.; Segura-Carretero, A.; Jones, P.J.H. Dietary high oleic canola oil supplemented with docosahexaenoic acid attenuates plasma proprotein convertase subtilisin kexin type 9 (PCSK9) levels in participants with cardiovascular disease risk: A randomized control trial. *Vasc. Pharmacol.* **2016**, *87*, 60–65. [CrossRef]
166. Graversen, C.B.; Lundbye-Christensen, S.; Thomsen, B.; Christensen, J.H.; Schmidt, E.B. Marine n-3 polyunsaturated fatty acids lower plasma proprotein convertase subtilisin kexin type 9 levels in pre- and postmenopausal women: A randomised study. *Vasc. Pharmacol.* **2016**, *76*, 37–41. [CrossRef]
167. Bradberry, J.C.; Hilleman, D.E. Overview of Omega-3 Fatty Acid Therapies. *PTJ Formul. Manag.* **2013**, *38*, 681–691.
168. Allaire, J.; Couture, P.; Leclerc, M.; Charest, A.; Marin, J.; Lépine, M.-C.; Talbot, D.; Tchernof, A.; Lamarche, B. A randomized, crossover, head-to-head comparison of eicosapentaenoic acid and docosahexaenoic acid supplementation to reduce inflammation markers in men and women: The Comparing EPA to DHA (ComparED) Study. *Am. J. Clin. Nutr.* **2016**, *104*, 280–287. [CrossRef]
169. Allaire, J.; Vors, C.; Tremblay, A.J.; Marin, J.; Charest, A.; Tchernof, A.; Couture, P.; Lamarche, B. High-Dose DHA Has More Profound Effects on LDL-Related Features Than High-Dose EPA: The ComparED Study. *J. Clin. Endocrinol. Metab.* **2018**, *103*, 2909–2917. [CrossRef]
170. Allaire, J.; Vors, C.; Harris, W.S.; Jackson, K.H.; Tchernof, A.; Couture, P.; Lamarche, B. Comparing the serum TAG response to high-dose supplementation of either DHA or EPA among individuals with increased cardiovascular risk: The ComparED study. *Br. J. Nutr.* **2019**, *121*, 1223–1234. [CrossRef]
171. Bjermo, H.; Iggman, D.; Kullberg, J.; Dahlman, I.; Johansson, L.; Persson, L.; Berglund, J.; Pulkki, K.; Basu, S.; Uusitupa, M.; et al. Effects of n-6 PUFAs compared with SFAs on liver fat, lipoproteins, and inflammation in abdominal obesity: A randomized controlled trial. *Am. J. Clin. Nutr.* **2012**, *95*, 1003–1012. [CrossRef]
172. Kathiresan, S.; Willer, C.J.; Peloso, G.M.; Demissie, S.; Musunuru, K.; E Schadt, E.; Kaplan, L.; Bennett, D.; Li, Y.; Tanaka, T.; et al. Common variants at 30 loci contribute to polygenic dyslipidemia. *Nat. Genet.* **2008**, *41*, 56–65. [CrossRef]
173. Yu, Z.; Huang, T.; Zheng, Y.; Wang, T.; Heianza, Y.; Sun, D.; Campos, H.; Qi, L. PCSK9 variant, long-chain n-3 PUFAs, and risk of nonfatal myocardial infarction in Costa Rican Hispanics. *Am. J. Clin. Nutr.* **2017**, *105*, 1198–1203. [CrossRef]
174. Maki, K.C.; Dicklin, M.R. Strategies to improve bioavailability of omega-3 fatty acids from ethyl ester concentrates. *Curr. Opin. Clin. Nutr. Metab. Care* **2019**, *22*, 116–123. [CrossRef]
175. Cuenoud, B.; Rochat, I.; Gosoniu, M.; Dupuis, L.; Berk, E.; Jaudszus, A.; Mainz, J.; Hafen, G.; Beaumont, M.; Cruz-Hernandez, C. Monoacylglycerol Form of Omega-3s Improves Its Bioavailability in Humans Compared to Other Forms. *Nutrients* **2020**, *12*, 1014. [CrossRef]
176. Mann, G.V.; Spoerry, A. Studies of a surfactant and cholesteremia in the Maasai. *Am. J. Clin. Nutr.* **1974**, *27*, 464–469. [CrossRef]
177. Ruscica, M.; Pavanello, C.; Gandini, S.; Macchi, C.; Botta, M.; Dall'Orto, D.; Del Puppo, M.; Bertolotti, M.; Bosisio, R.; Mombelli, G.; et al. Nutraceutical approach for the management of cardiovascular risk—A combination containing the probiotic Bifidobacterium longum BB536 and red yeast rice extract: Results from a randomized, double-blind, placebo-controlled study. *Nutr. J.* **2019**, *18*, 13. [CrossRef] [PubMed]

178. Zhou, S.L. Comparative analysis of lipid-lowering effect of Diao Xinxuekang and Xin nao shu tong. *Shandong Med. J.* **1997**, *37*.
179. Qu, L.; Li, D.; Gao, X.; Li, Y.; Wu, J.; Zou, W. Di'ao Xinxuekang Capsule, a Chinese Medicinal Product, Decreases Serum Lipids Levels in High-Fat Diet-Fed ApoE(-/-) Mice by Downregulating PCSK9. *Front. Pharmacol.* **2018**, *9*, 1170. [CrossRef] [PubMed]
180. Gai, Y.; Li, Y.; Xu, Z.; Chen, J. Pseudoprotodioscin inhibits SREBPs and microRNA 33a/b levels and reduces the gene expression regarding the synthesis of cholesterol and triglycerides. *Fitoterapia* **2019**, *139*, 104393. [CrossRef]
181. Guo, L.; Dial, S.; Shi, L.; Branham, W.; Liu, J.; Fang, J.-L.; Green, B.; Deng, H.; Kaput, J.; Ning, B. Similarities and differences in the expression of drug-metabolizing enzymes between human hepatic cell lines and primary human hepatocytes. *Drug Metab. Dispos.* **2010**, *39*, 528–538. [CrossRef]
182. Westerink, W.M.; Schoonen, W.G. Phase II enzyme levels in HepG2 cells and cryopreserved primary human hepatocytes and their induction in HepG2 cells. *Toxicol. Vitr.* **2007**, *21*, 1592–1602. [CrossRef]
183. Westerink, W.M.A.; Schoonen, W.G. Cytochrome P450 enzyme levels in HepG2 cells and cryopreserved primary human hepatocytes and their induction in HepG2 cells. *Toxicol. Vitr.* **2007**, *21*, 1581–1591. [CrossRef]
184. Shang, X.; Yuan, Z.-B. Determination of six effective components in Rheum by cyclodextrin modified micellar electrokinetic chromatography. *Yao Xue Xue Bao Acta Pharm. Sin.* **2002**, *37*, 798–801.
185. Li, J.; Ding, L.; Song, B.; Xiao, X.; Qi, M.; Yang, Q.; Yang, Q.; Tang, X.; Wang, Z.; Yang, L. Emodin improves lipid and glucose metabolism in high fat diet-induced obese mice through regulating SREBP pathway. *Eur. J. Pharmacol.* **2016**, *770*, 99–109. [CrossRef]
186. Wang, J.; Ji, J.; Song, Z.; Zhang, W.; He, X.; Li, F.; Zhang, C.-F.; Guo, C.-R.; Wang, C.; Yuan, C. Hypocholesterolemic effect of emodin by simultaneous determination of in vitro and in vivo bile salts binding. *Fitoterapia* **2016**, *110*, 116–122. [CrossRef]
187. Su, Z.-L.; Hang, P.-Z.; Hu, J.; Zheng, Y.-Y.; Sun, H.-Q.; Guo, J.; Liu, K.-Y.; Du, Z.-M. Aloe-emodin exerts cholesterol-lowering effects by inhibiting proprotein convertase subtilisin/kexin type 9 in hyperlipidemic rats. *Acta Pharmacol. Sin.* **2020**, 1–8. [CrossRef]
188. Maeng, H.-J.; Yoo, H.-J.; Kim, I.-W.; Song, I.-S.; Chung, S.-J.; Shim, C.-K. P-Glycoprotein–Mediated Transport of Berberine across Caco-2 Cell Monolayers. *J. Pharm. Sci.* **2002**, *91*, 2614–2621. [CrossRef]
189. Dooren, M.M.G.-V.; Ronden, J.E.; Soute, B.A.; Vermeer, C. Bioavailability of phylloquinone and menaquinones after oral and colorectal administration in vitamin K-deficient rats. *Biochem. Pharmacol.* **1995**, *50*, 797–801. [CrossRef]
190. Cohn, W.; Tenter, U.; Aebischer, C.; Schierle, J.; Schalch, W. Comparative multiple dose plasma kinetics of lycopene administered in tomato juice, tomato soup or lycopene tablets. *Eur. J. Nutr.* **2004**, *43*, 304–312. [CrossRef]
191. Lin, S.-P.; Chu, P.-M.; Tsai, S.-Y.; Wu, M.-H.; Hou, Y.-C. Pharmacokinetics and tissue distribution of resveratrol, emodin and their metabolites after intake of Polygonum cuspidatum in rats. *J. Ethnopharmacol.* **2012**, *144*, 671–676. [CrossRef]
192. Yu, J.; Guo, X.; Zhang, Q.; Peng, Y.; Zheng, J. Metabolite profile analysis and pharmacokinetic study of emodin, baicalin and geniposide in rats. *Xenobiotica* **2017**, *48*, 927–937. [CrossRef]
193. Macchi, C.; Sirtori, C.; Corsini, A.; Santos, R.; Watts, G.F.; Ruscica, M. A new dawn for managing dyslipidemias: The era of rna-based therapies. *Pharmacol. Res.* **2019**, *150*, 104413. [CrossRef]
194. Poli, A.; Barbagallo, C.M.; Cicero, A.F.; Corsini, A.; Manzato, E.; Trimarco, B.; Bernini, F.; Visioli, F.; Bianchi, A.; Canzone, G.; et al. Nutraceuticals and functional foods for the control of plasma cholesterol levels. An intersociety position paper. *Pharmacol. Res.* **2018**, *134*, 51–60. [CrossRef]
195. Fogacci, F.; Banach, M.; Mikhailidis, D.P.; Bruckert, E.; Toth, P.P.; Watts, G.F.; Reiner, Z.; Mancini, J.; Rizzo, M.; Mitchenko, O.; et al. Safety of red yeast rice supplementation: A systematic review and meta-analysis of randomized controlled trials. *Pharmacol. Res.* **2019**, *143*, 1–16. [CrossRef]
196. Ruscica, M.; Gomaraschi, M.; Mombelli, G.; Macchi, C.; Bosisio, R.; Pazzucconi, F.; Pavanello, C.; Calabresi, L.; Arnoldi, A.; Sirtori, C.R.; et al. Nutraceutical approach to moderate cardiometabolic risk: Results of a randomized, double-blind and crossover study with Armolipid Plus. *J. Clin. Lipidol.* **2014**, *8*, 61–68. [CrossRef]

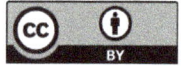

© 2020 by the authors. Licensee MDPI, Basel, Switzerland. This article is an open access article distributed under the terms and conditions of the Creative Commons Attribution (CC BY) license (http://creativecommons.org/licenses/by/4.0/).

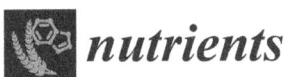

Review

The Effect of Natural Antioxidants in the Development of Metabolic Syndrome: Focus on Bergamot Polyphenolic Fraction

Cristina Carresi [1,*], Micaela Gliozzi [1], Vincenzo Musolino [1], Miriam Scicchitano [1], Federica Scarano [1], Francesca Bosco [1], Saverio Nucera [1], Jessica Maiuolo [1], Roberta Macrì [1], Stefano Ruga [1], Francesca Oppedisano [1], Maria Caterina Zito [1], Lorenza Guarnieri [1], Rocco Mollace [1,2], Annamaria Tavernese [1,2], Ernesto Palma [1,3], Ezio Bombardelli [1,3], Massimo Fini [3,4] and Vincenzo Mollace [1,3]

[1] Institute of Research for Food Safety & Health IRC-FSH, University Magna Graecia, 88100 Catanzaro, Italy; micaela.gliozzi@gmail.com (M.G.); xabaras3@hotmail.com (V.M.); miriam.scicchitano@hotmail.it (M.S.); federicascar87@gmail.com (F.S.); boscofrancesca.bf@libero.it (F.B.); saverio.nucera@hotmail.it (S.N.); jessicamaiuolo@virgilio.it (J.M.); robertamacri85@gmail.com (Roberta Macrì); rugast1@gmail.com (S.R.); oppedisanof@libero.it (F.O.); mariacaterina.zito@studenti.unicz.it (M.C.Z.); lorenzacz808@gmail.com (L.G.); rocco.mollace@gmail.com (Rocco Mollace); an.tavernese@gmail.com (A.T.); palma@unicz.it (E.P.); ezio.bombardelli@plantexresearch.it (E.B.); mollace@libero.it (V.M.)
[2] Department of Medicine, Chair of Cardiology, University of Rome Tor Vergata, 00133 Roma, Italy
[3] Nutramed S.c.a.r.l., Complesso Ninì Barbieri, Roccelletta di Borgia, 88021 Catanzaro, Italy; massimo.fini@sanraffaele.it
[4] IRCCS San Raffaele Pisana, 00163 Roma, Italy
* Correspondence: carresi@unicz.it; Tel.: +00-39-09613694128; Fax: 0039-0961-3695-737

Received: 22 March 2020; Accepted: 15 May 2020; Published: 21 May 2020

Abstract: Metabolic syndrome (MetS) represents a set of clinical findings that include visceral adiposity, insulin-resistance, high triglycerides (TG), low high-density lipoprotein cholesterol (HDL-C) levels and hypertension, which is linked to an increased risk of developing type 2 diabetes mellitus (T2DM) and atherosclerotic cardiovascular disease (ASCVD). The pathogenesis of MetS involves both genetic and acquired factors triggering oxidative stress, cellular dysfunction and systemic inflammation process mainly responsible for the pathophysiological mechanism. In recent years, MetS has gained importance due to the exponential increase in obesity worldwide. However, at present, it remains underdiagnosed and undertreated. The present review will summarize the pathogenesis of MetS and the existing pharmacological therapies currently used and focus attention on the beneficial effects of natural compounds to reduce the risk and progression of MetS. In this regard, emerging evidence suggests a potential protective role of bergamot extracts, in particular bergamot flavonoids, in the management of different features of MetS, due to their pleiotropic anti-oxidative, anti-inflammatory and lipid-lowering effects.

Keywords: metabolic syndrome; plant extracts; natural antioxidant; polyphenols; bergamot

1. Introduction

Among the so called non-communicable diseases, which represent the major cause of morbidity and mortality worldwide, Metabolic syndrome (MetS) can be considered the real scourge globally [1]. It is variously known as Raven syndrome, insulin resistance syndrome, plurimetabolic syndrome and some others. MetS has been increasingly recognized as one of the important contributors to the pandemic of ASCVD and T2DM, which represent a serious clinical and public health problem [2]. Through the years, several definitions of MetS have been suggested. In the United States, the National

Cholesterol Treatment Program Adult Treatment Panel III (NCEP–ATP III) published a clinically applicable definition for MetS in 2001, which was revised in 2005 establishing lower waist circumference thresholds and fasting blood glucose levels [3]. According to the NCEP ATP III definition, which is the most widely applied criteria to date, MetS is identified if three or more of the following five criteria are present: waist circumference over 40 inches (men) or 35 inches (women), blood pressure over 130/85 mmHg, fasting TG level over 150 mg/dL, fasting HDL-C level less than 40 mg/dL (men) or 50 mg/dL (women) and fasting blood sugar over 100 mg/dL (Table 1). The distinctive features of MetS included abdominal obesity, atherogenic dyslipidemia (elevated TG, small low-density lipoprotein–LDL particles, low HDL-C), elevated blood pressure, insulin resistance (with or without glucose intolerance), endothelial dysfunction and pro-thrombotic and pro-inflammatory states [4]. Often, the incidence of MetS parallels the incidence of obesity and/or T2DM. MetS is also associated with non-alcoholic fatty liver disease state (NAFLD), which has been defined as the hepatic manifestation of MetS. It was observed that MetS and NAFLD often coexist and about 90% of NAFLD patients show more than one component of MetS [5]. Indeed, some common pathophysiological features, such as increased TG, blood pressure, glucose and lower HDL levels underlying the development of NAFLD and MetS have been identified [6]. Moreover, several scientific reports have clearly recognized insulin resistance as a key factor in the pathophysiology of both diseases [5,7]. The incidence of MetS varies according to age, gender, socioeconomic status, ethnic background and criteria used for diagnosis. Several studies published in the past years reported that about one-quarter of adult manifest MetS criteria in multiple ethnic backgrounds [8]. Hence, considering the origin of Mets as a cluster of individual risk factors for disease and its spread worldwide, an accurate diagnosis to forecast the risk is crucial. The main purpose is to counteract the different components of MetS with therapeutic lifestyle changes (TLCs) and pharmacologic therapies to prevent disease, above all CVD and diabetes. In addition, there is growing interest in the use of naturally occurring compounds to reduce the risk and progression of MetS. In particular, in the last decade, interesting studies highlighted the beneficial effects of various natural antioxidants and their possible mechanisms of action for managing MetS.

Among these, bergamot has recently been studied. Bergamot (*Citrus bergamia* Risso et Poiteau) is an endemic plant growing in Calabria (Southern Italy). Already around 1660, the essence of bergamot was used as a pain reliever and, a little later, as fragrance. Bergamot has always played an important role in Calabrian economy as the main source for the production of the essential oil used in the cosmetic industry. It has been also traditionally used in the gastronomic field and in the pre-operative natural disinfection. Bergamot possesses a profile of flavonoids and glycosides, such as neoeriocitrin, neohesperidin, naringin, rutin and poncirin, which can be considered unique in its various forms (essential oil, hydro-alcoholic extract and fruit juice), and it differs from other citrus fruits not only for the composition of its flavonoids but also for their particularly high juice content [9,10]. Recent scientific data well identified the strong anti-oxidative and anti-inflammatory effects as well as interestingly hypolipidemic and hypocholesterolemic properties shedding a new light on its use as nutraceutical.

Table 1. Diagnostic criteria for metabolic syndrome.

Clinical Measure	WHO 1998	EGIR 1999	ATP III 2001	IDF 2005	AHA/NHLBI 2005
Criteria	Insulin Resistance + any other 2	Insulin Resistance + any other 2	Any other 3 of 5	Increased WC (population specific) + any other 2	Any other 3 of 5
Insulin Resistance	IGT/IFG/IR	Plasma insulin < 75th percentile	-	-	-
Blood Glucose	IFG/IGT/T2DM	IFG/IGT (excludes diabetes)	≥ 110 mg/gL (includes diabetes)	≥ 100 mg/gL	≥ 100 mg/gL (includes diabetes)
Dyslipidemia	TG ≥ 150 mg/dL HDL-C Men < 35mg/dL Women < 39mg/dL	TG ≥ 150 mg/dL HDL-C < 39mg/dL	TG ≥ 150 mg/dL HDL-C Men < 40 mg/dL Women < 50 mg/dL	TG ≥ 150 mg/dL or on TG treatment HDL-C Men < 40 mg/dL Women < 50 mg/dL or HDL treatment	TG ≥ 150 mg/dL or on TG treatment HDL-C Men < 40 mg/dL Women < 50 mg/dL or HDL treatment
Blood Pressure	≥ 140/90 mmHg	≥ 140/90 mmHg or on treatment	≥ 130/85 mmHg or on treatment	≥ 130/85 mmHg or on treatment	≥ 130/85 mmHg or on treatment
Obesity	Waist:Hip (W:H) ratio Man > 0,9 Women > 0,85 and/or BMI > 30 Kg/m²	WC Men ≥ 94 cm Women ≥ 80 cm	WC Men ≥ 102 cm Women ≥ 88 cm	WC ≥ 94 cm	WC Men ≥ 102 cm Women ≥ 88 cm
Other	Microalbuminuria	-	-	-	-

ATP, Adult Treatment Panel; BMI, Body Mass Index; EGIR, European Group for Study of Insulin Resistance; HDL-C, High Density Lipoprotein Cholesterol; IDF, International Diabetes Federation; IFG, Impaired Fasting Glucose; IGT, Impaired Glucose Tolerance; IR, Insulin Resistance; TG, Triglycerides; T2DM, Type 2 Diabetes Mellitus; WC, Waist Circumference; WHO, World Health Organization; -: no reference values have been reported.

2. Pathogenesis of Metabolic Syndrome

Several theories have been put forward to describe a common underlying mechanistic pathway for MetS. Whether the distinct features of MetS can be considered as distinct pathologies or are expression of a common disease is still under debate. Among the main factors contributing to the onset of MetS, lifestyle factors such as overeating and lack of physical activity have been identified. It has been suggested that visceral adiposity represents the main pathological condition that leads to the activation of most of the pathways involved in MetS [11,12]. According to this hypothesis, the high caloric intake could be considered one of the casual factors in the progression of MetS. Among the studied mechanisms involved in the development of MetS and in its transition to ASCVD and/or T2DM, insulin resistance, neurohumoral activation and chronic inflammation have been reported (Figure 1). Visceral fat has a gene expression pattern associated with higher risk of developing insulin resistance and producing smaller low-density lipoprotein cholesterol (LDL-C) size, increased LDL-C and very low–density lipoprotein (VLDL) and reduced HDL particle numbers [13]. In predisposed individuals, insulin-resistance condition leads to hyperinsulinemia, enhancing the hormone-sensitive lipase activity [14]. This condition triggers an additional lipolysis of stored TG from adipocytes raising the release of free fatty acids (FFAs) [14]. Circulating FFAs, in turn, inhibit the anti-lipolytic effect of insulin, creating a vicious cycle [15]. The increased amount of FFAs to the liver enhance their hepatic esterification to TG resulting in increased VLDL production, hypertriglyceridemia and reduction in plasma HDL-C [16]. Additional TG are further transferred to LDL, which become the main substrate for hepatic lipase resulting in more atherogenic small dense LDL (sdLDL) particles more prone to oxidation and uptake into the arterial wall [17]. With an impaired hepatic metabolism of cholesterol and excess circulating FFAs, gluconeogenesis is increased leading to hyperglycemia [18]. Several studies identified the mechanism of action underlying FFAs accumulation and muscle insulin resistance. Indeed, FFAs, converted to diacylglycerides (DAGs) and ceramides in the liver, trigger protein kinase C (PKC) activity and inhibit the protein kinase B (PKB or Akt) leading to insulin resistance [19]. This clinical condition often leads to the onset of T2DM since pancreatic β-cell function collapses trying to overcome resistance [20]. Moreover, insulin resistance is involved in the development of hypertension through different mechanisms of action. Partially, the increased circulating FFAs enhance reactive oxygen species (ROS) production, which in turn reduce the bioavailability of nitric oxide (NO) leading to increased vascular tone, vasoconstriction and elevated blood pressure [21]. Additional mechanisms involved in the development of hypertension include the effect of adipose tissue–derived cytokines [22] and hyperactivity of the renin-angiotensin-aldosterone system (RAAS) as it was observed in obese patients [23]. Visceral adipose tissue, which is considered as an active endocrine organ, synthesizes significantly high amounts of bioactive molecules, adipocytokines, which regulate inflammation process, immune function and also insulin sensitivity, blood pressure homeostasis, glucose and lipid metabolism [24]. It is well known that adipocyte products secrete monocyte chemoattractant protein-1 (MCP-1), tumor necrosis factor (TNF)-α and interleukin (IL)-6, which cause infiltration of macrophages into adipose tissue contributing to the onset of MetS [25]. In turn, TNF-α signaling activates intracellular kinases, such as c-Jun N-terminal kinase (JNK) and inhibitor of kappa B kinase (IKK), which increase serine phosphorylation of insulin receptor substrate-1 (IRS-1) impairing insulin-induced glucose uptake [26]. In an insulin resistance condition, the inhibition of Akt, due to phosphoinositide 3-kinase (PI3K) downregulation, leads to disruption of glucose transporter type 4 (GLUT-4) translocation to the surface membrane of skeletal muscle cells inhibiting glucose uptake [26]. Moreover, Akt inhibition triggers the activation of the transcription factor forkhead box protein O1 (Foxo1), which increases the expression of key enzymes of gluconeogenesis, leading to hyperglycemia [14]. Furthermore, high levels of TNF-α and IL-6 exacerbate inflammation through activation of the pro-inflammatory transcription factor nuclear factor kappa-light-chain-enhancer of activated B cells (NF-κB) [25]. NF-κB increases the release of cytokines and chemokines, the recruitment of monocytes and neutrophils to the tissues [27] and upregulates vascular cell adhesion molecules (VCAM) on endothelial cells, which leads to foam cell formation and atherosclerosis [28].

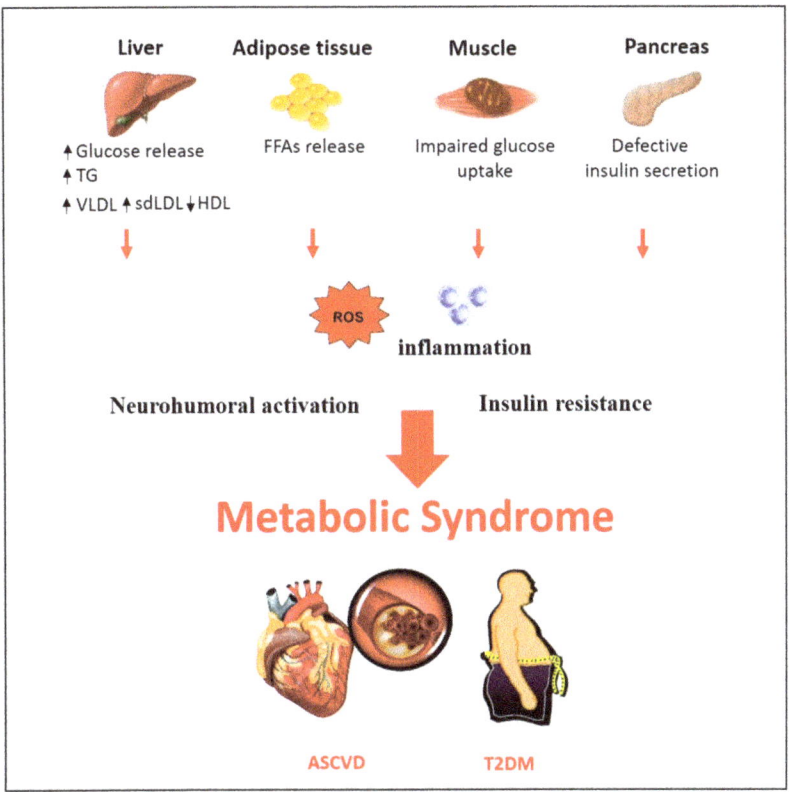

Figure 1. Pathogenesis of Metabolic syndrome. Pathophysiological mechanisms in metabolic syndrome. ASCVD, Atherosclerotic Cardiovascular Disease; FFAs, Free Fatty Acids; HDL, High Density Lipoprotein; sdLDL, small dense low-density Lipoprotein; TG, Triglycerides; T2DM, Type 2 Diabetes Mellitus; VLDL, very-low-density Lipoprotein.

Clinical Management of MetS components

The treatment of patients with MetS includes different approaches that involve lifestyle and dietary changes for weight loss and pharmacological interventions to treat atherogenic dyslipidemia and hypertension in order to decrease ASCVD and T2DM events. As described, many patients with MetS are obese because of high-calorie intake and unnecessary amount of calories. In these patients, weight loss through lifestyle modification and physical activity represent a key strategy. In a recent review, 11 randomized controlled studies of lifestyle interventions showed that the rate of patients recovered from MetS was approximately 2-fold over controls with a reduction in blood pressure, TG, waist circumference, and fasting glucose levels [29]. Dietary recommendations have been published in the American Heart Association/National Heart, Lung and Blood Institute (AHA/NHLBI) update on the NCEP criteria. According to it, fat intake should be 25% or less of calories, with reduced levels of saturated and trans fats, cholesterol intake, sodium and simple sugars [20]. A lifestyle consisting in both balanced diet and exercise is recommended as the first line treatment for MetS [30]. Weight reduction and maintenance of weight are essential and helpful in improving all the components of MetS. The Mediterranean and DASH (Dietary Approaches to Stop Hypertension) diets have demonstrated to be successful in reducing weight and improving MetS components [31,32]. Mediterranean diet, mainly based on the consumption of monounsaturated fatty acids from olives and olive oil, wholegrain cereals, fruits, vegetables, low-fat dairy, fish and nuts, has been associated with an improvement of cardiovascular outcomes decreasing oxidative stress and inflammation and improving endothelial function [33]. In addition, the *Prevención con Dieta Mediterránea* trial (Predimed) reported interesting results supporting the beneficial effects of Mediterranean diet in preventing diabetes and MetS [34]. It was shown that just an ounce of extra virgin olive oil added to the usual western type diet reduced the incidence of MetS and hypertension [34]. Interestingly, it was also observed that the molecular mechanisms underlying the beneficial effects involve the polyphenols contained in the Mediterranean diet, which cause the reduction of ROS-mediated activation of NF-κB, matrix metalloproteinases (MMPs) and cyclooxygenase-2 (COX-2) [21].

Beyond the application of these strategies, pharmacological interventions are used. Major traditional drugs include the use of metformin, which is, to date, the most effective and sole antidiabetic drug whose mechanism of action seems to mimic the effect of exercise [35]. Another widely used traditional drug is statin (3-hydroxy-3-methylglutaryl coenzyme A (HMG-CoA) reductase inhibitor), a potent cholesterol lowering drug with a strong effect mediated by the inhibition of the rate limiting step in the mevalonate synthesis. Statin is often used as a monotherapy or in association with other drugs targeted to decrease LDL-C levels [36]. Moreover, fibrates (a class of synthetic peroxisome proliferator-activated receptors (PPARs) agonists) are considered one of the main choice drugs in the treatment of patients with atherogenic dyslipidemia. Indeed, fibrates are effective in reducing TG levels more than 50% and increasing total HDL-C levels up to 25-30% [37]. Their different pharmacological properties have also been observed in several clinical trials carried out on patients with combined hyperlipidemia, diabetic dyslipidemia and NAFLD as well in combination therapy with statins [38–40]. Antiplatelet therapy is frequently used to reduce prothrombotic risk, and insulin sensitizers are administered to decrease the risk of diabetes [36]. Obese patients are treated with angiotensin converting enzyme inhibitor or angiotensin receptor blocker in presence of an increased RAAS activity [23]. To counteract salt sensitivity, the use of diuretics is acknowledged and, in some cases, recommended [23]. Although the available drugs are both safe and very effective in the treatment of the individual features of MetS, the prolonged use of more concurrent drugs could lead to serious side effects such as myopathy, pancreatitis, and thrombotic events [37,41]. However, the description of each individual therapy is beyond the scope of this review. Instead, in addition to approved pharmacological therapies, there is growing interest in the use of naturally occurring compounds as alternative strategies that could be effective in counteracting multiple components of MetS maybe avoiding the onset of side effects. Here, we describe some natural remedies useful in the management of subjects with MetS.

3. Natural remedies in the management of Metabolic Syndrome

Many natural remedies, which include plant extracts, spices, herbs and essential oils, have interesting therapeutic potential in the treatment of patients with MetS, which could be harnessed to create newer therapeutic modalities. Among the many existing so-called functional foods, effective in preventing MetS, berberine is of particular importance. It is a benzylisoquinoline alkaloid of the protoberberine type found in an array of plants (es. *Rhizoma coptidis*). Berberine is widely used in traditional Chinese medicine for its anti-microbial properties and has shown pharmacological biocompounds that include anti-inflammatory and antioxidant activities [42]. From twenty-seven randomized controlled clinical trials, it was reported that berberine treatment has significant therapeutic effects on patients with T2DM, hyperlipidemia and hypertension [43] In these patients, berberine reduces fasting blood glucose, postprandial plasma glucose and systolic blood pressure [43]. Furthermore, lower TG, total cholesterol (TC) and LDL-C levels were observed together with higher HDL-C levels [43]. Some recent studies have confirmed that the application of berberine effectively regulates blood glucose and lipids, ameliorates insulin resistance, inhibits inflammatory response [44] as well as reduces waist circumference, TG levels and systolic blood pressure in patients with MetS [45]. Moreover, berberine treatment results in the inhibition of human preadipocyte differentiation and leptin and adiponectin secretion. These processes are accompanied by downregulation of PPARγ2, CCAAT-enhancer-binding proteins (C/EBPα), adiponectin and leptin mRNA expression [46]. Interestingly, Jiayu Lin et al. have shown that berberine improves metabolic function in a mouse model fed with high fat diet (HFD) [47]. Indeed, in the animals treated with berberine, an increased energy metabolism and glucose tolerance was observed. In addition, the up-regulation of thermogenesis genes (uncoupling protein 1-UCP1, and phosphor signal transducer and activator of transcription 3-p-STAT3) and the reduction of pro-inflammatory cytokines (IL-6, TNFα and MCP1) and macrophages were observed in the white adipose tissue leading to a reduction of apoptotic gene expression [47]. Berberine also exerts an insulin sensitizing action, similar to that of metformin and thiazolidinediones, in obese and diabetic C57BLKS/J-$Lepr^{db}$/$Lepr^{db}$ male mice and in Wistar rats fed with HFD, which is mediated, at least in part, by AMP associated protein kinase activity [48]. One of the main drawbacks of berberine is its poor oral bioavailability, considered to be less than 1%, due to its low aqueous solubility [49]. In this regard, different pharmaceutical formulations such as microemulsion [50] and anhydrous reverse micelle system [51] have been developed to enhance its bioavailability. Despite low bioavailability and low plasma levels, high tissue distribution of berberine and its active metabolites has been observed [52]. Berberine mainly accumulates in the liver, followed by distribution in several other organs and finally in fat where it remains relatively stable for 48h [52]. Several studies performed on animal models and humans have shown that berberine undergoes demethylation in the phase I of liver metabolism followed by conjugation with glucuronic acid or sulfuric acid in phase II [53]. After oral administration, berberine and its metabolites are excreted in bile, urine and feces [54]. The safety profile of berberine has been widely studied in several human reports [55,56]. Some interactions of berberine with traditional drugs have been identified. Among others, clear synergistic effects between berberine and doxorubicin [57] or fluconazole [58] have been documented. Moreover, berberine when co-administered with L-DOPA exerts an antagonist action [59], while the concomitant use of tetradine enhances its hypoglycemic effect [60].

In recent years, another extensively studied natural antioxidant compound was curcumin [1,7-bis(4-hydroxy-3-methoxyphenyl)-1,6-heptadiene-3,5-dione]. It is the principal curcuminoid present in the *Curcuma longa*, a plant traditionally used in Asia as a natural remedy for several pathologies [61]. Much scientific evidence has been collected about curcumin including clinical trials of patients with MetS and in-depth studies on experimental models of obesity. A randomized, double-blind, placebo-controlled trial evaluated the lipid-lowering effects of curcumin in patients with MetS [62]. The study has shown that the intake of curcumin extract is associated with increased levels of HDL-C and reduced levels of LDL-C and TG. Moreover, in a subgroup of patients, it was also observed a reduced TC/HDL-C ratio [62]. Some other preliminary data have shown that a bioavailable form of curcumin ameliorates weight management in overweight people with MetS [63]. Curcumin also improves MetS in an experimental model of HFD fed rats [64]. The study demonstrated that curcumin significantly improves body mass, systolic blood pressure as well as serum levels of glucose, insulin, leptin, TC, TG, uric acid and malonildialdehyde (MDA) [64]. In addition, curcumin enhances catalase activity and strongly downregulates the expression level of TNF-α and NF-κB in hepatocytes [64]. Indeed, it is well described that curcumin inhibits the degradation of IκBα and the activation of IKK, related to NF-κB activation, leading to the suppression of inflammatory biomarkers, such as COX-2 and vascular endothelial growth factor (VEGF) in HFD fed rats [65]. Some other data have shown that curcumin downregulates the expression of different pro-inflammatory adipocytokines, such as chemokines (MCP-1, MCP-4) and interleukins (IL-1, IL-6, and IL-8), regulated by NF-κB activity, in adipose tissue isolated from obese mice [66]. Moreover, curcumin seems to be involved in the suppression of Jun NH2-terminal kinase (JNK), extracellular signal-regulated kinase1/2 (ERK1/2) and p38MAPK activities as it is shown in an in vitro model of 3T3-L1 adipocytes [67]. It was also proven that curcumin interrupts leptin signaling [68] and activates PPAR-γ in rat hepatic stellate cell growth [69], and it is able to increase adiponectin expression in a mouse model of obesity and diabetes [70]. Interestingly, curcumin also inhibits the wnt/β-catenin pathway, which is closely related to the onset of obesity [71]. In vitro and in vivo evaluation have shown that curcumin interferes to wnt/β-catenin pathway through different potential mechanisms such as downregulation of the transcription coactivator p300 [71] or inhibition of glycogen synthase kinase (GSK)-3β, which directly causes the phosphorylation of β-catenin [72]. Several animal and human studies have provided some information about the oral bioavailability of curcumin. In particular, Yang K et al. revealed that the oral bioavailability of curcumin in the plasma of rats treated with 500 mg/kg is only about 1%, suggesting that higher doses are necessary to observe some beneficial effects [73]. Interestingly, recent scientific advances in the development of new pharmaceutical formulations like liposome, polymeric nanoparticles, lipid-complexes and others have shown an increase in the bioavailability and in the activity of curcumin improving its beneficial effects [74]. Pharmacokinetics studies revealed that curcumin undergoes a biotransformation process in gut and liver producing curcumin glucuronides, sulphates or reduced molecules such as hexahydrocurcumin [75]. Intravenous injection of curcumin in mice suggests a tissue specific accumulation in particular in liver, lung, spleen and brain [76]. Curcumin metabolites, like curcumin glucuronide and curcumin sulphate, were also identified in plasma and urine of patients treated with at least 3600 milligrams of curcumin [77]. After oral administration, approximately 75% of curcumin metabolites are excreted in the feces [78]. No toxic effects were observed after oral administration of curcumin [77].

Among other natural remedies, Cinnamon (*Cinnamonium verum*), derived from the inner bark of many varieties of evergreen trees, is commonly used in Chinese and Indian traditional medicines [79]. Cinnamon extracts have shown anti-inflammatory and antioxidant properties as well as an interesting insulin-like activity [79]. In a randomized placebo-controlled trial, it was observed a significant improvement in fasting blood glucose, blood pressure and body composition in subjects with MetS treated with an aqueous extract of cinnamon [80]. Furthermore, a recent review, which collected 8 clinical trials that used *Cinnamomum cassia* in aqueous or powder form, reported a significant improvement of glycemic control in different animal models, in patients with pre-diabetes condition and in diabetic ones [81]. Interestingly, it was shown that cinnamon exerts its anti-diabetic activity through different molecular mechanisms including insulin receptor (IR) auto-phosphorlylation and de-phosphorylation, GLUT-4 receptor synthesis and translocation, modulation of hepatic glucose metabolism interfering with pyruvate kinase (PK) and phosphenol pyruvate carboxikinase (PEPCK) activities. This, in turn, alters the expression of PPARγ and inhibition of intestinal glucosidases [81]. The ability of Cinnamon in improving glycemic control and lipid levels was also described in an in vitro model of mouse 3T3-L1 adipocytes [82]. In particular, the study has shown a significant increase in mRNA and protein levels of IR, GLUT-4 and tristetraprolin in mouse 3T3-L1 adipocytes treated with cinnamon extract and polyphenols [82]. Recent data about the bioavailability and pharmacokinetics of cinnamaldehyde, one of the main active components derived from cinnamon, were collected. After oral administration, the bioavailability of cinnamaldehyde was approximatively 20% [83]. Pharmacokinetics studies have shown a well distribution of cinnamaldehyde and its metabolites throughout the body [84]. After oral administration, cinnamaldehyde metabolized into cinnamic acid mainly in the liver but also in stomach and small intestine [85]. Moreover, cinnamaldehyde can be converted into cinnamyl alcohol, being more susceptible to β-oxidation as their cinnamic acid derivatives [86]. It is suggested that the consumption of cinnamaldehyde should be limited to the dose related to the acceptable daily intake. Higher doses of cinnamaldehyde probably lead to toxic effects such as genotoxicity and hepatotoxicity [84]. The bioavailability and pharmacokinetics data about the other major cinnamon constituents, such as cinnamon polyphenols, cinnamic acid and eugenol have to be clarified.

Also noteworthy is capsaicin, which represents the major active constituent of chilly and constitutes, together with dihydrocapsaicin, about 90% of the capsaicinoids present in fruits belonging to the *Capsicum genus* [87]. Some epidemiologic data have shown that the consumption of foods high in capsaicin, improves metabolic and inflammatory status of adipose tissue and liver suggesting that dietary capsaicin is associated with lower incidence of obesity and/or MetS [88]. It was observed that the effects of capsaicin are mainly due to its agonist action on transient receptor potential cation channel subfamily V member 1 (TRPV1) [88]. Indeed, TRPV1 knockout mice fed a HFD become more obese and more resistant to insulin and leptin compared to the wild-type mice fed a HFD [89]. Capsaicin acts on the TRPV1 and PPARα receptors reducing metabolic dysregulation through an increase in expression levels of adiponectin and its receptor in an experimental model of obese mice [90]. Capsaicin is also able to increase liver X receptor (LXR) and pancreatic duodenal homeobox-1 (PDX-1) in the liver of streptozotocin-induced diabetic rats [91]. Both these proteins regulate glucose metabolism through modulation of GLUT-2, phosphoenolpyruvate carboxykinase and glucose 6-phosphatase expression levels, suggesting a role of capsaicin in gluconeogenesis inhibition and glycogen synthesis activation [91]. Several pharmacokinetics studies performed on experimental animal models reported that capsaicin is rapidly absorbed from the gastrointestinal lumen and detected in plasma 1h after oral administration. [92]. Chaiyasit et al. reported pharmacokinetics data obtained after oral administration of capsaicinoids in humans [93]. The results have shown capsaicin half-life in the plasma of approximatively 25 minutes and peak plasma concentration after 45 minutes. After less than 2h, no capsaicin was detected in the blood of the volunteers [93]. After oral administration, capsaicin and dihydrocapsaicin are mainly distributed in the liver and then in the kidney followed by the lung and rapidly metabolized within 24h. Most of the capsaicin is metabolized in the liver while a small amount was hydrolyzed in the small intestine [92]. Dihydrocapsaicin is metabolized to vanillyl alcohol, vanillic acid or vanillylamine as free forms or as their glucuronides and excreted in urine together with a small percentage of the unchanged form [92]. Limitations in the clinical use of capsaicin are related to its strong pungency and burning sensation. In this regard, several new pharmacological formulations have been designed such as chitosan microspheres, liposomes, nanoparticles or soft gel capsules able to bypass the release in the stomach [94–96]. Although several animal studies have provided evidence of the benefits of capsaicin in the treatment of MetS, less is known about the potential toxic effects.

Some data are available regarding carnosic acid, a phenolic diterpene synthesized by plants belonging to the *Lamiaceae* family (*Rosmarinus officinalis, Salvia officinalis*). Zhao et al. have shown that carnosic acid, the main active compound of plants, improves obesity and MetS features in an experimental model of HFD fed mice [97]. In addition to decreasing serum levels of TG, TC, insulin and glucose, carnosic acid is capable of inhibiting the expression levels of various pro-inflammatory cytokines such as IL-1β, IL-6 and TNF-α [98]. Moreover, it promotes the expression of anti-apoptotic protein B-cell lymphoma 2 (Bcl-2) and decreases the expression of pro-apoptotic protein Bcl-2-like *protein* 4 (Bax) and MMP-9 [98]. In an experimental animal study, the oral bioavailability of carnosic acid was 40%, and it was recorded 6h after administration, suggesting a slow absorption of the compound [99]. After oral administration, the main metabolites of carnosic acid such as glucuronide conjugates, carnosol and rosmanol as well as CA 12-methyl ether and 5,6,7,10- tetrahydro-7-hydroxyrosmariquinone were detected in gut, liver and plasma. It has been reported that most of the compounds persist in these tissues at significant concentrations for several hours. Carnosic acid and its metabolites are mainly excreted through the fecal route [100]. No side effects were observed both in animals treated with a single acute dose of carnosic acid and carnosol [101] and after sub-chronic consumption of the doses for 64 days suggesting a low toxicity of the extract [102] (Table 2).

Table 2. The main properties of different natural compounds.

Plant	Bioactive Component	Properties	In vitro/in vivo Models	Clinical Trials	References
Rosmarinus officinalis *Salvia officinalis*	Carnosic acid	↓ Body weight ↑ Insulin sensitivity ↓ Serum Glucose, TG, TC ↓ ALT, AST ↓ MDA, IL-1β, IL-6, TNF-α ↑ Bcl-2 ↓ Bax, MMP-9	- HFD fed mice		[34,35]
Cinnamomum verum *Cinnamomum cassia*	Cinnamaldehyde Polyphenols	Anti-inflammatory and antioxidant effects Insulin-like activity ↓ Fasting blood glucose and blood pressure ↑ IRβ, GLUT-4, TTP, GLP-1, PPAR-γ	- mouse 3T3-L1 adipocytes - High Fructose Diet fed mice - STZ-induced diabetic rats	- Pre-diabetes - MetS - T2DM	[36–39]
Capsicum genus	Capsaicin	↓ Fasting glucose ↑ Insulin sensitivity ↑ TG, Leptin ↑ Adiponectin ↓ Gluconeogenesis ↑ Glycogen synthesis ↓ TNF-α, MCP-1, IL-6 ↑ LXR, PDX-1 ↑ TRPV-1, GLUT-4, IRS-1 ↑ PPAR-α/PGC-1α	- TRPV1-KO mice fed with HFD - HFD fed mice - STZ-induced diabetic rats		[40–44]
Curcuma longa	Polyphenols	Anti-inflammatory and antioxidant effects ↑ Insulin sensitivity ↓ BMI, body fat, systolic blood pressure ↓ Plasma glucose ↓ NF-κB, COX-2, VEGF ↓ MCP-1, MCP-4, ILs, TNF-α ↓ JNK, ERK1/2, P38MAPK ↓ Wnt/β-catenin pathway ↓ TG, TC, Leptin ↑ Adiponectin ↓ Malondhyaleide ↑ PPAR-γ, Catalase activity	- mouse 3T3-L1 adipocytes - rat hepatic stellate cells - HFD fed mice - ob/ob C57Bl/6j mice - Balb/c mice - HFD fed rats - STZ-induced diabetic rats fed with HFD	- MetS	[45–56]

Table 2. Cont.

Plant	Bioactive Component	Properties	In vitro/in vivo Models	Clinical Trials	References
Rhizoma Coptidis	Berberine	Anti-inflammatory and antioxidant effects ↑ Insulin sensitivity ↑ Fasting glucose Plasma glucose, systolic blood pressure ↓ TG, TC, LDL-C ↑ HDL-C ↓ Leptin, adiponectin ↓ hs-CRP, IL-6, TNF-α, MCP-1 ↓ Macrophage recruitment ↑ Thermogenesis ↓ PPARγ2, C/EBPα, ↑ AMPK and GLUT-4	- mouse 3T3-L1 adipocytes - rat L6 myotubes - HFD fed mice - C57BLKS/J Lepr^{db}-Lepr^{db} mice - HFD fed rats	- T2DM - Hyperlipemia - Hypertension - MetS	[57–63]
Citrus bergamia Risso et Poiteau	BEO-NVF BPF	↓ SMC proliferation, LOX-1, p-PKB ↓ ROS, TBARS, MDA, Nitrotyrosine ↓ Serum glucose, TG, TC, LDL-C, VLDL-C ↑ HDL-C Re-arrangement of lipoprotein particles ↓ ALT, AST, γ-GT, ↓ Hs-CRP, TNF-α, JNK, p-P38 MAPK, ↓ Caspase-3, Cleaved- PARP ↓ Lipid transfer protein system ↓ Fibrogenic activity ↓ pCEH↓ Steatohepatitis, hepatocellular ballooning ↓ Sinusoidal fibrosis	- rat neointimal hyperplasia - hypercholesterolemic diet fed rats - NAFLD mice	-Hyperlipemia - MetS - NAFLD - T2DM	[66–72]
Cynara cardunculus	Cynaropicrin	↓ TNF-α, MDA ↓ ALT, AST, γ-GT, ALP ↓ Liver fibrosis ↑ SOD, GPx		- NAFLD - T2DM	[73]
Brassicaceae family Gramineae family	Coenzyme Q10	Antioxidant capacity, nephroprotective effect ↓ TG, TC, LDL-C, serum insulin ↑ β-cell Function ↑ Glucose metabolism	- db/db and dbH mice model of type 2 diabetic nephropathy - STZ-nicotinamide induced diabetic rats	- T2DM - MetS	Zozina V. I. et al. 2018 [74]

Table 2. Cont.

Plant	Bioactive Component	Properties	In vitro/in vivo Models	Clinical Trials	References
Vitis vinifera	Resveratrol	↓ BMI, waist circumference, insulin secretion ↓ Hs-CRP; TNF-α ↓ Malondhyaldeide ↓ Leptin, RAAS modulation ↓ Lipogenesis ↑ Lipolysis	- SGBS preadipocytes - human preadipocytes - adipose stem cells - high Fructose Diet fed rats - high Sucrose Diet fed rats - high-fat/cholesterol diet fed swine - IH-induced metabolic dysfunction in mice - insulin-resistant KKAy mice	- MetS	Hou C.Y. et al. 2019 [75]
Vaccinium myrtillus *Fragaria ananassa*	Anthocyanins	Anti-inflammatory and antioxidant effects Hypocholesterolemic effects ↓ TG, body weight, fat mass ↓ α-amylase and α-glucosidase activities ↓ Leptin ↓ MCP-1, ICAM-1, VCAM-1, NF-κB B ↑ PPARs	- HK-2 cells - HUVEC cells - STZ- induced diabetic rats - STZ- induced diabetic mice - db/db mice fed with HFD - obese Zucker rats - Dahl Salt-Sensitive rats	- MetS	Naseri R. et al. 2018 [76]
Oleaceae family (*Olea europaea* Linn.)	Oleuropein	Antioxidant effect ↑ Insulin sensitivity, glucose tolerance ↓ TG, TC, LDL-C ↑ SOD, GPx ↓ LpL, PPARγ, C/EBPα, SREBP-1c ↓ Leptin ↑ AMPK UCP-1 TRPV-1	- MSC from human bone marrow - 3T3-L1 adipocytes - C2C12 cells - Alloxan-induced diabetic rats - HFD fed mice and rats - PPARα null mice - BPA-induced hyperlipidemia and liver injury in rats	- Hyperchole sterolemia - Overweight	Ahamad J et al. 2019 [77]

↑: Increased. ↓: Decreased. ALP, Alkaline Phosphatase; ALT, Alanine Aminotransferase; AMPK, 5′ AMP-activated Protein Kinase; AST, Aspartate Aminotransferase; Bax, Bcl-2-like protein 4; Bcl-2, B-cell lymphoma 2; BEO-NVE, Non-Volatile Fraction of the Bergamot Essential Oil; BMI, Body Mass Index; BPA, Bisphenol A; BPF, Bergamot Polyphenolic Fraction; C/EBPα, CCAAT-Enhancer-Binding Protein-α; COX-2, Cyclooxygenase-2; ERK1/2, Extracellular signal-Regulated Kinase 1/2; GLP-1, Glucagon-Like Peptide-1; GLUT-4, Glucose Transporter Type 4; GPx, Glutathione Peroxidase; GSK-3β, Glycogen Synthase Kinase-3β; HDL-C, High Density Lipoprotein Cholesterol; HFD, High Fat Diet; Hs-CRP, High sensitivity C-Reactive Protein; ICAM-1, Intercellular Adhesion Molecule 1;IH, Intermittent Hypoxia; IL-1β (Interleukin-1β); IL-6, Interleukin:6; IRS-1, insulin receptor substrate-1; IRβ, Insulin Receptor- β; JNK, c-Jun N-terminal Kinase; LDL-C, Low Density Lipoprotein Cholesterol; LOX-1, Lectin-type Oxidized LDL receptor 1; LpL, Lipoprotein Lipase; LXR, Liver X Receptor; MCP-1, Monocyte Chemoattractant Protein-1; MDA, Malonildialdehyde; MetS, Metabolic Syndrome; MM-9, Matrix Metalloproteinase-9; NAFLD, Non Alcoholic Fatty Liver Disease; NF-κB, nuclear factor kappa-light-chain-enhancer of activated B cells; PARP, Poly(ADP-ribose) Polymerase; pCEH, pancreatic Cholesterol Ester Hydrolase; PDX-1, Pancreatic Duodenal homeobox-1; PGC-1α, PPAR-γ coactivator-1α; PPAR-γ, Peroxisome Proliferator-Activated Receptor- γ; p-PKB, phospho-Protein Kinase B; p-38 MAPK, p-38 Mitogen-Activated Protein Kinases; RAAS, Renin Angiotensin Aldosterone System; ROS, Reactive Oxygen Species; SMC, Smooth Muscle Cell; SOD, Superoxide Dismutase; SREBP-1c, Sterol Regulatory Element-Binding Protein-1c; STZ, Streptozotocin; TBARS, Thiobarbituric Acid Reactive Substances; TC, total Cholesterol; TG, Triglycerides; TNF-α, Tumor Necrosis Factor-alpha; TRPV-1, Transient Receptor Potential cation channel subfamily V member 1; TTP, Tristetraprolin; T2DM, Type 2 Diabetes Mellitus; UCP-1, Uncoupling Protein-1; VCAM-1, Vascular cell adhesion protein 1; VEGF, Vascular Endothelial Growth Factor; VLDL-C, Very-Low-Density Lipoprotein Cholesterol; γ-GT, Gamma-Glutamyl Transferase.

4. Citrus Bergamia

Bergamot (*Citrus bergamia* Risso et Poiteau) is an endemic plant growing in Calabria (Southern Italy). Bergamot possesses a profile of flavonoids and glycosides, such as neoeriocitrin, neohesperidin, naringin, rutin and poncirin, which can be considered unique in its various forms (essential oil, hydro-alcoholic extract and fruit juice), and it differs from other citrus fruits not only for the composition of its flavonoids but also for their particularly high juice content [9,10]. Emerging evidence suggests a potential protective role of bergamot flavonoids in the management of different features of MetS, due to their pleiotropic anti-oxidative, anti-inflammatory and lipid-lowering effects.

4.1. Preparation of Bergamot Polyphenolic Fraction

Bergamot juice can be concentrated by a patented method based on a preparative size exclusion chromatography, with polystyrene gel filtration, followed by eluate exsiccation to give rise to a polyphenol-enriched powder, BPF [103]. Briefly, bergamot juice was obtained from peeled-off fruits by industrial pressing and squeezing. Then, the juice was oil fraction-depleted by stripping, clarified by ultra-filtration and loaded on polystyrene resin columns absorbing polyphenol compounds of molecular weight between 300 and 600 Da. The polyphenol fractions obtained were thus eluted by a mild KOH solution. Next, the fitocomplex was neutralized by filtration on cationic resin at acidic pH. Finally, it was vacuum dried and minced to the desired particle size to obtain BPF powder. The following HPLC analysis performed on BPF powder has shown that flavonoids are over 200 times more concentrated than those contained in bergamot juice. It was also estimated that BPF contains over 45% flavonoids, of which 95% are flavanones and 5% flavones, as well as carbohydrates, pectins and other compounds. Specifically, titration for some BPF compounds was performed showing the percentage of neoeriocitrin (>9%), naringin (>11%), neohesperidin (>11%), melitidin (>1%) and brutieridin (>2%). In addition, toxicological analyses revealed the absence of known toxic compounds including heavy metal, pesticide, phthalate and sinephrine. Moreover, no mycotoxins and bacteria were detected after standard microbiological tests. [103].

4.2. Lipid-lowering and Anti-diabetic Effects of BPF

In the context of MetS, several beneficial effects of BPF have been detected both in clinical trials and in experimental models. In this regard, BPF has shown important properties when administered in patients suffering from isolated hypercholesterolemia, patients with hyperlipidemia (hypercholesterolemia and hypertriglyceridemia) and patients with mixed hyperlipidemia associated with hyperglycemia [103]. All patients received an oral dose of BPF (500 mg or 1000 mg) for 30 consecutive days. At the end of the treatment period, all patients have shown a strong reduction in TG, TC, LDL-C, blood glucose levels and a significant increase in HDL-C, which is dose-dependent. Interestingly, reduced excretion level of urinary mevalonate was reported suggesting a direct inhibitory action of BPF on HMG-CoA reductase activity. The latter evidence is probably due to the structural similarity to HMG-CoA reductase substrate shown by bruteridine and melitidine, which are 3-hydroxy-3-methylglutaryl derivatives of hesperetin and naringenin, respectively. Furthermore, BPF improves the impaired endothelium-mediated vasodilation in all treated patients. The reduction of all cholesterol parameters, due to BPF treatment, was also shown in a sub-group of patients with a relevant intolerance to statins [103]. Gliozzi and colleagues well demonstrated that the co-treatment with rosuvastatin (10 mg/daily/p.o.) and BPF (1000 mg/daily/p.o.) for 30 days significantly enhances the effect of rosuvastatin alone on serum lipemic profile of patients with hyperlipemia [104]. This effect is associated with significant reduction of MDA, lectin-type oxidized LDL receptor 1 (LOX-1) and p-PKB levels, suggesting a multi-action potential for BPF in patients on statin therapy [104]. In a work published in 2014, the same research group studied the effect of BPF on LDL small dense particles and NAFLD, another important biomarker for the development of cardiometabolic risk, in patients with MetS [105]. Interestingly, a significant reduction in serum TC, LDL-C and TG was shown in patients treated with BPF (650 mg, twice a day, p.o.) for 120 consecutive days. This effect is associated with a significant reduction of serum glucose, transaminases, gamma-glutamyl-transferase and inflammatory biomarkers such as TNF-α and C-reactive protein (CRP) [105]. Moreover, BPF is able of a substantial re-arrangement of lipoprotein particles. It reduces LDL small-size atherogenic particles and enhances large-size anti-atherogenic HDL particles [105].

In a randomized, placebo-controlled trial, performed on MetS patients with elevated atherogenic index of plasma (AIP) and moderate hyperglycemia, the efficacy of a new bergamot juice-derived formulation was reported [106]. Bergamot polyphenolic extract complex (BPE-C) is enriched with flavonoids, pectins and vitamin C. In patients treated with 650 or 1300 mg of BPE-C for 90 consecutive days, the clear improvement of dyslipidemia was confirmed, as previously reported [106]. In addition, a powerful reduction of AIP and the amelioration of insulin sensitivity accompanied by weight loss were observed. This evidence is associated with a significant reduction of circulating leptin and ghrelin and upregulation of adiponectin [106]. Recently, BPF novel phytosomal formulation (BPF phyto) was developed to reach a better absorption and tissue distribution of BPF in patients suffering from T2DM and mixed hyperlipemia [107]. After randomization, patients received BPF (650 mg/p.o.) or BPF Phyto (500 mg/p.o.) twice a day for 30 consecutive days. The data obtained well confirmed previous results showing the beneficial effects of BPF in improving lipid profile of patients undergoing MetS with elevated cardiometabolic risk [107].

The lipid-lowering and anticholesterolemic effects of BPF were previously observed in rat fed with hypercholesterolemic diet [103]. The data have shown that the administration of BPF for 30 days produces a significant reduction in TG, TC and LDL-C accompanied by moderate elevation of HDL-C. Moreover, in the BPF-treated group, a better epato-biliary turnover and cholesterol consumption was observed as suggested by increased levels of total bile acids and neutral sterols in fecal samples [103]. The beneficial properties of BPF in counteracting the detrimental features of NAFLD were studied in cafeteria (CAF) diet-induced rat model of MetS [108]. The results confirmed that BPF had a role in reducing serum TG, blood glucose and obesity. Moreover, BPF counteracts hepatic steatosis strongly decreasing the amount of lipid droplets in rat hepatocytes. BPF also prevents the pathogenic lipid accumulation by stimulating the autophagic process in the liver. Specifically, the phytocomplex exerts a potent induction of lipophagy, as documented by the higher levels of LC3II found in the lipid droplet (LD) subcellular fractions of BPF-expose livers [108].

Moreover, a detailed work published on Scientific Report in 2020 well demonstrated that BPF is able to improve dyslipidemia and different pathophysiological features in a diet-induced mouse model of NAFLD [109]. Interestingly, the results have shown that BPF improves glucose tolerance and insulin resistance as well as liver enzymes and dyslipidemia counteracting non-alcoholic steato-hepatitis (NASH) [109]. BPF is able to reduce oxidative stress markers along with JNK and p38 MAP kinase activity. BPF also prevents the exacerbation of inflammatory process and sinusoidal fibrosis in the liver [109]. In an in-depth study, a molecular mechanism partly responsible for the hypolipemic properties of BPF was also clarified [110]. In vivo data demonstrated that BPF prevents alteration of lipid profile in rats fed with hypercholesterolemic diet, reducing oxidative stress and ameliorating lipoprotein metabolism dysregulation [110]. This, in turn, restores the activity of acetyl-coenzyme A acetyltransferase (ACAT), lecithin cholesterol acyltransferase (LCAT), cholesteryl ester transfer protein (CETP) and paraxonoase-1 (PON1), an effect accompanied by the concomitant normalization of apolipoprotein A1 (Apo A1) and apolipoprotein B (Apo B) levels [110].

4.3. Antioxidant and Anti-Inflammatory Effects of BPF

The antioxidant effect of bergamot was initially observed by analyzing the potential activity of the non-volatile fraction of the bergamot essential oil (BEO-NVF) in an experimental model of neointima hyperplasia. Mollace et al. identified the highly significant effect of the antioxidant component of BEO-NVF on LOX-1 expression and ROS generation in a model of rat carotid artery injury [111]. The results have shown that balloon injury is associated with smooth muscle cell proliferation and neo-intima formation causing re-stenosis. These cells also reveal an increase in LOX-1 expression and generation of ROS. Interestingly, pre-treatment of rats with BEO-NVF decreases neo-intima formation, LOX-1 expression and ROS generation as well as the degree of stenosis [111]. The natural antioxidant and LOX-1 modulating properties of BEO-NVF appear to be promising for use in MetS to decrease endothelial dysfunction, smooth muscle cell proliferation and inflammation, all of which bridge the gap between MetS and ASCVD. Furthermore, BPF has shown robust antioxidant properties in a CAF diet-induced rat model of MetS ameliorating the plasmatic oxidative balance. In particular, data have shown an increase in the expression level of the antioxidant enzyme glutatione S-tranferasi P1 (GSTP1) and the inhibition of the pro-apoptotic markers caspase 8 and 9 [112]. Important evidence on the anti-inflammatory activity of BPF were collected in CAF diet-induced NASH rats. [113]. The study demonstrated the ability of BPF supplementation to decrease hepatic inflammation by reducing IL-6 and increasing anti-inflammatory IL-10 mRNA expression levels. These results correlate with fewer Kupffer cells, leukocytes infiltrating perivascular hepatic tissue and lower inflammatory foci score in CAF fed rats treated with BPF [113]. The reliable antioxidant and anti-inflammatory properties of bergamot polyphenols have also been studied in association with cynaropicrin, a sesquiterpene lactone of a guaianolide type isolated from artichoke (*Cynara cardunculus*) [114]. The phytocomplex, called Bergacyn, has been previously titrated in polyphenols derived from bergamot and artichoke. The percentage of titrated polyphenol coming from *Citrus bergamia* was > 19.5% while the one derived from *Cynara cardunculus* was >10%. Moreover, some compounds of Bergacyn have been titrated showing the percentage of neoeriocitrin (>4.5%), naringin (>5.5%), neohesperidin (>5.5%), melitidin (>1) and brutieridin (>2%). Musolino V. et al. well demonstrated the synergistic effect of Bergacyn on vascular inflammation and oxidative stress in a randomized, double blind, placebo controlled clinical study of patients with T2DM and NAFLD [114]. After 16 weeks of treatment with Bergacyn (300 mg/daily/p.o.), a significant improvement of NAFLD biomarkers (alanine aminotransferase-ALT, aspartate aminotransferase-AST, gamma-glutamyl transferase-γ-GT and alkaline phosphatase-ALP) as well as liver fibrosis biomarkers (hyaluronic acid-HA, type III precollagen-PC III and type IV collagen-IV-C) was shown in patients with T2DM [114]. These effects are associated with a substantial modulation of oxidative stress and inflammatory biomarkers. Indeed, an increase in glutathione peroxidase (GPx) and superoxide dismutase (SOD) levels and a reduction of MDA and TNF-α levels was shown [71]. Moreover, at the end of the experimental period, an improvement in endothelial dysfunction was observed, contributing to better NO-mediated reactive vasodilation [114] (Table 2, Figure 2).

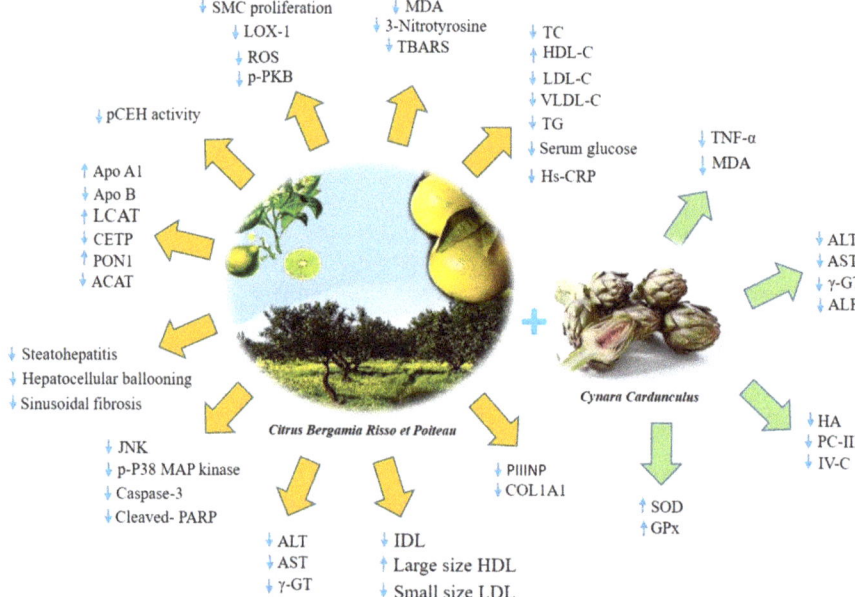

Figure 2. The molecular mechanisms involved in the beneficial effects of bergamot polyphenols. ACAT, Acetyl-Coenzyme A Acetyltransferase; ALP, Alkaline Phosphatase; ALT, Alanine Aminotransferase; Apo A1, Apolipoprotein A1; Apo B, Apolipoprotein B; AST, Aspartate Aminotransferase; CETP: Cholesteryl Ester Transfer Protein; COL1A1, Pro-Collagen type I; GPx, Glutathione Peroxidase; HA, hyaluronic acid; HDL-C, High Density Lipoprotein Cholesterol; Hs-CRP, High-sensitivity C-Reactive Protein; IDL, Intermediate Density Lipoprotein; JNK, c-Jun N-terminal Kinase; LCAT, Lecithin Cholesterol Acyltransferase; LDL-C, Low Density Lipoprotein Cholesterol; LOX-1, Lectin-type Oxidized LDL receptor 1; MDA, Malonildialdehyde; PARP, Poly(ADP-ribose) Polymerase; pCEH, pancreatic Cholesterol Ester Hydrolase; PC III, Pre-collagen type III; p-PKB, phospho- Protein Kinase B; PON1, Paraxonoase-1; PIIINP, Pro-Collagen III N-terminal propeptide; ROS, Reactive Oxygen Species; SMC, Smooth Muscle Cell; SOD, Superoxide Dismutase; TBARS, Thiobarbituric Acid Reactive Substances; TC, total Cholesterol; TG, Triglycerides; TNF-α, Tumor Necrosis Factor-alpha; VLDL-C, Very-Low-Density Lipoprotein Cholesterol; γ-GT, Gamma-Glutamyl Transferase; IV-C, Collagen type IV.

4.4. Bioavailability and Pharmacokinetics of BPF

Up to date, the oral bioavailability and pharmacokinetic of BPF has not been completely investigated. In the recent study of Musolino et al., oral bioavailability information of BPF has been collected. After 11 weeks of treatment, neoeriocitrin, naringin and neohesperidin have been detected in the serum of mice that received BPF by gavage, suggesting that those biocompounds are able to cross small intestine membrane [109]. Moreover, a recent pilot bioavailability study clarified how these compounds are modified after oral consumption of bergamot juice in healthy volunteers' biological fluids [115]. The authors demonstrated that flavonoids from *Citrus bergamia* undergo phase II conjugates metabolism (such as sulfate and glucuronides of hesperetin, naringenin and eriodictyol). They were detected at both 1h and 4h in the plasma samples of all the volunteers. The majority of conjugates were also detected in urine at 2h and 6h, accounting for the absorption profile observed in plasma [115]. Although it is unclear whether flavonoid metabolites retain some biological activity, their involvement in the modulation of intracellular responses is conceivable as has been observed for the sulfonated and methylated metabolites of resveratrol which retain, at least in part, the activity of the parent compound [116]. Toxicological studies revealing that BPF are absolutely safe, having been carried out according to EU Directive 2004/9/EC and Directive 2004/9/EC for Good Laboratory Practice Guidelines (GLP) as well as OECD Guidelines for Repeated Dose 28- and 90-day Oral Toxicity Study in Rodents [105]. In addition, comparable doses of bergacyn were used as reference protocol in terms of efficacy and safety profile in a study performed on diabetic patients [103,114].

4.5. Hypothesis on BPF Mechanisms of Action

The studies discussed above reveal the interesting pleiotropic effects of BPF due to its peculiar composition and the highest content of Citrus flavonoids. The molecular mechanisms underlying these effects are not fully known. However, the results obtained allow to identify some molecular mechanisms affected by BPF action.

The hypolipemic and anti-atherogenic effects of BPF are, at least in part, associated with the modulation of the activity of some enzymes responsible for cholesterol esterification reactions and lipid trafficking [110]. The improvement of lipoprotein metabolism is probably due to the restored activity of ACAT, LCAT, CETP and PON1 enzymes by BPF [110]. These enzymes differently contribute to the modification of plasma lipoprotein particle composition mediating cholesterol esterification within the cells (ACAT) [117] or in the plasma (LCAT) [118], lipid transfer in plasma compartment (CETP) [119] or through hydrolysis of lipid peroxides on LDL and HDL particles (PON1) [120]. BPF also interferes with the autophagic pathway preventing the pathogenic lipid accumulation [108]. Indeed, BPF strongly enhances autophagy in the liver upregulating the expression level of Beclin-1 and LC3II and reducing p62. Moreover, a potent induction of lipophagy, documented by the higher levels of LC3II, was found in the LD subcellular fractions of BPF-expose livers [108]. More recently, a direct action of BPF on MAPK, which represent a crucial regulator of glucose and fatty acids metabolism in all tissues, has been identified [109]. In particular, in pathological fatty liver, BPF induced modulation of JNK/p38 MAPKs represents the protective mechanism responsible for the amelioration of insulin sensitivity [109]. Furthermore, the reduction of liver inflammation and fibrosis is related to BPF direct inhibition of poly [ADP-ribose] polymerase 1 (PARP1), considered the direct suppressor of MAPK inhibitor mitogen-activated protein kinase-1 (MPK-1) [109]. It was also assumed that the reduction of serum and tissue cholesterol levels is due to the statin-like activity exerted by BPF. The structural similarity of bergamot polyphenols to HMG-CoA reductase substrate allows them to mimic the natural substrates of HMG-CoA and block the rate-limiting step in cholesterol synthesis [103]. The powerful antioxidant effects of BPF play a significant role in all the observed protective effects. BPF directly reduces lipid peroxidation biomarkers (TBARS) and MDA and strongly inhibits protein tyrosine nitration levels [104]. BPF also improves the activity of endogenous antioxidant enzymes such as SOD, GPx and GSTP1 [112,114]. The additive vaso-protective effect of BPF is closely related to its antioxidant property. BPF is able to reduce LOX-1 expression levels highly modulated in the development and progression of endothelial dysfunction to atherosclerosis [104]. The vaso-protective action of BPF is also associated with the increase in PKB phosphorylation providing protection against vascular atherogenic injury [104].

All together, these data add new insights into the beneficial role of bergamot and highlights the potential use of supplementation treatments of bergamot-extracts for reducing cardiometabolic disorders in patients with MetS. However, future research will be aimed to better clarify the molecular mechanisms underlying the several health effects described in this review. Moreover, although it is clear that several polyphenols contribute to the beneficial effects of BPF, the specific contribution of each of them still remains to be clarified. Furthermore, it would be of interest to assess the potential beneficial properties of other herbal compounds with BPF, which may enhance its effects. The identification of phytocomplexes with synergistic action can be useful in the management of different pathological features.

5. Conclusions

MetS represents a complex pathophysiologic condition whose main determinants are central adiposity, hypertension, high TG, low HDL-C and hyperglycemia. All these components are linked by a common mechanism of development of chronic inflammation that often leads to insulin-resistance. The overlap of multiple risk factors, in each disease state, increases the risk of ASCVD and development of T2DM. To date, the management of MetS components provides lifestyle recommendations including exercise, weight loss and Mediterranean diet consumption, as well as the use of traditional pharmacologic therapies. However, the use of the approved drugs is limited by various factors such as the onset of side effects due to prolonged treatment. Instead, there is growing interest in the use of naturally occurring compounds to reduce the risk and progression of MetS. This review collected some experimental evidence about the role of nutraceuticals in the management of the different components of MetS. Preclinical and clinical studies suggest that different natural compounds have beneficial effects against obesity and insulin resistance as well as against various complications resulting from these diseases. Interestingly, it has been shown how many nutraceuticals reduce serum level of glucose, insulin, TC, TG, normalize blood pressure and are capable of a substantial re-arrangement of lipoprotein particles ameliorating serum lipemic profile. Moreover, strong antioxidant and anti-inflammatory effects as well as anti-apoptotic effects have been demonstrated. Some of the studies also identified specific activity of natural compounds in glucose metabolism, adipogenesis and their interaction with wnt/β-catenin pathway, which is closely related to obesity. In particular, bergamot and artichoke extracts, in addition to the strong anti-inflammatory, antioxidant, hypolipidemic and hypocholesterolemic properties, have shown interesting effects against the key pathophysiological features of NAFLD.

These intriguing data shed new light on the potential use of nutraceuticals for preventing and/or reducing cardiometabolic risk in patients with MetS. However, more research, in particular clinical trials, is needed to further understand the link between natural compounds and chronic diseases and the molecular mechanisms underlying their beneficial effects.

Author Contributions: V.M. (Vincenzo Musolino) conceptualized and designed the manuscript; C.C. and V.M. (Vincenzo Musolino) wrote the manuscript; M.G. and V.M. (Vincenzo Mollace), M.S., F.S., F.B., S.N., J.M., R.M. (Roberta Macrì), S.R., F.O., M.C.Z., L.G., R.M. (Rocco Mollace), A.T., E.P., E.B. and M.F. participated in drafting the article and revising it critically. All authors have read and agreed to the published version of the manuscript.

Funding: The work has been supported by the public resources from the Italian Ministry of Research.

Acknowledgments: This work has been supported by PON-MIUR 03PE000_78_1 and PONMIUR 03PE000_78_2.

Conflicts of Interest: The authors declare no conflicts of interest.

References

1. Saklayen, M.G. The Global Epidemic of the Metabolic Syndrome. *Curr. Hypertens. Rep.* **2018**, *20*, 12. [CrossRef] [PubMed]
2. Sherling, D.H.; Perumareddi, P.; Hennekens, C.H. Metabolic Syndrome: Clinical and Policy Implications of the New Silent Killer. *J. Cardiovasc. Pharm. T* **2017**, *22*, 365–367. [CrossRef]
3. Expert Panel on Detection, Evaluation, and Treatment of High Blood Cholesterol in Adults. Executive summary of the third report of the national cholesterol education program (NCEP) expert panel on detection, evaluation, and treatment of high blood cholesterol in adults (adult treatment panel III). *JAMA* **2001**, *285*, 2486–2497.
4. Huang, P.L. Comprehensive definition for metabolic syndrome. *Dis. Model Mech.* **2009**, *2*, 231–237. [CrossRef] [PubMed]
5. Almeda-Valdes, P.; Aguilar-Olivos, N.; Uribe, M.; Méndez-Sánchez, N. Common features of the metabolic syndrome and nonalcoholic fatty liver disease. *Rev. Recent Clin. Trials* **2014**, *9*, 148–158. [CrossRef]
6. Castro-Martinez, M.G.; Banderas-Lares, D.Z.; Ramirez-Martinez, J.C.; Escobedo-de la Peña, J. Prevalence of nonalcoholic fatty liver disease in subjects with metabolic syndrome. *Cir. Cir.* **2012**, *80*, 128–133.
7. Paschos, P.; Paletas, K. Non alcoholic fatty liver disease and metabolic syndrome. *Hippokratia* **2009**, *13*, 9–19.

8. Gurka, M.G.; Filipp, S.L.; DeBoer, M.D. Geographical variation in the prevalence of obesity, metabolic syndrome, and diabetes among US adults. *Nutr. Diabetes* **2018**, *8*, 14. [CrossRef]
9. Gardana, C.; Nalin, F.; Simonetti, P. Evaluation of flavonoids and furanocoumarins from Citrus bergamia (Bergamot) juice and identification of new compounds. *Molecules* **2008**, *13*, 2220–2228. [CrossRef]
10. Salerno, R.; Casale, F.; Calandruccio, C.; Procopio, A. Characterization of flavonoids in Citrus bergamia (Bergamot) polyphenolic fraction by liquid chromatography-high resolution mass spectrometry (LC/HRMS). *Pharma Nutr.* **2016**, *4*, S1–S7. [CrossRef]
11. Matsuzawa, Y.; Funahashi, T.; Nakamura, T. The concept of metabolic syndrome: Contribution of visceral fat accumulation and its molecular mechanism. *J. Atheroscler. Thromb.* **2011**, *18*, 629–639. [CrossRef] [PubMed]
12. Pekgor, S.; Duran, C.; Berberoglu, U.; Eryilmaz, M.A. The Role of Visceral Adiposity Index Levels in Predicting the Presence of Metabolic Syndrome and Insulin Resistance in Overweight and Obese Patients. *Metab. Syndr. Relat. Disord.* **2019**, *17*, 296–302. [CrossRef] [PubMed]
13. Neeland, I.J.; Ayers, C.R.; Rohatgi, A.K.; Turer, A.T.; Berry, J.D.; Das, S.R.; Vega, G.L.; Khera, A.; McGuire, D.K.; Grundy, S.M.; et al. Associations of visceral and abdominal subcutaneous adipose tissue with markers of cardiac and metabolic risk in obese adults. *Obesity* **2012**, *21*, E439–E447. [CrossRef] [PubMed]
14. Czech, M.P. Insulin action and resistance in obesity and type 2 diabetes. *Nat. Med.* **2017**, *23*, 804–814. [CrossRef] [PubMed]
15. Boden, G.; Shulman, G.I. Free fatty acids in obesity and type 2 diabetes: Defining their role in the development of insulin resistance and beta-cell dysfunction. *Eur. J. Clin. Invest.* **2002**, *32*, 14–23. [CrossRef]
16. Nikolic, D.; Katsiki, N.; Montalto, G.; Isenovic, E.R.; Mikhailidis, D.P.; Rizzo, M. Lipoprotein subfractions in metabolic syndrome and obesity: Clinical significance and therapeutic approaches. *Nutrients* **2013**, *5*, 928–948. [CrossRef]
17. Subramanian, S.; Chait, A. Hypertriglyceridemia secondary to obesity and diabetes. *Biochim. Biophys. Acta* **2012**, *1821*, 819–825. [CrossRef]
18. Samuel, V.T.; Shulman, G.I. The pathogenesis of insulin resistance: Integrating signaling pathways and substrateflux. *J. Clin. Invest.* **2016**, *126*, 12–22. [CrossRef]
19. Stratford, S.; Hoehn, K.L.; Liu, F.; Summers, S.A. Regulation of insulin action by ceramide: Dual mechanisms linking ceramide accumulation to the inhibition of Akt/protein kinase B. *J. Biol. Chem.* **2004**, *279*, 36608–36615. [CrossRef]
20. Samson, S.L.; Garber, A.J. Metabolic Syndrome. *Endocrinol. Metab. Clin. N. Am.* **2014**, *43*, 1–23. [CrossRef]
21. Welty, F.K.; Alfaddagh, A.; Elajami, T.K. Targeting inflammation in metabolic syndrome. *Transl. Res.* **2016**, *167*, 257–280.
22. Reaven, G.M. Relationships among insulin resistance, type 2 diabetes, essential hypertension, and cardiovascular disease: Similarities and differences. *J. Clin. Hypertens.* **2011**, *13*, 238–243. [CrossRef] [PubMed]
23. Landsberg, L.; Aronne, L.J.; Beilin, L.J.; Burke, V.; Igel, L.I.; Lloyd-Jones, D.; Sowers, J. Obesity-related hypertension: Pathogenesis, cardiovascular risk, and treatment–a position paper of the Obesity Society and the American Society of Hypertension. *Obesity* **2013**, *21*, 8–24. [CrossRef] [PubMed]
24. Spite, M.; Claria, J.; Serhan, C.N. Resolvins, specialized proresolving lipid mediators, and their potential roles in metabolic diseases. *Cell Metab.* **2014**, *19*, 21–36. [CrossRef] [PubMed]
25. Donath, M.Y.; Shoelson, S.E. Type 2 diabetes as an inflammatory disease. *Nat. Rev. Immunol.* **2011**, *11*, 98–107. [CrossRef]
26. Zhang, J.; Gao, Z.; Yin, J.; Quon, M.J.; Ye, J. S6K directly phosphorylates IRS-1 on Ser-270 to promote insulin resistance in response to TNF-(alpha) signaling through IKK2. *J. Biol. Chem.* **2008**, *283*, 35375–35382. [CrossRef]
27. Serhan, C.N.; Gilroy, D.W.; Derek Ward, P.A. *Fundamentals of Inflammation*, 1st ed.; Cambridge University Press: Cambridge, UK, 2010.
28. Horrillo, R.; Gonzalez-Periz, A.; Martinez-Clemente, M.; Lopez-Parra, M.; Ferre, N.; Titos, E.; Morán-Salvador, E.; Deulofeu, R.; Arroyo, V.; Clària, J. 5- lipoxygenase activating protein signals adipose tissue inflammation and lipid dysfunction in experimental obesity. *J. Immunol.* **2010**, *184*, 3978–3987. [CrossRef]
29. Yamaoka, K.; Tango, T. Effects of lifestyle modification on metabolic syndrome: A systematic review and meta-analysis. *BMC Med.* **2012**, *10*, 138. [CrossRef]

30. National Cholesterol Education Program (NCEP) Expert Panel on Detection, Evaluation and Treatment of High Blood Cholesterol in Adults (Adult Treatment Panel III). Third Report of the National Cholesterol Education Program (NCEP) Expert Panel on Detection, Evaluation, and Treatment of High Blood Cholesterol in Adults (Adult Treatment Panel III) final report. *Circulation* **2002**, *106*(25), 3143–3421.
31. Potenza, M.V.; Mechanick, J.I. The metabolic syndrome: Definition, global impact, and pathophysiology. *Nutr. Clin. Pract.* **2009**, *24*, 560–577. [CrossRef]
32. Djousse, L.; Padilla, H.; Nelson, T.L.; Gaziano, J.M.; Mukamal, K.J. Diet and metabolic syndrome. *Endocr. Metab. Immune. Disord. Drug Targets* **2010**, *10*, 124–137. [CrossRef] [PubMed]
33. Esposito, K.; Marfella, R.; Ciotola, M.; Di Palo, C.; Giugliano, F.; Giugliano, G.; D'Armiento, M.; D'Andrea, F.; Giugliano, D. Effect of a mediterranean-style diet on endothelial dysfunction and markers of vascular inflammation in the metabolic syndrome: A randomized trial. *JAMA* **2004**, *292*, 1440–1446. [CrossRef] [PubMed]
34. Salas-salvado, J.; Bullo, M.; Estruch, R.; Covas, M.I.; Ibarrola-Jurado, N.; Corella, D.; Arós, F.; Gómez-Gracia, E.; Ruiz-Gutiérrez, V.; Romaguera, D.; et al. Prevention of diabetes with Mediterranean diet—A subgroup analysis of a randomized diet. *Ann. Intern. Med.* **2014**, *160*, 1–10. [CrossRef] [PubMed]
35. Wu, H.; Esteve, E.; Tremaroli, V.; Khan, M.T.; Caesar, R.; Mannerås-Holm, L.; Ståhlman, M.; Olsson, L.M.; Serino, M.; Planas-Fèlix, M.; et al. Metformin alters the gut microbiome of individual with treatment-naïve type 2 diabetes contributing to the therapeutics effects of the drug. *Nat. Med.* **2017**, *23*, 850–858. [CrossRef] [PubMed]
36. Grundy, S.M.; Cleeman, J.I.; Daniels, S.R.; Donato, K.A.; Eckel, R.H.; Franklin, B.A.; Gordon, D.J.; Krauss, R.M.; Savage, P.J.; Smith, S.C., Jr.; et al. American Heart Association, National Heart, Lung, and Blood Institute. Diagnosis and management of the metabolic syndrome: An american heart association/national heart, lung, and blood institute scientific statement. *Circulation* **2005**, *112*, 2735–2752. [CrossRef] [PubMed]
37. Malur, P.; Menezes, A.; DiNicolantonio, J.J.; O'Keefe, J.H.; Lavie, C.J. The Microvascular and Macrovascular Benefits of Fibrates in Diabetes and the Metabolic Syndrome: A review. *Mo. Med.* **2017**, *114*, 464–471.
38. Grundy, S.M.; Vega, G.L.; Yuan, Z.; Battisti, W.P.; Brady, W.E.; Palmisano, J. Effectiveness and tolerability of simvastatin plus fenofibrate for combined hyperlipidemia (the SAFARI trial). *Am. J. Cardiol.* **2005**, *15*, 462–468. [CrossRef]
39. Verges, B. Fenofibrate therapy and cardiovascular protection in diabetes: Recommendations after FIELD. *Curr. Opin. Lipidol.* **2006**, *17*, 653–658. [CrossRef]
40. Fernandez-Miranda, C.; Perez-Carreras, M.; Colina, F.; Lopez-Alonso, G.; Vargas, C.; Solis-Herruzo, J.A. A pilot trial of fenofibrate for the treatment of non-alcoholic fatty liver disease. *Dig. Liver Dis.* **2008**, *40*, 200–205. [CrossRef]
41. Sirtori, C.R. The pharmacology of statins. *Pharmacol. Res.* **2004**, *88*, 3–11. [CrossRef]
42. Kumar, A.; Chopra, K.; Mukherjee, M.; Pottabathini, R.; Dhull, D.K. Current knowledge and pharmacological profile of berberine: An update. *Eur. J. Pharmacol.* **2015**, *761*, 288–297. [CrossRef] [PubMed]
43. Lan, J.; Zhao, Y.; Dong, F.; Yan, Z.; Zheng, W.; Fan, J.; Sun, G. Meta-analysis of the effect and safety of berberine in the treatment of type 2 diabetes mellitus, hyperlipemia, and hy-pertension. *J. Ethnopharmacol.* **2015**, *161*, 69–81. [CrossRef] [PubMed]
44. Cao, C.; Su, M. Effects of berberine on glucose-lipid metabolism, inflammatory factors and insulin resistance in patients with metabolic syndrome. *Exp. Ther. Med.* **2019**, *17*, 3009–3014. [CrossRef] [PubMed]
45. Perez-Rubio, K.G.; Gonzalez-Ortiz, M.; Martinez-Abundis, E.; Robles-Cervantes, J.A.; Espinel-Bermudez, M.C. Effect of berberine administration on metabolic syndrome, insulin sensitivity, and insulin secretion. *Metab. Syndr. Relat. Disord.* **2013**, *11*, 366–369. [CrossRef] [PubMed]
46. Yang, J.; Yin, J.; Gao, H.; Xu, L.; Wang, Y.; Xu, L.; Li, M. Berberine improves insulin sensitivity by inhibiting fat store and adjusting adipokines profile in human preadipocytes and metabolic syndrome patients. *Evid. Based Complement. Alternat. Med.* **2012**, *2012*, 363845. [CrossRef]
47. Lin, J.; Cai, Q.; Liang, B.; Wu, L.; Zhuang, Y.; He, Y.; Lin, Y. Berberine, a traditional chinese medicine, reduces inflammation in adipose tissue, polarizes M2 macrophages, and increases energy expenditure in mice fed a high-fat diet. *Med. Sci. Monit.* **2019**, *25*, 87–97. [CrossRef]
48. Lee, Y.S.; Kim, W.S.; Kim, K.H.; Yoon, M.J.; Cho, H.J.; Shen, Y.; Ye, J.; Lee, C.H.; Oh, W.K.; Kim, C.T.; et al. Berberine, a natural plant product, activates AMP-activated protein kinase with beneficial metabolic effects in diabetic and insulin-resistant states. *Diabetes* **2006**, *55*, 2256–2264. [CrossRef]

49. Zhang, Y.; Cui, Y.L.; Gao, L.N.; Jiang, H.L. Effects of β-cyclodextrin on the intestinal absorption of berberine hydrochloride, a P-glycoprotein substrate. *Int. J. Biol. Macromol.* **2013**, *59*, 363–371. [CrossRef]
50. Gui, S.Y.; Wu, L.; Peng, D.Y.; Liu, Q.Y.; Yin, B.P.; Shen, J.Z. Preparation and evaluation of a microemulsion for oral delivery of berberine. *Pharmazie* **2008**, *63*, 516–519.
51. Wang, T.; Wang, N.; Song, H.; Xi, X.; Wang, J.; Hao, A.; Li, T. Preparation of an anhydrous reverse micelle delivery system to enhance oral bioavailability and antidiabetic efficacy of berberine. *Eur. J. Pharm. Sci.* **2011**, *44*, 127–135. [CrossRef]
52. Tan, X.S.; Ma, J.Y.; Feng, R.; Ma, C.; Chen, W.J.; Sun, Y.; Fu, J.; Huang, M.; He, C.Y.; Shou, J.; et al. Tissue distribution of berberine and its metabolites after oral administration in rats. *PLoS ONE* **2013**, *8*, e77969. [CrossRef] [PubMed]
53. Qiu, F.; Zhu, Z.; Kang, N.; Piao, S.; Qin, G.; Yao, X. Isolation and identification of urinary metabolites of berberine in rats and humans. *Drug Metab. Dispos.* **2008**, *36*, 2159–2165. [CrossRef]
54. Ma, J.Y.; Feng, R.; Tan, X.S.; Ma, C.; Shou, J.W.; Fu, J.; Huang, M.; He, C.Y.; Chen, S.N.; Zao, Z.X.; et al. Excretion of berberine and its metabolites in oral administration in rats. *J. Pharm. Sci.* **2013**, *102*, 4181–4192. [CrossRef] [PubMed]
55. Affuso, F.; Mercurio, V.; Fazio, V.; Fazio, S. Cardiovascular and metabolic effects of berberine. *World J. Cardiol.* **2010**, *2*, 71–77. [CrossRef] [PubMed]
56. Wei, W.; Zhao, H.; Wang, A.; Sui, M.; Liang, K.; Deng, H.; Ma, Y.; Zhang, Y.; Zhang, H.; Guan, Y. A clinical study on the short-term effect of berberine in comparison to metformin on the metabolic characteristics of women with polycystic ovary syndrome. *Eur. J. Endocrinol.* **2012**, *166*, 99–105. [CrossRef] [PubMed]
57. Tong, N.; Zhang, J.; Chen, Y.; Li, Z.; Luo, Y.; Zuo, H.; Zhao, X. Berberine sensitizes multiple human cancer cells to the anticancer effects of doxorubicin in vitro. *Oncol. Lett.* **2012**, *3*, 1263–1267. [CrossRef] [PubMed]
58. Quan, H.; Cao, Y.Y.; Xu, Z.; Zhao, J.X.; Gao, P.H.; Qin, X.F.; Jiang, Y.Y. Potent in vitro synergism of fluconazole and berberine chloride against clinical isolates of Candida albicans resistant to fluconazole. *Antimicrob. Agents Chemother.* **2006**, *50*, 1096–1099. [CrossRef]
59. Shin, K.S.; Choi, H.S.; Zhao, T.T.; Suh, K.H.; Kwon, I.H.; Choi, S.O.; Lee, M.K. Neurotoxic effects of berberine on long-term L-DOPA administration in 6-hydroxydopamine-lesioned rat model of Parkinson's disease. *Arch. Pharm. Res.* **2013**, *36*, 759–767. [CrossRef]
60. Zhang, C.H.; Yu, R.Y.; Liu, Y.H.; Tu, X.Y.; Tu, J.; Wang, J.S.; Xu, G.L. Interaction of baicalin with berberine for glucose uptake in 3T3-L1 adipocytes and HepG2 hepatocytes. *J. Ethnopharmacol.* **2014**, *151*, 864–872. [CrossRef]
61. Pulido-Moran, M.; Moreno-Fernandez, J.; Ramirez-Tortosa, J.; Ramirez-Tortosa, M. Curcumin and Health. *Molecules* **2016**, *21*, 264. [CrossRef]
62. Yang, Y.S.; Su, Y.F.; Yang, H.W.; Lee, Y.H.; Chou, J.I.; Ueng, K.C. Lipid-lowering effects of curcumin in patients with metabolic syndrome: A randomized, double-blind, placebo-controlled trial. *Phytother. Res.* **2014**, *28*, 1770–1777. [CrossRef] [PubMed]
63. Di Pierro, F.; Bressan, A.; Ranaldi, D.; Rapacioli, G.; Giacomelli, L.; Bertuccioli, A. Potential role of bioavailable curcumin in weight loss and omental adipose tissue decrease: Preliminary data of a randomized, controlled trial in overweight people with metabolic syndrome. Preliminary study. *Eur. Rev. Med. Pharmacol. Sci.* **2015**, *19*, 4195–4202. [PubMed]
64. Kelany, M.E.; Hakami, T.M.; Omar, A.H. Curcumin improves the metabolic syndrome in high-fructose-diet-fed rats: Role of TNF-α, NF-κB, and oxidative stress. *Can. J. Physiol. Pharmacol.* **2017**, *95*, 140–150. [CrossRef] [PubMed]
65. Aggarwal, B.B. Targeting inflammation-induced obesity and metabolic diseases by curcumin and other nutraceuticals. *Annu. Rev. Nutr.* **2010**, *30*, 173–199. [CrossRef]
66. Woo, H.M.; Kang, J.H.; Kawada, T.; Yoo, H.; Sung, M.K.; Yu, R. Active spice-derived components can inhibit inflammatory responses of adipose tissue in obesity by suppressing inflammatory actions of macrophages and release of monocyte chemoattractant protein-1 from adipocytes. *Life Sci.* **2007**, *80*, 926–931. [CrossRef]
67. Wang, S.L.; Li, Y.; Wen, Y.; Chen, Y.F.; Na, L.X.; Li, S.T.; Sun, C.H. Curcumin, a potential inhibitor of up-regulation of TNF-alpha and IL-6 induced by palmitate in 3T3-L1 adipocytes through NF-kappaB and JNK pathway. *Biomed. Environ. Sci.* **2009**, *22*, 32–39. [CrossRef]
68. Tang, Y.; Zheng, S.; Chen, A. Curcumin eliminates leptin's effects on hepatic stellate cell activation via interrupting leptin signalling. *Endocrinology* **2009**, *150*, 3011–3020. [CrossRef]

69. Xu, J.; Fu, Y.; Chen, A. Activation of peroxisome proliferator-activated receptor-gamma contributes to the inhibitory effects of curcumin on rat hepatic stellate cell growth. *Am. J. Physiol. Gastrointest. Liver Physiol.* **2003**, *285*, G20–G30. [CrossRef]
70. Weisberg, S.P.; Leibel, R.; Tortoriello, D.V. Dietary curcumin significantly improves obesity associated inflammation and diabetes in mouse models of diabesity. *Endocrinology* **2008**, *149*, 3549–3558. [CrossRef]
71. Ryu, M.J.; Cho, M.; Song, J.Y.; Yun, Y.S.; Choi, I.W.; Kim, D.E.; Park, B.S.; Oh, S. Natural derivatives of curcumin attenuate the Wnt/beta-catenin pathway through down-regulation of the transcriptional coactivator p300. *Biochem. Biophys. Res. Commun.* **2008**, *377*, 1304–1308. [CrossRef]
72. Bustanji, Y.; Taha, M.O.; Almasri, I.M.; Al-Ghussein, M.A.; Mohammad, M.K.; Alkhatib, H.S. Inhibition of glycogen synthase kinase by curcumin: Investigation by simulated molecular docking and subsequent in vitro/in vivo evaluation. *J. Enzyme Inhib. Med. Chem.* **2009**, *24*, 771–778. [CrossRef] [PubMed]
73. Yang, K.Y.; Lin, L.C.; Tseng, T.Y.; Wang, S.C.; Tsai, T.H. Oral bioavailability of curcumin in rat and the herbal analysis from Curcuma longa by LC-MS/MS. *J. Chromatogr B Anal Technol. Biomed. Life Sci.* **2007**, *53*, 183–189. [CrossRef] [PubMed]
74. Prasad, S.; Tyagi, A.K.; Aggarwal, B.B. Recent developments in delivery, bioavailability, absorption and metabolism of curcumin: The golden pigment from golden spice. *Cancer Res. Treat.* **2014**, *46*, 2–18. [CrossRef] [PubMed]
75. Pan, M.H.; Huang, T.M.; Lin, J.K. Biotransformation of curcumin through reduction and glucuronidation in mice. *Drug. Metab. Dispos. Biol. Fate Chem.* **1999**, *27*, 486–494. [PubMed]
76. Ryu, E.K.; Choe, Y.S.; Lee, K.-H.; Choi, Y.; Kim, B.-T. Curcumin and dehydrozingerone derivatives: Synthesis, radiolabeling, and evaluation for beta-amyloid plaque imaging. *J. Med. Chem.* **2006**, *49*, 6111–6119. [CrossRef]
77. Sharma, R.A.; Euden, S.A.; Platton, S.L.; Cooke, D.N.; Shafayat, A.; Hewitt, H.R.; Marczylo, T.H.; Morgan, B.; Hemingway, D.; Plummer, S.M.; et al. Phase I clinical trial of oral curcumin: Biomarkers of systemic activity and compliance. *Clin. Cancer Res.* **2004**, *10*, 6847–6854. [CrossRef]
78. Wahlstrom, B.; Blennow, G. A study on the fate of curcumin in the rat. *Acta Pharmacol. Toxicol.* **1978**, *43*, 86–92. [CrossRef]
79. Jayaprakasha, G.K.; Rao, L.J.M. Chemistry, biogenesis, and biological activities of Cinnamomum zeylanicum. *Crit. Rev. Food Sci. Nutr.* **2011**, *51*, 547–562. [CrossRef]
80. Ziegenfuss, T.N.; Hofheins, J.E.; Mendel, R.W.; Landis, J.; Anderson, R.A. Effects of a water-soluble cinnamon extract on body composition and features of the metabolic syndrome in pre-diabetic men and women. *J. Int. Soc. Sports Nutr.* **2006**, *3*, 45–53. [CrossRef]
81. Medagama, A.B. The glycaemic outcomes of Cinnamon, a review of the experimental evidence and clinical trials. *Nutr. J.* **2015**, *14*, 108. [CrossRef]
82. Cao, H.; Polansky, M.M.; Anderson, R.A. Cinnamon extract and polyphenols affect the expression of tristetraprolin, insulin receptor, and glucose transporter 4 in mouse 3T3-L1 adipocytes. *Arch. Biochem. Biophys.* **2007**, *459*, 214–222. [CrossRef] [PubMed]
83. Zhao, H.; Xie, Y.; Yang, Q.; Cao, Y.; Tu, H.; Cao, W.; Wang, S. Pharmacokinetic study of cinnamaldehyde in rats by gc-ms after oral and intravenous administration. *J. Pharm. Biomed. Anal.* **2014**, *89*, 150–157. [CrossRef] [PubMed]
84. Zhu, R.; Liu, H.; Liu, C.; Wang, L.; Ma, R.; Chen, B.; Li, L.; Niu, J.; Fu, M.; Zhang, D.; et al. Cinnamaldehyde in diabetes: A review of pharmacology, pharmacokinetics and safety. *Pharmacol. Res.* **2017**, *122*, 78–89. [CrossRef] [PubMed]
85. Chen, Y.; Ma, Y.; Ma, W. Pharmacokinetics and bioavailability of cinnamic acid after oral administration of ramulus cinnamomi in rats. *Eur. J. Drug Metab. Pharmacokinet.* **2009**, *34*, 51–56. [CrossRef]
86. Bickers, D.; Calow, P.; Greim, H.; Hanifin, J.M.; Rogers, A.E.; Saurat, J.H.; Sipes, I.G.; Smith, R.L.; Tagami, H. A toxicologic and dermatologic assessment of cinnamyl alcohol, cinnamaldehyde and cinnamic acid when used as fragrance ingredients. *Food Chem. Toxicol.* **2005**, *43*, 799–836. [CrossRef]
87. Zahra, N.; Alim-un-Nisa, I.K.; Hina, S.; Javed, A.; Inam, S.M.; Malik, S.M.; Arshad, F. Estimation of capsaicin in different chilli varieties using different extraction techniques and HPLC method: A review. *Pak. J. Food Sci.* **2016**, *26*, 54–60.
88. Panchal, S.K.; Bliss, E.; Brown, L. Capsaicin in Metabolic Syndrome. *Nutrients* **2018**, *10*, 630. [CrossRef]

89. Lee, E.; Jung, D.Y.; Kim, J.H.; Patel, P.R.; Hu, X.; Lee, Y.; Azuma, Y.; Wang, H.F.; Sitsilianos, N.; Shafiq, U.; et al. Transient receptor potential vanilloid type-1 channel regulates diet-induced obesity, insulin resistance, and leptin resistance. *FASEB J.* **2015**, *29*, 3182–3192. [CrossRef]
90. Kang, J.H.; Tsuyoshi, G.; Han, I.S.; Kawada, T.; Kim, Y.M.; Yu, R. Dietary Capsaicin Reduces Obesity-induced Insulin Resistance and Hepatic Steatosis in Obese Mice Fed a High-fat Diet. *Obesity* **2010**, *18*, 780–787. [CrossRef]
91. Zhang, S.; Ma, X.; Zhang, L.; Sun, H.; Liu, X.J. Capsaicin Reduces Blood Glucose by Increasing Insulin Levels and Glycogen Content Better than Capsiate in Streptozotocin-Induced Diabetic Rats. *Agric. Food Chem.* **2017**, *65*, 2323–2330. [CrossRef]
92. Rollyson, W.D.; Stover, C.A.; Brown, K.C.; Perry, H.E.; Tevenson, C.D.; McNees, C.A.; Ball, J.G.; Valentovic, M.A.; Dasgupta, P. Bioavailability of capsaicin and its implications for drug delivery. *J. Control Release* **2014**, *196*, 96–105. [CrossRef] [PubMed]
93. Chaiyasit, K.; Khovidhunkit, W.; Wittayalertpanya, S. Pharmacokinetic and the effect of capsaicin in Capsicum frutescens on decreasing plasma glucose level. *J. Med. Assoc. Thail.* **2009**, *92*, 108–113.
94. Tan, S.; Gao, B.; Tao, Y.; Guo, J.; Su, Z.Q. Antiobese effects of capsaicin-chitosan microsphere (CCMS) in obese rats induced by high fat diet. *J. Agric. Food Chem.* **2014**, *62*, 1866–1874. [CrossRef] [PubMed]
95. Zhu, Y.; Wang, M.; Zhang, J.; Peng, W.; Firempong, C.K.; Deng, W.; Wang, Q.; Wang, S.; Shi, F.; Yu, J.; et al. Improved oral bioavailability of capsaicin via liposomal nanoformulation: Preparation, in vitro drug release and pharmacokinetics in rats. *Arch. Pharm. Res.* **2015**, *38*, 512–552. [CrossRef]
96. Peng, W.; Jiang, X.Y.; Zhu, Y.; Omari-Siaw, E.; Deng, W.W.; Yu, J.N.; Xu, X.M.; Zhang, W.M. Oral delivery of capsaicin using MPEG-PCL nanoparticles. *Acta Pharmacol. Sin.* **2015**, *36*, 139–148. [CrossRef]
97. Zhao, Y.; Sedighi, R.; Wang, P.; Chen, H.; Zhu, Y.; Sang, S. Carnosic acid as a major bioactive component in rosemary extract ameliorates high-fat diet induced obesity and metabolic syndrome. *J. Agric. Food Chem.* **2015**, *63*, 4843–4852. [CrossRef]
98. Liu, Y.; Zhang, Y.; Hu, M.; Li, Y.H.; Cao, X.H. Carnosic acid alleviates brain injury through NF-κB-regulated inflammation and Caspase-3-associated apoptosis in high fat-induced mouse models. *Mol. Med. Rep.* **2019**, *20*, 495–504. [CrossRef]
99. Doolaege, E.H.A.; Raes, K.; De Vos, F.; Verhé, R.; De Smet, S. Absorption, distribution and elimination of carnosic acid, a natural antioxidant from rosmarinus officinalis, in rats. *Plant Foods Hum. Nutr.* **2011**, *66*, 196–202. [CrossRef]
100. Vaquero, M.R.; Villalba, R.G.; Larrosa, M.; Yánez-Gascon, M.J.; Fromentin, E.; Flanagan, J.; Roller, M.; Tomas-Barberan, F.A.; Espin, J.C.; Garcıa-Conesa, M.T. Bioavailability of the major bioactive diterpenoids in a rosemary extract: Metabolic profile in the intestine, liver, plasma, and brain of Zucker rats. *Mol. Nutr. Food Res* **2013**, *57*, 1834–1846. [CrossRef]
101. Anadón, A.; Martínez-Larrañaga, M.R.; Martínez, M.A.; Ares, I.; Garcia-Risco, M.R.; Senorans, F.J.; Reglero, G. Acute oral safety study of rosemary extracts in rats. *J. Food Prot.* **2008**, *71*, 790–795. [CrossRef]
102. Vaquero, M.R.; Yáñez-Gascón, M.J.; Villalba, R.G.; Larrosa, M.; Fromentin, E.; Ibarra, A.; Roller, M.; Tomas-Barberan, F.A.; Espín de Gea, J.C.; García-Conesa, M.T. Inhibition of Gastric Lipase as a Mechanism for Body Weight and Plasma Lipids Reduction in Zucker Rats Fed a Rosemary Extract Rich in Carnosic Acid. *PLoS ONE* **2012**, *7*, e39773. [CrossRef] [PubMed]
103. Mollace, V.; Sacco, I.; Janda, E.; Malara, C.; Ventrice, D.; Colica, C.; Visalli, V.; Muscoli, S.; Ragusa, S.; Muscoli, C.; et al. Hypolipemic and hypoglycaemic activity of bergamot polyphenols: From animal models to human studies. *Fitoterapia* **2011**, *82*, 309–316. [CrossRef] [PubMed]
104. Gliozzi, M.; Walker, R.; Muscoli, S.; Vitale, C.; Gratteri, S.; Carresi, C.; Musolino, V.; Russo, V.; Janda, E.; Ragusa, S.; et al. Bergamot polyphenolic fraction enhances rosuvastatin-induced effect on LDL-cholesterol, LOX-1 expression and protein kinase B phosphorylation in patients with hyperlipidemia. *Int. J. Cardiol.* **2013**, *170*, 140–145. [CrossRef] [PubMed]
105. Gliozzi, M.; Carresi, C.; Musolino, V.; Palma, E.; Muscoli, C.; Vitale, C.; Gratteri, S.; Muscianisi, G.; Janda, E.; Muscoli, S.; et al. The effect of bergamot-derived polyphenolic fraction on LDL small dense particles and non-alcoholic fatty liver disease in patients with metabolic syndrome. *Adv. Biol. Chem.* **2014**, *4*, 129–137. [CrossRef]

106. Capomolla, A.S.; Janda, E.; Paone, S.; Parafati, M.; Sawicki, T.; Mollace, R.; Ragusa, S.; Mollace, V. Atherogenic Index Reduction and Weight Loss in Metabolic Syndrome Patients Treated with A Novel Pectin-Enriched Formulation of Bergamot Polyphenols. *Nutrients* **2019**, *11*, 1271. [CrossRef] [PubMed]
107. Mollace, V.; Scicchitano, M.; Paone, S.; Casale, F.; Calandruccio, C.; Gliozzi, M.; Musolino, V.; Carresi, C.; Maiuolo, J.; Nucera, S.; et al. Hypoglycemic and Hypolipemic Effects of a New Lecithin Formulation of Bergamot Polyphenolic Fraction: A Double Blind, Randomized, Placebo-Controlled Study. *Endocr. Metab. Immune. Disord. Drug Targets* **2019**, *19*, 136–143. [CrossRef]
108. Parafati, M.; Lascala, A.; Morittu, V.M.; Trimboli, F.; Rizzuto, A.; Brunelli, E.; Coscarelli, F.; Costa, N.; Britti, D.; Ehrlich, J.; et al. Bergamot polyphenol fraction prevents nonalcoholic fatty liver disease via stimulation of lipophagy in cafeteria diet-induced rat model of metabolic syndrome. *J. Nutr. Biochem.* **2015**, *26*, 938–948. [CrossRef]
109. Musolino, V.; Gliozzi, M.; Scarano, F.; Bosco, F.; Scicchitano, M.; Nucera, S.; Carresi, C.; Ruga, S.; Zito, M.C.; Maiuolo, J.; et al. Bergamot polyphenols improve Dyslipidemia and pathophysiological features in a Mouse Model of non-Alcoholic fatty Liver Disease. *Sci. Rep.* **2020**, *10*, 2565. [CrossRef]
110. Musolino, V.; Gliozzi, M.; Nucera, S.; Carresi, C.; Maiuolo, J.; Mollace, R.; Paone, S.; Bosco, F.; Scarano, F.; Scicchitano, M.; et al. The effect of bergamot polyphenolic fraction on lipid transfer protein system and vascular oxidative stress in a rat model of hyperlipemia. *Lipids Health Dis.* **2019**, *18*, 115. [CrossRef]
111. Mollace, V.; Ragusa, S.; Sacco, I.; Muscoli, C.; Sculco, F.; Visalli, V.; Palma, E.; Muscoli, S.; Mondello, L.; Dugo, P.; et al. The protective effect of bergamot oil extract on lecitine-like oxyLDL receptor-1 expression in balloon injury-related neointima formation. *J. Cardiovasc. Pharmacol. Ther.* **2008**, *13*, 120–129. [CrossRef]
112. La Russa, D.; Giordano, F.; Marrone, A.; Parafati, M.; Janda, E.; Pellegrino, D. Oxidative Imbalance and Kidney Damage in Cafeteria Diet-Induced Rat Model of Metabolic Syndrome: Effect of Bergamot Polyphenolic Fraction. *Antioxidants* **2019**, *8*, 66. [CrossRef] [PubMed]
113. Parafati, M.; Lascala, A.; La Russa, D.; Mignogna, C.; Trimboli, F.; Morittu, V.M.; Riillo, C.; Macirella, R.; Mollace, V.; Brunelli, E.; et al. Bergamot Polyphenols Boost Therapeutic Effects of the Diet on Non-Alcoholic Steatohepatitis (NASH) Induced by "Junk Food": Evidence for Anti-Inflammatory Activity. *Nutrients* **2018**, *10*, 1604. [CrossRef] [PubMed]
114. Musolino, V.; Gliozzi, M.; Bombardelli, E.; Nucera, S.; Carresi, C.; Maiuolo, J.; Mollace, R.; Paone, S.; Bosco, F.; Scarano, F.; et al. The synergistic effect of Citrus bergamia and Cynara cardunculus extracts on vascular inflammation and oxidative stress in nonalcoholic fatty liver disease. *J. Tradit. Complement. Med.* **2020**, in press. [CrossRef]
115. Spigoni, V.; Mena, P.; Fantuzzi, F.; Tassotti, M.; Brighenti, F.; Bonadonna, R.C.; Del Rio, D.; Dei Cas, A. Bioavailability of Bergamot (Citrus bergamia) Flavanones and Biological Activity of Their Circulating Metabolites in Human Pro-Angiogenic Cells. *Nutrients* **2017**, *9*, 1328. [CrossRef] [PubMed]
116. Calamini, B.; Ratia, K.; Malkowski, M.G.; Cuendet, M.; Pezzuto, J.M.; Santarsiero, B.D.; Mesecar, A.D. Pleiotropic mechanisms facilitated by resveratrol and its metabolites. *Biochem. J.* **2010**, *429*, 273–282. [CrossRef] [PubMed]
117. Chang, T.Y.; Li, B.L.; Chang, C.C.Y.; Urano, Y. Acyl-coenzyme A: Cholesterol acyltransferases. *Am. J. Physiol. Endocrinol. Metab.* **2009**, *297*, E1–E9. [CrossRef]
118. Rousset, X.; Vaisman, B.; Amar, M.; Sethi, A.A.; Remaley, A.T. Lecithin: Cholesterol Acyltransferase: From Biochemistry to Role in Cardiovascular Disease. *Curr. Opin. Endocrinol. Diabetes Obes.* **2009**, *16*, 163–171. [CrossRef]
119. Barter, P.J.; Brewer, H.B., Jr.; Chapman, M.J.; Hennekens, C.H.; Rader, D.J.; Tall, A.R. Cholesteryl ester transfer protein: A novel target for raising HDL and inhibiting atherosclerosis. *Arterioscler. Thromb. Vasc. Biol.* **2003**, *23*, 160–167. [CrossRef]
120. Chistiakova, D.A.; Melnichenko, A.A.; Orekhov, A.N.; Bobryshev, Y.V. Paraoxonase and atherosclerosis-related cardiovascular diseases. *Biochimie* **2017**, *132*, 19–27. [CrossRef]

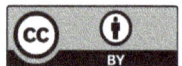

© 2020 by the authors. Licensee MDPI, Basel, Switzerland. This article is an open access article distributed under the terms and conditions of the Creative Commons Attribution (CC BY) license (http://creativecommons.org/licenses/by/4.0/).

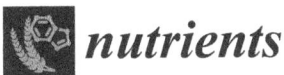

Review

The Role of Specific Components of a Plant-Based Diet in Management of Dyslipidemia and the Impact on Cardiovascular Risk

Elke A. Trautwein [1,*] and Sue McKay [2]

1. Trautwein Consulting, 58097 Hagen, Germany
2. Upfield Research & Development, 3071 JL Rotterdam, The Netherlands; Sue.Mckay@Upfield.com
* Correspondence: et@trautwein-consulting.com

Received: 4 August 2020; Accepted: 31 August 2020; Published: 1 September 2020

Abstract: Convincing evidence supports the intake of specific food components, food groups, or whole dietary patterns to positively influence dyslipidemia and to lower risk of cardiovascular diseases (CVD). Specific macro- and micro-components of a predominantly plant-based dietary pattern are vegetable fats, dietary fibers, and phytonutrients such as phytosterols. This review summarizes the current knowledge regarding effects of these components on lowering blood lipids, i.e., low-density lipoprotein cholesterol (LDL-C) and on reducing CVD risk. The beneficial role of a plant-based diet on cardiovascular (CV) health has increasingly been recognized. Plant-based dietary patterns include a Mediterranean and Nordic diet pattern, the dietary approaches to stop hypertension (DASH), and Portfolio diet, as well as vegetarian- or vegan-type diet patterns. These diets have all been found to lower CVD-related risk factors like blood LDL-C, and observational study evidence supports their role in lowering CVD risk. These diet patterns are not only beneficial for dyslipidemia management and prevention of CVD but further contribute to reducing the impact of food choices on environmental degradation. Hence, the CV health benefits of a predominantly plant-based diet as a healthy and environmentally sustainable eating pattern are today recommended by many food-based dietary as well as clinical practice guidelines.

Keywords: review; CVD; dyslipidemia; cardiovascular health; dietary fats; dietary fiber; phytosterols; plant-based diet; dietary pattern; sustainability

1. Introduction

Cardiovascular diseases (CVD), which include coronary heart disease (CHD), cerebrovascular disease (stroke), and peripheral vascular disease, are the most common non-communicable diseases globally, accounting for an estimated 31% of all deaths worldwide [1]. The underlying cause of CVD is atherosclerosis which is a progressive (and reversible) disease of the blood vessels. By managing risk factors associated with atherosclerosis it is possible to slow down (or reverse) the development of the disease and ultimately reduce the risk of CVD [2]. Underlying risk factors include elevated blood pressure, dyslipidemia, overweight/obesity, and type 2 diabetes mellitus (T2DM), as well as behavioral risk factors such as smoking, unhealthy diet, and physical inactivity [2]. Dyslipidemia is a metabolic abnormality leading to an increase in circulating concentrations of blood cholesterol (C) and triglycerides (TG). It is characterized by elevated low-density lipoprotein cholesterol (LDL-C), also known as hypercholesterolemia, and often combined with low concentrations of high-density lipoprotein cholesterol (HDL-C) and elevated TG, mainly as TG-rich lipoproteins (TRL) such as chylomicrons and very-low-density lipoprotein (VLDL).

Elevated LDL-C is a causal risk factor for CVD [3] and lowering LDL-C concentrations is the primary target for treatment and prevention of CVD [2]. Elevated TG, and especially TRL, are also treatment targets recommended in guidelines for the management of dyslipidemia [2].

Adopting a healthy diet and lifestyle should always be the cornerstone when seeking to lower LDL-C (and TG) concentrations [2]. Based on the severity of dyslipidemia and the total CVD risk score, additional pharmacological therapy may be recommended. With adequate changes in diet and lifestyle, about 80% of (premature) CVD mortality may be prevented [4].

The role of a healthy dietary pattern in the prevention of CVD has well been recognized [5–7]. Evidence supports the intake of specific nutrients, food groups, or certain dietary patterns to positively influence dyslipidemia and promote the prevention of CVD. A healthy dietary pattern is also a major determinant of environmental sustainability. Current food production practices contribute to environmental degradation in several ways, e.g., through greenhouse-gas emissions, fresh-water withdrawal, and land use [8]. Consequently, authorities are starting to adapt their food-based dietary guidelines to reflect a shift towards a predominantly plant-based diet. These recommendations aim to reduce the intake of animal-based foods for both health and environmental reasons [9,10].

Predominantly plant-based dietary patterns emphasize a higher intake of fruits, vegetables, legumes, whole-grain products, nuts, seeds, and vegetable oils and limited intake of foods from animal origin such as low- or non-fat dairy, lean meat, and fish [7]. Plant-based dietary patterns vary from flexitarian (with low consumption of meat) to pescatarian or lacto/ovo-vegetarian to vegan, where plant-based foods represent most or all the food in the diet.

In view of macronutrients, specific for a plant-based diet are the intake of more complex carbohydrates and plant-based proteins next to a lower total fat intake, especially fewer saturated and trans fats and more unsaturated fatty acids. Plant-based diets are also higher in dietary fiber (DF). In addition, they contain modest amount of phytosterols (PS) next to other bioactive plant-derived compounds often called phytonutrients, which are associated with positive health effects. This review focuses on PS because of their proven cholesterol-lowering effect which allows them to carry an authorized health claim. Other phytonutrients, such as polyphenols, lignans, and carotenoids, as well as vitamins like folic acid, are out of scope for this review.

This narrative review, based on evidence from reviews, systematic reviews, meta-analyses, and randomized controlled trials (RCTs) on CVD risk factors (LDL-C and on clinical endpoints) focuses on the beneficial effects of specific macro- and micro-components of a plant-based diet (vegetable fats, DF, and PS) in the management of dyslipidemia and the role of plant-based dietary patterns in cardiovascular (CV) health and briefly discusses aspects of environmental sustainability. Dietary fatty acids, DF, and PS have been reviewed in detail because of the proven evidence for cholesterol-lowering and CVD risk benefits and because they are specifically referred to in dietary recommendations for CVD prevention [2]. Literature databases like MEDLINE were used as the main sources for searching relevant literature.

While health benefits of these individual dietary components have been addressed in specific reviews and meta-analyses, the information provided in this review addresses them in the context of a plant-based diet/dietary pattern and contributes to a better understanding of the increasingly important role of a plant-based diet in the prevention of CVD. In the following sections, specific components of a plant-based diet in the management of dyslipidemia and prevention of CVD are discussed in detail.

2. Dietary Fats

2.1. Dietary Sources and Fat Quality

There is general consensus that fat quality, i.e., the fatty acid composition of dietary fat, is more important than fat quantity (total amount of fat) in the management of dyslipidemia and the prevention of CVD. The fat quality of foods is determined by the content of different fatty acids. Fat from animal origin such as fatty meat, butter, full-fat dairy, as well as the tropical oils coconut and palm oil, are typically rich in saturated fatty acids (SAFA). Meat and dairy foods are the main food sources of SAFA in Western diets [11]. In contrast, plant-based fats, i.e., vegetable oils, are generally rich in unsaturated fatty acids. Unsaturated fatty acids can be monounsaturated (MUFA), such as oleic acid and polyunsaturated (PUFA). Plant-based sources of PUFA are predominately n-6 (omega-6) fatty acids such as linoleic acid and some n-3 (omega-3) fatty acids such as α-linoleic acid. Very long-chain n-3 fatty acids such as eicosapentaenoic (EPA) and docosahexaenoic acid (DHA) come from marine sources (fish, fish oil, and algae). Trans fatty acids (TFA), unsaturated fatty acids with double bonds in the trans configuration, are naturally found in butter, full-fat dairy, and meat from ruminants like beef, sheep, and goat. Other sources of TFA are partially hydrogenated vegetable oils. TFA are commonly found in commercial baked goods like pastries, convenience foods, and battered or deep-fried foods. TFA from partially hydrogenated oils have been removed from many foods because of their adverse effects on blood lipids and CVD risk [12], leading to a substantial decrease in TFA intake, which is typically now less than 1% of energy [13]. TFA and SAFA raise LDL-C but TFA also lowers HDL-C concentrations and therefore has the most unfavorable effects amongst dietary fatty acids [12].

Based on dietary intake data, SAFA consumption is still higher and PUFA consumption lower than recommended [11,14]. For CVD prevention, it is recommended that a decrease in SAFA intake should be accompanied by an increase in PUFA intake, but this is not always achieved at a population level [14].

2.2. The Role of Saturated, Monounsaturated, and Polyunsaturated Fatty Acids on Blood Lipids and CVD Risk

Replacing SAFA with unsaturated fatty acids in the diet lowers LDL-C without affecting HDL-C and TG. The LDL-C lowering effect is larger when SAFA is replaced by PUFA compared to MUFA [15–17]. Replacing SAFA with carbohydrates, i.e., consuming a low-fat, high carbohydrate diet, lowers both LDL-C and HDL-C and raises fasting TG, and therefore does not improve the overall blood lipid profile [15,17]. The most beneficial effect on blood lipids is therefore achieved by replacing SAFA with unsaturated fats. Supplemental intake of the very long-chain n-3 PUFA (EPA and DHA), from fish oil have no substantial effect on LDL-C but dose-dependently lower TG concentrations [13].

In view of effects on CVD risk and clinical endpoints, both observational, i.e. prospective cohort studies and RCTs with clinical endpoints, have shown that reducing SAFA intake lowers the risk of CVD and CHD events. There is clear evidence that partial replacement of SAFA with unsaturated fatty acids, especially vegetable oil PUFA (mainly n-6 linoleic acid and the plant-based n-3 fatty acid α-linolenic acid) lowers the risk of CVD, mainly the risk of CHD [13,17]. There is insufficient or limited evidence for effects on CVD or CHD risk when SAFA is replaced by MUFA, carbohydrates, or proteins, and when the replacement nutrient is not specified [13]. Replacing 5% of total energy intake (% TE) of SAFA with PUFA was found to lower the risk of CHD by about 10%, while evidence is inconclusive due to lack of adequate studies to quantify the CHD risk benefit of MUFA [13,17]. More recently, data from two large cohort studies found a significantly lower CHD risk when 5% TE intake from SAFA, TFA, and refined carbohydrates was replaced by MUFA from plant sources (vegetable oils, nuts, and seeds), while replacement with MUFA from animal sources (red and processed meats and dairy foods) was not associated with lower CHD risk [18]. In addition, data from two other cohort studies has shown that replacing 5 g/day of dietary fats like margarine, mayonnaise, butter or dairy fat with a higher intake of olive oil, which is rich in MUFA, was associated with a 5–7% lower risk of CHD and total CVD [19]. The Prevención con Dieta Mediterránea (PREDIMED) trial also studied the effect of consuming MUFA, in the form of olive oil, as part of a Mediterranean (MED)-type diet on CVD outcomes. The MED-type diet supplemented with either extra-virgin olive oil or with nuts significantly lowered major CVD events by around 30% compared to a low-fat diet [20]. It should, however, be noted that these dietary patterns differ in more aspects than just dietary fat and fatty acid intake.

Even though marine n-3 PUFA are not the focus of this review, observational studies have consistently shown that higher intakes of fish, fish oil, and EPA and DHA is associated with lower risk of CVD, especially CHD risk, in the general population [13,21]. While evidence from RCTs for the primary prevention of CVD is weak, higher intakes of EPA and DHA have been shown to lower CVD risk in RCTs in secondary prevention [13,21].

An analysis based on prospective cohort studies has further shown that replacing SAFA with PUFA, MUFA, or whole-grain (high-quality) carbohydrates was associated with a lower CHD risk, while replacing SAFA with refined carbohydrates and sugars (low-quality carbohydrates) was not associated with CHD risk [22]. Furthermore, a higher PUFA intake was associated with a lower CHD risk compared to higher intakes of refined carbohydrate and sugar. These data support that PUFA-rich plant-based fats as well as whole grain products as part of a predominantly plant-based diet are beneficial for CV health.

For management of dyslipidemia not all plant-based fats are beneficial, especially not those that are rich in SAFA such as coconut oil. Despite the widespread popularity of coconut oil and its alleged health benefits, its consumption significantly raises LDL-C compared with other vegetable oils as summarized in a recent meta-analysis [23]. Thus, coconut oil should not be recommended as a healthy vegetable oil for CVD risk reduction, despite its HDL-C-raising effect [23,24].

In addition to the beneficial effects on dyslipidemia, emerging data also show that unsaturated fatty acids, especially n-6 PUFA, favorably affect blood glucose and insulin resistance, therefore helping to reduce the risk of T2DM, a risk factor for CVD [13,17].

2.3. Recommendations for Dietary Fat Intake

Quality of dietary fat intake is key for the prevention of CVD more so than quantity. Recommendations for total fat intake typically range from 20 to 35% TE; intakes exceeding 35–40%TE should be avoided as they are usually associated with an increased intake of SAFA [25,26]. Reducing SAFA intake to <10% TE and replacing SAFA with unsaturated fatty acids (MUFA and PUFA) is the recommendation in most food-based dietary guidelines aiming to prevent CVD [2,27,28]. Some guidelines advise SFA intake <7% TE, especially in the presence of hypercholesterolemia (Table 1) [2]. TFA increases the risk of CVD [2,28,29], and intake should be avoided (Table 1). Intake of n-3 PUFA, especially EPA and DHA, is not part of dietary recommendations to lower TC and LDL-C concentrations. Nevertheless, some guidelines do recommend an intake of 200–500 mg/day of EPA and DHA as part of a heart healthy diet [21] or advise 1 to 2 portions of fatty fish per week [30]. For specific TG-lowering, high doses (2–4 g/day) of n-3 fatty acid supplements are recommended either alone or as an adjunct to other lipid-lowering therapy [2,21,30].

2.4. Food-Based Dietary Guidelines and How a Plant-Based Diet Can Improve the Quality of Dietary Fat Intake

Food-based dietary guidelines advise a more plant-based diet and recommend eating less foods of animal origin such as meat, butter, and full-fat milk and cheese [9]. They also advise switching to leaner meat and low-fat dairy products and replacing animal fats with vegetable oils and vegetable oil-based fats. As a result, pre-dominantly plant-based diets typically deliver less total fat, especially less SAFA and TFA, more unsaturated fats, and more plant-based proteins, DF, micronutrients (vitamins and minerals), and phytonutrients. Regular fish consumption, especially fatty fish, is also advised as a part of a plant-based, heart-healthy dietary pattern.

Table 1. Impact of specific dietary changes in the management of dyslipidemia with focus on lowering low-density lipoprotein cholesterol (LDL-C) concentration.

Dietary Component	Specific Recommendation	Magnitude of Effect [1]	Strength (Level) of Evidence [2]
Dietary fat			
Reduce intake of saturated fatty acids (SAFA)	<10% of total energy intake (TE)<7% TE in the presence of hypercholesterolemia	++	***
Exchange SAFA with unsaturated fatty acids	Lower SAFA and increase intake of mono- (MUFA) and polyunsaturated fatty acids (PUFA)	++	***
Avoid intake of dietary trans fat	Reduce to <1%TE	++	***
Reduce intake of dietary cholesterol	<300 mg/day	+	**
Dietary fiber (DF)			
Increase total DF intake	25–40 g/day	++	***
Increase intake of soluble fibers, e.g., beta-glucan	≥7–13 g/day as part of total DF intake	++	***
Phytosterols	≥2 g/day	++	***

Modified based on the 2019 ESC/EAS guidelines for the management of dyslipidaemias [2]. [1,2] Magnitude of effect and strength of evidence refer to the impact of each dietary change on lowering TC and LDL-C concentrations. [1] Magnitude of effect: ++ = 5–10% reduction; + = <5% reduction. [2] Level of evidence: *** Data derived from multiple randomized clinical trials (RCTs) or meta-analyses; ** Data derived from a single RCT trial or from large non-randomized studies.

3. Dietary Fibers (DF)

3.1. Types of DF and Dietary Sources

DF consists of a wide range of plant-based compounds (carbohydrate polymers with ≤10 monomeric units) that vary in their physical and chemical properties. They have no nutritional value as such but play an important role in the regulation of different physiological functions in the body. DF are typically categorized into (water) soluble (SF) and insoluble fibers (IF) and are not hydrolyzed by digestive enzymes and hence not fully digested in the human gut [31]. IF include cellulose, hemi-celluloses, and lignin. They affect gut function by facilitating transit time of foods, normalizing bowel movements, increasing stool bulk, and preventing constipation. SF include pectin, beta-glucans, gums such as guar or konjac mannan, and mucilages like psyllium. They dissolve in water and form viscous gels in the gut lumen and so partially delay or reduce the absorption of carbohydrates, dietary fats, and cholesterol. IF are found mainly in vegetables, potatoes, nuts, and whole grain products such as wheat bran; sources of SF are vegetables, legumes, fruits such as apples, pears, citrus fruits, and cereals like oat and barley.

In addition to gut health, DF intake provides several health benefits and observational evidence has shown that a higher DF intake is associated with lower risk of CVD, T2DM, obesity, and certain forms of cancer [32,33].

Commonly, Western populations do not reach the recommended DF daily intakes. Grain-based foods contribute most to dietary DF intake with bread being by far the largest grain source followed by breakfast cereals. Vegetables, potatoes, and fruits also contribute substantially to DF intake [34].

In the context of this review, the beneficial effects of DF, and more specifically selected SF, on the risk of CVD and underlying risk factors such as dyslipidemia are detailed.

3.2. Effect of Specific DF on Blood Lipids and CVD Risk and Underlying Mechanism of Action

The first meta-analysis by Brown et al. [35] summarized the cholesterol-lowering effects of SF, i.e., oat products, psyllium, pectin, and guar gum. SF intake between 2–10 g/day was associated with modest but statistically significant decreases in TC and LDL-C, with no significant difference between the SF. Since then, several meta-analyses as discussed below have summarized the cholesterol-lowering effects of specific SF such as beta-glucan from oats and barley, psyllium, and glucomannan. A recent review found that increased DF intake significantly lowered TC and LDL-C, modestly but significantly decreased HDL-C, and had no effect on TG concentrations [36]. Further, there was no evidence that the type of DF, i.e., SF or IF or the way DF are administered, i.e., via supplements or foods, influenced the cholesterol-lowering effect [36].

Beta-glucan: Beta-glucan is a viscous SF found in oats, barley, edible mushrooms, and (baker's) yeast. A recent meta-analysis found that a median intake of 3.5 g/day of oat beta-glucan modestly lowered LDL-C by −0.19 mmol-L (95% CI: −0.23 to −0.14) or 4.2% and non-HDL-C by −0.20 mmol/L (95% CI: −0.26 to −0.15) or 4.8% compared with control diets [37]. An earlier meta-analysis found an LDL-C reduction of −0.25 mmol/L or 6% with a median daily intake of 5.1 g beta-glucan from oats [38].

Barley beta-glucan was also shown to lower blood cholesterol. A median intake of 6.5 and 6.9 g/day of barley beta-glucan, respectively, lowered LDL-C by −0.25 mmol/L (95% CI: −0.30 to −0.20) or 7% and non-HDL-C by −0.31 mmol/L (95% CI: −0.39 to −0.23) or 7% compared with control diets [39]. Similar effects were reported in a previous meta-analysis [39]. There was no clear dose–response relationship for barely beta-glucan [39], while a significant inverse association between dose and LDL-C lowering was found for oat-beta-glucan [37]. The established LDL-C lowering effect of beta-glucan, especially from oats, has resulted in approval of health claims for oat beta-glucan and its LDL-C lowering effect or CVD risk reduction benefit in Europe, USA, Canada, and Australia/New Zealand referring to an intake of at least 3 g/day of oat beta-glucan.

Psyllium: Psyllium is a viscous SF from the husk of the *Plantago ovata* seed and is a common fiber supplement. Two recent meta-analyses [40,41] found that daily intake of 10.2 g psyllium significantly lowered LDL-C by −0.28 mmol/L (95% CI: −0.21 to −0.31) [39] and -0.33 mmol/L (95% CI: −0.38 to −0.27) [40]; non-HDL-C was found to be lowered by −0.39 mmol/L (95% CI: −0.50 to −0.27) [41]. No clear dose–response relationship was observed, suggesting that the cholesterol-lowering benefit of psyllium intakes of ≥10 g/day will not result in bigger LDL-C lowering [41]. The recommended intake of psyllium for an optimal cholesterol-lowering and heart health benefit is 7 g/day SF from 10.2 g psyllium husk, based on the approved US FDA health claim.

Glucomannan: Glucomannan, also known as konjac mannan, is one of the most viscous DF. Its main source is the tuberous root of the konjac plant. Typically, glucomannan is consumed in the form of capsules next to some food formats like bars or biscuits. A recent meta-analysis found that daily intake of ~3 g glucomannan significantly lowered LDL-C by −0.35 mmol/L (95% CI: −0.46 to −0.25) or 10% and non-HDL-C by −0.32 mmol/L (95% CI: −0.46 to −0.19) or 7% [42]. There was no indication of a dose–response effect with glucomannan intakes between 2.0–15.1 g/day. An intake of 4 g/day glucomannan is the minimal dose of an approved health claim in Europe for maintaining a healthy blood cholesterol concentration.

Summarizing, an intake of 4–10 g/day of different types of SF is required to achieve a 5–10% reduction in LDL-C without substantially affecting HDL-C and TG concentrations.

SF with high viscosity and water-binding capacity form viscous gels in the intestinal lumen which decrease absorption of macronutrients as well as of cholesterol and bile acids and subsequent increased fecal excretion [32]. An impaired reabsorption and increased excretion of bile acids stimulates bile acids synthesis in the liver which consequently lowers circulating cholesterol concentrations in the blood. Furthermore, colonic fermentation of SF by gut bacteria produces short-chain fatty acids, and increased concentrations of circulating propionate may contribute to cholesterol lowering by decreasing cholesterol synthesis in the liver [32,43].

In view of the effects on CVD risk and clinical endpoints, observational studies have consistently shown that higher intakes of DF and dietary patterns high in DF are associated with a reduced risk of CVD as well as T2DM and obesity, also risk factors for CVD [32]. Meta-analyses of prospective cohort studies have shown a significant association between DF intake and lower risk of all-cause mortality [44] and mortality from CVD and CHD [43,44]. An additional DF intake of 7–10 g/day was inversely linked to a reduction in CVD mortality by 9% and CHD by 9–11% [44,45]. A recent umbrella review of systematic reviews and meta-analyses of observational studies concluded that there is convincing evidence that higher DF intake is associated with a lower risk of CVD, and particularly of coronary artery disease (CAD) and CVD-related death [33].

DF intake from cereals was significantly associated with lower CVD risk [43,44], while results for other fiber sources seem less conclusive. Kim and Je found that DF intake from legumes also showed an inverse association with CVD risk, while DF intake from vegetables and fruits failed to show an association [44]. Conversely, Threapleton et al. report an inverse association of vegetable fiber intake and CVD risk [44]. In particular, IF intake seems to be linked with lower risk of CVD while such a benefit was not convincingly seen for SF intake [44,45]. A recent prospective French cohort study supports that a higher intake of DF is associated with a decrease in CVD incidence and mortality. Both SFs and IFs were associated with lower risk of T2DM, while SFs were also associated with lower CVD risk. Amongst different DF sources, DFs from fruits were inversely associated with CVD risk [46]. Noteworthy, there are no RCTs on the effects of specific DF such as beta-glucan that have been shown that lowering LDL-C affects CVD outcomes.

3.3. Food-Based Dietary Guideline Recommendations for DF Intake

Recommendations for DF intake typically refer to total fiber intake. A healthy diet should contain more than 25 g/day of DF and most European countries recommend 25 and 30 g/day [34]. In the EFSA scientific opinion on dietary reference values, a DF intake of 25 g/day would be adequate for normal laxation in adults while intakes higher than 25 g/day would be necessary to reduce risk of CHD, T2DM, and to improve weight maintenance [34].

Usually, no recommendations are made for intakes of specific fiber types such as SF. Nevertheless, in view of approved health claims for maintaining or lowering blood cholesterol concentrations, daily intakes of 3 g beta-glucan from oats, oat bran, barley, or barley bran, 6 g pectin, 10 g guar gum, and 4 g glucomannan could be recommended. The 2019 ESC/EAS guidelines for the management of dyslipidemia recommend a DF intake of 25–40 g/day, including ≥7–13 g of SF, preferably from wholegrain products, e.g., oats and barley (Table 1) [2].

Adopting a predominantly plant-based diet helps to achieve the daily recommended intake of DF; in particular, vegan and vegetarian-type diets are rich in DF from various plant-based sources such as whole grains and seeds, legumes, vegetables and fruits, and nuts.

4. Phytosterols

4.1. Dietary Sources

Phytosterols (PS), comprising plant sterols and stanols, are compounds similar in structure and function to cholesterol. Principal PS are sitosterol, campesterol, and stigmasterol and their saturated counterparts sitostanol and campestanol. They occur naturally in all plant-based foods and are found in vegetable oils (especially unrefined oils), vegetable oil-based margarines, seeds, nuts, cereal grains, legumes, vegetables and fruits next to various foods and food supplements with added PS [47]. Daily intakes of PS with habitual diets typically range between 200 and 400 mg [48]. Consuming diets that emphasise plant-based foods results in higher PS intakes. With vegetarian- or vegan-type diets, PS intake can increase up to 600 mg/day [49]. With a MED-type diet such as the PREDIMED diet [20] or the dietary approaches to stop hypertension (DASH) diet [50], PS intakes of 500–550 mg/day can be achieved. Higher PS intakes such as a recommended intake of 2 g/day for LDL-C lowering [2] can only be achieved by consuming food products enriched with PS such as fat-based spreads and margarines, dairy-type foods like milk, yogurt, and yogurt drinks, or food supplements with added PS. A PS intake of about 2 g/day can be realized with the Portfolio diet through the consumption of a daily serving of a PS-added margarine next to consuming SF, soy, and other vegetable proteins and nuts, i.e., almonds [51].

4.2. Cholesterol-Lowering Efficacy and Underlying Mechanisms of Action

The TC and especially LDL-C lowering properties of PS in humans were discovered in the early 1950s [52]. Several meta-analyses have summarized their LDL-C lowering efficacy based on numerous RCTs [53–56]. The most recent meta-analysis including 124 clinical studies (with 201 study arms) concluded that PS intake significantly lowers LDL-C in a dose-dependent manner by 6–12% with intakes of 0.6–3.3 g/day without affecting HDL-C. [56]. PS intakes exceeding 3 g/day have only little additional benefit as the LDL-C lowering effect is expected to taper off because the underlying mechanism of action—inhibition of cholesterol absorption—is a saturable process. Nevertheless, RCTs with PS intakes greater than 4 g/day are limited; thus, it remains speculative whether the dose-response relationship would continue with higher PS intakes [56]. PS intake was also found to lower atherogenic apo-lipoproteins (apo) such as apo-B and apo-E and to increase anti-atherogenic apo-lipoproteins like apo-AI and apo-CII as summarized in a recent meta-analysis [57].

PS are effective in both healthy and diseased individuals and their LDL-C lowering benefit has been demonstrated in adults and children with familial hypercholesterolemia, in patients with T2DM, and individuals with the metabolic syndrome [58]. Furthermore, PS are shown to be effective in various types of food formats such as fat-based foods like spreads and margarines, dairy-type foods, and food supplements including capsules and tablets, thereby offering a variety of choices to achieve the recommended daily PS intake for a cholesterol-lowering benefit [47]. Intake occasion and frequency are critical factors for an optimal LDL-C lowering efficacy. Thus, PS should be consumed with a (main) meal and twice daily [47].

Meta-analyses have also found a significant TG-lowering effect whereby the effect was more pronounced in individuals with higher baseline TG concentrations [59]. Hence, PS offer a dual blood lipid benefit especially in individuals with dyslipidemia such as patients with T2DM or the metabolic syndrome [59].

Partial inhibition of intestinal absorption of (dietary and biliary) cholesterol is the key mechanism for the cholesterol-lowering effect of PS, with several underlying mechanisms including displacing cholesterol from mixed micelles due to limited capacity to embody sterols, interfering with transport-mediated processes of sterol uptake and stimulating cholesterol excretion via the transintestinal excretion [60]. An intake of 2 g/day of PS reduces cholesterol absorption by 30–40%, resulting in a subsequent 10% lowering of circulating LDL-C [61].

PS intake can also be a useful adjunct to lipid-lowering medication. Statins inhibit hepatic cholesterol synthesis and PS inhibit intestinal cholesterol absorption; thus, combining PS and statins leads to an additive LDL-C lowering effect [61,62]. Additional effects on LDL-C lowering have also been reported when combining PS with fibrates or with ezetimibe [61,63].

Although there are no RCTs showing the effects of long-term PS intake on CVD outcomes, e.g., CV events; it seems reasonable that PS intake may lower CVD risk based on the established LDL-C lowering effect.

4.3. Recommendations for PS Intake

Based on the proven plasma LDL-C lowering effect and the absence of adverse effects, consumption of 2 g/day PS as an adjunct to a healthy diet is one of the recommended dietary interventions for the management of dyslipidemia (Table 1) [2,64,65]. Foods with added PS may be considered i) for individuals with high serum cholesterol at intermediate or low global CVD risk who do not (yet) qualify for drug treatment, ii) as adjunct to drug (statin) therapy, in high- to very high-risk patients who fail to achieve LDL-C target goals or could not be treated with statins, and iii) in adults and children (>6 years) with familial hypercholesterolaemia, in line with current guidelines [2,61].

5. Combinations of Natural Lipid-Lowering Compounds as Part of a Heart-Healthy Diet

Combining PS (2 g/day) with different types of SF, e.g., 3 g/day oat beta-glucan has been shown to lead to additional LDL-C lowering when combined in a single food [66]. Further, a combination of 10 g/day psyllium and 2.6 g/day PS added to cookies leads to a substantial reduction in LDL-C [67].

In addition, the combination of 3.3 g/day PS with a healthy diet (low in total and saturated fat) shows an additive effect of PS to that of the diet alone [68]. By combining PS with other plant-based, cholesterol-lowering compounds or foods, further reductions in LDL-C can be achieved as observed with the Portfolio diet. This plant-based dietary pattern combines (per 2000 kcal energy intake) 20 g/day of viscous DF from oats, barley, psyllium, eggplant, okra, apples, oranges, or berries, about 50 g/day of plant protein from soy products or pulses (beans, peas, chickpeas, and lentils), 42 g/day of nuts (tree nuts such as almonds and peanuts), and 2 g/day PS in the form of a PS-enriched margarine [51,69]. Under controlled settings, an LDL-C lowering effect of 30% could be achieved with the Portfolio diet, an effect comparable to that achievable with a low-dose statin [51]. Based on a meta-analysis, the Portfolio dietary pattern significantly lowers LDL-C by -0.73 mmol/L (95% CI: -0.89 to -0.56) or by ~17%. Non-HDL-C, apo B, TC, TG, as well as systolic and diastolic blood pressure, were also significantly lowered [69].

A dual blood lipid lowering benefit of lowering both LDL-C and TG concentrations was achieved with the intake of 2 g/day PS and a minimum of 1 g/day EPA/DHA from fish oil [70].

6. The Impact of Plant-Based Dietary Patterns on CV and Planetary Health

6.1. Dietary Patterns and CV Health

Historically, dietary recommendations for CVD prevention focused on single nutrients like lowering SAFA or increasing DF intake, or on specific foods like eating more fish, whole grains, nuts, fruits, and vegetables, and less meat. Today, the focus is on the role of dietary patterns for the management of dyslipidemia and lowering CVD risk [71,72]. A healthy dietary pattern is typically described as a predominantly plant-based diet. Observational study evidence supports the beneficial effect of single plant-based foods as well as fatty fish, and the adverse effects of animal-based foods, on CVD risk [73,74]. Since foods are typically consumed in combinations, it is more reasonable to look at health benefits of a complete dietary pattern.

Several dietary patterns have been found to lower CVD outcomes and risk factors such as blood lipids, i.e., TC and LDL-C or blood pressure. These include traditional diets prevailing in the MED and in Nordic countries [75–79], dietary patterns intended to control CVD risk factors like the DASH diet [50] and Portfolio diet [51] as well as vegetarian- or vegan-type dietary patterns. A common characteristic of these dietary patterns is that they emphasize plant-based foods with reduced animal food consumption.

The MED dietary pattern refers to the traditional diet of Greece, Crete, and Southern Italy with (virgin) olive oil as the main dietary fat source as a key characteristic [72,75,78]. Further characteristics are summarized in Table 2. The Nordic diet emphasizes the intake of locally grown vegetables like cabbage and potatoes, whole grains and cereals such as oats, rye, and barley, locally grown seasonal fruits such as berries, next to rapeseed oil and fatty fish (Table 2) [72,77,78]. The DASH diet emphasizes amongst others higher intakes of vegetables, fruits and fat-free or low-fat dairy foods (Table 2) [50,79]. The Portfolio diet is a plant-based diet that emphasises the intake of four known cholesterol-lowering foods, i.e., viscous DF, plant proteins from soy and legumes, nuts, and PS (Table 2) [51,69]. The healthy vegetarian dietary pattern is based on a variety of vegetables, legumes, soy products, fruits, and whole grains, occasionally dairy foods, eggs, and fish, but no meat and poultry. A strict vegan dietary pattern excludes all animal-based foods (Table 2) [72,73,80].

6.2. Effect on Blood Lipids

Both observational studies and RCTs have found that dietary patterns emphasizing consumption of plant-based foods have beneficial effects on blood lipids, especially on TC and LDL-C.

Next to lowering systolic and diastolic blood pressure, for which the DASH diet was originally designed, the DASH diet was also found to lower TC and LDL-C. An umbrella review of systematic reviews and meta-analyses concluded that TC was lowered by −0.20 mmol/L (95% CI: −0.31, −0.10) and LDL-C by −0.10 mmol/L (95% CI: −0.20 to −0.01) without affecting HDL-C and TG [79,81]. The observed cholesterol-lowering benefit of the DASH diet may be attributable to the high intake of DF from the consumption of fruits, nuts, legumes, and whole grains, and the lower intake of saturated fat.

The Portfolio diet combining four recognized cholesterol-lowering foods/food components with a background diet low in total fat (≤30% TE) and saturated fat (<7% TE) and low in dietary cholesterol (<200 mg/day) led to clinically relevant benefits in lowering cholesterol and other CVD risk factors. A meta-analysis of RCTs has shown that TC was lowered by −0.81 mmol/L (95% CI: −0.98 to −0.64) or 12% and LDL-C by -0.73 mmol/L (95% CI: -0.89 to -0.56) or 17% [69]. Non-HDL-C was lowered by -0.83 mmol/L (95% CI: −1.03 to −0.64) or 14% and TG by −0.28 mmol/L (95% CI: −0.42 to −0.14 mmol/L) or 16%; all compared to a low total fat, low saturated fat, and low cholesterol diet. The LDL-C lowering effect of the Portfolio diet was found to be 21% in efficacy trials and 12% in effectiveness trials. Other CVD risk factors like systolic and diastolic blood pressure and C-reactive protein were also lowered [69].

Table 2. Healthy dietary patterns for the management of dyslipidemia and the prevention of cardiovascular diseases (CVD).

Healthy Dietary Pattern	Background/Definition	Key Characteristics
Mediterranean (MED) diet	Traditionally based on dietary patterns typical of Crete, Greece, and Southern Italy in the early 1960s. No uniform definition of a MED diet, but MED dietary patterns emphasize plant-based foods and olive oil as main dietary fat source. Modified versions were studied in the PREDIMED trial [1].	Eating plenty of fruits, vegetables, legumes, (whole) grains, nuts; olive oils as main oil for daily use; moderate intake of fish; poultry and dairy foods like yogurt and cheese; eating less red meat, meat products and sweets; allows wine (in moderation) with meals. The MED diet is high in dietary fat and especially monounsaturated fatty acids but low in saturated fat.
Nordic diet	A dietary pattern comparable to the MED diet that emphasises traditional, locally grown, and seasonal foods of the Nordic countries. Developed as a diet to address health concerns such as obesity and taking local food culture, environmental aspects, and sustainability into account [2].	Emphasizes locally grown, seasonal foods; eating plenty of fruits, e.g., berries, vegetables, e.g., cabbage, legumes, potatoes, whole grains, e.g., oats and rye breads, nuts, seeds, fish and seafood, low-fat dairy, rapeseed oil, and, in moderation, game meats, free-range eggs, cheese, and yogurt; rarely eating red meats and animal fats; avoiding sugar-sweetened beverages, added sugars, processed meats. The Nordic diet is especially rich in dietary fiber and low in sugar and sodium.
Dietary approaches to stop hypertension (DASH) diet	A prescribed dietary pattern originally developed to lower blood pressure as studied in the DASH clinical trials [3].	Eating plenty of fruits, vegetables, legumes, whole grains; including fat-free or low-fat dairy products, fish, poultry, nuts, seeds, and vegetable oils; limiting fatty meats, tropical oils, sweets, sugar-sweetened beverages. The DASH diet is low in saturated fat, dietary cholesterol, salt (sodium), and high in dietary fiber, potassium, and calcium.
Portfolio diet	A predominately plant-based, vegan-type diet developed to further include a portfolio of foods/food components that are known to lower total and LDL-cholesterol [4].	Eating a diet low in fat (≤30% of energy), especially saturated fat (<7% of energy), and high in fruits and vegetables with the addition of four plant-based, cholesterol-lowering foods: 50 g/day plant protein from various soy foods, legumes like beans, chickpeas, lentils; 45 g/day (about a handful) nuts such as peanuts, almonds; 20 g/day viscous soluble fiber from oats, barley, eggplant, okra, apples, berries, oranges, and psyllium; 2 g/day plant sterols from enriched foods such as spreads, dairy-type foods, or from supplements.
Vegetarian/vegan diet pattern	Dietary patterns of specific population groups that were adapted based on observational studies and randomized controlled trials.	Eating plenty of fruits, vegetables, legumes, whole grains, nuts and seeds, specific foods, e.g., soy products and excluding meat and poultry and partly also dairy foods, eggs, and fish; lacto/ovo-vegetarians eat eggs and dairy products; lacto-vegetarians consume dairy products, ovo-vegetarians eat eggs and pesco-vegetarians eat fish and seafood; vegans completely refrain of all animal-based foods including meat, poultry, eggs, dairy foods, and fish. Vegetarian/vegan diets are high in dietary fiber, and typically low in total and saturated fat, intake of n-3 fatty, acids, iron, and vitamin B_{12}.

Adapted in parts from Hemler and Hu, 2019 [74], Zampelas and Magriplis, 2019 [72], Magkos et al. 2020 [78]. [1] Estruch et al. [20], [2] Bere and Brug [76], [3] Appel et al. [50], [4] Jenkins et al. [51].

Following a MED or a Nordic dietary pattern is also associated with beneficial blood lipid effects. Based on a meta-analysis of RCTs, the Nordic diet lowered TC by −0.39 mmol/L (95% CI: −0.76 to −0.01) and LDL-C by −0.30 mmol/L (95% CI: −0.54 to −0.06) with no significant changes in HDL-C and TG [82,83]. Beneficial effects on reducing systolic and diastolic blood pressure were also seen [83]. The beneficial effects of the Nordic dietary pattern can be attributed to the high DF intake and the low intake of saturated fat. Likewise, the MED dietary pattern was found to significantly lower LDL-C by −0.07 mmol/L (95% CI: −0.13 to−0.01) and TG by −0.46 mmol/L (95%CI: −0.72 to −0.21) [83]. Small or no reductions in TC and/or LDL-C were reported in a recent review that compared a MED diet intervention vs. either no intervention or another dietary intervention in primary prevention of CVD [84]. Blood pressure is also modestly reduced by the MED diet, but effects are less than those observed with the Nordic diet [83].

Several meta-analyses addressed the effects of a vegetarian dietary pattern on blood lipids. Two meta-analyses of RCTs found that vegetarian diets significantly lowered TC by −0.32 to −0.36 mmol/L and LDL-C by −0.32 to −0.34 mmol/L [85,86]. HDL-C was also significantly lowered by −0.09 to −0.10 mmol/L while TG were not significantly altered [85,86]. Another recent meta-analysis of RCTs studying vegetarian diet patterns and lipid risk factors in T2DM found a reduction in LDL-C of −0.12 mmol/L (95% CI: −0.20 to 0.04) with no significant effects on HDL-C and TG [83]. Taken together, vegetarian diet patterns, particularly vegan diets, are associated with lower blood cholesterol concentrations. That vegetarian diets are low in total and especially saturated fat, low in dietary cholesterol, and particularly high in DF intake may explain their cholesterol-lowering effect. The higher intake of phytochemicals such as PS, phenolics compounds, and carotenoids with vegetarian/vegan diet patterns may further contribute to this effect.

6.3. Effects on CVD Risk and Outcomes

Evidence for beneficial effects of dietary patterns on CVD risk and related outcomes derives mostly from observational studies; RCTs that studied the effect of dietary patterns on CVD-related endpoints are rare or non-existent.

There is no direct evidence from observational studies for a CVD risk benefit, e.g., on CVD incidence or mortality of the Portfolio diet. Nevertheless, the combined effects of that dietary pattern on CVD risk factors such as LDL-C and blood pressure as observed in RCTs was assumed to decrease the estimated 10-year CHD risk by ~13% [69].

The DASH diet that is well-accepted for its blood pressure lowering effect was found to reduce CVD incidence by 20%, CHD incidence by 21%, and stroke incidence by 19% [79,83]. These CVD risk-related benefits are attributable to the substantial reductions in blood pressure and in other CVD risk factors, i.e., TC and LDL-C.

The effects of the MED diet on CVD risk have been assessed in several meta-analyses of observational studies. Rosato et al. [87] found in their meta-analysis of prospective studies a 19% lower risk for unspecified CVD, a 30% lower risk for CHD/acute myocardial infarction, a 27% lower risk for unspecified stroke, and 18% lower risk for ischemic stroke when comparing the highest vs. the lowest adherence to this dietary pattern based on a MED diet score [72,87]. Another meta-analysis of prospective studies reports a risk reduction (RR) in total CVD, CHD, and stroke mortality of 0.79 (95% CI: 0.77, 0.82), 0.83 (95% CI: 0.75, 0.92), and 0.87 (95% CI: 0.80, 0.96), respectively, next to a lower CHD incidence (RR: 0.73; 95% CI: 0.62, 0.86) and stroke incidence (RR: 0.80; 95% CI: 0.71, 0.90), comparing the highest vs. lowest categories of MED diet adherence [88]. A meta-analysis of three RCTs revealed that the MED diet is associated with a 38% lower risk of total CVD and a 35% lower risk of total myocardial infarction (MI) but a nonsignificant reduction in CVD mortality [83,88]. Especially the PREDIMED trial, a primary prevention RCT that investigated a modified MED diet supplemented with either extra virgin olive oil or nuts compared to a reduced-fat control diet, revealed an approximately 30% lower incidence of a composite of CVD endpoints (MI, stroke, and death from CV causes) with these MED diet patterns [20]. A re-analysis of the original outcome data assessing individual endpoints revealed a reduction in stroke incidence but little or no effect on total and CVD mortality or MI [20,84]. In their review, Rees et al. [84] concluded that there is still some uncertainty regarding the effects of a MED-style diet on clinical endpoints and CVD risk factors for both primary and secondary prevention.

Less, though more conflicting, evidence for CVD risk-related effects are reported for the Nordic diet. Adhering to a healthy Nordic diet was associated with a lower risk of CVD in men and women from the Danish Diet, Cancer and Health cohort [89,90] but not in women of the Swedish Women's Lifestyle and Health cohort [91]. A recent systematic review and meta-analysis of prospective studies assessing the Nordic diet reports a modest reduction in CVD risk (RR: 0.93; 95% CI, 0.88, 0.99) and stroke risk (RR: 0.87 95% CI, 0.77, 0.97) but not in CVD mortality [83].

Meta-analyses of observational study evidence support that a vegetarian diet pattern is associated with a 22% lower CHD mortality while no association was found for CVD or stroke mortality. Furthermore, vegetarian diets are associated with a 28% reduced risk of CHD [80,83]. These results are comparable to a previous meta-analysis reporting a 25% risk reduction in CHD incidence and mortality but no significant effects for CVD and stroke and all-cause mortality [92].

7. Dietary Patterns and Environmental Aspects

Dietary choices clearly contribute to the risk for developing CVD. Evidence supports the intake of specific nutrients, food groups, or certain dietary patterns to positively influence dyslipidemia and to promote the prevention of CVD. Next to their impact on CV health, dietary patterns also impact the environment in various ways. Plant-based dietary patterns have been shown to have a smaller impact on climate change (greenhouse-gas emissions), fresh-water use, cropland use (deforestation), and biodiversity loss [8,93] than consumption of animal-based foods such as (red and processed) meat. A recent global modeling study combined analyses of nutrient level, diet-related, and weight-related chronic disease mortality, and environmental impact in different sets of diet scenarios for more than 150 countries [94]. Four different energy-balanced diets were found to reduce environmental impact, nutrient deficiencies, and diet-related mortality. All four dietary patterns were predominately plant-based diets with limited red and processed meat intake. These patterns were described as flexitarian, pescatarian, vegetarian, and vegan diets [94].

It must be noted that not all plant-based diets are necessarily beneficial in view of diet-related chronic diseases such as CVD risk [74]. Observational evidence from cohort studies found that plant-based diets containing higher amounts of refined grains, juices/sugar-sweetened beverages, sweets, potatoes/fries were associated with an increased CHD risk, while plant-based diets including higher amounts of whole grains, fruits, vegetables, legumes, nuts, and vegetable oils were associated with lower risk of CHD [74,95]. While predominately plant-based diets have beneficial effects on CV risk, their impact on body weight and prevention or treatment of obesity are less clear [78]. Hence, consuming an energy-balanced diet in view of avoiding weight gain and obesity seems crucial.

There are several possibilities for adopting a predominately plant-based dietary pattern based on personal food taste and preference as well as individual needs. Characteristics for choosing a predominantly plant-based healthy diet are summarized in Table 3.

Table 3. Characteristics of a predominantly plant-based healthy diet for management of dyslipidemia and CVD prevention.

Foods and Food Group-Related Recommendations	
Eat more	
Vegetables	Eat plenty of vegetables * including a wide variety from all colors
Legumes	Choose from a variety of legumes and pulses
Fruits	Eat plenty of (fresh or frozen) fruits * including berries; limit intake of fruit juices
Nuts and seeds	Choose from a variety of unsalted tree nuts and peanuts
Whole grain	Eat a variety of whole grains such as whole grain bread, pasta, brown rice
Eat adequately/moderately	
Healthy fats	Limit saturated fats like butter, full-fat cheese, and cream; avoid trans fats; choose vegetable oils and fats (margarine) rich in unsaturated fatty acids
Milk and dairy foods	Choose no- or low-fat over full-fat milk, cheese, and other dairy foods
Fish and seafood	Choose sustainable varieties of fish and seafood
Poultry and eggs	Eat occasionally and choose products from welfare-oriented animal husbandry
Limit eating	
Meat	Eat less red and processed meats
Sweets and sugar-sweetened beverages	Limit intake of sweets and sugar-sweetened beverages
Nutrient-specific recommendations	
Reduce saturated fats by replacing them with mono- and polyunsaturated fats	SAFA should be replaced with MUFA or PUFA to reduce LDL-C.
Increase total dietary fiber (DF) intake and esp. intake of soluble DF	Consume 25-45 g of DF per day of which 5–15 g of soluble fibers from foods rich in these fibers for an LDL-C lowering effect
Limit salt intake	Limit salt intake of less than 5 g/day
Specific advice to further lower LDL-C	
Consider phytosterols as an adjunct to a healthy diet	Consume about 2 g/day phytosterols through foods/foods supplements with added phytosterols
Increase intake of soluble fiber such as beta-glucan from oat and barley	Consume about 3 g/day beta-glucan from foods like oat bran, oatmeal, barley flakes, pearl barley

Complied based on dietary recommendations described in Mach et al. [2], the UK Eat Well guide (https://www.gov.uk/government/publications/the-eatwell-guide), the 2015–2020 dietary guidelines for Americans [96]. * Plenty refers to 5 portions of fruits and vegetables per day.

8. Current Recommendations for a Healthy Dietary Pattern

The CV health benefits of certain dietary patterns have been recognized by numerous dietary and clinical practice guidelines. For instance, the DASH dietary pattern is recognized by the 2015–2020 dietary guidelines for Americans [96], the AHA/ACC guideline on lifestyle management to reduce cardiovascular risk [27], the Canadian Cardiovascular Society guidelines for the management of dyslipidemia [64], and by the ESC/EAS 2019 guidelines for the management of dyslipidaemias [2]. The Canadian Cardiovascular Society [64] also mentions the Portfolio diet as a healthy dietary pattern. Adopting a healthy MED diet pattern for the promotion of healthy eating and the prevention of CVD is acknowledged by the 2015–2020 dietary guidelines for Americans [96], the 2019 ACC/AHA guideline on the primary prevention of CVD [27], and by the ESC/EAS 2019 guidelines for the management of dyslipidaemias [2]. Eating a plant-based Nordic diet as a healthy alternative to the MED-dietary pattern is advocated by the Nordic nutrition recommendations [97]. A healthy vegetarian eating pattern is mentioned by the 2015–2020 dietary guidelines for Americans [96] and the Canadian Cardiovascular Society guidelines for the management of dyslipidemia [64].

Notably, the emphasis of eating a predominantly plant-based diet as a healthy eating pattern to prevent diet-related chronic diseases such as CVD is a common theme of many food-based dietary guidelines [9,96]. Another driving factor for recommending a more plant-based diet relates to environmental sustainability [8,9]. Nevertheless, the environmental aspects of dietary patterns are not yet widely addressed in food-based dietary guidelines, only a few countries have so far included environmental sustainability in their guidelines [78].

9. Conclusions

This review describes the beneficial effects of specific macro- and micro-components of a plant-based diet (vegetable fats, DF, and PS) in the management of dyslipidemia and CVD prevention. Moreover, the role of common plant-based dietary patterns in CV health is discussed.

The protective effect of predominately plant-based dietary patterns such as the MED and Nordic diet or the DASH and Portfolio diet on CVD risk and related risk factors, e.g., LDL-C, is associated with specific plant-based foods which are known for their CV health benefits [72,74–76,79]. These foods include fruits, vegetables, legumes, whole grains, nuts, and seeds [73,74]. Plant-based foods are typically rich in unsaturated fatty acids, DF, plant proteins and various micronutrients like vitamins and phytonutrients such as PS and polyphenols; they are low in saturated fats and often low in energy density compared to foods from animal sources [74]. The beneficial effects of these plant-based food components are explained by different underlying mechanisms which influence the development of CVD either directly or indirectly by influencing risk factors such as dyslipidaemia. For instance, replacing saturated fats in the diet with unsaturated fatty acids like MUFA and PUFA is known to lower LDL-C [13,16]. Observational studies and RCTs with clinical endpoints have further shown that replacing SAFA with especially vegetable oil PUFA lowers the risk of CVD, mainly the risk of CHD [13,17] whereas evidence for effects on CVD or CHD risk when SAFA is replaced by MUFA, carbohydrates, or proteins is insufficient or limited [13]. DF, especially viscous SF like beta-glucan, reduce the intestinal absorption of cholesterol and re-absorption of bile acids and produce short-chain fatty acids in the colon which may affect hepatic cholesterol synthesis, all contributing to a LDL-C-lowering effect [43]. Observational studies have shown a significant association between DF intake and lower risk of all-cause mortality [44] and mortality from CVD and CHD [43,44]. PS also inhibit intestinal cholesterol absorption resulting in lower circulating concentrations of LDL-C [61]. Although there are no RCTs showing the effects of long-term intake of specific DF like beta-glucan or PS on CVD outcomes, e.g., CV events, it seems reasonable that their intake may lower CVD risk based on the established LDL-C lowering effect. Replacing animal protein with plant protein has also been shown to lower LDL-C [98].

Noteworthy, not all plant-based dietary patterns are equally effective in lowering CVD risk as not all plant-based foods have beneficial CV effects [74,95]. Hence, the quality of plant-based foods and food components plays an important role. For instance, a dietary pattern with more refined grains than whole grains or more sugars-sweetened foods and beverages have been linked with a higher CVD risk. The same dietary patterns for which a positive impact on dyslipidemia and the prevention of CVD has been shown can also help reduce the impact of food choices on environmental degradation [8]. Hence, shifting to a more plant-based dietary pattern will not only improve CV health but will also be more environmentally sustainable. While plant-based, e.g., vegetarian, dietary patterns are generally perceived positively because of their benefits on health (CVD prevention) and the environment, there are also several barriers that hinder the switch to, and maintenance of a plant-based diet. Common barriers include health concerns that a plant-based diet may lack specific nutrients, reluctance to change dietary behavior, and enjoyment of eating meat and animal-based foods [99,100].

A limitation of this narrative review is that only selected macro- and micro components of a plant-based diet are described while other components such as vitamins and other phytonutrients like polyphenols with proposed CV benefits were not considered. Nevertheless, dietary fatty acids, DF, and PS were chosen because of their proven evidence for LDL-C-lowering and CVD risk benefits and because they are specifically referred to in dietary recommendations for CVD prevention [2]. While health benefits of these individual dietary components have been addressed before, this review addresses them in the context of a plant-based dietary pattern. As mostly observational study evidence is available on CVD risk and clinical endpoints, more evidence from RCTs demonstrating such benefits for these dietary components in the context of a plant-based diet would be desirable, despite the challenges of carrying out long-term, controlled dietary intervention studies.

Author Contributions: E.A.T. was responsible for the conception of the review. E.A.T and S.M. contributed to the literature search, E.A.T. wrote the manuscript, and S.M. provided critical input; both authors approved the final version for submission. All authors have read and agreed to the published version of the manuscript.

Funding: This work received no external funding except that the publication costs were funded by Upfield.

Conflicts of Interest: S.M. is employed by Upfield. Upfield markets plant-based consumer goods such as margarines and spreads including foods products with added phytosterols. E.A.T. works as a consultant for Upfield. The authors declare no further conflict of interest.

References

1. Cardiovascular diseases (CVDs). Available online: https://www.who.int/news-room/fact-sheets/detail/cardiovascular-diseases-(cvds) (accessed on 29 June 2020).
2. Mach, F.; Baigent, C.; Catapano, A.L.; Koskinas, K.C.; Casula, M.; Badimon, L.; Chapman, M.J.; De Backer, G.G.; Delgado, V.; Ference, B.A.; et al. ESC Scientific Document Group. 2019 ESC/EAS Guidelines for the management of dyslipidaemias: Lipid modification to reduce cardiovascular risk. *Eur. Heart J.* **2020**, *41*, 111–188. [CrossRef] [PubMed]
3. Ference, B.A.; Ginsberg, H.N.; Graham, I.; Ray, K.K.; Packard, C.J.; Bruckert, E.; Hegele, R.A.; Krauss, R.M.; Raal, F.J.; Schunkert, H.; et al. Low density lipoproteins cause atherosclerotic cardiovascular disease. 1. Evidence from genetic, epidemiologic, and clinical studies. A consensus statement from the European Atherosclerosis Society Consensus Panel. *Eur. Heart J.* **2017**, *38*, 2459–2472. [CrossRef] [PubMed]
4. Piepoli, M.F.; Hoes, A.W.; Agewall, S.; Albus, C.; Brotons, C.; Catapano, A.L.; Cooney, M.T.; Corra, U.; Cosyns, B.; Deaton, C.; et al. Authors Task Force, M. 2016 European Guidelines on cardiovascular disease prevention in clinical practice: The Sixth Joint Task Force of the European Society of Cardiology and Other Societies on Cardiovascular Disease Prevention in Clinical Practice (constituted by representatives of 10 societies and by invited experts) Developed with the special contribution of the European Association for Cardiovascular Prevention & Rehabilitation (EACPR). *Eur. Heart J.* **2016**, *37*, 2315–2381.
5. Hu, F.B.; Willet, W. C Optimal diets for prevention of coronary heart disease. *JAMA* **2002**, *288*, 2569–2578. [CrossRef]
6. Dalen, J.-E.; Devries, S. Diets to Prevent Coronary Heart Disease 1957–2013: What Have We Learned? *Am. J. Med.* **2014**, *127*, 364–369. [CrossRef] [PubMed]
7. Yu, E.; Malik, V.S.; Hu, F.B. Cardiovascular Disease Prevention by Diet Modification. JACC Health Promotion Series. *J. Am. Coll. Cardiol.* **2018**, *72*, 914–926. [CrossRef] [PubMed]
8. Willett, W.; Rockström, J.; Loken, B.; Springmann, M.; Lang, T.; Vermeulen, S.; Garnett, T.; Tilman, D.; DeClerck, F.; Wood, A.; et al. Food in the Anthropocene: The EAT-Lancet Commission on healthy diets from sustainable food systems. *Lancet* **2019**, *393*, 447–492. [CrossRef]
9. Bechthold, A.; Boeing, H.; Tetens, I.; Schwingshackl, L.; Nothlings, U. Perspective: Food-based dietary guidelines in Europe. Scientific concepts, current status, and perspectives. *Adv. Nutr.* **2018**, *9*, 544–560. [CrossRef]
10. Clark, M.A.; Springmann, M.; Hill, J.; Tilman, D. Multiple health and environmental impacts of foods. *PNAS* **2019**, *116*, 23357–23362. [CrossRef]
11. Eilander, A.; Harika, R.K.; Zock, P.L. Intake and sources of dietary fatty acids in Europe: Are current population intakes of fats aligned with dietary recommendations? *Eur. J. Lipid Sci. Technol* **2015**, *117*, 1370–1377. [CrossRef]
12. Mensink, R.P.; Katan, M.B. Effect of dietary trans fatty acids on high-density and low-density lipoprotein cholesterol levels in healthy subjects. *N. Engl. J. Med.* **1990**, *323*, 439–445. [CrossRef] [PubMed]
13. Zock, P.L.; Blom, W.A.M.; Nettleton, J.A.; Hornstra, G. Progressing Insights into the Role of Dietary Fats in the Prevention of Cardiovascular Disease. *Curr. Cardiol. Rep.* **2016**, *18*, 111. [CrossRef] [PubMed]
14. Harika, R.K.; Eilander, A.; Alssema, M.; Osendarp, S.J.; Zock, P.L. Intake of fatty acids in general populations worldwide does not meet dietary recommendations to prevent coronary heart disease: A systematic review of data from 40 countries. *Ann. Nutr. Metab.* **2013**, *63*, 229–238. [CrossRef] [PubMed]

15. Mensink, R.P. *Effects of Saturated Fatty Acids on Serum Lipids and Lipoproteins: A Systematic Review and Regression Analysis*; World Health Organization: Geneva, Switzerland, 2016.
16. Schwingshackl, L.; Bogensberger, B.; Benčič, A.; Knüppel, S.; Boeing, H.; Hoffmann, G. Effects of oils and solid fats on blood lipids: A systematic review and network meta-analysis. *J. Lipid Res.* **2018**, *59*, 1771–1782. [CrossRef]
17. The Scientific Advisory Committee on Nutrition (SACN). Report on Saturated Fats and Health 2019. Available online: https://www.gov.uk/government/publications/saturated-fats-and-health-sacn-report (accessed on 31 August 2020).
18. Zong, G.; Li, Y.; Sampson, L.; Dougherty, L.W.; Willett, W.C.; Wanders, A.J.; Alssema, M.; Zock, P.L.; Hu, F.B.; Sun, Q. Monounsaturated fats from plant and animal sources in relation to risk of coronary heart disease among US men and women. *Am. J. Clin. Nutr.* **2018**, *107*, 445–453. [CrossRef]
19. Guasch-Ferré, M.; Liu, G.; Li, Y.; Sampson, L.; Manson, J.E.; Salas-Salvadó, J.; Martínez-González, M.A.; Stampfer, M.J.; Willett, W.C.; Sun, Q.; et al. Olive Oil Consumption and Cardiovascular Risk in U.S. Adults. *J. Am. Coll. Cardiol.* **2020**, *75*, S0735–S1097. [CrossRef]
20. Estruch, R.; Ros, E.; Salas-Salvadó, J.; Covas, M.I.; Corella, D.; Arós, F.; Gómez-Gracia, E.; Ruiz-Gutiérrez, V.; Fiol, M.; Lapetra, J.; et al. Retraction and Republication: Primary Prevention of Cardiovascular Disease with a Mediterranean Diet. *N Engl. J. Med.* **2013**, *368*, 1279–1290, Retraction and Republication in: *N. Engl. J. Med.* **2018**, *378*(25), 2441–2442. [CrossRef]
21. Innes, J.K.; Calder, P.C. Marine Omega-3 (N-3) Fatty Acids for Cardiovascular Health: An Update for 2020. *Int. J. Mol. Sci.* **2020**, *21*, 1362. [CrossRef]
22. Li, Y.; Hruby, A.; Bernstein, A.M.; Ley, S.H.; Wang, D.D.; Chiuve, S.E.; Sampson, L.; Rexrode, K.M.; Rimm, E.B.; Willett, W.C.; et al. Saturated fats compared with unsaturated fats and sources of carbohydrates in relation to risk of coronary heart disease: A Prospective Cohort Study. *J. Am. Coll. Cardiol.* **2015**, *66*, 1538–1548. [CrossRef]
23. Neelakantan, N.; Seah, J.Y.H.; van Dam, R.M. The Effect of Coconut Oil Consumption on Cardiovascular Risk Factors: A Systematic Review and Meta-Analysis of Clinical Trials. *Circulation* **2020**, *141*, 803–814. [CrossRef]
24. Eyres, L.; Eyres, M.F.; Chisholm, A.; Brown, R.C. Coconut oil consumption and cardiovascular risk factors in humans. *Nutr. Rev.* **2016**, *74*, 267–280. [CrossRef] [PubMed]
25. FAO/WHO. *Fats and D-atty Acids in Human Nutrition*; Report of an expert consultation, Food and Nutrition Paper; Food and Agriculture Organisation of the United Nations: Rome, Italy, 2010.
26. Vannice, G.; Rasmussen, H. Position of the academy of nutrition and dietetics: Dietary fatty acids for healthy adults. *J. Acad. Nutr. Diet.* **2014**, *114*, 136–153. [CrossRef] [PubMed]
27. Eckel, R.H.; Jakicic, J.M.; Ard, J.D.; de Jesus, J.M.; Houston Miller, N.; van Hubbard, S.; Lee, I.-M.; Lichtenstein, A.:H.; Loria, C.M.; Millen, B.E.; et al. AHA/ACC guideline on lifestyle management to reduce cardiovascular risk: A report of the American College of Cardiology/American Heart Association Task Force on Practice Guidelines. *J. Am. Coll. Cardiol.* **2014**, *63*, 2960–2984. [CrossRef] [PubMed]
28. Sacks, F.M.; Lichtenstein, A.H.; Wu, J.H.Y.; Appel, L.J.; Creager, M.A.; Kris-Etherton, P.M.; Miller, M.; Rimm, E.B.; Rudel, L.L.; Robinson, J.G.; et al. Dietary Fats and Cardiovascular Disease. A Presidential Advisory from the American Heart Association. *Circulation* **2017**, *136*, e1–e23. [CrossRef] [PubMed]
29. Mozaffarian, D.; Aro, A.; Willett, W.C. Health effects of trans-fatty acids: Experimental and observational evidence. *Eur. J. Clin. Nutr.* **2009**, *63*, S5–S21. [CrossRef]
30. Rimm, E.B.; Appel, L.J.; Chiuve, S.E.; Djoussé, L.; Engler, M.B.; Kris-Etherton, P.M.; Mozaffarian, D.; Siscovick, D.S.; Lichtenstein, A.H. American Heart Association Nutrition Committee of the Council on Lifestyle and Cardiometabolic Health; Council on Epidemiology and Prevention; Council on Cardiovascular Disease in the Young; Council on Cardiovascular and Stroke Nursing; and Council on Clinical Cardiology. Seafood Long-Chain n-3 Polyunsaturated Fatty Acids and Cardiovascular Disease: A Science Advisory from the American Heart Association. *Circulation* **2018**, *138*, e35–e47.
31. Evans, C.E.L. Dietary fibre and cardiovascular health: A review of current evidence and policy. *Proc. Nutr. Soc.* **2020**, *79*, 61–67. [CrossRef]
32. Anderson, J.W.; Baird, P.; Davis, R.H.J.; Ferreri, S.; Knudtson, M.; Koraym, A.; Waters, V.; Williams, C.L. Health benefits of dietary fiber. *Nutr. Rev.* **2009**, *67*, 188–205. [CrossRef]

33. Veronese, N.; Solmi, M.; Caruso, M.G.; Giannelli, G.; Osella, A.R.; Evangelou, E.; Maggi, S.; Fontana, L.; Stubbs, B.; Tzoulaki, I. Dietary fiber and health outcomes: An umbrella review of systematic reviews and meta-analyses. *Am. J. Clin. Nutr.* **2018**, *107*, 436–444. [CrossRef]
34. Stephen, A.M.; Champ, M.M.; Cloran, S.J.; Fleith, M.; van Lieshout, L.; Mejborn, H.; Burley, V.J. Dietary fibre in Europe: Current state of knowledge on definitions, sources, recommendations, intakes and relationships to health. *Nutr. Res. Rev.* **2017**, *30*, 149–190. [CrossRef]
35. Brown, L.; Rosner, B.; Willett, W.C.; Sacks, F.M. Cholesterol-lowering effects of dietary fiber: A meta-analysis. *Am. J. Clin. Nutr.* **1999**, *69*, 30–42. [CrossRef] [PubMed]
36. Harley, L.; May, M.D.; Loveman, E.; Colquitt, J.L.; Rees, K. Dietary fibre for the primary prevention of cardiovascular disease. *Cochrane Database Syst. Rev.* **2016**, *7*, CD011472.
37. Ho, H.V.; Sievenpiper, J.L.; Zurbau, A.; Blanco Mejia, S.; Jovanovski, E.; Au-Yeung, F.; Jenkins, A.L.; Vuksan, V. The effect of oat β-glucan on LDL-cholesterol, non-HDL-cholesterol and apoB for CVD risk reduction: A systematic review and meta-analysis of randomised-controlled trials. *Br. J. Nutr.* **2016**, *116*, 1369–1382. [CrossRef]
38. Whitehead, A.; Beck, E.J.; Tosh, S.; Wolever, T.M. Cholesterol lowering effects of oat beta-glucan: A meta-analysis of randomized controlled trials. *Am. J. Clin. Nutr* **2014**, *100*, 1413–1421. [CrossRef]
39. Ho, H.V.; Sievenpiper, J.L.; Zurbau, A.; Blanco Mejia, S.; Jovanovski, E.; Au-Yeung, F.; Jenkins, A.L.; Vuksan, V. A systematic review and meta-analysis of randomized controlled trials of the effect of barley β-glucan on LDL-C, non-HDL-C and apoB for cardiovascular disease risk reduction. *Eur. J. Clin. Nutr.* 2016; 70, 1239–1245, Erratum in *Eur J. Clin. Nutr.* **2016**, *70*(11), 1340.
40. Wei, Z.; Wang, H.; Chen, X.; Wang, B.; Rong, Z.; Wang, B.; Su, B.; Chen, H. Time- and dose-dependent effect of psyllium on serum lipids in mild-to-moderate hypercholesterolemia: A meta-analysis of controlled clinical trials. *Eur. J. Clin. Nutr.* **2009**, *63*, 821–827. [CrossRef] [PubMed]
41. Jovanovski, E.; Yashpal, S.; Komishon, A.; Zurbau, A.; Blanco Mejia, S.; Ho, H.V.T.; Li, D.; Sievenpiper, J.; Duvnjak, L.; Vuksan, V. Effect of psyllium (Plantago ovata) fiber on LDL cholesterol and alternative lipid targets, non-HDL cholesterol and apolipoprotein B: A systematic review and meta-analysis of randomized controlled trials. *Am. J. Clin. Nutr.* **2018**, *108*, 922–932. [CrossRef] [PubMed]
42. Ho, H.V.T.; Jovanovski, E.; Zurbau, A.; Blanco Mejia, S.; Sievenpiper, J.L.; Au-Yeung, F.; Jenkins, A.L.; Duvnjak, L.; Leiter, L.; Vuksan, V. A systematic review and meta-analysis of randomized controlled trials of the effect of konjac glucomannan, a viscous soluble fiber, on LDL cholesterol and the new lipid targets non-HDL cholesterol and apolipoprotein B. *Am. J. Clin. Nutr.* **2017**, *105*, 1239–1247. [CrossRef]
43. Theuwissen, E.; Mensink, R.P. Water-soluble dietary fibers and cardiovascular disease. *Physiol. Behav.* **2008**, *94*, 285–292. [CrossRef]
44. Kim, Y.; Je, Y. Dietary fibre intake and mortality from cardiovascular disease and all cancers: A meta-analysis of prospective cohort studies. *Arch. Cardiovasc. Dis.* **2016**, *109*, 39–54. [CrossRef]
45. Threapleton, D.E.; Greenwood, D.C.; Evans, C.E.; Cleghorn, C.L.; Nykjaer, C.; Woodhead, C.; Cade, J.E.; Gale, C.P.; Burley, V.J. Dietary fibre intake and risk of cardiovascular disease: Systematic review and meta-analysis. *BMJ* **2013**, *347*, f6879. [CrossRef]
46. Partula, V.; Deschasaux, M.; Druesne-Pecollo, N.; Latino-Martel, P.; Desmetz, E.; Chazelas, E.; Kesse-Guyot, E.; Julia, C.; Fezeu, L.K.; Galan, P.; et al. Associations between consumption of dietary fibers and the risk of cardiovascular diseases, cancers, type 2 diabetes, and mortality in the prospective NutriNet-Santé cohort. *Am. J. Clin. Nutr.* **2020**, *112*, 195–207. [CrossRef] [PubMed]
47. Trautwein, E.A.; Vermeer, M.A.; Hiemstra, H.; Ras, R.T. LDL-cholesterol lowering of plant sterols and stanols-which factors influence their efficacy? *Nutrients* **2018**, *10*, 1262. [CrossRef] [PubMed]
48. Ras, R.T.; van der Schouw, Y.T.; Trautwein, E.A.; Sioen, I.; Dalmeijer, G.W.; Zock, P.L.; Beulens, J.W. Intake of phytosterols from natural sources and risk of cardiovascular disease in the European prospective investigation into cancer and nutrition-the Netherlands (epic-nl) population. *Eur. J. Prev. Cardiol.* **2015**, *22*, 1067–1075. [CrossRef] [PubMed]
49. Jaceldo-Siegl, K.; Lutjohann, D.; Sirirat, R.; Mashchak, A.; Fraser, G.E.; Haddad, E. Variations in dietary intake and plasma concentration of plant sterols across plant-based diets among north American adults. *Mol. Nutr. Food Res.* **2017**, *61*. [CrossRef]

50. Appel, L.J.; Moore, T.J.; Obarzanek, E.; Vollmer, W.M.; Svetkey, L.P.; Sacks, F.M.; Bray, G.A.; Vogt, T.M.; Cutler, J.A.; Windhauser, M.M.; et al. A clinical trial of the effects of dietary patterns on blood pressure. DASH Collaborative Research Group. *N. Engl. J. Med.* **1997**, *336*, 1117–1124. [CrossRef]
51. Jenkins, D.J.; Kendall, C.W.; Marchie, A.; Faulkner, D.A.; Wong, J.M.; de Souza, R.; Emam, A.; Parker, T.L.; Vidgen, E.; Trautwein, E.A.; et al. Direct comparison of a dietary portfolio of cholesterol-lowering foods with a statin in hypercholesterolemic participants. *Am. J. Clin. Nutr.* **2005**, *81*, 380–387. [CrossRef]
52. Pollak, O.J. Reduction of blood cholesterol in man. *Circulation* **1953**, *7*, 702–706. [CrossRef]
53. Katan, M.B.; Grundy, S.M.; Jones, P.; Law, M.; Miettinen, T.A.; Paoletti, R. Efficacy and safety of plant stanols and sterols in the management of blood cholesterol levels. *Mayo Clin. Proc.* **2003**, *78*, 965–978. [CrossRef]
54. Demonty, I.; Ras, R.T.; Van der Knaap, H.C.M.; Duchateau, G.S.M.J.; Meijer, L.; Zock, P.L.; Geleijnse, J.M.; Trautwein, E.A. Continuous dose-response relationship of the LDL-cholesterol-lowering effect of phytosterol intake. *J. Nutr.* **2009**, *139*, 271–284. [CrossRef]
55. Musa-Veloso, K.; Poon, T.H.; Elliot, J.A.; Chung, C. A comparison of the LDL-cholesterol lowering efficacy of plant stanols and plant sterols over a continuous dose range: Results of a meta-analysis of randomized, placebo-controlled trials. *Prostaglins Leukot. Essent. Fat. Acids* **2011**, *85*, 9–28. [CrossRef]
56. Ras, R.T.; Geleijnse, J.M.; Trautwein, E.A. LDL-cholesterol-lowering effect of plant sterols and stanols across different dose ranges: A meta-analysis of randomised controlled studies. *Br. J. Nutr.* **2014**, *112*, 214–219. [CrossRef] [PubMed]
57. Ghaedi, E.; Kord-Varkaneh, H.; Mohammadi, H.; Askarpour, M.; Miraghajani, M. Phytosterol Supplementation Could Improve Atherogenic and Anti-Atherogenic Apolipoproteins: A Systematic Review and Dose-Response Meta-Analysis of Randomized Controlled Trials. *J. Am. Coll. Nutr.* **2020**, *39*, 82–92. [CrossRef] [PubMed]
58. Plat, J.; Mackay, D.; Baumgartner, S.; Clifton, P.M.; Gylling, H.; Jones, P.J. Progress and prospective of plant sterol and plant stanol research: Report of the Maastricht meeting. *Atherosclerosis* **2012**, *225*, 521–533. [CrossRef] [PubMed]
59. Trautwein, E.A.; Koppenol, W.P.; de Jong, A.; Hiemstra, H.; Vermeer, M.A.; Noakes, M.; Luscombe-Marsh, N.D. Plant sterols lower LDL-cholesterol and triglycerides in dyslipidemic individuals with or at risk of developing type 2 diabetes; a randomized, double-blind, placebo-controlled study. *Nutr. Diabetes* **2018**, *8*, 30. [CrossRef] [PubMed]
60. De Smet, E.; Mensink, R.P.; Plat, J. Effects of plant sterols and stanols on intestinal cholesterol metabolism: Suggested mechanisms from past to present. *Mol. Nutr. Food Res.* **2012**, *56*, 1058–1072. [CrossRef]
61. Gylling, H.; Plat, J.; Turley, S.; Ginsberg, H.N.; Ellegård, L.; Jessup, W.; Jones, P.J.; Lütjohann, D.; März, W.; Masana, L.; et al. For the European Atherosclerosis Society Consensus Panel on Phytosterols. Plant sterols and plant stanols in the management of dyslipidaemia and prevention of cardiovascular disease. *Atherosclerosis* **2014**, *232*, 346–360. [CrossRef]
62. Han, S.; Jiao, J.; Xu, J.; Zimmermann, D.; Actis-Goretta, L.; Guan, L.; Zhao, Y.; Qin, L. Effects of plant stanol or sterol-enriched diets on lipid profiles in patients treated with statins: Systematic review and meta-analysis. *Sci. Rep.* **2016**, *6*, 31337. [CrossRef]
63. Gomes, G.B.; Zazula, A.D.; Shigueoka, L.S.; Fedato, R.A.; da Costa, A.B.; Guarita-Souza, L.C.; Baena, C.P.; Olandoski, M.; Faria-Neto, J.R. A Randomized Open-Label Trial to Assess the Effect of Plant Sterols Associated with Ezetimibe in Low-Density Lipoprotein Levels in Patients with Coronary Artery Disease on Statin Therapy. *J. Med. Food* **2017**, *20*, 30–36. [CrossRef]
64. Anderson, T.J.; Grégoire, J.; Pearson, G.J.; Barry, A.R.; Couture, P.; Dawes, M.; Francis, G.A.; Genest, J.J.; Grover, S.; Gupta, M.; et al. 2016 Canadian cardiovascular society guidelines for the management of dyslipidemia for the prevention of cardiovascular disease in the adult. *Can. J. Cardiol.* **2016**, *32*, 1263–1282. [CrossRef]
65. Expert Dyslipidemia Panel of the International Atherosclerosis Society. An International Atherosclerosis Society Position Paper: Global recommendations for the management of dyslipidemia—Full report. *J. Clin. Lipidol* **2014**, *8*, 29–60. [CrossRef] [PubMed]
66. Ferguson, J.J.; Stojanovski, E.; MacDonald-Wicks, L.; Garg, M.L. High molecular weight oat β-glucan enhances lipid-lowering effects of phytosterols. A randomised controlled trial. *Clin. Nutr.* **2020**, *39*, 80–89. [CrossRef] [PubMed]

67. Shrestha, S.; Volek, J.S.; Udani, J.; Wood, R.J.; Greene, C.M.; Aggarwal, D.; Contois, J.H.; Kavoussi, B.; Fernandez, M.L. A combination therapy including psyllium and plant sterols lowers LDL cholesterol by modifying lipoprotein metabolism in hypercholesterolemic individuals. *J. Nutr.* **2006**, *136*, 2492–2497. [CrossRef] [PubMed]
68. Chen, S.C.; Judd, J.T.; Kramer, M.; Meijer, G.W.; Clevidence, B.A.; Baer, D.J. Phytosterol intake and dietary fat reduction are independent and additive in their ability to reduce plasma LDL cholesterol. *Lipids* **2009**, *44*, 273–281. [CrossRef] [PubMed]
69. Chiavaroli, L.; Nishi, S.K.; Khan, T.A.; Braunstein, C.R.; Glenn, A.J.; Mejia, S.B.; Rahelić, D.; Kahleová, H.; Salas-Salvadó, J.; Jenkins, D.J.A.; et al. Portfolio Dietary Pattern and Cardiovascular Disease: A Systematic Review and Meta-analysis of Controlled Trials. *Prog. Cardiovasc. Dis.* **2018**, *61*, 43–53. [CrossRef]
70. Blom, W.A.M.; Koppenol, W.P.; Hiemstra, H.; Stojakovic, T.; Scharnagl, H.; Trautwein, E.A. A low-fat spread with added plant sterols and fish omega-3 fatty acids lowers serum triglyceride and LDL-cholesterol concentrations in individuals with modest hypercholesterolaemia and hypertriglyceridaemia. *Eur. J. Nutr.* **2019**, *58*, 1615–1624. [CrossRef]
71. Hu, F.B. Dietary pattern analysis: A new direction in nutritional epidemiology. *Curr. Opin. Lipidol.* **2002**, *13*, 3–9. [CrossRef]
72. Zampelas, A.; Magriplis, E. Dietary patterns and risk of cardiovascular diseases: A review of the evidence. *Proc. Nutr. Soc.* **2020**, *79*, 68–75. [CrossRef]
73. Bechthold, A.; Boeing, H.; Schwedhelm, C.; Hoffmann, G.; Knuppel, S.; Iqbal, K.; De Henauw, S.; Michels, N.; Devleesschauwer, B.; Schlesinger, S.; et al. Food groups and risk of coronary heart disease, stroke and heart failure: A systematic review and dose-response meta-analysis of prospective studies. *Crit. Rev. Food Sci. Nutr.* **2019**, *59*, 1071–1090. [CrossRef]
74. Hemler, E.C.; Hu, F.B. Plant-Based Diets for Cardiovascular Disease Prevention: All Plant Foods Are Not Created Equal. *Curr. Atheroscler. Rep.* **2019**, *21*, 18. [CrossRef]
75. Shen, J.; Wilmot, K.A.; Ghasemzadeh, N.; Molloy, D.L.; Burkman, G.; Mekonnen, G.; Gongora, M.C.; Quyyumi, A.A.; Sperling, L.S. Mediterranean Dietary Patterns and Cardiovascular Health. *Annu. Rev. Nutr.* **2015**, *35*, 425–449. [CrossRef] [PubMed]
76. Bere, E.; Brug, J. Towards health-promoting and environmentally friendly regional diets-a Nordic example. *Public Health Nutr.* **2009**, *12*, 91–96. [CrossRef] [PubMed]
77. Adamsson, V.; Reumark, A.; Cederholm, T.; Vessby, B.; Risérus, U.; Johansson, G. What is a healthy Nordic diet? Foods and nutrients in the NORDIET study. *Food Nutr. Res.* **2012**, *56*, 18189. [CrossRef] [PubMed]
78. Magkos, F.; Tetens, I.; Bügel, S.G.; Felby, C.; Schacht, S.R.; Hill, J.O.; Ravussin, E.; Astrup, A. A Perspective on the Transition to Plant-Based Diets: A Diet Change May Attenuate Climate Change, but Can It Also Attenuate Obesity and Chronic Disease Risk? *Adv. Nutr.* **2020**, *11*, 1–9. [CrossRef] [PubMed]
79. Chiavaroli, L.; Viguiliouk, E.; Nishi, S.K.; Blanco Mejia, S.; Raheli´c, D.; Kahleová, H.; Salas-Salvadó, J.; Kendall, C.W.; Sievenpiper, J.L. DASH Dietary Pattern and Cardiometabolic Outcomes: An Umbrella Review of Systematic Reviews and Meta-Analyses. *Nutrients* **2019**, *11*, 338. [CrossRef] [PubMed]
80. Glenn, A.J.; Viguiliouk, E.; Seider, M.; Boucher, B.A.; Khan, T.A.; Blanco Mejia, S.; Jenkins, D.J.A.; Kahleová, H.; Raheli´c, D.; Salas-Salvadó, J. Relation of Vegetarian Dietary Patterns with Major Cardiovascular Outcomes: A Systematic Review and Meta-Analysis of Prospective Cohort Studies. *Front. Nutr.* **2019**, *6*, 80. [CrossRef] [PubMed]
81. Siervo, M.; Lara, J.; Chowdhury, S.; Ashor, A.; Oggioni, C.; Mathers, J.C. Effects of the Dietary Approach to Stop Hypertension (DASH) diet on cardiovascular risk factors: A systematic review and meta-analysis. *Br. J. Nutr.* **2015**, *113*, 1–15. [CrossRef]
82. Ramezani-Jolfaie, N.; Mohammadi, M.; Salehi-Abargouei, A. The effect of healthy Nordic diet on cardio-metabolic markers: A systematic review and meta-analysis of randomized controlled clinical trials. *Eur. J. Nutr.* **2018**, *58*, 2159–2174. [CrossRef]
83. Kahleova, H.; Salas-Salvadó, J.; Rahelić, D.; Kendall, C.W.; Rembert, E.; Sievenpiper, J.L. Dietary Patterns and Cardiometabolic Outcomes in Diabetes: A Summary of Systematic Reviews and Meta-Analyses. *Nutrients* **2019**, *11*, 2209. [CrossRef]
84. Rees, K.; Takeda, A.; Martin, N.; Ellis, L.; Wijesekara, D.; Vepa, A.; Das, A.; Hartley, L.; Stranges, S. Mediterranean-style diet for the primary and secondary prevention of cardiovascular disease. *Cochrane Database Syst. Rev.* **2019**, *3*. [CrossRef]

85. Wang, F.; Zheng, J.; Yang, B.; Jiang, J.; Fu, Y.; Li, D. Effects of Vegetarian Diets on Blood Lipids: A Systematic Review and Meta-Analysis of Randomized Controlled Trials. *J. Am. Heart Assoc.* **2015**, *4*, e002408. [CrossRef]
86. Yokoyama, Y.; Levin, S.M.; Barnard, N.D. Association between plant-based diets and plasma lipids: A systematic review and meta-analysis. *Nutr. Rev.* **2017**, *75*, 683–698. [CrossRef] [PubMed]
87. Rosato, V.; Temple, N.J.; La Vecchia, C.; Castellan, G.; Tavani, A.; Guercio, V. Mediterranean diet and cardiovascular disease: A systematic review and meta-analysis of observational studies. *Eur. J. Nutr.* **2019**, *58*, 173–191. [CrossRef] [PubMed]
88. Becerra-Tomás, N.; Mejía, S.B.; Viguiliouk, E.; Khan, T.; Kendall, C.W.; Kahleova, H.; Raheli´c, D.; Sievenpiper, J.L.; Salas-Salvadó, J. Mediterranean diet, cardiovascular disease and mortality in diabetes: A systematic review and meta-analysis of prospective cohort studies and randomized clinical trials. *Crit. Rev. Food Sci. Nutr.* **2019**, 1–21. [CrossRef] [PubMed]
89. Gunge, V.B.; Andersen, I.; Kyrø, C.; Hansen, C.P.; Dahm, C.C.; Christensen, J.; Tjønneland, A.; Olsen, A. Adherence to a healthy Nordic food index and risk of myocardial infarction in middle-aged Danes: The diet, cancer and health cohort study. *Eur. J. Clin. Nutr.* **2017**, *71*, 652–658. [CrossRef] [PubMed]
90. Hansen, C.P.; Overvad, K.; Kyrø, C.; Olsen, A.; Tjønneland, A.; Johnsen, S.P.; Jakobsen, M.U.; Dahm, C.C. Adherence to a Healthy Nordic Diet and Risk of Stroke: A Danish Cohort Study. *Stroke* **2017**, *48*, 259–264. [CrossRef] [PubMed]
91. Roswall, N.; Sandin, S.; Scragg, R.; Löf, M.; Skeie, G.; Olsen, A.; Adami, H.O.; Weiderpass, E. No association between adherence to the healthy Nordic food index and cardiovascular disease amongst Swedish women: A cohort study. *J. Intern. Med.* **2015**, *278*, 531–541. [CrossRef]
92. Dinu, M.; Abbate, R.; Gensini, G.F.; Casini, A.; Sofi, F. Vegetarian, vegan diets and multiple health outcomes: A systematic review with meta-analysis of observational studies. *Crit. Rev. Food Sci. Nutr.* **2017**, *57*, 3640–3649. [CrossRef]
93. Nelson, M.E.; Hamm, M.W.; Hu, F.B.; Abrams, S.A.; Griffin, T.S. Alignment of healthy dietary patterns and environmental sustainability: A systematic review. *Adv. Nutr.* **2016**, *7*, 1005–1025. [CrossRef]
94. Springmann, M.; Wiebe, K.; Mason-D'Croz, D.; Sulser, T.B.; Rayner, M.; Scarborough, P. Health and nutritional aspects of sustainable diet strategies and their association with environmental impacts: A global modelling analysis with country-level detail. *Lancet Planet. Health* **2018**, *2*, e451–e61. [CrossRef]
95. Satija, A.; Bhupathiraju, S.N.; Spiegelman, D.; Chiuve, S.E.; Manson, J.E.; Willett, W.; Rexrode, K.M.; Rimm, E.B.; Hu, F.B. Healthful and unhealthful plant based diets and the risk of coronary heart disease in U.S. adults. *J. Am. Coll. Cardiol.* **2017**, *70*, 411–422. [CrossRef]
96. U.S. Department of Health and Human Services and U.S. Department of Agriculture. 2015–2020 Dietary Guidelines for Americans, 8th ed.; December 2015. Available online: http://health.gov/dietaryguidelines/2015/guidelines/ (accessed on 31 August 2020).
97. Nordic Council of Ministers. *Nordic Nutrition Recommendations 2012: Integrating Nutrition and Physical Activity*, 5th ed.; Nordic Council of Ministers: Copenhagen, Denmark, 2014.
98. Li, S.S.; Blanco Mejia, S.; Lytvyn, L.; Stewart, S.E.; Viguiliouk, E.; Ha, V.; de Souza, R.J.; Leiter, L.A.; Kendall, C.W.C.; Jenkins, D.J.A.; et al. Effect of Plant Protein on Blood Lipids: A Systematic Review and Meta-Analysis of Randomized Controlled Trials. *J. Am. Heart Assoc.* **2017**, *6*, e006659. [CrossRef] [PubMed]
99. Corrin, T.; Papadopoulos, A. Understanding the attitudes and perceptions of vegetarian and plant-based diets to shape future health promotion programs. *Appetite* **2017**, *109*, 40–47. [CrossRef] [PubMed]
100. Fehér, A.; Gazdecki, M.; Véha, M.; Szakály, M.; Szakály, Z. A Comprehensive Review of the Benefits of and the Barriers to the Switch to a Plant-Based Diet. *Sustainability* **2020**, *12*, 4136.

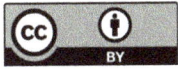

© 2020 by the authors. Licensee MDPI, Basel, Switzerland. This article is an open access article distributed under the terms and conditions of the Creative Commons Attribution (CC BY) license (http://creativecommons.org/licenses/by/4.0/).

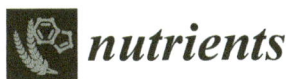

Review

Beyond Fish Oil Supplementation: The Effects of Alternative Plant Sources of Omega-3 Polyunsaturated Fatty Acids upon Lipid Indexes and Cardiometabolic Biomarkers—An Overview

Heitor O. Santos [1],*, James C. Price [2] and Allain A. Bueno [2]

1 School of Medicine, Federal University of Uberlandia (UFU), Uberlandia 38408-100, Brazil
2 College of Health, Life and Environmental Sciences, University of Worcester, Worcester WR2 6AJ, UK; prij2_16@uni.worc.ac.uk (J.C.P.); a.bueno@worc.ac.uk (A.A.B.)
* Correspondence: heitoroliveirasantos@gmail.com

Received: 27 September 2020; Accepted: 14 October 2020; Published: 16 October 2020

Abstract: Cardiovascular diseases remain a global challenge, and lipid-associated biomarkers can predict cardiovascular events. Extensive research on cardiovascular benefits of omega-3 polyunsaturated fatty acids (n3-PUFAs) is geared towards fish oil supplementation and fish-rich diets. Nevertheless, vegetarianism and veganism are becoming more popular across all segments of society, due to reasons as varied as personal, ethical and religious values, individual preferences and environment-related principles, amongst others. Due to the essentiality of PUFAs, plant sources of n3-PUFAs warrant further consideration. In this review, we have critically appraised the efficacy of plant-derived n3-PUFAs from foodstuffs and supplements upon lipid profile and selected cardiometabolic markers. Walnuts and flaxseed are the most common plant sources of n3-PUFAs, mainly alpha-linolenic acid (ALA), and feature the strongest scientific rationale for applicability into clinical practice. Furthermore, walnuts and flaxseed are sources of fibre, potassium, magnesium, and non-essential substances, including polyphenols and sterols, which in conjunction are known to ameliorate cardiovascular metabolism. ALA levels in rapeseed and soybean oils are only slight when compared to flaxseed oil. *Spirulina* and *Chlorella*, biomasses of cyanobacteria and green algae, are important sources of n3-PUFAs; however, their benefits upon cardiometabolic markers are plausibly driven by their antioxidant potential combined with their n3-PUFA content. In humans, ALA is not sufficiently bioconverted into eicosapentaenoic and docosahexaenoic acids. However, evidence suggests that plant sources of ALA are associated with favourable cardiometabolic status. ALA supplementation, or increased consumption of ALA-rich foodstuffs, combined with reduced omega-6 (n6) PUFAs intake, could improve the n3/n6 ratio and improve cardiometabolic and lipid profile.

Keywords: alpha-linolenic acid; flaxseed; lipids; omega-3; walnuts

1. Introduction

Cardiovascular diseases remain a major Public Health concern, with lipid-associated biomarkers being trusted predictors of major cardiovascular events [1,2]. Added to the pharmacological strategies and conscious effort to improve the patients' lifestyle by adequate nutrition and physical activity, nutraceutical strategies which include certain supplements, herbal extracts and functional foods, may be a helpful complementary approach for individuals with cardiovascular disease and dyslipidaemia [3–9].

The dietary replacement of saturated fats for polyunsaturated fatty acids (PUFAs) has shown beneficial effects upon lipid profile [10], as well as long-term protective benefits against major cardiovascular events and associated clinical complications [11,12]. For decades, omega-3 polyunsaturated fatty acids (n3-PUFAs) from either marine sources or fish oil (FO) supplementation were broadly referred to in cardiology guidelines [13–15]. For example, amongst several clinical investigations, Sagara et al. in 2011 showed that 2 g of DHA daily for five weeks improved blood pressure and lipid profile in a sample population of 38 middle-age men with hypertension and hypercholesterolaemia [16].

On the other hand, however, Manger et al. in 2010 did not find a significant trend in reduced risk of coronary events with increased consumption of n3-PUFAs from fish and fish supplements. Nonetheless, Manger argues that their sample population had a high intake of n3-PUA to begin with, and possibly the lack of association could have been attributed to a ceiling effect of n3-PUFAs [17]. Interestingly, a robust meta-analysis published in 2018, which included 79 Randomized Control Trials (RCTs) and a total of 112,059 participants, showed that n3-PUFAs supplementation actually did not show significantly greater efficacy on reducing the occurrence of cardiovascular events [18]. Such results must be interpreted carefully due to factors such as methodology employed, varied sample population investigated, other factors beyond the scope of the study, and a potential risk for bias. At the same time, it has also been demonstrated that plant sources of n3-PUFAs have shown some potential against cardiovascular events and dyslipidaemia [18].

The findings on fish consumption and FO supplementation upon cardiovascular health do not disregard the merit of investigating the usefulness of plant-derived n3-PUFAs in clinical practice. Studies on the potential efficacy of plant-derived n3-PUFAs become further justified as dramatic reductions of fish stocks have been reported in the North Atlantic Ocean and Mediterranean Sea [19,20]. In the present review, we have critically appraised the efficacy of plant-derived n3-PUFAs from foodstuffs, as well as its supplementation, upon the modulation of lipid profile and selected cardiometabolic markers. More specifically, we searched for the effects of chia seeds, flaxseeds, walnuts, as well as *Spirulina* and *Chlorella*. As those foodstuffs are gaining more popularity, a phenomenon possibly attributed to the increased awareness of environmental issues related to overfishing, combined with the increasing trend towards veganism, vegetarianism and flexitarianism across all segments of society, it is of greatest interest to clarify the clinical potential of plant sources of n3-PUFAs.

2. Methods

We employed the electronic databases Pubmed/Medline and Google Scholar to identify relevant publications. Randomised Controlled Trials (RCTs) written in English were the chosen sources of results as a means of translating current research findings into clinical practice. Preferred Reporting Items for Systematic Reviews and Meta-Analyses (PRISMA) guidelines [21] were used to evaluate and select the RCTs.

Limited to RCTs, we searched for plant sources of ALA by using the following combinations of Medical Subject Heading (MeSH) keywords: ("Chia Seeds" OR "Flaxseeds" OR "Hemp Seeds" OR "Walnuts" OR "Seaweeds" OR "*Spirulina*" OR "*Chlorella*") AND ("LDL-C" OR "Low-Density Lipoprotein Cholesterol" OR "Total Cholesterol" OR "Triglycerides" OR "HDL-C" OR "Low-Density Lipoprotein Cholesterol" OR "Blood Pressure" OR "Cardiovascular Disease" OR "Cardiometabolic Risk" OR "Inflammatory Biomarkers" OR "Proinflammatory Cytokines"). The period covered in the search included inception to August 2020. Summary findings from the selected papers are presented in Supplementary Tables S1–S3. After perusal of such findings, we discussed key aspects and manually expanded the review by selecting further articles that have investigated nutrition facts, mechanisms of action and clinical applications.

As the number and robustness of clinical studies that have investigated the metabolic effects of plant-derived n3-PUFAs are only a fraction of those that employed FO, we have also summarized in Supplementary Table S4 the outcomes of 38 selected FO supplementation studies identified using the key terms listed above and published in the last five years, with a combined sample population of 4136 individuals. The evidence gathered confirms that whilst some studies did show improvements in metabolic biomarkers after FO supplementation, some others did not.

3. Metabolic Pathways

3.1. Conversion of ALA in Humans

Not only the insufficient intake of dietary n3-PUFAs, but also the inefficient elongation and desaturation of ALA to eicosapentaenoic acid (EPA) and docosahexaenoic acid (DHA) in humans, result in low n3 long chain-PUFA content in blood and other peripheral tissues [22,23]. Accordingly, North America, Central and South America, and Africa, are geographical examples where EPA and DHA concentrations are endemically low [24]. More specifically, the intake of n3-PUFAs in the average USA population is low or very low [14].

Approximately only 5% of ALA is converted to EPA whilst less than 0.5% is converted to DHA in humans, although mammals have the essential enzymes used in this pathway [25–27]. A proof-of-concept study published in 2010 showed in newborn infants that only approximately 0.04% of ALA administered was elongated and desaturated to circulating EPA, whilst the subsequent conversion of EPA to DHA was comparatively more efficient [28]. The very low ALA to EPA bioconversion ratio identified in that study does not account for the EPA that was actually incorporated into solid tissues, but it does confirm the suggestion that even large amounts of dietary ALA will probably have negligible effects on plasma DHA levels [27].

Moreover, the conversion of ALA to EPA and subsequently DHA appears to be more efficient in women than in men, a phenomenon that could probably be explained by a possibly advantageous action of oestrogens in protecting the mother and the lactating child. Gender difference is a factor to be considered before making dietary recommendations for n3-PUFAs intake [25].

3.2. n3-PUFAs Versus n6-PUFAs

The inefficient bioconversion of ALA to EPA and DHA becomes more evident when considering that n3 and omega-6 (n6) PUFAs, although in much different concentrations in the typical westernized diet, compete almost equally for the same enzymatic pathway that elongates and desaturates the precursors ALA and linoleic acid (LA) to EPA and arachidonic acid (AA), respectively [29]. On the other hand however, potential roles for ALA in human health that may be independent of its bioconversion onto DHA have been proposed [27].

Experimental evidence alludes to a slower enzymatic metabolism of n3-PUFAs in relation to n6-PUFAs [30]. Therefore, focus on ALA intake is paramount for human health, but similarly important is the adequate intake of LA, as not to imbalance the n6/n3 ratio. Typical westernized diets show abundance of meats and poultry alongside deep-fried foodstuffs, an important dietary characteristic that favours high LA intake.

As seen in Figure 1, dietary sources of n6-PUFAs lead to raised levels of AA, culminating in increased synthesis of pro-inflammatory eicosanoids. Dietary sources of n3-PUFAs, in turn, allow the synthesis of anti-inflammatory eicosanoids. Increased n3-PUFA concomitant to decreased n6-PUFA decreases the AA content in platelets, vascular endothelial cells and vascular wall macrophages, thus reducing AA-derived pro-inflammatory mediators [31]. Cyclooxygenases (COX) and lipoxygenases (LOX) convert AA to prostaglandin E2, thromboxane A2, prostaglandin I2 and leukotriene B4, amongst other pro-inflammatory eicosanoids, whilst the same enzymatic pathways convert EPA to prostaglandin E3, thromboxane A3, prostaglandin I3 and leukotriene B5, amongst other anti-inflammatory eicosanoids [32–34].

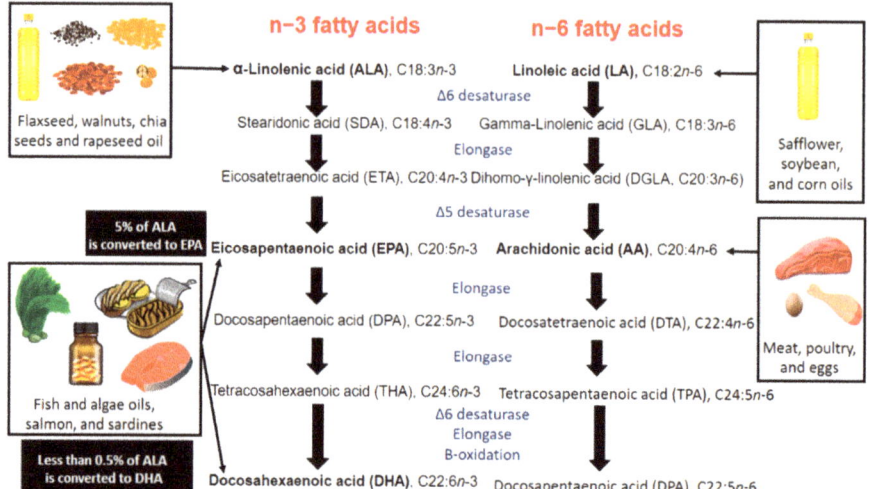

Figure 1. Whilst the main dietary sources of the n3-PUFAs EPA and DHA are fatty fish (e.g., salmon and sardines) and algae, the n3 precursor ALA is found mainly in walnuts, chia seeds, flaxseeds, and rapeseed oil. Likewise, meat, poultry and eggs are important sources of the n6-PUFAs AA, and its n6 precursor LA is found mainly in safflower, sunflower, soybean and corn oils [35–37]. ALA and LA are converted by desaturases and elongases to EPA and AA, respectively, and subsequently converted in a series of complex enzymatic reactions to the longer forms DHA and n6-docosapentaenoic (n6-DPA), respectively [38,39].

3.3. Cardiometabolic Pathways

It has been observed in vitro that ALA is associated with decreased expression levels of vascular cell adhesion molecule-1 (VCAM-1), interleukin 6 (IL-6), proliferating cell nuclear antigen (PCNA), macrophage marker M3/84 (mac-3) and stearoyl-CoA desaturase-1 (SCD-1) [40]. Indirect effects of ALA upon cardiometabolic pathways have also been observed; ALA bioconversion to DPA is associated with decreased expression levels of COX-1, COX-2 and tumour necrosis factor-alpha (TNF-α), whilst its bioconversion to EPA and DHA is associated with decreased expression levels of peroxisome proliferator-activated receptor gamma (PPAR-γ) [40].

Given that such results have also been identified in aortic tissue [41], it is reasonable to speculate that the positive effects of ALA are driven by attenuation of inflammation, cell proliferation and oxidation [40]. In a more optimistic, long-term speculative scenario, such ALA-induced effects could retard the progression, or even promote an amelioration, of the atherosclerotic state.

ALA administration to primary cultured endothelial cells induced inhibitions of NAD-dependent deacetylase sirtuin-3 (SIRT3) reduction, superoxide dismutase 2 (SOD2) hyperacetylation, and mitochondrial reactive oxygen species (ROS) overproduction, alongside restoration of autophagic flux under damage induced by treatment with angiotensin II plus TNFα [42,43]. Such effects, apparently attributed to ALA, are in line with mitigation of endothelial dysfunction and experimental hypertension [42].

It is known that n3-PUFAs have the capacity to decrease liver triglyceride (TG) synthesis by competitive inhibition of 1,2 diglyceride acyltransferase (DAT), at the same time suppressing the activity of sterol regulatory element-binding protein 1c (SREBP-1c)—A protein that regulates the expression of genes involved in fatty acid and TG synthesis—and also to increase β-oxidation in adipose tissue [44,45]. Regarding the latter, the high affinity of n3-PUFAs for peroxisome proliferator-activated receptor alpha (PPAR-α) leads to a greater synthesis of enzymes involved in lipid catabolism, thus favoring not only fatty acid β-oxidation in peripheral tissues but also catabolism of circulating TG in chylomicrons and very low-density lipoprotein cholesterol (VLDL-C) [44,46,47]. Moreover, substrates for TG synthesis are also decreased by reduced transport of non-esterified fatty acids to hepatocytes, consequently reducing VLDL-C synthesis [44,48]. Nonetheless, as the majority of the cardiometabolic pathways so far elucidated are based on experimental data [40–43], a more thorough, critical and applied appraisal of the effects of ALA is needed before any general conclusions can be made.

4. Alternative Plant Sources of n3-PUFAs

4.1. Nuts and Seeds

4.1.1. Nutrition Facts

Nuts and seeds are important sources of ALA and also micronutrients, polyphenolic compounds, sterols and fibres, which are protective elements against the exacerbation of chronic diseases [49–51]. For instance, nuts and seeds that are sources of ALA also contain a considerable amount of calcium, magnesium, and potassium (Table 1), which are fundamental macrominerals for cardiovascular health, mainly in the management of hypertension [52–56]. Furthermore, nuts and seeds are a source of protein. Although at lower levels as compared to animal-derived protein in terms of needs for muscle hypertrophy, the consumption of nuts and seeds is inversely correlated with cardiovascular events and mortality, as demonstrated by recent studies [57,58].

Table 1. Nutrition facts of ALA-containing seeds.

Food Item, one Ounce /≈28 g [FDC ID]	Energy (kcal)	Protein (g)	Total Lipid (g)	Total Fiber (g)	CHO (g)	Ca (mg)	Mg (mg)	K (mg)	LA, 18:2, n-6 (g)	ALA, 18:3, n-3 (g)	n-6 /n-3 Ratio
Chia seeds [170554]	136	4.63	8.60	9.75	11.79	176.68	93.8	113.96	1.63	4.99	0.32
Hemp seed [170148]	155	8.83	13.65	1.12	2.42	19.6	196	366	7.68	2.80	2.74
Flaxseed [169414]	150	5.12	11.80	7.64	8.08	71.4	109.76	227.64	1.65	6.38	0.25
Walnuts [784410]	183.12	4.26	18.25	1.9	3.83	27.44	44.24	123.48	10.8	2.54	4.25

Adapted from the United States Department of Agriculture (USDA) database [59]. ALA, alpha-linolenic acid; CA, calcium; CHO, carbohydrate by difference; FDC, FoodData Central; K, potassium; LA, linoleic acid; Mg, Magnesium.

Regarding the ALA content of nuts and seeds, one ounce (28 g) of flaxseed, chia seeds, hemp seed or walnuts exceeds the Adequate Intake (AIs) for ALA, which is 1.1 g/day for women and 1.6 g/day for men, and 1.4 g/day and 1.3 g/day during pregnancy and lactation, respectively [59,60]. In one ounce, there are 6.38 g (398% and 580% of AIs for men and women) of ALA in flaxseed, 4.99 g (175% and 254% of AIs for men and women) in chia seeds, 2.80 g (312% and 453% of AIs for men and women) in hemp seed, 2.54 g (159% and 230% of AIs for men and women) in walnuts (Table 1).

4.1.2. Walnuts

Walnuts are an important source of ALA [61,62]. A 2-years follow-up study recruited 236 elderly subjects, segregated into two groups: a control group without nut consumption, and an intervention group in which 15% of the approximate daily energy intake consisted of walnuts, at approximately 30–60 g/day of walnuts [63]. The researchers found a reduction of 8.5 mmHg in the systolic blood pressure, whose baseline levels were >125 mmHg; however, no changes were observed in diastolic blood pressure. In the same study, the participants who consumed walnuts required lower dosages of antihypertensive drugs as compared to the control participants. The blood pressure of all participants in that study was monitored by the 24-h ambulatory blood pressure monitoring, which is considered the gold standard in the diagnosis of hypertension [64]. In contrast, a recent meta-analysis [65] did not support walnut consumption per se as a blood pressure-lowering strategy. Despite being a meta-analysis, that study [65] may have had a few limitations due to heterogeneity. The results of Domènech et al. [63] provide what appears to be reliable evidence, based mainly on its long-term duration and sample size.

Le et al. [66] recruited 213 overweight and obese women to a weight loss study, and offered one of the three following dietary regimens: a walnut-rich diet which consisted of 35% energy from fat and 45% energy from carbohydrates, or a low-fat (20%) high-carbohydrate (65%) diet, or a high-fat (35%) low-carbohydrate (45%) diet. After six months of intervention, high-density lipoprotein cholesterol (HDL-C) levels were significantly increased ($p < 0.05$) in the walnut-rich group (from ≈60 to ≈63 mg/dL), whilst a small decrease was observed in the low-fat (from ≈60 to ≈57 mg/dL) and low-carbohydrate (from ≈58 to ≈57 mg/dL) groups.

Interestingly, Fatahi et al. [67] randomised 99 overweight and obese women into three low energy-diet groups: the first group consisted of 300 g/week of fatty fish such as salmon, avoiding the intake of plant sources of n3-PUFAs; the second group consisted of 18 walnuts/week, avoiding the intake of fish and other plant sources of n3-PUFAs; the third group consisted of 150 g fatty fish and nine walnuts/week, avoiding the intake of other sources of n3-PUFAs. After 12 weeks of dietary intervention, as compared to the fish-only group and walnut-only group, the fish + walnut group showed better metabolic profile overall, evidenced by greater increase in HDL-C (+3.6 mg/dL) levels, followed with greater decrease in systolic blood pressure (−5 mmHg), fasting blood glucose (−12 mg/dL), low-density lipoprotein cholesterol (LDL-C) (−6 mg/dL), high-sensitivity C-reactive protein (hs-CRP) (−0.51 mg/L), D-dimer (−0.45 mg/dL), fibrinogen (−22 mg/dL), alanine aminotransferase (ALT) (−6 IU/L), aspartate aminotransferase (AST) (−6 IU/L), TNF-α (−0.08 ng/mL) and IL-6 (−1.6 ng/mL).

4.1.3. Flaxseed

Flaxseed is an important source of ALA, and a few trials have identified beneficial effects of flaxseed intake upon lipid indexes and cardiometabolic biomarkers. In a study recruiting 21 patients with coronary artery disease [68], a pivotal population to ascertain the magnitude of a cardiometabolic intervention, the daily consumption of 30 g flaxseed for 12 weeks promoted better outcomes as compared to the control group in increasing flow-mediated dilation (5.1 vs. −0.55% change from baseline for the flaxseed and control groups, respectively), whilst decreasing the inflammatory status by reducing the levels of CRP (−1.18 mg/L), IL-6 (−7.65 pg/mL), and TNF-α (−34.73 pg/mL). Importantly, no significant change in body weight was observed in either groups [68], which appears to be a very relevant result as it suggests that flaxseed may improve cardiovascular parameters independently of weight loss.

In a systematic review and meta-analysis of RCTs with 1502 patients across 32 studies, flaxseed or its derivatives (whole or ground flaxseed, flaxseed oil, or lignan supplements) reduced the concentrations of hs-CRP (weighted mean difference (WMD): −0.75; 95% CI −1.19, −0.31) and TNF-α (WMD: −0.38; 95% CI −0.75, −0.01) but did not change IL-6 levels. Flaxseed was tested in the form of whole flaxseed, golden flaxseed, flaxseed oil, and lignan supplements at dosages ranging from 360 mg to 60 g, for 2 to 12 weeks, with an averaged intervention period of approximately 10 weeks [69].

A recently published clinical trial recruited 41 women suffering with polycystic ovary syndrome, randomly segregated into two groups, group 1 subjected to lifestyle changes (American Heart Association recommendations + >30 min moderate to intense activity 3x/week) plus 30 g/day brown flaxseed flour in salad, yogurt or cold drinks, and group 2 subjected to the same lifestyle changes only, for 12 weeks [70]. The authors found that the flaxseed group showed significant improvements in insulin, homeostasis model assessment of insulin resistance (HOMA-IR), TG, hs-CRP, IL-6, leptin, HDL-C and adiponectin, as compared to the non-flaxseed group [70].

In a RCT recruiting 100 eligible patients suffering with non-alcoholic fatty liver disease (NAFLD), Yari et al. [71] found that 30 g flaxseed daily plus positive lifestyle interventions for 12 weeks decreased serum concentrations of total cholesterol (TC) (−31.71 mg/dL), TG (−61.33 mg/dL),

LDL-C (−22.64 mg/dL), ALT (−11.12 U/L), AST (−5.37 U/L) and gamma-glutamyltransferase (−11.54 U/L), results that were not matched in the group submitted to positive lifestyle interventions only. It should be noted however that both groups showed reductions in BMI (30.37 ± 4.42 to 28.05 ± 3.89 kg/m^2 in the flaxseed plus lifestyle improvement group, and 33.37 ± 5.56 to 32.42 ± 5.98 in the lifestyle improvement only group) as well as the intensity of hepatic steatosis, a result most likely attributed to decreased energy intake in both groups (2379.41 ± 473.74 to 2117.47 ± 378.46, and 2424.45 ± 470.89 to 1966.39 ± 449.52 kcal, respectively). Such findings reinforce the hypothesis of beneficial effects of flaxseed independently of changes in energy intake and body composition.

In a mirrored RCT [72], this time recruiting 98 patients suffering with metabolic syndrome, the same researchers from the previously mentioned study [71] observed comparable results, in which 30 g flaxseed plus positive lifestyle interventions for 12 weeks reduced by 76% the prevalence of metabolic syndrome, whilst the lifestyle intervention only group had this parameter reduced by 36.4% (p = 0.013 for the difference between groups). Likewise, both groups reduced their calorie intake before versus after, but without differences between them (2423.04 ± 468.98 to 2198.76 ± 455.47 and 2410.26 ± 451.87 to 2079.89 ± 465.46 for flaxseed and control groups, respectively).

4.2. Oils

4.2.1. Lipid Profile of Oils

Oils rich in ALA are a powerful tool to investigate the effects of ALA within a less complex matrix. Despite the presence of other fatty acids and fat-soluble compounds in the oil, the removal of fibre, vitamins, especially water-soluble ones, and water-soluble matter surely minimize the effects of confounding variables. Flaxseed, walnut, and rapeseed oils are, respectively, the main sources of ALA. Soybean oil is often considered a small to reasonable source of ALA, once research into its fatty acid composition has shown ALA concentrations ranging from 2.7% to 7.8% [73,74]. The n6-PUFAs content is nonetheless crucial when contemplating the n3 content of plant oils, as sunflower, corn, walnut, cottonseed, soybean, and peanut oils are important sources of n6-PUFAs (Table 2).

Table 2. ALA content and principal nutrition facts of selected edible oils.

Oil Type, 1 Tablespoon/13.6 g [FDC ID]	Energy (kcal)	Total Lipid (g)	Vitamin E (mg)	Saturated Fats (g)	Monounsaturated Fats (g)	Polyunsaturated Fats (g)	LA, 18:2/n-6 (g)	ALA, 18:3 n-3 (g)	n-6/n-3 Ratio
Flaxseed oil [789037]	120	13.6	0.064	1.22	2.51	9.23	1.95	7.26	0.26
Walnut oil [789048]	120	13.6	0.054	1.24	3.1	8.61	7.19	1.41	5.09
Rapeseed oil [172336]	120	13.6	2.38	1.01	8.64	3.82	2.58	1.24	2.08
Soybean oil [789045]	120	13.6	1.11	2.13	3.1	7.85	6.93	0.92	7.53
Corn oil [789035]	122	13.6	1.94	1.76	3.75	7.44	7.28	0.158	46.07
Olive oil [789038]	120	13.6	1.94	1.86	9.85	1.42	1.32	0.103	12.81
Cottonseed oil [789036]	120	13.6	4.8	3.52	2.42	7.06	7	0.027	259.25
Coconut oil [789034]	121	13.5	0.015	11.2	0.861	0.231	0.229	0.003	76.33
Peanut oil [789039]	120	13.6	2.12	2.28	6.24	4.32	4.32	0	-
Almond oil [789033]	120	13.6	5.33	1.12	9.51	2.37	2.37	0	-
Sunflower oil [789047]	120	13.6	5.59	1.4	2.65	8.94	8.94	0	-

Highest to lowest sources of ALA among common oils used for cooking. In addition, the main sources of LA can be noted, which are sunflower, corn, walnut, cottonseed, soybean, and peanut oils, respectively. Adapted from the United States Department of Agriculture (USDA) database [59].

4.2.2. Flaxseed Oil

A RCT investigated the effects of either 25 mL/d flaxseed oil or 25 mL/d sunflower oil administered for seven weeks to 60 patients suffering with metabolic syndrome [75]. Serum IL-6 levels decreased significantly in both groups (9.37 to 7.90 pg/mL, $p < 0.001$ for flaxseed oil, and 9.22 to 8.48 pg/mL, $p < 0.006$ for sunflower oil), but the flaxseed oil group presented a greater reduction (p = 0.017).

Given that that was a dosage considered high, it is worth mentioning that no side effects were reported in either group [75]. Interestingly, in a study recruiting 60 women with gestational diabetes [76], the daily supplementation for 6 weeks with 2 g/day flaxseed oil capsules, which contained 800 mg/day ALA, reduced the concentrations of TG (−40.5 mg/dL), TC (−22.7 mg/dL), insulin (−2.2 µIU/mL), and hs-CRP (−1.3 mg/L), as compared to a matched group that received sunflower oil capsules. The flaxseed oil-receiving group also showed upregulated LDL receptor, downregulated IL-1 and TNF-α gene expression, decreased malondialdehyde levels and increased total nitrite and total glutathione levels.

In a recent study [77] recruiting 59 overweight and obese adults with stage I hypertension without pharmacological treatment, 10 g of refined cold-pressed flaxseed oil (4.7 g ALA) for 12 weeks decreased fasting free fatty acid (−58 µmol/L) and TNF-α (−0.14 pg/mL) plasma concentrations. In contrast, no changes were found in other metabolic risk markers (e.g., serum glucose and TG levels) nor vascular function markers (e.g., brachial artery flow-mediated vasodilation, carotid-to-femoral pulse wave velocity, and retinal microvascular calibres) before versus after testing, both on fasting and postprandially. We consider this result to be extremely relevant for our critical discussion, as the ALA intake in that study was about three to five times higher than the recommended daily intake and, even so, it failed to improve cardiovascular markers. Furthermore, the volunteers of that study not only had obesity or overweight and stage I hypertension, their average age was 60 ± 8 years, a finding that is positively associated with vascular ageing, which by definition poses a greater risk for hypertension and atherosclerotic disease than the more traditional risk factors, including lipid and glucose levels, smoking and sedentary lifestyle [78].

The Omega-3 Index (O3I) reflects the relative percentage amount of EPA and DHA in erythrocyte membranes, and is considered a surrogate biomarker for cardiovascular events [79]. Cao et al. investigated in individuals with low baseline n3-PUFA levels the effects of supplementation with fish oil or flaxseed oil upon O3I [80]. Cao found that supplementing 2.1 g/day FO (1296 mg EPA + 864 mg DHA) for eight weeks increased the O3I from 4.3% to 7.8% ($p < 0.001$), followed by a gradual decline to 5.7% and to 3.8% at 4 and 16 weeks after the end of the supplementation period, respectively. On the other hand, supplementation with flaxseed oil (3510 mg ALA + 900 mg LA/d) for the same period, in turn, did not significantly change the O3I, but it did increase not only EPA but also n3-docosapentaenoic acid (DPA) [80], a fatty acid that sits in between EPA and DHA in the elongation desaturation pathway.

It can be argued that the study of Cao et al. [80] did not cover a period of supplementation that would allow maximum incorporation and saturation of supplemented PUFAs into erythrocyte membranes, therefore not raising the O3I to its maximum achievable level. A O3I higher than 8% has been proposed to be favourable against cardiovascular events, whilst ≤ 4% is interpreted as low [24,79,81]. Accordingly, the benefits of ALA as a mitigator of cardiometabolic events can be supported by its role as a substrate for EPA. The latter is a well-known element against pro-inflammatory pathways in the cardiovascular system.

4.2.3. Soybean Oil

Despite having an obviously different fatty acid profile as compared to FO, soybean oil, unarguably, is a source of some ALA, and a few studies have already demonstrated a mild but relatively positive potential for soybean oil. For example, in treated hepatitis C patients ($n = 52$), 6000 mg/day FO or a soybean oil control for 12 weeks significantly decreased serum insulin levels (17.1 to 10.9 µIU/mL $p = 0.001$, 12.6 to 10.6 µIU/mL $p = 0.011$ for FO and soybean oil groups, respectively) and HOMA values (3.8 to 2.4 $p = 0.002$, 3.1 to 3.0 $p = 0.046$ for FO and soybean oil groups, respectively) when comparing baseline versus end-of-intervention. The FO group was clearly more efficient; however, differences between both groups ($p = 0.016$ for insulin levels and $p = 0.015$ for HOMA-IR values) have been observed [82].

In a small controlled clinical trial recruiting 16 hypercholesterolaemic women in a 10 weeks intervention, participants received an amount of soybean oil that consisted of 20% of their energy intake in a weight-maintaining diet with <300 mg/day of cholesterol [83]. The control group consisted of the same participants in a weight-maintaining diet with <300 mg/day of cholesterol for eight weeks but no soybean oil. As compared to the eight-week control period, TC, HDL-C, LDL-C and small dense low-density lipoprotein-cholesterol (sdLDL-C) levels were reduced at the end of the 10 week-soybean oil intervention period [83]. Furthermore, the sdLDL oxidation lag time was reduced after soybean oil consumption. In addition to the unfavourable cardiovascular conditions of maintaining low HDL-C levels, the former is linked to the pathophysiology of atherosclerotic disease due to the damage potential of sdLDL-C subclasses, especially in their oxidised form, on arterial structures [6].

4.2.4. Rapeseed Oil

In a meta-analysis of 27 RCTs [84], consumption of rapeseed oil was associated with reductions of approximately 7.24 mg/dL in TC (95% CI, −12.1 to −2.7) and of approximately 6.4 mg/dL in LDL-C (95% CI, −10.8 to −2) serum levels, as compared to sunflower oil and saturated fat. No changes were observed in TG nor HDL-C. Overall, the daily dose of rapeseed oil ranged from 12 to 50 g for 21 to 180 days. Most trials in that meta-analysis addressed individuals with lipid disorders and patients with heart disease, type 2 diabetes mellitus, obesity, metabolic syndrome, or non-alcoholic fatty liver disease. Importantly, the trials were under isocaloric conditions and, thus, partially avoided the bias of weight loss and its relationship with amelioration of lipid indices [84]. A clinical trial study in well-controlled conditions, recruiting 10 healthy men aged 25.3 ± 1 years, found that 24 h lipid oxidation was more pronounced when the participants received rapeseed oil-enriched meals for the duration of the study, as compared to a matched meal enriched with palm oil, a source of saturated fat [85].

It is well known that replacing dietary saturated fats with monounsaturated fatty acids (MUFAs) and PUFAs can reduce overall mortality [86]. The United Kingdom Scientific Advisory Committee on Nutrition in 2019 concluded that the recommendation for the population average contribution of saturated fat to total calorie intake should remain at no more than 10% of total dietary intake, and that reducing intakes of saturated fats reduces the risk of cardiovascular and heart disease events [87].

The alleged cholesterol-lowering properties of rapeseed oil could be attributed not only to its ALA content, but also possibly combined with its MUFA composition. Approximately 56% of the total fatty acids in rapeseed oil are MUFAs, with oleic acid as the most abundant one, at 54.5% of the total fatty acids, approximately [88]. The abundance of oleic acid in rapeseed oil may support its beneficial properties, as it has been shown that oleic acid elicits improvement on lipids and lipoproteins, as well as reduced risk of cardiovascular disease in humans [89]. The ALA content in rapeseed oil, in turn, is estimated at approximately 6 to 10% of total fatty acids [59,90,91]. Interestingly however, a study found a much lower ALA content in rapeseed oil, $\approx$1.2% [92].

A critical interpretation of published studies will see that other plant sources of MUFAs and PUFAs may show positive results in comparison to rapeseed oil. For instance, the consumption of sesame oil was more favourable for glycaemic control markers when compared to rapeseed oil in a recent RCT recruiting individuals with type 2 diabetes mellitus [91]. In that study, rapeseed oil increased serum fasting blood glucose ($+7.72 \pm 3.15$ mg/dL, $p < 0.05$), whilst sesame oil decreased serum insulin (-6.00 ± 1.72 mIU/mL, $p < 0.05$) levels in a nine-week intervention period. The dietary recommendation was based on 30–32% of the total energy intake from fats but, despite the predominance of oil intake in each intervention, we noticed that the authors did not present in their study the exact or estimated amount of oil consumed. Some of the strengths of the study include its design, a triple-blind, cross-over clinical trial with 92 subjects completing all treatment periods, which were composed of four-week run-in and four-week wash-out periods based on sunflower oil.

4.3. Seaweed

4.3.1. Lipid Profile of Seaweed

The use of seaweed for cooking and as a food supplement is gaining more popularity worldwide [93,94]. As a functional food, seaweed is a vegetarian source of n3-PUFAs, protein, and micronutrients [95]. Spirulina and chlorella are commercially available biomass extracts of cyanobacteria and green algae respectively, designed to attend a growing demand [96]. Both spirulina and chlorella are often claimed to be valuable sources of n3-PUFAs; however, the accuracy of such statement needs to be clarified in context, as to obtain approximately 2 to 3 g of total lipids from these microalgae it is necessary to ingest approximately 28 g of it in its powdered form. The total lipid content can be practically zero in supplemental dosages (≈3 g/day) [59].

Chlorella minutissima UTEX 2219 and UTEX 2341 feature 3.3% and 31.3% EPA, respectively, of the total fatty acid content, but DHA was not detected in either strain [97]. In a fatty acid profile analysis of *Spirulina platensis* from seven commercially available products, EPA and DHA were detected in only two samples, contributing with 1.79% and 7.70%, and 2.28% and 2.88%, respectively, of the total fatty acids [98]. Similarly to flaxseed and nuts, whether the effects of dietary intervention with seaweed are attributed to its n3-PUFAs per se remain to be investigated, as the food matrix should be considered. *Spirulina* and *Chlorella* contain not only macro and micronutrients but also other compounds with antioxidant properties which may play a role in positive health outcomes [99–101].

4.3.2. Clinical Findings

A meta-analysis published in 2016 [102] found that in general the daily consumption of 1 to 10 g *Spirulina* led to significant improvements in lipid profile by reducing TC in ≈47 mg/dL (95% CI: −67.31 to −26.22), LDL-C in ≈41 mg/dL (95% CI: −60.62 to −22.03), TG in ≈44 mg/dL (95% CI: −50.22 to −38.24), whilst increasing HDL-C in ≈6 mg/dL (95% CI: 2.37–9.76). Seven placebo-controlled clinical trials with duration of 2–4 months were included in that meta-analysis, and the population appraised consisted of patients with diabetes, cardiac diseases, nephrotic syndrome and HIV infection, illnesses whose pathophysiologies are related to dyslipidaemia [103–105]. Seemingly, an effective and practical dose was about 4 g/day of *Spirulina*, which can be administered in capsules or powder [102]. Nevertheless, as discussed above, we believe that the n3-PUFAs content in *Spirulina* was not the sole player in yielding such outcomes.

Supplementation with 300 mg/day of *Chlorella* for 8 weeks decreased TNF-α levels, in comparison with the placebo group, in a RCT of 70 patients with NAFLD [106]. An 8 week-long RCT investigating 44 women suffering with primary dysmenorrhea and supplemented with 1500 mg/day *Chlorella* found a significant reduction in hs-CRP levels (from 2590.00 ± 1801.66 to 974.21 ± 292.85 ng/mL), as compared to the control group [107].

In a Japanese sample population, 40 daily tablets of *Chlorella* were provided to 17 individuals with borderline high fasting blood glucose, TC, and TG levels, as well as to 17 healthy individuals [108]. After 16 weeks of supplementation, the researchers found reductions in body fat percentage, serum TC, and fasting blood glucose levels in both groups [108]. In our view however, that study appears to show a few limitations that should be considered in the context of a broader clinical scenario. The researchers did not measure food intake, there was no matched control group, and body fat percentage was obtained through bioelectrical impedance, which as a method of body composition analysis has some limitations [109]. Lastly, *Chlorella* supplementation was used in an impracticable dosage that, although it may be tested, cannot be translated into a broader clinical recommendation. As 40 tablets were ingested together with a considerable volume of fluid every day, probably this posology in itself with fluid may have resulted in lower food intake due to stomach filling.

5. Population

Type 2 diabetes, obesity, dyslipidaemia and hypertension, conditions that we have attempted to address in the present study, are related to a pro-inflammatory state [110–113]. The evidence so far available suggests that the consumption of ALA-rich foodstuffs may attenuate the levels of inflammation-associated biomarkers. More importantly however, the consumption of ALA food sources appears to be associated with reduced incidence of cardiovascular events. Further long-term RCTs are imperative to further elucidate such preliminary findings.

In the context of liver diseases, NAFLD particularly, lifestyle improvement is a cornerstone in ameliorating the disease. We have identified studies that showed beneficial effects of ALA interventions in patients with NAFLD [71,84]. Accordingly, a favourable nutritional support based on ALA food sources could be considered in therapies for NAFLD patients in cases of low frequency of fatty fish intake or absence of FO supplementation.

Food sources of ALA may also be relevant during pregnancy and lactation due not only to their rich nutritional composition but also due to a thoroughly justified need to avoid complex herbal supplement mixtures that may jeopardize the health of the mother and of the child. Additionally, plant sources of n3-PUFAs could be seen as an option for pregnant women who do not tolerate fatty fish and for those who suffer with nausea and with hyperemesis gravidarum, relatively common manifestations during the gestational period [114,115]. The amount and profile of n3-PUFAs ingested by the lactating mother is paramount for infant health, as the mother's diet directly reflects upon her milk fatty acid profile [116].

Exclusively vegan diets are to be examined carefully due to the risk of n3-PUFAs deficiency. Apart from a lower intake of total and saturated fats, another characteristic of exclusively vegan diets is a higher proportional intake of n6-PUFAs, when compared to omnivorous and vegetarian diets [110,117]. For those reasons, recommendations for vegan diets that include appropriate amounts of ALA, necessarily combined with a balanced n3/n6 ratio, are paramount for the maintenance of long-term health.

It is widely accepted that peanut and peanut butter have been speculated by the layperson and by some health practitioners as friendly components of the exclusively vegan diet. Careful consideration however should be exercised regarding the amounts of peanut and peanut butter consumed, as a pilot study observed in 14 exercise-trained healthy individuals with an average age of 30 years that the daily consumption of approximately 103 g of peanut butter for 4 weeks led to changes in body composition, markedly increased body fat content [118]. Such results only confirm that careful calorie counting is pivotal when adding a new source of lipids to the diet plan, regardless of whether those are considered healthy food items. Furthermore, peanut is particularly rich in LA and virtually absent of ALA (Table 2).

6. Decision-Making Practice

A diet poor in n3-PUFAs and rich in n6-PUFAs in the long term leads to inflammation and increased risk of diseases, including cardiovascular diseases [119]. If the patient does not comply with a diet that includes fatty fish or FO supplements, ALA-rich foods are important to at least partially supply some of the n3 requirement, at the same time reducing the LA bioavailability. Furthermore, some individuals in society may choose not to adhere to food supplementation, be it because of added costs, dietary choices such as veganism and vegetarianism, the wish to avoid polypharmacy if they are already taking medicine tablets, or due to personal values. Such lifestyle choices and circumstances further emphasize the need for a careful nutritional planning that includes sources of n3-PUFAs.

Along those lines, some period supplementing FO and followed by some period incrementing plant sources of n3-PUFAs may be an example of what would be a "periodized" loading of n3 status. Such hypothesis can be sustained due to the incorporation of n3-PUFAs into cell membranes, which occurs over a few months after supplementation, whilst the period appears to be longer for decreasing n3 status than the progress of storage. In the case of the study of Cao et al. [80] for example, two months of FO supplementation was sufficient to almost achieve a reasonable n3 state, which was maintained by one month afterwards but returning to the same baseline level after 16 weeks of interruption. We believe that a "periodized" FO supplementation regimen could be conceivable two to three times a year for one to four months, followed with nutritional counselling and observing the intake of foodstuffs rich in ALA in the period without the FO supplementation, hoping to provide a better n3-DPA level. Nutritional advice however will always be tailored to the individual's needs and preferences, such as frequency of consumption of fatty fish and food sources of ALA, patient's income, and any coexisting morbidity. As nutritional strategy for individuals who, for one reason or another, do not eat fish nor take FO supplementation, adding in ALA-rich foods, e.g., flaxseed and chia seeds, or adding their oils within a dietary plan, alongside a careful consideration to dietary sources of n6-PUFAs, in itself seems to be paramount for long term overall health.

7. Perspectives

In the present study we focused on the effects of ALA found naturally in foodstuffs, seeds, nuts and oils, instead of isolated ALA supplementation. Further clinical research is urgently required to broaden the current knowledge of the potential of ALA upon cardiometabolic dysregulations and cardiometabolic protection. Well-designed RCTs could certainly minimize the residual confounding variables caused by other nutrients.

The limitations of our study, as well as of other studies that have investigated ALA cardiometabolic effects specifically, are many. Ultimately however, although the current study provides some insights in a real-world prescription-based intervention, we also encourage the execution of meta-analyses to expand the current knowledge of specific nutrients in specific populations, in an attempt to find ideal dose-responses, as well as to continuously update guidelines in nutrition and cardiology.

8. Conclusions

In case of suspected insufficient n3 status, such as in individuals with low intake of fatty fish, those who do not take FO supplement, and in vegan individuals with very narrow dietary habits, alternative plant sources of n3-PUFAs may be candidates for partially attending the n3 metabolic demands. Although plant sources of n3-PUFAs are less impactful on EPA and DHA levels, evidence suggests that those are foodstuffs positively associated with favourable cardiometabolic outcomes, which could be triggered by other plant components, in synergy with ALA. Not only ALA in isolation, but its proposed effect in combination with other plant fatty acids and other plant components such as fibre, potassium, magnesium, and non-essential substances, e.g., polyphenols and sterols, may be the players in yielding benefits in cardiovascular metabolism.

Consumption of walnuts and flaxseed seems to be the main plant sources of n3-PUFAs with strong scientific basis for translation into clinical practice. Regarding oil intake, we believe that flaxseed oil is more advantageous than walnut oil, because the former's ALA content is five times greater than that of the latter, which in turn, can be considered the second principal source of ALA. Although several studies have alluded to rapeseed and soybean oils as ALA sources, their ALA amount is slight when compared to flaxseed oil, so that a usual oil serving must be considered in order not to exceed the daily energy requirement in an attempt to achieve an optimal level of ALA. Regarding seaweed, *Spirulina* and *Chlorella* have gained attention but there are no discernible studies corroborating a relevant amount of n3-PUFAs in usual doses of supplementation. Seemingly, the benefits of seaweed over cardiometabolic markers appear to be driven by their antioxidant content.

The introduction of ALA-rich foods is a cornerstone for individuals looking for n3 sources beyond fish and fish oil. It is nevertheless of greatest concern that the proposal to increase the consumption of ALA ought to be integrated with a controlled calorie intake and controlled n6-PUFAs intake, since both of them can be raised concomitantly, thus ensuing in untoward effects such as increased fat mass and cardiometabolic dysregulations.

Supplementary Materials: The following are available online at http://www.mdpi.com/2072-6643/12/10/3159/s1, Table S1: Identification of RCTs that investigated the effects of nuts and seeds rich in ALA through the database search, Table S2: Identification of RCTs that investigated the effects of ALA-rich oils through the database search, Table S3: Identification of RCTs that investigated the effects of seaweed through the database search, Table S4: Identification of recent RCTs that investigated the effects of fish oil supplementation through the database search.

Author Contributions: Conceptualization, H.O.S.; methodology, H.O.S., J.C.P.; writing—original draft preparation, H.O.S.; funding acquisition, A.A.B.; supervision, A.A.B. All authors have read and agreed to the published version of the manuscript.

Funding: The authors are grateful to the University of Worcester for funding the publication fees.

Conflicts of Interest: The authors declare no conflict of interest.

References

1. Emerging Risk Factors Collaboration; Di Angelantonio, E.; Gao, P.; Pennells, L.; Kaptoge, S.; Caslake, M.; Thompson, A.; Butterworth, A.S.; Sarwar, N.; Wormser, D.; et al. Lipid-related markers and cardiovascular disease prediction. *JAMA* **2012**, *307*, 2499–2506. [PubMed]
2. Rapsomaniki, E.; Timmis, A.; George, J.; Pujades-Rodriguez, M.; Shah, A.D.; Denaxas, S.; White, I.R.; Caulfield, M.J.; E Deanfield, J.; Smeeth, L.; et al. Blood pressure and incidence of twelve cardiovascular diseases: Lifetime risks, healthy life-years lost, and age-specific associations in 1.25 million people. *Lancet* **2014**, *383*, 1899–1911. [CrossRef]
3. Santos, H.O.; Macedo, R.C.O. Cocoa-induced (Theobroma cacao) effects on cardiovascular system: HDL modulation pathways. *Clin. Nutr. ESPEN* **2018**, *27*, 10–15. [CrossRef] [PubMed]
4. Santos, H.O.; da Silva, G.A.R. To what extent does cinnamon administration improve the glycemic and lipid profiles? *Clin. Nutr. ESPEN* **2018**, *27*, 1–9. [CrossRef]
5. Santos, H.O.; Bueno, A.A.; Mota, J.F. The effect of artichoke on lipid profile: A review of possible mechanisms of action. *Pharmacol. Res.* **2018**, *137*, 170–178. [CrossRef] [PubMed]
6. Santos, H.O.; Earnest, C.P.; Tinsley, G.M.; Izidoro, L.F.M.; Macedo, R.C.O. Small dense low-density lipoprotein-cholesterol (sdLDL-C): Analysis, effects on cardiovascular endpoints and dietary strategies. *Prog. Cardiovasc. Dis.* **2020**, *63*, 503–509. [CrossRef]
7. Santos, H.O.; Kones, R.; Rumana, U.; Earnest, C.P.; Izidoro, L.F.M.; Macedo, R.C.O. Lipoprotein(a): Current Evidence for a Physiologic Role and the Effects of Nutraceutical Strategies. *Clin. Ther.* **2019**, *41*, 1780–1797. [CrossRef]
8. Wang, P.; Zhang, Q.; Hou, H.; Liu, Z.; Wang, L.; Rasekhmagham, R.; Kord-Varkaneh, H.; Santos, H.O.; Yao, G. The effects of pomegranate supplementation on biomarkers of inflammation and endothelial dysfunction: A meta-analysis and systematic review. *Complement. Ther. Med.* **2020**, *49*, 102358. [CrossRef]
9. Santos, H.O.; Genario, R.; Gomes, G.K.; Schoenfeld, B.J. Cherry intake as a dietary strategy in sport and diseases: A review of clinical applicability and mechanisms of action. *Crit. Rev. Food Sci. Nutr.* **2020**, 1–14. [CrossRef]
10. E Ramsden, C.; Zamora, D.; Majchrzak-Hong, S.; Faurot, K.R.; Broste, S.K.; Frantz, R.P.; Davis, J.M.; Ringel, A.; Suchindran, C.M.; Hibbeln, J.R. Re-evaluation of the traditional diet-heart hypothesis: Analysis of recovered data from Minnesota Coronary Experiment (1968–73). *BMJ* **2016**, *353*, i1246. [CrossRef]
11. Marklund, M.; Wu, J.H.; Imamura, F.; Del Gobbo, L.C.; Fretts, A.; De Goede, J.; Shi, P.; Tintle, N.; Wennberg, M.; Aslibekyan, S.; et al. Biomarkers of Dietary Omega-6 Fatty Acids and Incident Cardiovascular Disease and Mortality. *Circulation* **2019**, *139*, 2422–2436. [CrossRef] [PubMed]
12. Wu, J.H.Y.; Marklund, M.; Imamura, F.; Tintle, N.; Korat, A.V.A.; De Goede, J.; Zhou, X.; Yang, W.-S.; Otto, M.C.D.O.; Kröger, J.; et al. Omega-6 fatty acid biomarkers and incident type 2 diabetes: Pooled analysis of individual-level data for 39 740 adults from 20 prospective cohort studies. *Lancet Diabetes Endocrinol.* **2017**, *5*, 965–974. [CrossRef]
13. Skulas-Ray, A.C.; Wilson, P.W.; Harris, W.S.; Brinton, E.A.; Kris-Etherton, P.M.; Richter, C.K.; Jacobson, T.A.; Engler, M.B.; Miller, M.; Robinson, J.G.; et al. Omega-3 Fatty Acids for the Management of Hypertriglyceridemia: A Science Advisory From the American Heart Association. *Circulation* **2019**, *140*, e673–e691. [CrossRef] [PubMed]
14. Kris-Etherton, P.M.; Harris, W.S.; Appel, L.J. Fish consumption, fish oil, omega-3 fatty acids, and cardiovascular disease. *Circulation* **2002**, *106*, 2747–2757. [CrossRef] [PubMed]

15. Weylandt, K.H.; Serini, S.; Chen, Y.Q.; Su, H.M.; Lim, K.; Cittadini, A.; Calviello, G. Omega-3 Polyunsaturated Fatty Acids: The Way Forward in Times of Mixed Evidence. *BioMed Res. Int.* **2015**, *2015*, 143109. [CrossRef] [PubMed]
16. Sagara, M.; Njelekela, M.; Teramoto, T.; Taguchi, T.; Mori, M.; Armitage, L.; Birt, N.; Birt, C.; Yamori, Y. Effects of docosahexaenoic Acid supplementation on blood pressure, heart rate, and serum lipids in Scottish men with hypertension and hypercholesterolemia. *Int. J. Hypertens.* **2011**, *2011*, 809198. [CrossRef]
17. Manger, M.S.; Strand, E.; Ebbing, M.; Seifert, R.; Refsum, H.; Nordrehaug, J.E.; Nilsen, D.W.; A Drevon, C.; Tell, G.S.; Øyvind, B.; et al. Dietary intake of n-3 long-chain polyunsaturated fatty acids and coronary events in Norwegian patients with coronary artery disease. *Am. J. Clin. Nutr.* **2010**, *92*, 244–251. [CrossRef]
18. Abdelhamid, A.S.; Brown, T.J.; Brainard, J.S.; Biswas, P.; Thorpe, G.C.; Moore, H.J.; Deane, K.H.; Summerbell, C.D.; Worthington, H.V.; Song, F.; et al. Omega-3 fatty acids for the primary and secondary prevention of cardiovascular disease. *Cochrane Database Syst. Rev.* **2018**, *7*, CD003177.
19. Hilborn, R.; Amoroso, R.O.; Anderson, C.M.; Baum, J.K.; Branch, T.A.; Costello, C.; De Moor, C.L.; Faraj, A.; Hively, D.; Jensen, O.P.; et al. Effective fisheries management instrumental in improving fish stock status. *Proc. Natl. Acad. Sci. USA* **2020**, *117*, 2218–2224. [CrossRef]
20. Jackson, J.B. The future of the oceans past. *Philos. Trans. R. Soc. B Biol. Sci.* **2010**, *365*, 3765–3778. [CrossRef]
21. Moher, D.; Liberati, A.; Tetzlaff, J.; Altman, D.G.; Prisma Group. Preferred reporting items for systematic reviews and meta-analyses: The PRISMA statement. *PLoS Med.* **2009**, *6*, e1000097. [CrossRef]
22. Anderson, B.M.; Ma, D.W. Are all n-3 polyunsaturated fatty acids created equal? *Lipids Health Dis.* **2009**, *8*, 33. [CrossRef] [PubMed]
23. Rapoport, S.I.; Rao, J.S.; Igarashi, M. Brain metabolism of nutritionally essential polyunsaturated fatty acids depends on both the diet and the liver. *Prostaglandins Leukot. Essent. Fat. Acids* **2007**, *77*, 251–261. [CrossRef] [PubMed]
24. Stark, K.D.; Van Elswyk, M.E.; Higgins, M.R.; Weatherford, C.A.; Salem, N., Jr. Global survey of the omega-3 fatty acids, docosahexaenoic acid and eicosapentaenoic acid in the blood stream of healthy adults. *Prog. Lipid Res.* **2016**, *63*, 132–152. [CrossRef] [PubMed]
25. Burdge, G.C. Metabolism of alpha-linolenic acid in humans. *Prostaglandins Leukot. Essent. Fat. Acids* **2006**, *75*, 161–168. [CrossRef] [PubMed]
26. Pawlosky, R.J.; Hibbeln, J.R.; Novotny, J.A.; Salem, N., Jr. Physiological compartmental analysis of alpha-linolenic acid metabolism in adult humans. *J. Lipid Res.* **2001**, *42*, 1257–1265.
27. Plourde, M.; Cunnane, S.C. Extremely limited synthesis of long chain polyunsaturates in adults: Implications for their dietary essentiality and use as supplements. *Appl. Physiol. Nutr. Metab.* **2007**, *32*, 619–634. [CrossRef]
28. Lin, Y.H.; Llanos, A.; Mena, P.; Uauy, R.; Salem, N.; Jr Pawlosky, R.J. Compartmental analyses of 2H5-alpha-linolenic acid and C-U-eicosapentaenoic acid toward synthesis of plasma labeled 1, 6n-3 in newborn term infants. *Am. J. Clin. Nutr.* **2010**, *92*, 284–293. [CrossRef]
29. Lin, Y.H.; Salem, N., Jr. Whole body distribution of deuterated linoleic and alpha-linolenic acids and their metabolites in the rat. *J. Lipid Res.* **2007**, *48*, 2709–2724. [CrossRef]
30. Wada, M.; Delong, C.J.; Hong, Y.H.; Rieke, C.J.; Song, I.; Sidhu, R.S.; Yuan, C.; Warnock, M.; Schmaier, A.H.; Yokoyama, C.; et al. Enzymes and receptors of prostaglandin pathways with arachidonic acid-derived versus eicosapentaenoic acid-derived substrates and products. *J. Biol. Chem.* **2007**, *282*, 22254–22266. [CrossRef]
31. Kromhout, D.; Yasuda, S.; Geleijnse, J.M.; Shimokawa, H. Fish oil and omega-3 fatty acids in cardiovascular disease: Do they really work? *Eur. Heart J.* **2012**, *33*, 436–443. [CrossRef] [PubMed]
32. Back, M. Omega-3 fatty acids in atherosclerosis and coronary artery disease. *Future Sci. OA* **2017**, *3*, FSO236. [CrossRef] [PubMed]
33. Fischer, R.; Konkel, A.; Mehling, H.; Blossey, K.; Gapelyuk, A.; Wessel, N.; Von Schacky, C.; Dechend, R.; Muller, D.N.; Rothe, M.; et al. Dietary omega-3 fatty acids modulate the eicosanoid profile in man primarily via the CYP-epoxygenase pathway. *J. Lipid Res.* **2014**, *55*, 1150–1164. [CrossRef] [PubMed]
34. Balogun, K.A.; Cheema, S.K. Cardioprotective Role of Omega-3 Polyunsaturated Fatty Acids Through the Regulation of Lipid Metabolism. In *Pathophysiology and Pharmacotherapy of Cardiovascular Disease*; Adis: Cham, Switzerland, 2015; pp. 563–588.

35. Micha, R.; Khatibzadeh, S.; Shi, P.; Fahimi, S.; Lim, S.; Andrews, K.G.; Engell, R.E.; Powles, J.; Ezzati, M.; Mozaffarian, D.; et al. Global, regional, and national consumption levels of dietary fats and oils in 1990 and 2010: A systematic analysis including 266 country-specific nutrition surveys. *BMJ* **2014**, *348*, g2272. [CrossRef] [PubMed]
36. Blasbalg, T.L.; Hibbeln, J.R.; Ramsden, C.E.; Majchrzak, S.F.; Rawlings, R.R. Changes in consumption of omega-3 and omega-6 fatty acids in the United States during the 20th century. *Am. J. Clin. Nutr.* **2011**, *93*, 950–962. [CrossRef] [PubMed]
37. Hibbeln, J.R.; Nieminen, L.R.; Blasbalg, T.L.; Riggs, J.A.; Lands, W.E. Healthy intakes of n-3 and n-6 fatty acids: Estimations considering worldwide diversity. *Am. J. Clin. Nutr.* **2006**, *83*, 1483S–1493S. [CrossRef]
38. Cranmer-Byng, M.M.; Liddle, D.M.; De Boer, A.A.; Monk, J.M.; Robinson, L.E. Proinflammatory effects of arachidonic acid in a lipopolysaccharide-induced inflammatory microenvironment in 3T3-L1 adipocytes in vitro. *Appl. Physiol. Nutr. Metab.* **2015**, *40*, 142–154. [CrossRef]
39. Zivkovic, A.M.; Telis, N.; German, J.B.; Hammock, B.D. Dietary omega-3 fatty acids aid in the modulation of inflammation and metabolic health. *Calif. Agric.* **2011**, *65*, 106–111. [CrossRef]
40. Francis, A.A.; Deniset, J.F.; Austria, J.A.; Lavalleé, R.K.; Maddaford, G.G.; Hedley, T.E.; Dibrov, E.; Pierce, G.N. Effects of dietary flaxseed on atherosclerotic plaque regression. *Am. J. Physiol. Circ. Physiol.* **2013**, *304*, H1743–H1751. [CrossRef]
41. Dupasquier, C.M.C.; Dibrov, E.; Kneesh, A.L.; Cheung, P.K.M.; Lee, K.G.Y.; Alexander, H.K.; Yeganeh, B.K.; Moghadasian, M.H.; Pierce, G.N. Dietary flaxseed inhibits atherosclerosis in the LDL receptor-deficient mouse in part through antiproliferative and anti-inflammatory actions. *Am. J. Physiol. Circ. Physiol.* **2007**, *293*, H2394–H2402. [CrossRef]
42. Li, G.; Wang, X.; Yang, H.; Zhang, P.; Wu, F.; Li, Y.; Zhou, Y.; Zhang, X.; Ma, H.; Zhang, W.; et al. alpha-Linolenic acid but not linolenic acid protects against hypertension: Critical role of SIRT3 and autophagic flux. *Cell Death Dis.* **2020**, *11*, 83. [CrossRef] [PubMed]
43. Ren, J.; Chung, S.H. Anti-inflammatory effect of alpha-linolenic acid and its mode of action through the inhibition of nitric oxide production and inducible nitric oxide synthase gene expression via NF-kappaB and mitogen-activated protein kinase pathways. *J. Agric. Food Chem.* **2007**, *55*, 5073–5080. [CrossRef] [PubMed]
44. Calvo, M.J.; Martínez, M.S.; Torres, W.; Chávez-Castillo, M.; Luzardo, E.; Villasmil, N.; Salazar, J.; Velasco, M.; Bermúdez, V. Omega-3 polyunsaturated fatty acids and cardiovascular health: A molecular view into structure and function. *Vessel Plus* **2017**, *1*, 116–128. [CrossRef]
45. Backes, J.; Anzalone, D.; Hilleman, D.; Catini, J. The clinical relevance of omega-3 fatty acids in the management of hypertriglyceridemia. *Lipids Health Dis.* **2016**, *15*, 118. [CrossRef]
46. Zuniga, J.; Cancino, M.; Medina, F.; Varela, P.; Vargas, R.; Tapia, G.; Videla, L.A.; Fernández, V. N-3 PUFA supplementation triggers PPAR-alpha activation and PPAR-alpha/NF-kappaB interaction: Anti-inflammatory implications in liver ischemia-reperfusion injury. *PLoS ONE* **2011**, *6*, e28502. [CrossRef]
47. Hardwick, J.P.; Osei-Hyiaman, D.; Wiland, H.; Abdelmegeed, M.A.; Song, B.J. PPAR/RXR Regulation of Fatty Acid Metabolism and Fatty Acid omega-Hydroxylase (CYP4) Isozymes: Implications for Prevention of Lipotoxicity in Fatty Liver Disease. *PPAR Res.* **2009**, *2009*, 952734. [CrossRef]
48. Jump, D.B.; Lytle, K.A.; Depner, C.M.; Tripathy, S. Omega-3 polyunsaturated fatty acids as a treatment strategy for nonalcoholic fatty liver disease. *Pharmacol. Ther.* **2018**, *181*, 108–125. [CrossRef]
49. Reynolds, A.; Mann, J.; Cummings, J.; Winter, N.; Mete, E.; Te Morenga, L. Carbohydrate quality and human health: A series of systematic reviews and meta-analyses. *Lancet* **2019**, *393*, 434–445. [CrossRef]
50. Del Bo, C.; Bernardi, S.; Marino, M.; Porrini, M.; Tucci, M.; Guglielmetti, S.; Cherubini, A.; Carrieri, B.; Kirkup, B.M.; Kroon, P.A.; et al. Systematic Review on Polyphenol Intake and Health Outcomes: Is there Sufficient Evidence to Define a Health-Promoting Polyphenol-Rich Dietary Pattern? *Nutrients* **2019**, *11*, 1355.
51. Ros, E.; Hu, F.B. Consumption of plant seeds and cardiovascular health: Epidemiological and clinical trial evidence. *Circulation* **2013**, *128*, 553–565. [CrossRef]
52. Anderson, J.J.; Kruszka, B.; Delaney, J.A.; He, K.; Burke, G.L.; Alonso, A.; Bild, D.E.; Budoff, M.; Michos, E.D. Calcium Intake From Diet and Supplements and the Risk of Coronary Artery Calcification and its Progression Among Older Adults: 10-Year Follow-up of the Multi-Ethnic Study of Atherosclerosis (MESA). *J. Am. Hear. Assoc.* **2016**, *5*, e003815. [CrossRef] [PubMed]

53. Budoff, M.J.; Young, R.; Burke, G.L.; Carr, J.J.; Detrano, R.; Folsom, A.R.; Kronmal, R.; Lima, J.A.C.; Liu, K.; McClelland, R.L.; et al. Ten-year association of coronary artery calcium with atherosclerotic cardiovascular disease (ASCVD) events: The multi-ethnic study of atherosclerosis (MESA). *Eur. Heart J.* **2018**, *39*, 2401–2408. [CrossRef] [PubMed]
54. Kanbay, M.; Bayram, Y.; Solak, Y.; Sanders, P.W. Dietary potassium: A key mediator of the cardiovascular response to dietary sodium chloride. *J. Am. Soc. Hypertens.* **2013**, *7*, 395–400. [CrossRef] [PubMed]
55. Reid, I.R.; Birstow, S.M.; Bolland, M.J. Calcium and Cardiovascular Disease. *Endocrinol. Metab.* **2017**, *32*, 339–349. [CrossRef]
56. Rosique-Esteban, N.; Guasch-Ferre, M.; Hernandez-Alonso, P.; Salas-Salvado, J. Dietary Magnesium and Cardiovascular Disease: A Review with Emphasis in Epidemiological Studies. *Nutrients* **2018**, *10*, 168. [CrossRef]
57. Zhubi-Bakija, F.; Bajraktari, G.; Bytyçi, I.; Mikhailidis, D.P.; Henein, M.Y.; Latkovskis, G.; Rexhaj, Z.; Zhubi, E.; Banach, M.; Alnouri, F.; et al. The impact of type of dietary protein, animal versus vegetable, in modifying cardiometabolic risk factors: A position paper from the International Lipid Expert Panel (ILEP). *Clin. Nutr.* **2020**. [CrossRef]
58. Shan, Z.; Guo, Y.; Hu, F.B.; Liu, L.; Qi, Q. Association of Low-Carbohydrate and Low-Fat Diets with Mortality Among US Adults. *JAMA Intern. Med.* **2020**, *180*, 513. [CrossRef]
59. United States Department of Agriculture. *USDA National Nutrient Database for Standard Reference*; USDA: Washington, DC, USA, 2015.
60. Institute of Medicine FaNB. *Dietary Reference intakes for Energy, Carbohydrate, Fiber, Fat, Fatty Acids, Cholesterol, Protein, and Amino Acids (Macronutrients)*; National Academy Press: Washington, DC, USA, 2005.
61. Yang, L.; Guo, Z.; Qi, S.; Fang, T.; Zhu, H.; Santos, H.O.; Wong, C.H.; Qiu, Z. Walnut intake may increase circulating adiponectin and leptin levels but does not improve glycemic biomarkers: A systematic review and meta-analysis of randomized clinical trials. *Complement. Ther. Med.* **2020**, *52*, 102505. [CrossRef]
62. Fang, Z.; Dang, M.; Zhang, W.; Wang, Y.; Kord-Varkaneh, H.; Nazary-Vannani, A.; Santos, H.O.; Tan, S.C.; Clark, C.C.; Zanghelini, F.; et al. Effects of walnut intake on anthropometric characteristics: A systematic review and dose-response meta-analysis of randomized controlled trials. *Complement. Ther. Med.* **2020**, *50*, 102395. [CrossRef]
63. Domènech, M.; Serra-Mir, M.; Roth, I.; Freitas-Simoes, T.; Valls-Pedret, C.; Cofán, M.; López, A.; Sala-Vila, A.; Calvo, C.; Rajaram, S.; et al. Effect of a Walnut Diet on Office and 24-Hour Ambulatory Blood Pressure in Elderly Individuals. *Hypertension* **2019**, *73*, 1049–1057. [CrossRef]
64. Peixoto, A.J. Practical Aspects of Home and Ambulatory Blood Pressure Monitoring. *Methodist DeBakey Cardiovasc. J.* **2015**, *11*, 214–218. [CrossRef] [PubMed]
65. Li, J.; Jiang, B.; HOS Santos, D.; Singh, A.; Wang, L. Effects of walnut intake on blood pressure: A systematic review and meta-analysis of randomized controlled trials. *Phytother. Res.* **2020**. [CrossRef] [PubMed]
66. Le, T.; Flatt, S.W.; Natarajan, L.; Pakiz, B.; Quintana, E.L.; Heath, D.D.; Rana, B.K.; Rock, C.L. Effects of Diet Composition and Insulin Resistance Status on Plasma Lipid Levels in a Weight Loss Intervention in Women. *J. Am. Hear. Assoc.* **2016**, *5*, e002771. [CrossRef]
67. Fatahi, S.; Haghighatdoost, F.; Larijani, B.; Azadbakht, L. Effect of Weight Reduction Diets Containing Fish, Walnut or Fish plus Walnut on Cardiovascular Risk Factors in Overweight and Obese Women. *Arch. Iran. Med.* **2019**, *22*, 574–583. [PubMed]
68. Khandouzi, N.; Zahedmehr, A.; Mohammadzadeh, A.; Sanati, H.R.; Nasrollahzadeh, J. Effect of flaxseed consumption on flow-mediated dilation and inflammatory biomarkers in patients with coronary artery disease: A randomized controlled trial. *Eur. J. Clin. Nutr.* **2019**, *73*, 258–265. [CrossRef] [PubMed]
69. Rahimlou, M.; Jahromi, N.B.; Hasanyani, N.; Ahmadi, A.R. Effects of Flaxseed Interventions on Circulating Inflammatory Biomarkers: A Systematic Review and Meta-Analysis of Randomized Controlled Trials. *Adv. Nutr.* **2019**, *10*, 1108–1119. [CrossRef] [PubMed]
70. Haidari, F.; Banaei-Jahromi, N.; Zakerkish, M.; Ahmadi, K. The effects of flaxseed supplementation on metabolic status in women with polycystic ovary syndrome: A randomized open-labeled controlled clinical trial. *Nutr. J.* **2020**, *19*, 8. [CrossRef]
71. Yari, Z.; Cheraghpour, M.; Alavian, S.M.; Hedayati, M.; Eini-Zinab, H.; Hekmatdoost, A. The efficacy of flaxseed and hesperidin on non-alcoholic fatty liver disease: An open-labeled randomized controlled trial. *Eur. J. Clin. Nutr.* **2020**, 1–13. [CrossRef]

72. Yari, Z.; Cheraghpour, M.; Hekmatdoost, A. Flaxseed and/or hesperidin supplementation in metabolic syndrome: An open-labeled randomized controlled trial. *Eur. J. Nutr.* **2020**, 1–12. [CrossRef]
73. Alves, A.Q.; Da Silva, V.A.; Góes, A.J.S.; Silva, M.S.; De Oliveira, G.G.; Bastos, I.V.G.A.; Neto, A.G.D.C.; Alves, A.J. The Fatty Acid Composition of Vegetable Oils and Their Potential Use in Wound Care. *Adv. Ski. Wound Care.* **2019**, *32*, 1–8. [CrossRef]
74. Kim, J.; Kim, D.N.; Lee, S.H.; Yoo, S.H.; Lee, S. Correlation of fatty acid composition of vegetable oils with rheological behaviour and oil uptake. *Food Chem.* **2010**, *118*, 398–402. [CrossRef]
75. Akrami, A.; Makiabadi, E.; Askarpour, M.; Zamani, K.; Hadi, A.; Mokari-Yamchi, A.; Babajafari, S.; Faghih, S.; Hojhabrimanesh, A. A Comparative Study of the Effect of Flaxseed Oil and Sunflower Oil on the Coagulation Score, Selected Oxidative and Inflammatory Parameters in Metabolic Syndrome Patients. *Clin. Nutr. Res.* **2020**, *9*, 63–72. [CrossRef] [PubMed]
76. Jamilian, M.; Tabassi, Z.; Reiner, Ž.; Panahandeh, I.; Naderi, F.; Aghadavood, E.; Amirani, E.; Taghizadeh, M.; Shafabakhsh, R.; Satari, M.; et al. The effects of n-3 fatty acids from flaxseed oil on genetic and metabolic profiles in patients with gestational diabetes mellitus: A randomised, double-blind, placebo-controlled trial. *Br. J. Nutr.* **2020**, *123*, 792–799. [CrossRef] [PubMed]
77. Joris, P.J.; Draijer, R.; Fuchs, D.; Mensink, R.P. Effect of alpha-linolenic acid on vascular function and metabolic risk markers during the fasting and postprandial phase: A randomized placebo-controlled trial in untreated (pre-)hypertensive individuals. *Clin. Nutr.* **2020**, *39*, 2413–2419. [CrossRef]
78. Jani, B.; Rajkumar, C. Ageing and vascular ageing. *Postgrad. Med. J.* **2006**, *82*, 357–362. [CrossRef]
79. Harris, W.S.; Sands, S.A.; Windsor, S.L.; Ali, H.A.; Stevens, T.L.; Magalski, A.; Porter, C.B.; Borkon, A.M. Omega-3 fatty acids in cardiac biopsies from heart transplantation patients: Correlation with erythrocytes and response to supplementation. *Circulation* **2004**, *110*, 1645–1649. [CrossRef]
80. Cao, J.; Schwichtenberg, K.A.; Hanson, N.Q.; Tsai, M.Y. Incorporation and clearance of omega-3 fatty acids in erythrocyte membranes and plasma phospholipids. *Clin. Chem.* **2006**, *52*, 2265–2272. [CrossRef]
81. Hals, P.A.; Wang, X.; Piscitelli, F.; Di Marzo, V.; Xiao, Y.F. The time course of erythrocyte membrane fatty acid concentrations during and after treatment of non-human primates with increasing doses of an omega-3 rich phospholipid preparation derived from krill-oil. *Lipids Health Dis.* **2017**, *16*, 16. [CrossRef] [PubMed]
82. Freire, T.O.; Boulhosa, R.S.S.B.; Oliveira, L.P.M.; De Jesus, R.P.; Cavalcante, L.N.; Lemaire, D.C.; Toralles, M.B.P.; Lyra, L.G.C.; Lyra, A.C. n-3 polyunsaturated fatty acid supplementation reduces insulin resistance in hepatitis C virus infected patients: A randomised controlled trial. *J. Hum. Nutr. Diet.* **2016**, *29*, 345–353. [CrossRef] [PubMed]
83. Utarwuthipong, T.; Komindr, S.; Pakpeankitvatana, V.; Songchitsomboon, S.; Thongmuang, N. Small dense low-density lipoprotein concentration and oxidative susceptibility changes after consumption of soybean oil, rice bran oil, palm oil and mixed rice bran/palm oil in hypercholesterolaemic women. *J. Int. Med. Res.* **2009**, *37*, 96–104. [CrossRef] [PubMed]
84. Ghobadi, S.; Hassanzadeh-Rostami, Z.; Mohammadian, F.; Zare, M.; Faghih, S. Effects of Canola Oil Consumption on Lipid Profile: A Systematic Review and Meta-Analysis of Randomized Controlled Clinical Trials. *J. Am. Coll. Nutr.* **2019**, *38*, 185–196. [CrossRef]
85. Yajima, K.; Iwayama, K.; Ogata, H.; Park, I.; Tokuyama, K. Meal rich in rapeseed oil increases 24-h fat oxidation more than meal rich in palm oil. *PLoS ONE* **2018**, *13*, e0198858. [CrossRef] [PubMed]
86. Wang, D.D.; Li, Y.; Chiuve, S.E.; Stampfer, M.J.; Manson, J.E.; Rimm, E.B.; Willett, W.C.; Hu, F.B. Association of Specific Dietary Fats with Total and Cause-Specific Mortality. *JAMA Intern. Med.* **2016**, *176*, 1134–1145. [CrossRef] [PubMed]
87. The Scientific Advisory Committee on Nutrition. *Saturated Fats and Health: SACN Report*; SACN: Vissenbjerg, Denmark, 2019.
88. Vehovský, K.; Stupka, R.; Zadinová, K.; Šprysl, M.; Okrouhlá, M.; Lebedová, N.; Mlyneková, E.; Čítek, J. Effect of dietary rapeseed and soybean oil on growth performance, carcass traits, and fatty acid composition of pigs. *Rev. Bras. Zootec.* **2019**, *48*, 48. [CrossRef]
89. Bowen, K.J.; Kris-Etherton, P.; West, S.G.; A Fleming, J.; Connelly, P.W.; Lamarche, B.; Couture, P.; A Jenkins, D.J.; Taylor, C.G.; Zahradka, P.; et al. Diets Enriched with Conventional or High-Oleic Acid Canola Oils Lower Atherogenic Lipids and Lipoproteins Compared to a Diet with a Western Fatty Acid Profile in Adults with Central Adiposity. *J. Nutr.* **2019**, *149*, 471–478. [CrossRef]

90. Zambiazi, R.C.; Przybylski, R.; Zambiazi, M.W.; Mendonça, C.B. Fatty acid composition of vegetable oils and fats. *Bol. Cent. Pesqui. Process. Aliment.* **2007**, *25*, 111–120.
91. Raeisi-Dehkordi, H.; Amiri, M.; Zimorovat, A.; Moghtaderi, F.; Zarei, S.; Forbes, S.C.; Salehi-Abargouei, A. The effects of canola oil compared with sesame and sesame-canola oil on glycemic control and liver function enzymes in patients with type 2 diabetes: A 3-way randomized triple-blind cross-over clinical trial. *Diabetes/Metab. Res. Rev.* **2020**, e3399. [CrossRef]
92. Orsavova, J.; Misurcova, L.; Ambrozova, J.V.; Vicha, R.; Mlcek, J. Fatty Acids Composition of Vegetable Oils and Its Contribution to Dietary Energy Intake and Dependence of Cardiovascular Mortality on Dietary Intake of Fatty Acids. *Int. J. Mol. Sci.* **2015**, *16*, 12871–12890. [CrossRef]
93. Khan, M.I.; Shin, J.H.; Kim, J.D. The promising future of microalgae: Current status, challenges, and optimization of a sustainable and renewable industry for biofuels, feed, and other products. *Microb. Cell Factories* **2018**, *17*, 36. [CrossRef]
94. Kent, M.; Welladsen, H.M.; Mangott, A.; Li, Y. Nutritional evaluation of Australian microalgae as potential human health supplements. *PLoS ONE* **2015**, *10*, e0118985. [CrossRef]
95. Panahi, Y.; Darvishi, B.; Jowzi, N.; Beiraghdar, F.; Sahebkar, A. Chlorella vulgaris: A Multifunctional Dietary Supplement with Diverse Medicinal Properties. *Curr. Pharm. Des.* **2016**, *22*, 164–173. [CrossRef] [PubMed]
96. Andrade, L.M.; Andrade, C.J.; Dias, M.; Nascimento, C.A.O.; Mendes, M.A. Chlorella and spirulina microalgae as sources of functional foods, nutraceuticals, and food supplements; an overview. *MOJ Food Process. Technol.* **2018**, *6*, 45–58. [CrossRef]
97. Vazhappilly, R.; Chen, F. Eicosapentaenoic Acid and Docosahexaenoic Acid Production Potential of Microalgae and Their Heterotrophic Growth. *J. Am. Oil Chem. Soc.* **1998**, *75*, 393–397. [CrossRef]
98. Diraman, H.; Koru, E.; Dibeklioglu, H. Fatty Acid Profile of Spirulina platensis Used as a Food Supplement. *Isr. J. Aquac.* **2009**, *61*, 134–142.
99. Deng, R.; Chow, T.J. Hypolipidemic, antioxidant, and antiinflammatory activities of microalgae Spirulina. *Cardiovasc. Ther.* **2010**, *28*, e33–e45. [CrossRef]
100. Lee, S.H.; Kang, H.J.; Lee, H.J.; Kang, M.H.; Park, Y.K. Six-week supplementation with Chlorella has favorable impact on antioxidant status in Korean male smokers. *Nutrition* **2010**, *26*, 175–183. [CrossRef]
101. Dartsch, P.C. Antioxidant potential of selected Spirulina platensis preparations. *Phytother. Res.* **2008**, *22*, 627–633. [CrossRef]
102. Serban, M.-C.; Sahebkar, A.; Dragan, S.; Stoichescu-Hogea, G.; Ursoniu, S.; Andrica, F.; Banach, M. A systematic review and meta-analysis of the impact of Spirulina supplementation on plasma lipid concentrations. *Clin. Nutr.* **2016**, *35*, 842–851. [CrossRef]
103. Goldberg, I.J. Clinical review 124: Diabetic dyslipidemia: Causes and consequences. *J. Clin. Endocrinol. Metab.* **2001**, *86*, 965–971. [CrossRef]
104. Lo, J. Dyslipidemia and lipid management in HIV-infected patients. *Curr. Opin. Endocrinol. Diabetes Obes.* **2011**, *18*, 144–147. [CrossRef]
105. Mikolasevic, I.; Zutelija, M.; Mavrinac, V.; Orlic, L. Dyslipidemia in patients with chronic kidney disease: Etiology and management. *Int. J. Nephrol. Renov. Dis.* **2017**, *10*, 35–45. [CrossRef] [PubMed]
106. Ebrahimi-Mameghani, M.; Sadeghi, Z.; Abbasalizad Farhangi, M.; Vaghef-Mehrabany, E.; Aliashrafi, S. Glucose homeostasis, insulin resistance and inflammatory biomarkers in patients with non-alcoholic fatty liver disease: Beneficial effects of supplementation with microalgae Chlorella vulgaris: A double-blind placebo-controlled randomized clinical trial. *Clin. Nutr.* **2017**, *36*, 1001–1006. [CrossRef] [PubMed]
107. Haidari, F.; Homayouni, F.; Helli, B.; Haghighizadeh, M.H.; Farahmandpour, F. Effect of chlorella supplementation on systematic symptoms and serum levels of prostaglandins, inflammatory and oxidative markers in women with primary dysmenorrhea. *Eur. J. Obstet. Gynecol. Reprod. Biol.* **2018**, *229*, 185–189. [CrossRef]
108. Mizoguchi, T.; Takehara, I.; Masuzawa, T.; Saito, T.; Naoki, Y. Nutrigenomic studies of effects of Chlorella on subjects with high-risk factors for lifestyle-related disease. *J. Med. Food* **2008**, *11*, 395–404. [CrossRef] [PubMed]
109. Khalil, S.F.; Mohktar, M.S.; Ibrahim, F. The theory and fundamentals of bioimpedance analysis in clinical status monitoring and diagnosis of diseases. *Sensors* **2014**, *14*, 10895–10928. [CrossRef]
110. Rogerson, D. Vegan diets: Practical advice for athletes and exercisers. *J. Int. Soc. Sports Nutr.* **2017**, *14*, 36. [CrossRef]

111. Ellulu, M.S.; Patimah, I.; Khaza'ai, H.; Rahmat, A.; Abed, Y. Obesity and inflammation: The linking mechanism and the complications. *Arch. Med. Sci.* **2017**, *13*, 851–863. [CrossRef]
112. Esteve, E.; Ricart, W.; Fernandez-Real, J.M. Dyslipidemia and inflammation: An evolutionary conserved mechanism. *Clin. Nutr.* **2005**, *24*, 16–31. [CrossRef]
113. Nishi, M.; Seki, M. Degree of infiltration and prognosis of early cancer of the stomach; with special reference to early cancer with elevated lesion. *Naika Intern. Med.* **1970**, *26*, 102–116.
114. Chan, R.L.; Olshan, A.F.; Savitz, D.A.; Herring, A.H.; Daniels, J.L.; Peterson, H.B.; Martin, S.L. Maternal influences on nausea and vomiting in early pregnancy. *Matern. Child Health J.* **2011**, *15*, 122–127. [CrossRef]
115. McCarthy, F.P.; Lutomski, J.E.; Greene, R.A. Hyperemesis gravidarum: Current perspectives. *Int. J. Women's Health* **2014**, *6*, 719–725.
116. Barrera, C.; Valenzuela, A.; Chamorro, R.; Bascuñán, K.; Sandoval, J.; Sabag, N.; Valenzuela, F.; Valencia, M.-P.; Puigrredon, C.; Valenzuela, A. The Impact of Maternal Diet during Pregnancy and Lactation on the Fatty Acid Composition of Erythrocytes and Breast Milk of Chilean Women. *Nutrients* **2018**, *10*, 839. [CrossRef] [PubMed]
117. Clarys, P.; Deliens, T.; Huybrechts, I.; Deriemaeker, P.; Vanaelst, B.; De Keyzer, W.; Hebbelinck, M.; Mullie, P. Comparison of nutritional quality of the vegan, vegetarian, semi-vegetarian, pesco-vegetarian and omnivorous diet. *Nutrients* **2014**, *6*, 1318–1332. [CrossRef] [PubMed]
118. Antonio, J.; Axelrod, C.; Ellerbroek, A.; Carson, C.; Burgess, V.; Silver, T.; Peacock, C.A. The Effect of Peanut Butter Overfeeding in Trained Men and Women: A Pilot Trial. *J. Exerc. Nutr.* **2018**, *1*, 5–6.
119. Russo, G.L. Dietary n-6 and n-3 polyunsaturated fatty acids: From biochemistry to clinical implications in cardiovascular prevention. *Biochem. Pharmacol.* **2009**, *77*, 937–946. [CrossRef] [PubMed]

Publisher's Note: MDPI stays neutral with regard to jurisdictional claims in published maps and institutional affiliations.

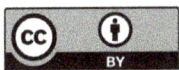

© 2020 by the authors. Licensee MDPI, Basel, Switzerland. This article is an open access article distributed under the terms and conditions of the Creative Commons Attribution (CC BY) license (http://creativecommons.org/licenses/by/4.0/).

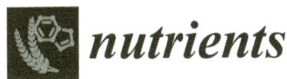

Article

Association between Three Low-Carbohydrate Diet Scores and Lipid Metabolism among Chinese Adults

Li-Juan Tan, Seong-Ah Kim and Sangah Shin *

Department of Food and Nutrition, Chung-Ang University, Gyeonggi-do 17546, Korea; tanlijuan88@cau.ac.kr (L.-J.T.); sakim8864@gmail.com (S.-A.K.)
* Correspondence: ivory8320@cau.ac.kr; Tel.: +82-31-670-3259; Fax: +82-31-675-1381

Received: 23 April 2020; Accepted: 29 April 2020; Published: 3 May 2020

Abstract: This study investigated the blood lipid levels of 5921 Chinese adults aged >18 years using data from the China Health and Nutrition Survey 2009. Diet information was collected through 3 day, 24 h recalls by trained professionals. The low-carbohydrate diet (LCD) score was determined according to the percentage of energy obtained from carbohydrate, protein, and fat consumption. Dyslipidemia was defined when one or more of the following abnormal lipid levels were observed: high cholesterol levels, high triglyceride levels, and low high-density lipoprotein cholesterol levels. Multivariate adjusted odds ratios (ORs) and their 95% confidence intervals (95% CIs) were calculated using logistic regression models. After adjusting the confounding variables, in males, the OR of hypercholesterolemia was 1.87 (95% CI, 1.23–2.85; p for trend = 0.0017) and the OR of hypertriglyceridemia was 1.47 (95% CI, 1.04–2.06; p for trend = 0.0336), on comparing the highest and lowest quartiles of the LCD score. The animal-based LCD score showed a similar trend. The OR of hypercholesterolemia was 2.15 (95% CI, 1.41–3.29; p for trend = 0.0006) and the OR of hypertriglyceridemia was 1.51 (95% CI, 1.09–2.10; p for trend = 0.0156). However, there was no significant difference between plant-based LCD scores and dyslipidemia. In females, lipid profiles did not differ much among the quartiles of LCD scores—only the animal-based LCD score was statistically significant with hypercholesterolemia. The OR of hypercholesterolemia was 1.64 (95% CI, 1.06–2.55), on comparing the highest and lowest quartiles of the LCD score. In conclusion, a higher LCD score, indicating lower carbohydrate intake and higher fat intake, especially animal-based fat, was significantly associated with higher odds of hypercholesterolemia and hypertriglyceridemia in Chinese males. Future studies investigating the potential mechanisms by which macronutrient types and sex hormones affect lipid metabolism are required.

Keywords: LCD score; CHNS; dyslipidemia; dietary factor; plant based; animal based; Chinese adults

1. Introduction

With an increasing prevalence worldwide, dyslipidemia has become a public health problem. Dyslipidemia is a well-known important risk factor for cardiovascular disease (CVD) and metabolic syndrome [1]. In 2012, the mortality rate of chronic non-communicable diseases in China was 533 per 100,000, including 272 deaths caused by cardiovascular and cerebrovascular diseases [2]. In the past 30 years, with rapid economic development and improvement in the standard of living in China, the blood lipid levels in the Chinese population have gradually increased, and the prevalence of dyslipidemia has increased significantly. In 2012, the prevalence of hypercholesterolemia was 4.9%, which is 69% higher than in 2002 (2.9%); the overall prevalence of dyslipidemia in Chinese adults was 40.4% in 2012, which was significantly higher than that in 2002 (18.6%) [2]. This indicates that the health care burden of dyslipidemia and its related diseases has consistently increased in the past decade.

Dyslipidemia is a disease characterized by elevated total cholesterol (TC) and/or triglyceride (TG) levels or a low high-density lipoprotein cholesterol (HDL-C) level, which contributes to the development of coronary heart disease and stroke [1]. According to the data reported by the Chinese Center for Disease Control and Prevention in 2015, 26.4% of ischemic heart disease cases in China are attributed to hypercholesterolemia, which is one component of dyslipidemia. Secondary dyslipidemia accounts for most dyslipidemia cases and is associated with lifestyle factors or medical conditions that interfere with blood lipid levels over time. Among these influencing factors, obesity (specifically abdominal obesity), alcohol consumption, and high-fat diets (specifically, high saturated and trans-fatty acid intakes) are well-known risk factors of dyslipidemia, as confirmed by several previous studies [3–5].

Carbohydrates significantly contribute to the total energy intake, particularly in the Chinese population who use rice and wheat as their staple food. At present, several studies have assessed the effect of carbohydrate intake on dyslipidemia [6–10]. Moreover, most of these studies have been conducted in European and American populations, and a few Asian studies have been conducted in the Korean population [9,10]. A study assessing the effect of carbohydrate intake on dyslipidemia in the Chinese native population has not been conducted yet.

The concept of and calculations to determine the low-carbohydrate diet (LCD) score have been introduced in detail previously [9,11,12]. In summary, participants with the highest scores have the lowest carbohydrate intakes. In 1992, the percentage of energy intake from carbohydrates in urban and rural residents in China was 66.2%, which decreased to 55.0% in 2012 according to The Report on the Status of Nutrition and Chronic Diseases of Chinese residents (2015). Therefore, it is of epidemiological value to study the effect of carbohydrate intake on dyslipidemia in the Chinese population. The present study used the low-carbohydrate diet (LCD) score to examine the association between LCD and dyslipidemia and its components in Chinese adults. Further, we identified the association by source foods (plant based and animal based).

2. Materials and Methods

2.1. Study Population

Data were obtained from the China Health and Nutrition Survey (CHNS), which used a multistage, random cluster sampling process to select samples from 15 provinces in China [13]. The sample scheme is reported in detail elsewhere [13]. Data on fasting blood glucose levels were first collected in 2009 (N = 9549). In the CHNS, the information was collected by trained interviewers to assure compliance and quality of data. The CHNS dataset and the Institutional Review Board information are available on the official website of the CHNS (https://www.cpc.unc.edu/projects/china). Participants provided written informed consent for inclusion in this study.

This study used one round of survey data from 2009. Participants aged less than 18 years (n = 1160) were excluded. Subsequently, we excluded 54 participants with insufficient blood sample data (i.e., TC, HDL-C, low-density lipoprotein cholesterol [LDL-C], TG, and fasting plasma glucose levels) and 22 participants with implausible energy intake (<800 kcal/day or >6000 kcal/day for males; <600 kcal/day or >4000 kcal/day for females) [14]. Additionally, we excluded participants taking medications for hypertension, diabetes, and myocardial infarction and participants who reported a medical history of heart attack, stroke, or diabetes (n = 2392). Finally, a total of 5921 participants (2743 males and 3178 females) were included in this study. A flowchart of the selection process of the study population is shown in Figure 1.

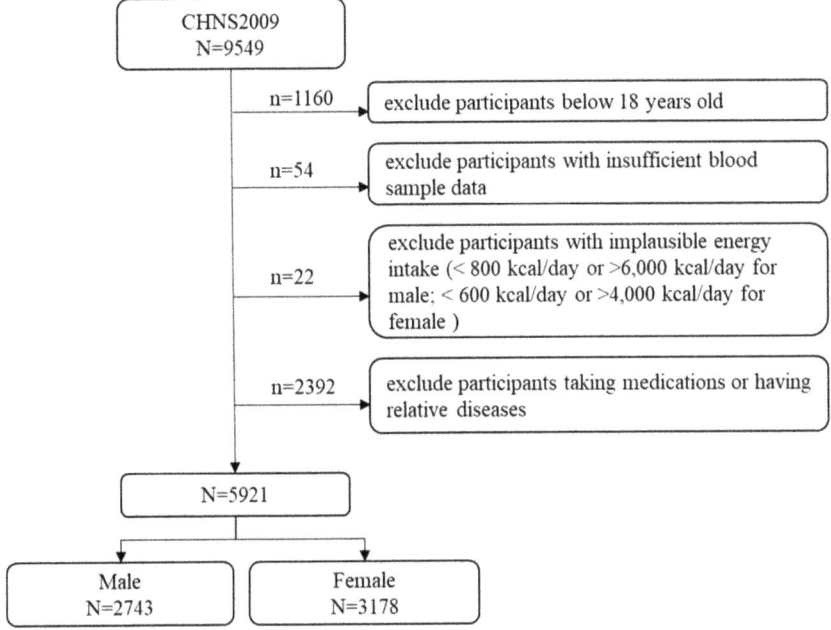

Figure 1. Selection process for the study population in the 2009 China Health and Nutrition Survey (CHNS).

2.2. Dietary Assessment and Calculation of the Low-Carbohydrate Diet Score

The 3 day, 24 h dietary recalls were used to assess the dietary intake of each participant. The quantities and types of food and beverages consumed during the past 24 h were determined from the participants. The interviewers measured the participants' dietary intake with picture aids and food models during household interviews. The participants' energy and nutrient intakes were calculated using the China Food Composition Table (FCT) (FCT 2002 edition and FCT 2004 edition).

To evaluate LCD based on the method used by Halton et al. [11], we referred to the concept of the LCD score. According to the percentage of energy from carbohydrate, protein, and fat consumption, the participants were ranked separately and were subsequently divided into 11 groups. Using the assignment method by Halton et al., the highest score (LCD score = 30) group had the lowest carbohydrate intake and the highest fat and protein intakes, while the lowest score (LCD score = 0) group had the highest carbohydrate intake and the lowest fat and protein intakes. To facilitate the analysis, we further calculated the scores for animal-based food (the percentage of energy from carbohydrate, animal protein, and animal fat consumption) and plant-based food (the percentage of energy from carbohydrate, plant protein, and plant fat consumption) in a similar manner. The division of animal- and plant-based food is based on the FCT 2002 and FCT 2004 editions. Table 1 presents the percentages used to determine the LCD score, animal-based LCD score, and plant-based LCD score. According to the scores (from low to high), the participants were divided into four groups according to gender.

Table 1. Energy percent of macronutrients used in calculating the low-carbohydrate diet (LCD) scores, animal-based LCD scores, and plant-based LCD scores of Chinese adults, China Health and Nutrition Survey.

	Total Carbohydrate	Total Protein	Total Fat	Animal-Based Protein	Animal-Based Fat	Plant-Based Protein	Plant-Based Fat
			Median of Energy% (Minimum–Maximum) [1]				
0	83.11 (80.80–93.06)	10.43 (4.92–11.00)	4.57 (1.94–6.20)	0.00 (0.00–0.84)	0.00 (0.00–1.36)	5.79 (2.19–6.44)	1.68 (0.66–1.91)
1	78.85 (77.09–80.78)	11.44 (11.00–11.81)	8.00 (6.20–9.45)	1.47 (0.85–1.94)	2.68 (1.37–4.14)	6.89 (6.44–7.25)	2.06 (1.91–2.26)
2	75.50 (73.95–77.07)	12.13 (11.81–12.45)	11.11 (9.48–12.47)	2.39 (1.94–2.77)	5.66 (4.14–7.09)	7.57 (7.25–7.83)	2.47 (2.26–2.67)
3	72.53 (71.14–73.95)	12.77 (12.45–13.04)	13.77 (12.47–14.83)	3.14 (2.77–3.49)	8.31 (7.09–9.41)	8.09 (7.83–8.32)	2.92 (2.67–3.17)
4	69.98 (68.61–71.14)	13.31 (13.04–13.55)	15.92 (14.84–17.03)	3.83 (3.49–4.17)	10.61 (9.42–11.66)	8.54 (8.32–8.80)	3.44 (3.17–3.70)
5	67.35 (66.01–68.60)	13.83 (13.55–14.12)	18.23 (17.04–19.36)	4.57 (4.17–4.97)	12.71 (11.66–13.83)	9.04 (8.80–9.32)	3.96 (3.70–4.27)
6	64.87 (63.51–66.01)	14.48 (14.12–14.85)	20.41 (19.36–21.60)	5.35 (4.97–5.81)	15.03 (13.84–16.05)	9.61 (9.32–9.91)	4.62 (4.27–5.00)
7	62.21 (60.69–63.50)	15.29 (14.86–15.76)	22.82 (21.61–24.04)	6.24 (5.81–6.77)	17.22 (16.06–18.66)	10.24 (9.91–10.58)	5.48 (5.00–6.08)
8	59.05 (57.36–60.69)	16.27 (15.76–16.88)	25.47 (24.04–27.10)	7.32 (6.77–7.95)	20.13 (18.66–21.76)	10.96 (10.58–11.42)	6.90 (6.08–7.84)
9	55.16 (52.49–57.34)	17.66 (16.88–18.74)	29.08 (27.10–31.37)	8.76 (7.96–9.95)	23.77 (21.76–26.54)	11.95 (11.42–12.62)	9.04 (7.84–10.67)
10	48.74 (17.49–52.48)	20.47 (18.74–35.75)	35.23 (31.37–64.22)	11.72 (9.96–28.77)	30.26 (26.54–63.15)	13.44 (12.62–35.02)	13.49 (10.68–37.60)

[1] The overlap of values in parentheses is due to rounding the values to the second decimal place. Energy from diet total carbohydrate, total protein, total fat, animal protein, animal fat, plant protein, and plant fat is shown according the score assigned to the 11 groups after ranking the participants' macronutrient intake, respectively.

Simultaneously, based on the study by Kim et al. [9], when comparing the acceptable macronutrient distribution range (AMDR) for carbohydrates as recommended by the Chinese Dietary Reference Intakes (CDRIs) Handbook (2013), the participants in each quartile were divided into three groups according to the percentage of energy from carbohydrates: lower (<50%), standard (50–65%), and higher (>65%). Moreover, we adjusted the carbohydrate intake criteria according to previous research criteria [15,16]: low-carbohydrate diet (<40%), moderate-carbohydrate diet (40–65%), and high-carbohydrate diet (>65%). Finally, fat intake in each quartile was also determined in our study on comparing the AMDR using the fat intake criteria from the CDRIs Handbook: lower (<20%), standard (20–30%), and higher (>30%).

2.3. Determination of Dyslipidemia

Dyslipidemia is diagnosed when one or more of the following abnormal lipid levels are observed: high cholesterol levels (hypercholesterolemia), high triglyceride levels (hypertriglyceridemia), and low HDL-C levels based on the Guidelines for the Prevention and Treatment of Dyslipidemia in China (2007) [2]. Hypercholesterolemia is a disease characterized by increased TC levels in fasting serum (>240 mg/dL (6.22 mmol/L)) or increased LDL-C levels (>160 mg/dL (4.10 mmol/L). Hypertriglyceridemia is a disease characterized by increased TG levels in fasting serum (200 mg/dL (2.26 mmol/L)), and low HDL-C levels is a disease characterized by decreased HDL-C levels (<40 mg/dL (1.04 mmol/L)) [2].

2.4. Assessment of Other Variables

Body mass index (BMI) was obtained by dividing the body weight by the square of the height (kg/m^2). Participants were divided into four groups based on their BMI values: underweight (BMI < 18.5 kg/m^2), normal weight (≥18.5 kg/m^2 and <24 kg/m^2), overweight (≥24 kg/m^2 and <28 kg/m^2), and obese (BMI ≥ 28 kg/m^2) according to the Guidelines for the Prevention and Control of Overweight and Obesity in Chinese Adults (2003). Sociodemographic variables such as age, gender, and income level and lifestyle variables such as alcohol consumption, smoking status, and physical activity level (PAL) were obtained using well-validated questionnaires distributed by trained interviewers. Information regarding alcohol consumption was divided into two groups according to frequency: "yes" (consumed alcohol more than once in the past year) or "no." Information regarding smoking status was divided into three groups: "current smoker" (still smoking), "past smoker" (previously smoking but currently not smoking), or "never smoker".

PAL included the following three domains: transportation activities, occupational activities, and sports. PAL was measured in terms of metabolic equivalent of task (MET) minutes in each week [17,18], which were converted using the time spent on each activity. The MET scores for each activity were based on the 2011 Compendium of Physical Activities. Physical activity was also divided into three categories: light PAL (<600 MET minutes/wk), moderate PAL (≥600 MET minutes/wk and <3000 MET minutes/wk), and vigorous PAL (≥3000 MET minutes/wk) [18,19].

The area of residence was categorized into "rural" and "urban". According to the results of the questionnaire, "urban neighborhood" (primary sampling units = 36) and "suburban neighborhoods" (primary sampling units = 36) were classified as "urban"; "towns" (primary sampling units) and "rural villages" (primary sampling units = 108) were classified as "rural". Other covariates that were defined in the model included age (years), educational level (less than primary school, middle school, technical school, college, or university or above), and ethnicity (Han, other ethnicities).

2.5. Statistical Analyses

Participants' general characteristics, such as age, income level, BMI, obesity, alcohol consumption, smoking status, PAL, and nutrient intake were analyzed using the generalized linear model and chi-square test for continuous and categorical variables, respectively, according to the quartiles of LCD scores based on gender. Moreover, all results for the continuous variables are presented as the mean ± standard error, and the results for the categorical variables are presented as n (%). After adjusting for potential confounding variables (including age, educational level, body mass index, ethnicity, physical activity level, alcohol consumption, smoking status, and individual income), logistic regression models were used to calculate the odds ratios (ORs) of dyslipidemia and their 95% confidence intervals (95% CIs). All statistical analyses were performed using the Statistical Analysis System software version 9.4. A p value < 0.05 was considered statistically significant.

3. Results

Table 2 shows the general characteristics of the participants according to LCD score quartiles based on gender. The male and female LCD median scores both ranged from 5.00 in the lowest quartile (Q1) to 25.00 in the highest quartile (Q4). Moreover, participants with higher LCD scores had higher income levels, lived in urban areas, consumed alcohol, performed more physical activity, and had higher educational levels compared to participants in Q1 (all p < 0.05). Males in Q4 were more likely to have obesity (p < 0.05). Further, regarding lipid profiles, participants with higher LCD scores had higher levels of TC and LDL-C. Furthermore, males in Q4 had higher levels of TG than males in Q1 (all p < 0.05).

Macronutrient intake was assessed according to LCD score quartiles based on gender (Table 3). Carbohydrate intake was decreased and protein and fat intakes were increased according to the LCD score. Interestingly, intake of plant-based protein was decreasing according to the LCD score.

In Table 4, carbohydrate and fat intakes are presented according to the quartiles of the LCD score. Compared with the AMDR for carbohydrates as recommended by the CDRIs Handbook, only 34.85% of males and 36.25% of females consumed carbohydrates within the recommended level, whereas 58.95% of males and 58.34% of females consumed carbohydrates above the recommended level. None of the participants consumed carbohydrates below the recommended level in Q1. In total, 56.58% and 57.49% of males and females, respectively, had lower fat intake than the AMDR, and most of these participants were assigned to Q1 and Q2. According to previous research criteria, 39.7% of males and 40.59% of females consumed moderate-carbohydrate diets, whereas only 1.35% of males and 1.07% of females adhered to a LCD. All participants in Q1 consumed high-carbohydrate diets. Even in Q4, 94.88% of males and 95.87% of females consumed moderate-carbohydrate diets, whereas only 5.12% of males and 4.13% of females adhered to a LCD.

The multivariate adjusted ORs and their 95% CIs for the components of dyslipidemia according to the LCD score quartiles based on gender are summarized in Table 5. Male participants with higher LCD scores had a higher risk of hypercholesterolemia (OR, 1.87; 95% CI, 1.23–2.85) than those in Q1 (p for trend = 0.0017) after adjusting for age, educational level, BMI, ethnicity, PAL, alcohol consumption, smoking status, and income level. Meanwhile, a similar significant association between the LCD scores and hypertriglyceridemia was observed in males (OR, 1.47; 95% CI, 1.04–2.06) on comparison with participants in Q1 (p for trend = 0.0336) after adjusting for the mentioned confounding variables previously. However, in females, there were no significant associations between the ORs for dyslipidemia and LCD scores in comparison to the participants in Q1.

Table 6 illustrates the multivariate adjusted ORs and their 95% CIs for the components of dyslipidemia according to the animal- and plant-based LCD score quartiles based on gender. Comparing the fourth and the first animal-based LCD score quartiles, the multivariate ORs for hypercholesterolemia were 2.15 (95% CI, 1.41–3.29; p for trend = 0.0006) and the multivariate ORs for hypertriglyceridemia were 1.51 (95% CI, 1.09–2.10; p for trend = 0.0156) in males. In females, there was a borderline linear trend for hypercholesterolemia from the first quartile to the fourth quartile (p for trend = 0.0651). Regarding the plant-based LCD score, there was no significant linear trend for dyslipidemia from the first quartile to the fourth quartile both in males and females.

Table 2. General characteristics of Chinese adults according to the quartiles (Q) of the low-carbohydrate diet (LCD) scores, China Health and Nutrition Survey. [1]

	Male					Female				
	Q1	Q2	Q3	Q4	p Value [2]	Q1	Q2	Q3	Q4	p Value [2]
N	669	735	656	683		824	794	786	774	
LCD Score (Median) [3]	5	12	18	25		5	12	19	25	
LCD Range (Min-Max)	0–8	9–15	16–21	22–30		0–8	9–15	16–21	22–30	
Age (Years)	49.41 ± 0.57	49.07 ± 0.55	47.94 ± 0.58	48.45 ± 0.57	0.1171	48.88 ± 0.50	48.42 ± 0.52	48.46 ± 0.51	47.46 ± 0.53	0.0001
Age Groups (Years)					0.5199					0.0570
18–29	73 (10.91)	72 (9.8)	79 (12.04)	81 (11.86)		71 (8.62)	84 (10.58)	91 (11.58)	105 (13.57)	
30–39	107 (15.99)	137 (18.64)	117 (17.84)	121 (17.72)		126 (15.29)	142 (17.88)	140 (17.81)	146 (18.86)	
40–49	144 (21.52)	170 (23.13)	162 (24.7)	143 (20.94)		216 (26.21)	188 (23.68)	197 (25.06)	202 (26.1)	
50–59	170 (25.41)	181 (24.63)	158 (24.09)	185 (27.09)		214 (25.97)	197 (24.81)	190 (24.17)	168 (21.71)	
≥60	175 (26.16)	175 (23.81)	140 (21.34)	153 (22.4)		197 (23.91)	183 (23.05)	168 (21.37)	153 (19.77)	
Area of Residence [4]					<0.0001					<0.0001
Rural	481 (88.26)	436 (74.53)	338 (67.74)	312 (59.54)		692 (85.33)	547 (89.53)	431 (76.42)	356 (68.2)	
Individual Net Income [5]					<0.0001					<0.0001
High	242 (44.9)	328 (56.65)	324 (65.72)	380 (72.66)		192 (32.32)	229 (41.49)	278 (53.56)	335 (62.5)	
BMI (kg/m²) [6]	22.59 ± 0.12	22.93 ± 0.12	23.31 ± 0.13	23.67 ± 0.13	<0.0001	23.12 ± 0.12	23.22 ± 0.12	23.18 ± 0.12	23.07 ± 0.12	0.7209
Weight Status [6]					<0.0001					0.6930
Overweight	178 (26.61)	213 (28.98)	191 (29.12)	237 (34.7)		229 (27.79)	227 (28.59)	221 (28.12)	214 (27.65)	
Obese	33 (4.93)	53 (7.21)	62 (9.45)	74 (10.83)		76 (9.22)	73 (9.19)	66 (8.4)	61 (7.88)	
Alcohol Consumption [7]					<0.0001					<0.0001
Yes	398 (59.49)	431 (58.64)	421 (64.18)	474 (69.40)		54 (6.55)	65 (8.2)	68 (8.65)	109 (14.08)	
Smoking Status [8]					0.6072					0.5605
Current Smokers	393 (58.74)	429 (58.45)	381 (58.08)	407 (59.59)		16 (1.94)	21 (2.65)	17 (2.16)	18 (2.33)	
Physical Activity [9]					<0.0001					<0.0001
Light	193 (29.07%)	238 (33.06%)	252 (39.44%)	295 (43.96%)		132 (16.26%)	170 (21.6%)	151 (19.56%)	160 (21.16%)	
Moderate	105 (15.81%)	109 (15.14%)	115 (18%)	147 (21.91%)		285 (35.1%)	325 (41.3%)	365 (47.28%)	399 (52.78%)	
Heavy	366 (55.12)	373 (51.81)	272 (42.57)	229 (34.13)		395 (48.65)	292 (37.1)	256 (33.16)	197 (26.06)	
Educational Level [10]					<0.0001					<0.0001
≥Technical School	330 (49.33)	412 (56.05)	371 (56.55)	371 (54.32)		292 (35.44)	328 (41.31)	344 (43.77)	355 (45.87)	
Lipid Profile										
Total Cholesterol (mg/dL)	178.61 ± 1.35	185.21 ± 1.38	188.43 ± 1.44	193.09 ± 1.55	<0.0001	183.88 ± 1.33	189.64 ± 1.43	188.17 ± 1.34	190.74 ± 1.44	0.0019
Triglycerides (mg/dL)	129.27 ± 3.9	154.15 ± 5.5	159.85 ± 5.33	171.46 ± 6.45	<0.0001	132.03 ± 3.96	134.81 ± 3.5	125.88 ± 2.97	124.87 ± 3.47	0.0538
HDL-C (mg/dL)	55.7 ± 0.76	53.76 ± 0.6	52.74 ± 0.57	54.04 ± 0.75	0.0531	57.6 ± 0.53	57.6 ± 0.67	58.21 ± 0.67	58.49 ± 0.52	0.1939
LDL-C (mg/dL)	110.44 ± 1.67	111.59 ± 1.32	115.63 ± 1.37	116.99 ± 1.52	0.0003	112.19 ± 1.22	117.19 ± 1.33	116.39 ± 1.24	118.06 ± 1.32	0.0029

[1] All statistical analyses accounted for the sampling design of the national surveys in the 2009 wave. Values are presented as the mean ± standard error, median, or n (%). [2] p values were calculated using the generalized linear model for continuous variables and the χ^2 test for categorical variables. [3] The LCD scores range from a minimum of zero to a maximum of 30; a low LCD score indicates weaker adherence, whereas a high score indicates greater adherence and higher protein and fat intake. [4] Classified by "rural" and "urban" according to the questionnaire. [5] Classified into "low", "middle", "high" according to the file from National Development and Reform Commission. [6] Determined by body mass index: underweight (<18.5 kg/m²), normal weight (≥18.5 kg/m² and <24 kg/m²), overweight (≥24 kg/m² and <28 kg/m²), and obesity (≥28 kg/m²) according to the Guidelines for the Prevention and Control of Overweight and Obesity in Chinese Adults (2006). [7] "Yes" indicated drank alcohol over the past year. [8] "Past" indicated that the person has smoked over their lifetime but has not smoked recently, and "current" indicated that the person still smokes. [9] "Heavy" indicated the metabolic equivalent of task (MET) hours per week ≥ 3000, "moderate" indicated MET ≥ 600 and <3000, and "light" indicated MET < 600 according to the 2011 Compendium of Physical Activities. [10] Divided into four groups: "less than primary school", "middle school", "technical school", and "college or university".

Table 3. Macronutrient intake and energy percent according to the LCD score based on gender, China Health and Nutrition Survey. [1]

	Male					Female				
	Q1	Q2	Q3	Q4	p Value [2]	Q1	Q2	Q3	Q4	p Value
N	669	735	656	683		824	794	786	774	
Food and Nutrient Intake										
Total Energy (kcal/d)	2348.78 ± 24.71	2339.9 ± 24.4	2425.81 ± 27.17	2370.44 ± 25.56	0.1879	1990.64 ± 20.69	1979.7 ± 20.09	2030.83 ± 20.8	1934.02 ± 19.56	0.2027
Carbohydrate (g/d)	406.71 ± 5.15	348.69 ± 3.85	327.59 ± 4.12	258.65 ± 3.46	<0.0001	335.28 ± 3.87	299.59 ± 3.5	270.45 ± 3.04	220.35 ± 2.72	<0.0001
Protein (g/d)	61.09 ± 0.78	66.93 ± 0.81	75.26 ± 0.99	83.03 ± 1.11	<0.0001	50.63 ± 0.60	57.87 ± 0.72	62.53 ± 0.75	70.56 ± 0.87	<0.0001
Fat (g/d)	20.85 ± 0.52	34.9 ± 0.57	52.65 ± 1.05	63.06 ± 0.97	<0.0001	16.82 ± 0.37	29.45 ± 0.49	42.55 ± 0.66	52.39 ± 0.82	<0.0001
Energy from Carbohydrates (%)										
Total	79.28 ± 0.15	70.72 ± 0.12	63.16 ± 0.18	53.31 ± 0.25	<0.0001	79.36 ± 0.14	70.79 ± 0.12	63.21 ± 0.14	53.84 ± 0.24	<0.0001
Energy from Protein (%)										
Total	11.93 ± 0.06	13.64 ± 0.07	14.64 ± 0.1	17.41 ± 0.13	<0.0001	12.00 ± 0.05	13.74 ± 0.07	14.72 ± 0.09	17.48 ± 0.11	<0.0001
Animal-Based	1.82 ± 0.06	4.15 ± 0.07	5.76 ± 0.09	8.86 ± 0.13	<0.0001	1.75 ± 0.05	4.05 ± 0.07	5.84 ± 0.08	8.7 ± 0.12	<0.0001
Plant-Based	10.1 ± 0.08	9.49 ± 0.08	8.89 ± 0.1	8.55 ± 0.11	<0.0001	10.25 ± 0.07	9.69 ± 0.08	8.89 ± 0.08	8.78 ± 0.11	<0.0001
Energy from Fat (%)										
Total	8.8 ± 0.16	15.64 ± 0.17	22.2 ± 0.25	29.28 ± 0.25	<0.0001	8.63 ± 0.14	15.46 ± 0.16	22.07 ± 0.2	28.68 ± 0.25	<0.0001
Animal Based	4.77 ± 0.17	11.12 ± 0.2	16.63 ± 0.29	22.54 ± 0.31	<0.0001	4.46 ± 0.15	10.51 ± 0.2	16.84 ± 0.25	22.06 ± 0.3	<0.0001
Plant Based	4.03 ± 0.09	4.52 ± 0.11	5.57 ± 0.17	6.74 ± 0.2	<0.0001	4.17 ± 0.08	4.95 ± 0.12	5.23 ± 0.13	6.62 ± 0.17	<0.0001

[1] All statistical analyses accounted for the sampling design of the national surveys in the 2009 wave. Values are presented as the mean ± standard error. [2] p values were calculated using the generalized linear model for continuous variables.

Table 4. Carbohydrate and fat intakes among Chinese adults according to the quartiles (Q) of the low-carbohydrate diet scores, China Health and Nutrition Survey. [1]

	Male						Female					
	Total	Q1	Q2	Q3	Q4	p Value [2]	Total	Q1	Q2	Q3	Q4	p Value [2]
Compliance with AMDR [3] for Carbohydrates Recommended by the CDRI 2013 [4]												
Low (<50%)	170 (6.20)	0 (0)	0 (0)	13 (1.98)	157 (22.99)	<0.0001	172 (5.41)	0 (0)	0 (0)	6 (0.76)	166 (21.45)	<0.0001
Moderate	956 (34.85)	0 (0)	20 (2.72)	410 (62.50)	526 (77.01)		1152 (36.25)	0 (0)	36 (4.53)	508 (64.63)	608 (78.55)	
High (>65%)	1617 (58.95)	669 (100)	715 (97.28)	233 (35.52)	0 (0)		1854 (58.34)	824 (100)	758 (95.47)	272 (34.61)	0 (0)	
Dietary Classification Based on the Amount of Carbohydrates Consumed [5]												
Low (<40%)	37 (1.35)	0 (0)	0 (0)	2 (0.30)	35 (5.12)	<0.0001	34 (1.07)	0 (0)	0 (0)	2 (0.25)	32 (4.13)	<0.0001
Moderate	1089 (39.70)	0 (0)	20 (2.72)	421 (64.18)	648 (94.88)		1290 (40.59)	0 (0)	36 (4.53)	512 (65.14)	742 (95.87)	
High (>65%)	1617 (58.95)	669 (100)	715 (97.28)	233 (35.52)	0 (0)		1854 (58.34)	824 (100)	758 (95.47)	272 (34.61)	0 (0)	
Compliance with AMDR [3] for Fat Recommended by the CDRI 2013 [4]												
Low (<20%)	1552 (56.58)	669 (100)	600 (81.63)	245 (37.35)	38 (5.56)	<0.0001	1827 (57.49)	824 (100)	656 (82.62)	294 (37.40)	53 (6.85)	<0.0001
Moderate	848 (30.92)	0 (0)	135 (18.37)	348 (53.05)	365 (53.44)		1007 (31.69)	0 (0)	138 (17.38)	435 (55.34)	434 (56.07)	
High (>30%)	343 (12.50)	0 (0)	0 (0)	63 (9.60)	280 (41.00)		344 (10.82)	0 (0)	0 (0)	57 (7.25)	287 (37.08)	

[1] All statistical analyses accounted for the sampling design of the national surveys in the 2009 wave. Values are presented as n (%). [2] p values were calculated by χ^2 test for categorical variables. [3] AMDR = acceptable macronutrient distribution range. [4] CDRI 2013 = Chinese Dietary Reference Intakes (CDRIs) Handbook (2013); the AMDR for carbohydrates recommended by the CDRI is 50–65%. [5] Classification of the dietary carbohydrate level based on the previous modified criteria: low-carbohydrate diet, <40% of energy; moderate-carbohydrate diet, 40–65% energy; high-carbohydrate diet, >65% of energy.

Table 5. Multivariate adjusted odds ratios (ORs) for dyslipidemia according to the quartiles (Q) of the low-carbohydrate diet (LCD) scores of Chinese adults, China Health and Nutrition Survey.[1]

LCD Score	Male					Female				
	Q1	Q2	Q3	Q4	p Value for Trend [2]	Q1	Q2	Q3	Q4	p Value for Trend [2]
	OR (95% CI)					OR (95% CI)				
Hypercholesterolemia [3]										
N (%)	55 (8.22)	79 (10.75)	86 (13.11)	103 (15.08)		85 (10.32)	109 (13.73)	106 (13.49)	110 (14.21)	
Adjusted Model [4]	1.00	1.28	1.64	1.87	0.0017	1.00	1.46	1.36	1.42	0.1455
		(0.84–1.97)	(1.07–2.51)	(1.23–2.85)			(0.99–2.14)	(0.91–2.03)	(0.93–2.14)	
Hypertriglyceridemia [5]										
N (%)	105 (15.7)	154 (20.95)	146 (22.26)	159 (23.28)		119 (14.44)	126 (15.87)	113 (14.38)	113 (14.6)	
Adjusted Model [4]	1.00	1.24	1.25	1.47	0.0336	1.00	1.04	1.00	1.10	0.7060
		(0.89–1.72)	(0.89–1.76)	(1.04–2.06)			(0.73–1.49)	(0.69–1.45)	(0.72–1.60)	
Low High-Density Lipoprotein Cholesterol [6]										
N (%)	88 (13.15)	117 (15.92)	123 (18.75)	121 (17.72)		74 (8.98)	62 (7.81)	52 (6.62)	56 (7.24)	
Adjusted Model [4]	1.00	1.10	1.21	1.14	0.4427	1.00	0.87	0.48	0.87	0.1638
		(0.77–1.58)	(0.84–1.75)	(0.78–1.65)			(0.56–1.36)	(0.28–0.82)	(0.55–1.40)	

[1] All statistical analyses accounted for the sampling design of the national surveys in the 2009 wave. Values are presented as n (%) or ORs (95%CIs). [2] p for trend values were calculated using the generalized linear model. [3] Hypercholesterolemia was defined as a total cholesterol level $\geq$ 6.22 mmol/L (240 mg/dL) on fasting blood glucose test, low-density lipoprotein cholesterol level $\geq$ 4.14 mmol/L (160 mg/dL). [4] Adjusted for age, educational level, body mass index, ethnicity, physical activity level, alcohol consumption, smoking status, and individual income. [5] Hypertriglyceridemia was defined as a triglyceride level $\geq$ 2.26 mmol/L (200 mg/dL). [6] A low high-density lipoprotein cholesterol (HDL-C) level was defined as a HDL-C level < 1.04 mmol/L (40 mg/dL).

Table 6. Multivariate adjusted odds ratios (ORs) for dyslipidemia according to the quartiles (Q) of animal-based and plant-based low-carbohydrate diet (LCD) scores of Chinese adults, China Health and Nutrition Survey.

	Male					Female				
	Q1	Q2	Q3	Q4	p Value for Trend [1]	Q1	Q2	Q3	Q4	p Value for Trend [1]
	OR (95% CI)					OR (95% CI)				
Animal-Based LCD Score [2]										
N	708	671	697	667		777	835	821	745	
Hypercholesterolemia [3]										
N (%)	56 (7.91)	79 (11.77)	88 (12.63)	100 (14.99)		83 (10.68)	111 (13.29)	114 (13.89)	102 (13.69)	
Adjusted Model [4]	1.00	1.66 (1.08–2.54)	1.8 (1.17–2.77)	2.15 (1.41–3.29)	0.0006	1.00	1.64 (1.10–2.44)	1.41 (0.93–2.13)	1.64 (1.06–2.55)	0.0651
Hypertriglyceridemia [5]										
N (%)	127 (17.94)	133 (19.82)	144 (20.66)	160 (23.99)		116 (14.93)	126 (15.09)	123 (14.98)	106 (14.23)	
Adjusted Model [4]	1.00	1.01 (0.72–1.40)	1.04 (0.74–1.45)	1.51 (1.09–2.10)	0.0156	1.00	1.09 (0.76–1.56)	1.13 (0.77–1.64)	0.94 (0.63–1.41)	0.8828
Low High-Density Lipoprotein Cholesterol [6]										
N (%)	46 (6.50)	64 (9.54)	73 (10.47)	78 (11.69)		70 (9.01)	92 (11.02)	96 (11.69)	89 (11.95)	
Adjusted Model [4]	1.00	0.97 (0.68–1.39)	1.08 (0.75–1.54)	1.06 (0.73–1.52)	0.6618	1.00	0.77 (0.49–1.22)	0.79 (0.49–1.28)	0.63 (0.37–1.08)	0.1101
Plant-Based LCD Score [2]										
N	736	617	634	756		776	899	767	736	
Hypercholesterolemia [3]										
N (%)	95 (12.91)	69 (11.18)	68 (10.73)	91 (12.04)		96 (12.37)	125 (13.9)	83 (10.82)	106 (14.40)	
Adjusted Model [4]	1.00	0.81 (0.55–1.20)	0.72 (0.48–1.07)	0.82 (0.56–1.18)	0.2929	1.00	1.15 (0.80–1.67)	0.81 (0.55–1.21)	0.98 (0.67–1.46)	0.5608
Hypertriglyceridemia [5]										
N (%)	145 (19.70)	122 (19.77)	141 (22.24)	156 (20.63)		102 (13.14)	132 (14.68)	125 (16.30)	112 (15.22)	
Adjusted Model [4]	1.00	0.86 (0.62–1.20)	0.95 (0.69–1.32)	0.77 (0.56–1.06)	0.1386	1.00	1.1 (0.76–1.60)	1.23 (0.85–1.79)	1.35 (0.92–1.97)	0.0951
Low High-Density Lipoprotein Cholesterol [6]										
N (%)	85 (11.55)	57 (9.24)	46 (7.26)	73 (9.66)		84 (10.82)	107 (11.90)	66 (8.60)	90 (12.23)	
Adjusted Model [4]	1.00	0.76 (0.52–1.09)	0.88 (0.62–1.25)	0.92 (0.66–1.30)	0.8642	1.00	1.31 (0.82–2.12)	1.1 (0.67–1.80)	1.21 (0.73–2.00)	0.6380

[1] p for trend values were calculated using the generalized linear model. [2] The LCD scores range from a minimum of zero to a maximum of 30; a low LCD score indicates weaker adherence, whereas a high score indicates greater adherence and higher protein and fat intakes. [3] Hypercholesterolemia was defined as a total cholesterol level ≥ 6.22 mmol/L (240 mg/dL) or a fasting blood glucose test, low-density lipoprotein cholesterol level ≥ 4.14 mmol/L (160 mg/dL). [4] Adjusted for age, educational level, ethnicity, body mass index, physical activity level, alcohol consumption, smoking status, and individual income. [5] Hypertriglyceridemia was defined as a triglyceride level ≥ 2.26 mmol/L (200 mg/dL). [6] A low high-density lipoprotein cholesterol (HDL-C) level was defined as a HDL-C level < 1.04 mmol/L (40 mg/dL).

4. Discussion

Using the CHNS 2009, the present study examined the impact of dietary carbohydrate intake on dyslipidemia and its components using the LCD scores. It was found that higher LCD scores were significantly associated with higher intake of legumes, nuts, fish, and other non-carbohydrate food sources, consistent with the results of an improved carbohydrate quality index from an original study [20] (Table A1). Furthermore, in the present study, it was also found that participants with higher LCD scores lived in urban areas, had high income, consumed alcohol, performed light physical activity, and had higher educational levels. Among these, the PAL and drinking status have been widely studied and confirmed as important factors on lipid metabolism [4,21,22]. Due to their inescapable impact, in the present study, we adjusted PAL and drinking status as covariables in the multivariate model to minimize their impact, improve the validity of research results and focus on the analyses of the impact of diet on lipid metabolism. In the follow-up study, we will consider PAL and drinking status as exposure factors in order to study their impact on lipid metabolism.

Furthermore, it was found that a higher LCD score was significantly associated with a higher risk of hypercholesterolemia and hypertriglyceridemia in males after adjusting for eight confounding variables. These observations are consistent with the observations noted in a series of studies comprising Chinese adults [1,14]. Furthermore, higher animal-based LCD scores were also associated with a higher risk of hypercholesterolemia and hypertriglyceridemia in males and with a borderline increase in TC levels in females, while the plant-based LCD score was statistically insignificant in males and females.

We grouped the participants according to the quartiles of the LCD scores and there was a clear dose–response relationship between dietary macronutrients and the components of dyslipidemia, specifically for carbohydrates. In our study, the higher the LCD score, the lower the carbohydrate intake, the higher the fat intake, and the higher the risk of hypercholesterolemia and hypertriglyceridemia in males.

A previous study [14] reported that males with the highest carbohydrate intake (>68.2% of energy) had a significantly lower TC level after adjusting for several confounding variables. This result was consistent with the result of the present study, in which participants with high LCD scores had a higher risk of hypercholesterolemia than participants with lower LCD scores.

The effect of the LCD score on lipid metabolism can be analyzed from the perspective of a low-carbohydrate and high-fat diet using our results in Table 4. According to Volek et al. [16], carbohydrates are considered as the main source of energy and glucose in the general diet, and they directly or indirectly regulate the distribution of excessive dietary nutrients through insulin to regulate lipolysis and lipoprotein assembly and processing. Thus, carbohydrates affect the association between dietary intake of saturated fat and circulating lipid levels.

Furthermore, the group with high LCD scores obtained a higher percentage of energy from fat, as shown in Table 4. Moreover, 41% and 37.08% of male and female participants in Q4 had a high-fat diet, respectively, resulting in an increase in the serum TC and LDL-C levels [23,24]. Hence, the higher the LCD score, the higher the odds of hypercholesterolemia.

Recent studies have focused not only on the quantities of fat and carbohydrate intake but also on the quality of fat and carbohydrates. In our study, participants with higher LCD scores consumed less cereals and tubers, which are the main sources of dietary carbohydrates. Nuts contain high levels of unsaturated fatty acids [25], and various animal products have different saturated, polyunsaturated, and trans-fatty acid levels [16,26]. Limiting the intake of certain forms of carbohydrates is the preferred dietary strategy for improving cardiovascular health. Dietary fiber, which is a form of carbohydrate, reduces the risk of atherosclerosis and CVD [27]. Several types of fatty acids and their intake also have different effects on lipid metabolism [28,29]. Moreover, according to Acosta-Navarro et al. [30], higher consumption of an animal-based diet leads to higher TC levels. Hence, animal-based LCD scores were associated with differences in TC levels according to gender in this study. In both males and females, higher animal-based LCD scores were significantly associated with a higher risk of hypercholesterolemia, while the plant-based LCD score showed no statistical significance. This result is inconsistent with the result of a previous study [31], mainly because the previous study, which assessed plant-based diets, emphasized not eating meat or eating less meat. However, in our study, the plant-based LCD score refers to the percentages of protein and fat that the participants consumed from plant-sourced foods during the 3 day diet survey, and the participants themselves were not prohibited from eating meat (Table 1).

The difference between males and females in statistical significance according to our results is possibly attributed to the different body fat distributions and hormonal differences between males and females. In normal-weight individuals, significant differences are observed in lipid and fat distributions between males and females [32]. Serum TG levels are relatively lower and HDL-C levels are higher in females than in males (Table 2), due to the differences in gender hormones and body fat distribution [33,34]. Additionally, the response to a high-fat diet in terms of lipoproteins has a gender dimorphism [35]. These findings indicate that the effect of a high-fat diet on serum HDL-C levels is more significant in females than in males, as confirmed in our study, and a multivariate adjusted OR for HDL-C levels was also observed in our study (Table 5, OR, 0.48; 95% CI, 0.28–0.82).

This study based on the CHNS indicates that higher LCD scores result in a higher risk of hypercholesterolemia and hypertriglyceridemia in males, but we cannot exactly determine the amount and type of carbohydrate or fat intake using LCD scores. Therefore, the comprehensive effect of several macronutrients in the general diet on lipid metabolism should be further considered.

Although the data collection of CHNS 2009 is a little dated, the CHNS is a study that constitutes a wide age range and large sample size after adjusting for a comprehensive range of potential confounding variables. The analysis results of the representative datasets are reliable and can be extended to the general Chinese population. To the best of our knowledge, this is the first study to use LCD scores to study the risk of dyslipidemia among Chinese adults. Compared to a food frequency questionnaire, a 24 h recall is more accurate and has a lower estimation bias [13].

However, this study has several limitations. First, since this is a cross-sectional study, we were not able to determine the causal association between dietary macronutrients and the risk of dyslipidemia. Second, the dataset assessed dietary intake using 3 day, 24 h recalls, which may have a relatively limited correction for the internal differences among the participants and may be affected by seasons. Third, as we assessed confounding variables, such as PAL, using a questionnaire, bias may exist. Finally, although we adjusted for confounding variables, there are still unknown variables that can influence the results. Hence, larger-scale prospective studies are required to determine the association between LCD and dyslipidemia.

5. Conclusions

In conclusion, among Chinese males, the group with higher LCD scores has a higher fat intake (especially animal-based fat), a diet pattern that is closer to a LCD, and greater odds of hypercholesterolemia and hypertriglyceridemia. We advise that people should pay more attention to the proportion of macronutrients in their diet, especially animal-based fat. The association between LCD score and dyslipidemia is significantly complex. In the future, careful attention should be paid to the quality of macronutrients for preventing dyslipidemia in the Chinese population. Further prospective studies and those involving detailed dietary nutrient intake evaluations are required to verify these findings in Chinese and other populations.

Author Contributions: Conceptualization, L.-J.T.; methodology, L.-J.T.; software, L.-J.T.; formal analysis, L.-J.T.; data curation, L.-J.T.; writing–original draft preparation, L.-J.T.; writing–review and editing, S.S.; visualization, S.-A.K.; supervision, S.S.; project administration, S.S. All authors have read and agreed to the published version of the manuscript.

Funding: This work was supported by the National Research Foundation of Korea (NRF) grant funded by the Korea government (MSIT) (No.2020R1C1C1014286). MSIT: Ministry of Science and ICT.

Acknowledgments: This study uses data from the CHNS. We thank the National Institute for Nutrition and Health, China Center for Disease Control and Prevention, Carolina Population Center (P2C HD050924, T32 HD007168), the University of North Carolina at Chapel Hill, the NIH (R01-HD30880, DK056350, R24 HD050924, and R01-HD38700), and the NIH Fogarty International Center (D43 TW009077, D43 TW007709) for their financial support for CHNS data collection and analysis from 1989 to 2015 and future surveys. We also thank the China–Japan Friendship Hospital and the Ministry of Health for support for the CHNS 2009, the Chinese National Human Genome Center at Shanghai since 2009, and Beijing Municipal Center for Disease Prevention and Control since 2011.

Conflicts of Interest: The authors declare no conflict of interest.

Appendix A

Table A1. Food intake and energy percent according to the LCD score based on gender, China Health and Nutrition Survey. [1]

	Male					Female				
	Q1	Q2	Q3	Q4	p Value [2]	Q1	Q2	Q3	Q4	p Value [2]
Cereals and Cereal Products (g/d)	524.31 ± 6.72	452.56 ± 6.42	410.25 ± 5.91	363.64 ± 6.14	<0.0001	437.56 ± 5.50	371.6 ± 4.96	335.49 ± 4.36	302.09 ± 4.57	<0.0001
Energy (%)	80.14 ± 0.43	69.63 ± 0.46	61.44 ± 0.46	48.30 ± 0.53	0.028	78.61 ± 0.45	67.74 ± 0.47	60.48 ± 0.45	47.44 ± 0.46	0.0133
Tubers, Starches, and Products (g/d)	39.88 ± 2.43	31.80 ± 2.10	27.68 ± 1.88	23.16 ± 1.69	<0.0001	39.15 ± 2.32	31.23 ± 1.90	28.62 ± 1.79	18.20 ± 1.29	<0.0001
Energy (%)	1.81 ± 0.12	1.58 ± 0.11	1.35 ± 0.10	1.15 ± 0.09	0.0032	2.21 ± 0.14	1.78 ± 0.12	1.65 ± 0.11	1.15 ± 0.08	0.0114
Dried Legumes and Legume Products (g/d)	36.84 ± 2.51	60.6 ± 3.06	60.99 ± 2.61	85.67 ± 3.67	<0.0001	31.50 ± 1.81	54.85 ± 2.61	60.24 ± 2.49	75.57 ± 3.01	<0.0001
Energy (%)	2.00 ± 0.15	3.68 ± 0.23	4.10 ± 0.21	5.81 ± 0.31	<0.0001	2.08 ± 0.13	3.84 ± 0.22	4.42 ± 0.21	6.25 ± 0.28	<0.0001
Vegetables and Vegetable Products (g/d)	354.03 ± 7.28	336.73 ± 7.24	348.92 ± 6.51	326.41 ± 5.86	0.0309	317.29 ± 6.07	319.35 ± 6.66	318.82 ± 6.30	319.58 ± 5.33	0.8755
Energy (%)	4.08 ± 0.14	3.88 ± 0.11	4.33 ± 0.14	4.41 ± 0.13	0.084	4.50 ± 0.17	4.47 ± 0.14	4.63 ± 0.13	5.10 ± 0.13	0.0052
Fungi and Algae (g/d)	2.63 ± 0.49	6.03 ± 0.90	6.84 ± 0.69	9.40 ± 0.92	0.0266	2.02 ± 0.32	5.86 ± 0.68	6.84 ± 0.64	9.54 ± 1.07	0.0128
Energy (%)	0.07 ± 0.01	0.13 ± 0.02	0.22 ± 0.03	0.26 ± 0.03	0.0017	0.07 ± 0.01	0.15 ± 0.02	0.25 ± 0.03	0.39 ± 0.04	0.0069
Fruits and Fruit Products (g/d)	27.41 ± 3.07	42.63 ± 3.66	47.69 ± 3.42	55.96 ± 4.13	0.1291	43.58 ± 3.70	57.49 ± 3.90	59.40 ± 3.84	75.05 ± 4.51	0.0068
Energy (%)	0.74 ± 0.16	0.89 ± 0.08	1.07 ± 0.09	1.22 ± 0.09	0.141	1.20 ± 0.11	1.49 ± 0.11	1.55 ± 0.10	1.97 ± 0.12	0.0315
Nuts and Seeds (g/d)	1.96 ± 0.35	4.34 ± 0.64	5.01 ± 0.74	9.76 ± 1.16	<0.0001	2.57 ± 1.03	3.54 ± 0.50	3.79 ± 0.64	6.95 ± 0.92	0.0613
Energy (%)	0.32 ± 0.06	0.74 ± 0.10	0.83 ± 0.11	1.94 ± 0.21	<0.0001	0.34 ± 0.08	0.72 ± 0.10	0.66 ± 0.09	1.43 ± 0.15	<0.0001
Meat and Meat Products (g/d)	42.37 ± 1.89	77.43 ± 2.53	106.72 ± 2.73	136.24 ± 3.45	<0.0001	31.29 ± 1.33	62.51 ± 1.89	84.96 ± 2.30	112.16 ± 2.67	<0.0001
Energy (%)	6.37 ± 0.26	11.06 ± 0.31	16.10 ± 0.37	20.81 ± 0.48	<0.0001	5.35 ± 0.21	10.85 ± 0.30	15.31 ± 0.35	20.03 ± 0.43	<0.0001
Poultry and Poultry Products (g/d)	8.20 ± 0.98	15.16 ± 1.31	19.07 ± 1.41	36.52 ± 2.25	<0.0001	6.16 ± 0.69	13.38 ± 1.13	16.21 ± 1.15	29.27 ± 1.67	<0.0001
Energy (%)	0.51 ± 0.06	1.05 ± 0.09	1.37 ± 0.11	2.79 ± 0.18	<0.0001	0.46 ± 0.05	1.05 ± 0.09	1.34 ± 0.10	2.61 ± 0.16	<0.0001
Milk and Milk Products (g/d)	1.42 ± 0.53	6.32 ± 1.52	11.52 ± 1.82	25.68 ± 3.11	<0.0001	3.14 ± 0.79	6.25 ± 1.21	13.61 ± 1.75	30.38 ± 2.65	<0.0001
Energy (%)	0.05 ± 0.02	0.22 ± 0.05	0.35 ± 0.06	0.91 ± 0.12	<0.0001	0.11 ± 0.03	0.22 ± 0.04	0.58 ± 0.09	1.30 ± 0.13	<0.0001
Eggs and Egg Products (g/d)	22.05 ± 1.17	28.28 ± 1.29	35.17 ± 1.51	37.91 ± 1.69	<0.0001	19.01 ± 0.95	27.97 ± 1.26	29.73 ± 1.33	37.49 ± 1.56	<0.0001
Energy (%)	1.37 ± 0.07	1.86 ± 0.08	2.42 ± 0.10	2.80 ± 0.13	<0.0001	1.41 ± 0.07	2.21 ± 0.09	2.41 ± 0.10	3.25 ± 0.13	<0.0001
Fish, Shellfish, and Mollusks (g/d)	19.55 ± 1.67	33.10 ± 2.14	38.16 ± 2.13	69.07 ± 3.31	<0.0001	14.94 ± 1.21	26.13 ± 1.81	32.44 ± 1.77	57.22 ± 2.83	<0.0001
Energy (%)	0.61 ± 0.05	1.18 ± 0.08	1.43 ± 0.08	2.84 ± 0.17	<0.0001	0.56 ± 0.04	1.04 ± 0.07	1.38 ± 0.08	2.66 ± 0.13	<0.0001
Fast Food (g/d)	5.70 ± 0.95	16.01 ± 1.79	24.82 ± 2.24	35.78 ± 3.03	<0.0001	8.49 ± 1.08	16.48 ± 1.97	19.65 ± 1.59	23.98 ± 1.76	<0.0001
Energy (%)	0.78 ± 0.12	2.01 ± 0.21	3.29 ± 0.29	4.66 ± 0.37	<0.0001	1.24 ± 0.15	2.35 ± 0.24	3.21 ± 0.27	4.07 ± 0.31	<0.0001
Beverages (g/d)	0.61 ± 0.39	3.40 ± 1.25	10.04 ± 3.03	12.92 ± 3.04	0.0042	0.43 ± 0.24	3.14 ± 0.83	3.90 ± 0.95	10.56 ± 3.10	0.0097
Energy (%)	0.02 ± 0.01	0.14 ± 0.06	0.23 ± 0.06	0.43 ± 0.11	0.0001	0.01 ± 0.01	0.17 ± 0.06	0.18 ± 0.05	0.23 ± 0.06	0.0429

[1] All statistical analyses accounted for the sampling design of the national surveys in the 2009 wave. Values are presented as the mean ± standard error. Energy of every kind of food referred to the China Food Composition Table (FCT) (FCT 2002 edition and FCT 2004 edition). [2] p values were calculated using the generalized linear model.

References

1. Pan, L.; Yang, Z.; Wu, Y.; Yin, R.-X.; Liao, Y.-H.; Wang, J.; Gao, B.; Zhang, L. The prevalence, awareness, treatment and control of dyslipidemia among adults in China. *Atherosclerosis* **2016**, *248*, 2–9. [CrossRef]
2. ZHAO, S.-P.; LU, G.-P. 2016 Chinese guidelines for the management of dyslipidemia in adults. *J. Geriatr.'Cardiol.* **2018**, *15*, 1–29. [CrossRef]
3. Paccaud, F.; Schlüter-Fasmeyer, V.; Wietlisbach, V.; Bovet, P. Dyslipidemia and abdominal obesity. *J. Clin. Epidemiol.* **2000**, *53*, 393–400. [CrossRef]
4. Shen, Z.; Munker, S.; Wang, C.; Xu, L.; Ye, H.; Chen, H.; Xu, G.; Zhang, H.; Chen, L.; Yu, C.; et al. Association between alcohol intake, overweight, and serum lipid levels and the risk analysis associated with the development of dyslipidemia. *J. Clin. Lipidol.* **2014**, *8*, 273–278. [CrossRef] [PubMed]
5. Bendsen, N.T.; Chabanova, E.; Thomsen, H.S.; Larsen, T.M.; Newman, J.; Stender, S.; Dyerberg, J.; Haugaard, S.B.; Astrup, A. Effect of trans fatty acid intake on abdominal and liver fat deposition and blood lipids: A randomized trial in overweight postmenopausal women. *Nutr. Diabetes* **2011**, *1*, e4. [CrossRef]
6. Ma, Y.; Li, Y.; Chiriboga, D.E.; Olendzki, B.; Hébert, J.R.; Li, W.; Leung, K.; Hafner, A.R.; Ockene, I.S. Association between carbohydrate intake and serum lipids. *J. Am. Coll. Nutr.* **2006**, *25*, 155–163. [CrossRef] [PubMed]
7. Merchant, A.T.; Anand, S.S.; Kelemen, L.E.; Vuksan, V.; Jacobs, R.; Davis, B.; Teo, K.; Yusuf, S.; for the SHARE and SHARE-AP Investigators. Carbohydrate intake and HDL in a multiethnic population. *Am. J. Clin. Nutr.* **2007**, *85*, 225–230. [CrossRef]
8. Layman, D.; Boileau, R.A.; Erickson, D.J.; Painter, J.E.; Shiue, H.; Sather, C.; Christou, D.D. A Reduced Ratio of Dietary Carbohydrate to Protein Improves Body Composition and Blood Lipid Profiles during Weight Loss in Adult Women. *J. Nutr.* **2003**, *133*, 411–417. [CrossRef] [PubMed]
9. Kim, S.-A.; Lim, K.; Shin, S. Associations between Low-Carbohydrate Diets from Animal and Plant Sources and Dyslipidemia among Korean Adults. *J. Acad. Nutr. Diet.* **2019**, *119*, 2041–2054. [CrossRef] [PubMed]
10. Song, S.; Song, W.; Song, Y. Dietary carbohydrate and fat intakes are differentially associated with lipid abnormalities in Korean adults. *J. Clin. Lipidol.* **2017**, *11*, 338–347.e3. [CrossRef]
11. Halton, T.L.; Willett, W.C.; Liu, S.-M.; Manson, J.E.; Albert, C.M.; Rexrode, K.M.; Hu, F.B. Low-Carbohydrate-Diet Score and the Risk of Coronary Heart Disease in Women. *N. Engl. J. Med.* **2006**, *355*, 1991–2002. [CrossRef]
12. Fung, T.T.; Van Dam, R.M.; Hankinson, S.E.; Stampfer, M.; Willett, W.C.; Hu, F.B. Low-carbohydrate diets and all-cause and cause-specific mortality: Two cohort studies. *Ann. Intern. Med.* **2010**, *153*, 289–298. [CrossRef] [PubMed]
13. Zhang, B.; Zhai, F.Y.; Du, S.F.; Popkin, B.M. The China Health and Nutrition Survey, 1989–2011. *Obes. Rev.* **2014**, *15*, 2–7. [CrossRef] [PubMed]
14. Ma, Y.; Su, C.; Wang, H.; Wang, Z.; Liang, H.; Zhang, B. Relationship between carbohydrate intake and risk factors for cardiovascular disease in Chinese adults: Data from the China Health and Nutrition Survey (CHNS). *Asia Pac. J. Clin. Nutr.* **2019**, *28*, 520–532. [PubMed]
15. Cornier, M.-A.; Donahoo, W.T.; Pereira, R.; Gurevich, I.; Westergren, R.; Enerbäck, S.; Eckel, P.J.; Goalstone, M.L.; Hill, J.O.; Eckel, R.H.; et al. Insulin Sensitivity Determines the Effectiveness of Dietary Macronutrient Composition on Weight Loss in Obese Women. *Obes. Res.* **2005**, *13*, 703–709. [CrossRef]
16. Volek, J.S.; Fernandez, M.-L.; Feinman, R.D.; Phinney, S. Dietary carbohydrate restriction induces a unique metabolic state positively affecting atherogenic dyslipidemia, fatty acid partitioning, and metabolic syndrome. *Prog. Lipid Res.* **2008**, *47*, 307–318. [CrossRef]
17. Ainsworth, B.E.; Haskell, W.L.; Whitt, M.C.; Irwin, M.L.; Swartz, A.M.; Strath, S.J.; O'brien, W.L.; Bassett, D.R.; Schmitz, K.H.; Emplaincourt, P.O.; et al. Compendium of Physical Activities: An update of activity codes and MET intensities. *Med. Sci. Sports Exerc.* **2000**, *32*, S498–S516. [CrossRef]
18. Defina, L.F.; Radford, N.B.; Barlow, C.E.; Willis, B.L.; Leonard, D.; Haskell, W.L.; Farrell, S.W.; Pavlovic, A.; Abel, K.; Berry, J.D.; et al. Association of All-Cause and Cardiovascular Mortality with High Levels of Physical Activity and Concurrent Coronary Artery Calcification. *JAMA Cardiol.* **2019**, *4*, 174. [CrossRef]

19. McDowell, C.; Dishman, R.K.; Vancampfort, D.; Hallgren, M.; Stubbs, B.; MacDonncha, C.; Herring, M.P. Physical activity and generalized anxiety disorder: Results from The Irish Longitudinal Study on Ageing (TILDA). *Int. J. Epidemiol.* **2018**, *47*, 1443–1453. [CrossRef]
20. Martínez-González, M.A.; Fernandez-Lazaro, C.I.; Toledo, E.; Díaz-López, A.; Corella, D.; Goday, A.; Romaguera, D.; Vioque, J.; Alonso-Gómez, Á.M.; Wärnberg, J.; et al. Carbohydrate quality changes and concurrent changes in cardiovascular risk factors: A longitudinal analysis in the PREDIMED-Plus randomized trial. *Am. J. Clin. Nutr.* **2019**, *111*, 291–306. [CrossRef]
21. Goldberg, L.; Elliot, D. The Effect of Exercise on Lipid Metabolism in Men and Women. *Sports Med.* **1987**, *4*, 307–321. [CrossRef]
22. Van De Wiel, A. The Effect of Alcohol on Postprandial and Fasting Triglycerides. *Int. J. Vasc. Med.* **2011**, *2012*, 1–4. [CrossRef] [PubMed]
23. Blackburn, G.L.; Phillips, J.C.; Morreale, S. Physician's guide to popular low-carbohydrate weight-loss diets. *Clevel. Clin. J. Med.* **2001**, *68*, 761. [CrossRef] [PubMed]
24. Lichtenstein, A.H.; Appel, L.J.; Brands, M.; Carnethon, M.; Daniels, S.; Franch, H.; Franklin, B.; Kris-Etherton, P.; Harris, W.S.; Howard, B.; et al. Diet and Lifestyle Recommendations Revision 2006. *Circulation* **2006**, *114*, 82–96. [CrossRef] [PubMed]
25. Brufau, G.; Boatella, J.; Rafecas, M.; Rafecas, M. Nuts: Source of energy and macronutrients. *Br. J. Nutr.* **2006**, *96*, S24–S28. [CrossRef]
26. Zhao, J.; Xing, Q. Fatty Acid Composition in Different Animal Products. *Wei Sheng Yan Jiu* **2018**, *47*, 254–259.
27. Soliman, G. Dietary Fiber, Atherosclerosis, and Cardiovascular Disease. *Nutrients* **2019**, *11*, 1155. [CrossRef]
28. Shih, C.W.; Hauser, M.; Aronica, L.; Rigdon, J.; Gardner, C.D. Changes in blood lipid concentrations associated with changes in intake of dietary saturated fat in the context of a healthy low-carbohydrate weight-loss diet: A secondary analysis of the Diet Intervention Examining the Factors Interacting with Treatment Success (DIETFITS) trial. *Am. J. Clin. Nutr.* **2019**, *109*, 433–441. [CrossRef]
29. Fernández-Martínez, E.; Lira-Islas, I.G.; Cariño-Cortés, R.; Soria-Jasso, L.E.; Pérez-Hernández, E.; Pérez-Hernández, N. Dietary chia seeds (*Salvia hispanica*) improve acute dyslipidemia and steatohepatitis in rats. *J. Food Biochem.* **2019**, *43*, e12986. [CrossRef]
30. Acosta-Navarro, J.C.; Oki, A.; Antoniazzi, L.; Bonfim, M.A.C.; Hong, V.A.D.C.; Gaspar, M.C.D.A.; Sandrim, V.; Nogueira, A. Consumption of animal-based and processed food associated with cardiovascular risk factors and subclinical atherosclerosis biomarkers in men. *Revista da Associação Médica Brasileira* **2019**, *65*, 43–50. [CrossRef]
31. Yokoyama, Y.; Levin, S.M.; Barnard, N.D. Association between plant-based diets and plasma lipids: A systematic review and meta-analysis. *Nutr. Rev.* **2017**, *75*, 683–698. [CrossRef] [PubMed]
32. Patwardhan, V.; Khadilkar, A.; Chiplonkar, S.; Khadilkar, V. Dyslipidemia and Fat Distribution in Normal Weight Insulin Resistant Men. *J. Assoc. Phys. India* **2019**, *67*, 26–29.
33. Freedman, D.S.; Jacobsen, S.; Barboriak, J.J.; Sobocinski, K.A.; Anderson, A.J.; Kissebah, A.H.; Sasse, E.A.; Gruchow, H.W. Body fat distribution and male/female differences in lipids and lipoproteins. *Circulation* **1990**, *81*, 1498–1506. [CrossRef] [PubMed]
34. Park, J.H.; Lee, M.H.; Shim, J.-S.; Choi, D.P.; Song, B.M.; Lee, S.W.; Choi, H.; Kim, H.C. Effects of Age, Sex, and Menopausal Status on Blood Cholesterol Profile in the Korean Population. *Korean Circ. J.* **2015**, *45*, 141–148. [CrossRef]
35. Knopp, R.H.; Paramsothy, P. Gender Differences in Lipoprotein Metabolism and Dietary Response: Basis in Hormonal Differences and Implications for Cardiovascular Disease. *Curr. Atherocler. Rep.* **2005**, *7*, 472–479. [CrossRef]

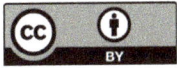

© 2020 by the authors. Licensee MDPI, Basel, Switzerland. This article is an open access article distributed under the terms and conditions of the Creative Commons Attribution (CC BY) license (http://creativecommons.org/licenses/by/4.0/).

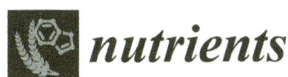

Article

Low Serum Vitamin B12 Levels Are Associated with Adverse Lipid Profiles in Apparently Healthy Young Saudi Women

Sara Al-Musharaf [1,2,*], Ghadeer S. Aljuraiban [1], Syed Danish Hussain [2], Abdullah M. Alnaami [2], Ponnusamy Saravanan [3,4,*] and Nasser Al-Daghri [2]

1. Department of Community Health Sciences, College of Applied Medical Sciences, King Saud University, Riyadh 11451, Saudi Arabia; galjuraiban@ksu.edu.sa
2. Chair for Biomarkers of Chronic Diseases, Riyadh Biochemistry Department, College of Science, King Saud University, Riyadh 11451, Saudi Arabia; danishhussain121@gmail.com (S.D.H.); aalnaami@yahoo.com (A.M.A.); ndaghri@ksu.edu.sa (N.A.-D.)
3. Population, Evidence and Technologies, Division of Health Sciences, Warwick Medical School, University of Warwick, Coventry CV2 2 DX, UK
4. Academic Department of Diabetes, Endocrinology and Metabolism, George Eliot Hospital, Nuneaton CV10 7DJ, UK
* Correspondence: salmosharruf@ksu.edu.sa (S.A.-M.); P.Saravanan@warwick.ac.uk (P.S.); Tel.: +966-55-424-3033 (S.A.-M.); +44-2476865329 (P.S.)

Received: 12 July 2020; Accepted: 6 August 2020; Published: 10 August 2020

Abstract: An abnormal lipid profile is an independent risk factor for cardiovascular diseases. The relationship between vitamin B12 deficiency and lipid profile is inconclusive, with most studies conducted in unhealthy populations. In this study, we aimed to assess the relationship between serum vitamin B12 levels and lipid profiles in a cross-sectional study that included 341 apparently healthy Saudi women, aged 19–30 years, from different colleges at King Saud University, Saudi Arabia. Sociodemographic, anthropometric, biochemical, and lifestyle data were collected, including diet and physical activity. Serum vitamin B12 deficiency was defined as serum B12 level of <148 pmol/L. The prevalence of vitamin B12 deficiency was approximately 0.6%. Using multivariable linear regression models, serum vitamin B12 levels were found to be inversely associated with total cholesterol (B = −0.26; $p < 0.001$), low-density lipoprotein cholesterol levels (B = −0.30; $p < 0.001$), and triglyceride (B = −0.16; $p < 0.01$) after adjusting for potential confounders, while obesity indices of body mass index, central obesity, and fat percentage showed no association. Therefore, we conclude that low serum vitamin B12 levels are independently associated with abnormal lipid profiles in healthy young Saudi women. Further interventional studies are needed to determine whether improving serum vitamin B12 levels in a healthy population can improve lipid profiles.

Keywords: vitamin B12; lipid profile; healthy; Saudi Arabia

1. Introduction

Micronutrient deficiencies contribute to the development of many metabolic chronic diseases and are of great importance in global health research, especially in the Middle East [1,2]. Vitamin B12, also known as cobalamin, is a water-soluble vitamin [3] that plays an important role in many cellular functions, such as erythropoiesis, DNA synthesis, and lipid and carbohydrate metabolism [3–5]. Vitamin B12 deficiency can develop because of malabsorption, genetic polymorphisms, or low dietary intake [3,6], and it has been associated with health issues ranging from mild fatigue to severe neurological impairment [3,5,7]. According to the World Health Organization (WHO), women of childbearing age are considered a high-risk group for vitamin B12 deficiency [8] and the risk of B12 deficiency may increase by 10%–20% from preconception to early pregnancy [9].

Globally, the prevalence of vitamin B12 deficiency ranges between 2.5% and 40% [6,10,11]. Prevalence among women of childbearing age has been measured at around 12% in the United Kingdom [12] and 34% in Canada [13]. A systematic review showed that during pregnancy, up to 20%–30% of women can be affected by B12 deficiency during all three trimesters, with higher rates among some ethnic groups [14]. The limited number of studies conducted in Arabian countries have suggested that the prevalence of vitamin B12 deficiency ranges from 6% to 30% among diabetes and high-risk populations, respectively [15,16].

Observational studies have shown an inverse association between vitamin B12 intake and metabolic disorders, including body mass index (BMI) [17], insulin resistance [18], type 2 diabetes mellitus (T2DM) [19], adverse lipid profile [20], and cardiovascular diseases (CVDs) [21–23]. Animal studies suggest that maternal low B12 levels may be causally linked to adverse lipid profiles in offspring [21]. In addition, vitamin B12 deficiency among pregnant women has been associated with gestational diabetes mellitus [24] and impaired cardiometabolic health of offspring [25]. One suggested mechanism through which vitamin B12 is linked to these disorders is via plasma total homocysteine (tHcy). Both vitamin B12 deficiency and CVDs have been linked to high tHcy concentration [26,27]. tHcy disturbs phospholipid metabolism by affecting the assembly or secretion of very low-density lipoprotein (VLDL), leading to abnormal lipid levels [28]. Other studies have suggested an independent role of vitamin B12, possibly via gene expression involved in lipogenesis [23,29] and inflammation [30]. However, a systematic review of seven prospective cohort studies showed limited and inconclusive results on the role of B12 on CVDs [29], although this could be due to the presence of confounders and the health status of the study samples.

It is important to note that Arabian women of childbearing age have a high risk of metabolic syndrome (29%) [31], prediabetes (40%), and T2DM (35%) [32]. At present, and to the best of our knowledge, no previous studies from the Middle East have assessed vitamin B12 status in relation to lipid profiles in apparently healthy women of childbearing age. Hence, cross-sectional associations of serum vitamin B12 levels and lipid profile indices were investigated using objective measures and detailed dietary data in apparently healthy young women living in Saudi Arabia.

2. Materials and Methods

2.1. Study Design, Population, and Sample Size

In this study, we included 355 randomly selected women aged between 19 and 30 years with no history of medical issues from different colleges at King Saud University (KSU), Riyadh, Saudi Arabia. Study recruitment was carried out between January and March 2019. Students were invited to participate and were randomly selected from three colleges (sciences, humanities, and medical colleges). Of the 355 women initially selected, 14 individuals were excluded (pregnancy; non-Saudi ethnic group; previous diagnosis of gastrointestinal disorders; anemia; malabsorption; any known chronic conditions such as thyroid disorders, diabetes mellitus, malignancies, and chronic obstructive pulmonary disease; arthritis; and consumption of vitamin B12 supplements or medications with known effects on serum vitamin B12 levels, such as metformin and proton pump inhibitors). The remaining 341 participants provided written informed consent. Among them, 118 (34.6%) were from the humanities college, 112 (32.9%) were from the science college, and 111 (32.6%) were from the medical college. Permission was also obtained for data collection and blood sample stock storage in a biobank at the Chair for Biomarkers of Chronic Diseases (CBCD) laboratories. Ethical approval for this study was obtained from the institutional review board (IRB) of King Khalid University Hospital, Riyadh (IRB number: E-19-3625). The sample size was calculated to identify the relationship between vitamin B12 and lipid profile. At an estimated effect size of 0.20 [33], 95% power, and 95% confidence interval, the required sample size to calculate the correlation between vitamin B12 and triglycerides is 262 subjects. However, to account for a 10% dropout, the minimum sample size was considered 288 subjects. The final sample size in this study was 341.

2.2. Biochemical Assessment

Fasting blood was collected after a 10-h overnight fast. A 10 mL sample of venous blood (5 mL serum and 5 mL whole blood) was drawn from the cubital vein. The samples were packaged and transported in a portable refrigerator to the CBCD at KSU. All the samples were aliquoted and stored in a freezer at −80 °C for subsequent analyses.

2.2.1. Lipid Profile and Glucose

Serum total cholesterol (TC), high-density lipoprotein cholesterol (HDL-C), triglyceride (TG), and glucose levels were measured by a colorimetric method using an automated chemistry analyzer (Konelab, ThermoFisher, Finland). The intra- and interassay coefficients of variation (CVs) were TC: 0.7% and 1.5%; HDL-C: 0.6% and 1.2%; TG: 0.9% and 1.8%; and glucose: 0.8% and 2.6%. LDL cholesterol (LDL-C) was calculated using the Friedewald formula [34]. The following thresholds were considered abnormal: TG $\geq$ 1.7 mmol/L [35], HDL-C < 1.29 mmol/L [36], TC > 5.172 mmol/L, and LDL-C $\geq$ 3.36 mmol/L [37]. Abnormalities in any one of these parameters are considered indicative of dyslipidemia [38]. Impaired fasting glucose was classified as a glucose level of $\geq$ 5.6 mmol/L [39].

2.2.2. Vitamin B12

Serum vitamin B12 levels were determined using an electrochemiluminescent immunoassay using a Roche Cobas e411 immunoassay analyzer (Roche Diagnostics, Germany). Vitamin B12 deficiency was defined as a serum vitamin B12 level of <148 pmol/L [40] and insufficiency as <221 pmol/L. The intra- and interassay CVs were 2.9% and 4.1%, respectively.

2.3. Dietary Assessment

The Saudi Food and Drug Administration's food frequency questionnaire was used to measure vitamin B12 intake over the past year [41]. The official Arabic language version of the questionnaire was used to interview individuals. A list of 133 food items was included in the questionnaire and a close-ended approach was used. Nine answer options were provided for each close-ended question, with consumption frequency choices given as follows: never or less than once a month, 1–3 times per month, once a week, 2–4 times per week, 5–6 times per week, once a day, 2–3 times per day, 4–5 times per day, or 6+ times per day. In addition, the questionnaire included open-ended questions, at the end, to gather information about other food items that were not listed. It also included questions regarding the types of cooking fat used, visible fat consumption, and salt and vitamin consumption [41]. The nutritional values of the items were based on the Saudi Food Composition Tables for 1996, McCance and Widdowson's Composition of Foods Integrated Dataset for 2015, and the 12th edition of the Concise New Zealand Food Composition Tables from 2016 [41–43]. In addition, we used another validated questionnaire, "vitamin B12 food questionnaire", that had been specifically developed to measure vitamin B12 intake from food and beverages [43]. Thus, both questionnaires were integrated to capture the most accurate picture of vitamin B12 intake. The recommended dietary allowance (RDA) for vitamin B12 in adults is 2.4 mcg/day to define adequate daily intake [3].

2.4. Clinical Assessment

Anthropometric data were obtained using standard procedures. Weight and height without shoes and heavy clothing were recorded to the nearest 0.2 kg and 0.5 cm, respectively, using an appropriate international standard scale (Digital Pearson Scale, ADAM Equipment Inc., Danbury, CT, USA). BMI (kg/m^2) was calculated as weight in kilograms divided by height in meters squared. According to the WHO [44], individuals can be categorized into four groups based on BMI: underweight (<18.5 kg/m^2), normal weight (18.5–24.9 kg/m^2), overweight (25.0–29.9 kg/m^2), and obese ($\geq$30 kg/m^2). Waist and hip circumferences were measured according to WHO procedures. Female participants with a waist circumference of >88 cm were classified as having central obesity, which substantially increased the risk of metabolic complications [45]. Waist-to-hip ratios (WHRs) were obtained by dividing the mean waist circumference by the mean hip circumference. The InBody 770 body composition analyzer (USA, Cerritos, CA, USA) was used for assessing the fat percentage of participants.

2.5. Other Risk Factors

All participants were interviewed via a general health history questionnaire that solicited information regarding their sociodemographic background (income and living region) along with family medical history [46]. They were then interviewed using the global physical activity questionnaire (GPAQ).

Physical Activity Questionnaire

GPAQ version 2.0 was used to assess physical activity [47], covering several components of physical activity, such as intensity, duration, and frequency, in addition to assessing three domains in which physical activity is performed: occupational physical activity, transport-related physical activity, and physical activity during discretionary or leisure time [48]. This study used the official Arabic version of the GPAQ, which has been used previously for a college-aged Saudi population [47].

2.6. Statistical Analysis

Data were analyzed using the SPSS version 23.0 statistical software. The normality of all quantitative variables was tested before performing the analysis. Descriptive statistics (means, standard deviations, medians, quartiles, frequencies, and percentages) were used to quantify the continuous and categorical variables. Data were presented in tertiles of vitamin B12: tertile 1, $\leq$333.05 pmol/L; tertile 2 ranged from 333.1 to 482.2 pmol/L; and tertile 3, >482.2 pmol/L. Log transformation was used prior to conducting parametric testing. Associations between serum vitamin B12 levels and selected parameters were analyzed using Pearson's correlation. Multivariate linear and logistic regression models were used to assess the association between serum vitamin B12 levels and the lipid profile per (1 SD = 176.5 pmol/L) of vitamin B12. The models were adjusted for age, BMI, WHR, glucose, income, physical activity, and family history of dyslipidemia and heart disease. $p < 0.05$ was considered to indicate significance.

3. Results

3.1. Baseline Characteristics by Vitamin B12 Tertiles

The mean age and BMI of participants were 20.7 ± 1.5 years and 23.6 ± 5.2 kg/m^2, respectively. In total, 14% of participants were overweight, while 14.9% were obese. Moreover, 3.5% of the total participants had central obesity. About 23% and 30.6% of the participants had a family history of dyslipidemia and heart disease, respectively. The demographic characteristics of the participants (e.g., clinical history, income, vitamin B12 intake, physical activity levels) are presented by tertiles of vitamin B12 (Table 1).

Participants with higher serum vitamin B12 levels (tertile 3) had lower levels of TC, LDL-C, and TG levels as well as TC/HDL, TG/HDL, and LDL/HDL ratios compared to participants with a lower serum vitamin B12 level (tertile 1) (Table 1). Macronutrients, energy, and water intake did not show any differences between the three groups (Table S1).

The median serum vitamin B12 concentration was 398.9 pmol/L. The prevalence of vitamin B12 deficiency was 0.6% (2/341) and insufficiency was 5.6% (19/341). Of the participants, 15.9% had high TC levels, 18.6% had high LDL-C levels, and 82.4% had dyslipidemia (Figure 1).

Table 1. Characteristics of study participants according to vitamin B12 tertiles.

Parameters	Total	Tertile 1	Tertile 2	Tertile 3	p-Value
N	341	114	113	114	
Age (years)	20.7 ± 1.5	20.7 ± 1.6	20.9 ± 1.8	20.7 ± 1.2	0.40
BMI (kg/m^2)	23.6 ± 5.2	23.9 ± 5.6	23.5 ± 4.7	23.7 ± 5.4	0.85
Waist circumference (cm)	71.1 ± 10.4	72.1 ± 11.0	69.7 ± 9.3	71.4 ± 10.7	0.22
Hip circumference (cm)	99.5 ± 11.7	100.1 ± 10.7	98.7 ± 13.1	99.5 ± 11.1	0.66
Waist/hip ratio	0.72 ± 0.06	0.72 ± 0.07	0.70 ± 0.05 [A]	0.72 ± 0.06	0.03
Fat (%)	36.9 ± 8.2	37.1 ± 8.1	36.8 ± 8.0	37.3 ± 8.1	0.91
Family history of dyslipidemia	8 (2.3)	2 (1.8)	5 (4.4)	1 (0.9)	0.19
Family history of hyperlipidemia	129 (37.8)	42 (36.8)	50 (44.2)	37 (32.5)	0.19
Family history of heart disease	104 (30.6)	39 (34.2)	35 (31.0)	30 (26.5)	0.55
Income level (<10,000 SAR)	70 (20.5)	26 (22.8)	24 (21.2)	20 (17.5)	0.60
Vitamin B12 intake (mcg/day)	6.9 (4.4–10.8)	6.3 (3.5–10.1)	6.8 (4.9–9.9)	8.3 (4.8–11.6) [A]	0.02
Adequate vitamin B12 (≥2.4 mcg/day)	323 (94.7)	102 (89.5)	109 (96.5)	112 (98.2) [A]	0.01
Median B12 levels	398.9 (305.8–534.6)	269.1 (243.0–305.8)	398.9 (361.0–448.3) [A]	596.6 (534.6–683.7) [AB]	<0.001
GPAQ score (MET-minute/week) [#]	504.0 (160.0–1240.0)	600.0 (200.0–1620.0)	560.0 (160.0–1200.0)	400.0 (180.0–940.0)	0.18
Biochemical characteristics					
Fasting glucose (mmol/L)	4.6 ± 1.0	4.6 ± 1.0	4.6 ± 1.1	4.7 ± 0.9	0.77
TC (mmol/L)	3.8 ± 1.4	4.3 ± 1.6	3.8 ± 1.4 [A]	3.3 ± 1.2 [A]	<0.001
HDL-C (mmol/L)	1.0 ± 0.4	1.0 ± 0.3	1.0 ± 0.4	1.1 ± 0.4	0.34
LDL-Cl (mmol/L)	2.4 ± 1.2	2.8 ± 1.3	2.3 ± 1.0 [A]	2.0 ± 0.9 [A]	<0.001
TG (mmol/L)	0.8 ± 0.4	0.9 ± 0.5	0.7 ± 0.4 [A]	0.7 ± 0.4 [A]	<0.001
TC/HDL ratio	3.9 ± 1.6	4.6 ± 2.0	3.8 ± 1.4 [A]	3.3 ± 1.0 [A]	<0.001
TG/HDL ratio	0.9 ± 0.6	1.0 ± 0.6	0.8 ± 0.8	0.7 ± 0.4 [A]	<0.01
LDL-C/HDL-C	2.4 ± 1.4	3.0 ± 1.7 [A]	2.4 ± 1.2 [A]	2.0 ± 0.9	<0.001

Note: data presented as mean ± SD for normal variables and median (IQR) for non-normal variables; [#] indicates non-normal variables; superscript A and B indicates significance from tertile 1 and tertile 2, respectively; p-values were obtained from ANOVA and Kruskal–Wallis H tests for normal and non-normal variables, respectively; significance is set at p < 0.05. GPAQ; global physical activity questionnaire.

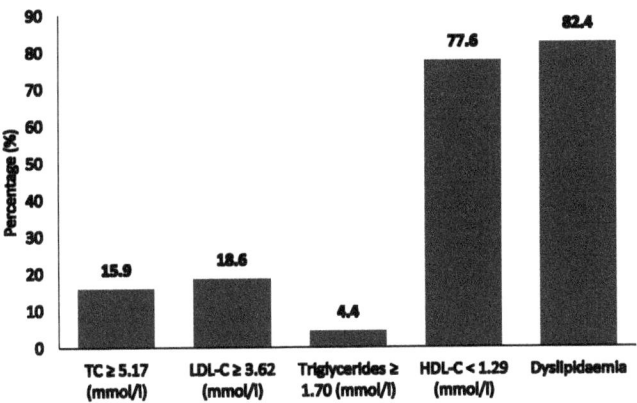

Figure 1. Prevalence of abnormal lipid parameters and dyslipidemia.

3.2. Serum Vitamin B12 Levels and Lipid Profile

Pearson's correlation showed significant inverse associations between serum vitamin B12 levels and the lipid profile parameters, with the exception of HDL-C (Figure 2). Linear regression analyses showed that the serum vitamin B12 level was independently and inversely associated with TC, TG, LDL-C levels, LDL/HDL ratio, TC/HDL ratio, and TG/HDL ratio after adjusting for confounders (Table 2). One SD increase in serum vitamin B12 levels (176.5 pmol/L) reduced TC, TG, and LDL-C by 0.38, 0.07, and 0.34 pmol/L, respectively (Table 2). Multiple logistic regression found that serum vitamin B12 level was inversely related to dyslipidemia but was not significant when adjusted for all confounders. The results were similar when BMI was replaced by either height and WHR, height and fat percentage, or height and central obesity (Table S2).

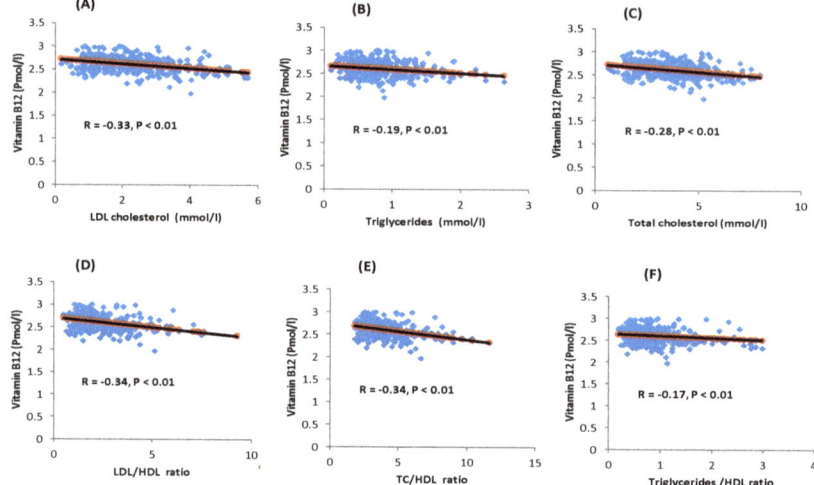

Figure 2. Associations between serum vitamin B12 levels and lipid parameters. (**A**) Association between serum vitamin B12 levels and LDL-C; (**B**) Association between serum vitamin B12 levels and triglycerides; (**C**) Association between serum vitamin B12 levels and total cholesterol; (**D**) Association between serum vitamin B12 levels and LDL/HDL ratio; (**E**) Association between serum vitamin B12 levels and TC/HDL ratio; and (**F**) Association between serum vitamin B12 levels and Triglyceride/HDL ratio. Note: the *p*-value was obtained from the Pearson correlation test.

Table 2. Associations between vitamin B12 and lipid profile per 1 SD vitamin B12; $n = 341$.

Parameters	Model 1			Model 2		
	B ± SE/OR	B (S)/95%CI	*p*-Value	B ± SE	B (S)/95%CI	*p*-Value
Total cholesterol (mmol/L)	−0.39 ± 0.08	−0.27	<0.0001	−0.38 ± 0.07	−0.26	<0.0001
Triglycerides (mmol/L)	−0.07 ± 0.02	−0.17	<0.01	−0.07 ± 0.02	−0.16	<0.01
LDL-C (mmol/L)	−0.35 ± 0.06	−0.30	<0.0001	−0.34 ± 0.06	−0.30	<0.0001
HDL-C (mmol/L)	0.01 ± 0.02	0.04	0.51	0.01 ± 0.02	0.04	0.48
LDL/HDL ratio	−0.41 ± 0.07	−0.30	<0.0001	−0.41 ± 0.07	−0.30	<0.0001
TC/HDL ratio	−0.48 ± 0.09	−0.30	<0.0001	−0.47 ± 0.09	−0.29	<0.0001
Triglyceride/HDL ratio	−0.09 ± 0.04	−0.14	0.02	−0.08 ± 0.04	−0.13	0.02
Dyslipidemia *	0.75	0.56–1.00	0.05	0.74	0.55–1.01	0.06

Note: data presented as B ± SE and odds ratio for continuous and categorical variables were obtained from linear and logistic regression models, respectively; the lipid profile was the dependent variable. Model 1 adjusted for age, BMI, physical activity, income, family history of hyperlipidemia, and heart disease; Model 2 adjusted for Model 1 and glucose. $p < 0.05$ was considered significant. * indicates categorical variables; $p < 0.05$ is considered significant.

4. Discussion

In a cohort of young women living in Saudi Arabia, we found that serum vitamin B12 levels were inversely associated with the lipid profile (TC, LDL-C, and TG levels), TC/HDL, TG/HDL, and LDL/HDL ratios. The relationship persisted after adjusting for potential confounding factors. The prevalence of dyslipidemia was considered high (around 82%) based on the standard definitions.

To the best of our knowledge, no previous studies have analyzed the prevalence of vitamin B12 deficiency within an apparently healthy young Saudi population. The prevalence of vitamin B12 deficiency found in the current study was 0.6% (insufficiency, 5.5%), which is lower than that reported in other studies in Saudi Arabia and other Arabian countries (i.e., between 6% and 30%) [15,16]. This might be because the high estimated intake of vitamin B12 in our study sample was higher than in others [49]. Nearly 95% of our participants took adequate daily doses of vitamin B12. In addition, some studies from Arabian countries focus on older age groups and patients with diabetes [15,16]. These patients would likely have been on metformin, a commonly used drug for the treatment of diabetes, which is known to cause lower serum vitamin B12 levels [50].

Our findings were consistent with observations in other samples. In a comparative study of patients with T2DM living in the United Kingdom and India, Adaikalakoteswari et al. found that serum vitamin B12 level was independently and inversely associated with levels of TGs and the TC/HDL ratio [33]. Similarly, another cross-sectional study of 300 patients with coronary artery disease reported that serum vitamin B12 level was inversely associated with dyslipidemia as well as TG and VLDL levels and positively associated with HDL-C levels, but was not associated with TC or LDL-C levels [22]. Our study extends this observation to young women in Saudi Arabia. Previous studies have shown that lipid profile ratios are better indicators of CVD than each variable alone [51,52]. Therefore, our observation highlights the importance of understanding the relationship between lipid profile and vitamin B12.

To date, only a few studies have investigated the association of serum vitamin B12 levels with lipid profile in apparently healthy individuals. In a prospective cohort that involved 421 healthy Korean individuals followed up for 12 years, serum vitamin B12 levels were not associated with dyslipidemia or any atherosclerotic events. However, the mean serum vitamin B12 level among Korean individuals was higher than those in other population samples previously studied [53]. Nevertheless, as hypertriglyceridemia is associated with higher rates of gestational diabetes and macrosomia [54], our findings are important as these are observations from young women of child-bearing age. In addition, serum vitamin B12 levels (along with folate) have been linked with adverse pregnancy outcomes [24] and higher insulin resistance in offspring [25].

The mechanism by which vitamin B12 deficiency is associated with the lipid profile may involve elevated plasma tHcy concentrations and affects phospholipid metabolism; this, in turn, causes the high secretion of VLDL, leading to abnormal lipid levels [28]. Another proposed mechanism involves gene expression related to lipogenesis [23,29] and inflammation [30]. The mechanism underlying the relationship with the lipid profile can be further explained by the fact that vitamin B12 acts as a coenzyme in the conversion of methylmalonyl-CoA to succinyl-CoA [55,56]. This reaction is blocked if there are low serum vitamin B12 levels, resulting in methylmalonyl-CoA accumulation, which inhibits the rate-limiting enzyme of fatty acid oxidation [57] and thereby causes lipogenesis.

The current study has the following strengths. First, it involves healthy young women, a group that had not been previously investigated. Second, the extensive data collected in our study on sociodemographic, medical history, dietary information, and physical activity may help identify other important confounding or mediating variables in the association between B12 levels and lipid profiles. However, several limitations are presented in our study. First, it employed a cross-sectional design; therefore, no causal inferences can be made. Second, only the serum vitamin B12 level was used to assess the B12 status. We did not include methylmalonic acid or tHcy levels, indicators of tissue-level B12 deficiency. However, serum vitamin B12 levels have been previously shown to be valid indicators of B12 status in individuals as well as in epidemiological settings [58]. Third, the use of the FFQ and GPAQ questionnaires may have led to recall bias.

In conclusion, we found a high prevalence of dyslipidemia in apparently healthy young women in Saudi Arabia. While it is reassuring to find adequate intake of B12 in this population, our finding of an inverse association between B12 and adverse lipid profile is concerning and warrants further studies. These studies should focus on understanding the mechanisms of the relationship between serum vitamin B12 levels and adverse lipid profiles.

Supplementary Materials: The following are available online at http://www.mdpi.com/2072-6643/12/8/2395/s1, Table S1: Dietary intake of study participants by vitamin B12 tertiles, Table S2: Associations between vitamin B12 and lipid profile.

Author Contributions: Conceptualization, S.A.-M. and P.S.; data curation, A.M.A.; formal analysis, S.D.H. and A.M.A.; methodology, S.A.-M. and P.S.; project administration, P.S. and N.A.-D.; supervision, G.S.A. and N.A.-D.; writing—original draft, S.A.-M.; writing—review and editing, G.S.A. and P.S. All authors have read and agreed to the published version of the manuscript.

Funding: This research was funded by Deanship of Scientific Research at King Saud University, grant number RG-1441-346. P.S. was supported in part by the Medical Research Council, UK grants MR/N006232/1 and MR/R020981/1.

Acknowledgments: The authors extend their appreciation to the Deanship of Scientific Research at King Saud University for funding this work through research group no. RG-1441-346.

Conflicts of Interest: The authors declare no conflicts of interest.

References

1. Zalaket, J.; Wehbe, T.; Jaoude, E.A. Vitamin B12 Deficiency in Diabetic Subjects Taking Metformin: A Cross Sectional Study in a Lebanese Cohort. *J. Nutr. Intermed. Metab.* **2018**, *11*, 9–13. [CrossRef]
2. Al-Daghri, N.M.; Al-Attas, O.S.; Alokail, M.S.; Alkharfy, K.M.; Yakout, S.M.; Aljohani, N.J.; Alfawaz, H.A.; Al-Ajlan, A.S.M.; Sheshah, E.S.; Al-Yousef, M.; et al. Lower Vitamin D Status is More Common Among Saudi Adults with Diabetes Mellitus Type 1 Than in Non-diabetics. *BMC Public Health* **2014**, *14*, 153. [CrossRef]
3. Institute of Medicine (US) Standing Committee on the Scientific Evaluation of Dietary Reference Intakes. *Dietary Reference Intakes for Thiamin, Riboflavin, Niacin, Vitamin b6, Folate, Vitamin b12, Pantothenic Acid, Biotin, and Choline*; National Academies Press: Washington, DC, USA, 1998.
4. Saravanan, P.; Yajnik, C.S. Role of Maternal Vitamin B12 on the Metabolic Health of the Offspring: A Contributor to the Diabetes Epidemic? *Br. J. Diabetes Vasc. Dis.* **2010**, *10*, 109–114. [CrossRef]
5. Rolfes, S.R.; Pinna, K.; Whitney, E. *Understanding Normal and Clinical Nutrition*, 9th ed.; Cengage Learning: Boston, MA, USA, 2012; pp. 321–365. ISBN1 084006845X. ISBN2 9780840068453.
6. Palacios, G.; Sola, R.; Barrios, L.; Pietrzik, K.; Castillo, M.J.; González-Gross, M. Algorithm for the Early Diagnosis of Vitamin B12 Deficiency in Elderly People. *Nutr. Hosp.* **2013**, *28*, 1447–1452. [CrossRef] [PubMed]
7. Mccombe, P.A.; Mcleod, J.G. The Peripheral Neuropathy of Vitamin B12 Deficiency. *J. Neurol. Sci.* **1984**, *66*, 117–126. [CrossRef]
8. de Benoist, B. Conclusions of a WHO Technical Consultation on Folate and Vitamin B12 Deficiencies. *Food Nutr. Bull.* **2008**, *29*, S238–S244. [CrossRef] [PubMed]
9. Murphy, M.M.; Molloy, A.M.; Ueland, P.M.; Fernandez-Ballart, J.D.; Schneede, J.; Arija, V.; Scott, J.M. Longitudinal Study of the Effect of Pregnancy on Maternal and Fetal Cobalamin Status in Healthy Women and Their Offspring. *J. Nutr.* **2007**, *137*, 1863–1867. [CrossRef]
10. Bailey, R.L.; Carmel, R.; Green, R.; Pfeiffer, C.M.; Cogswell, M.E.; Osterloh, J.D.; Sempos, C.T.; Yetley, E.A. Monitoring of Vitamin B-12 Nutritional Status in the United States by Using Plasma Methylmalonic Acid and Serum Vitamin B-12. *Am. J. Clin. Nutr.* **2011**, *94*, 552–561. [CrossRef]
11. Green, R.; Allen, L.H.; Bjørke-Monsen, A.-L.; Brito, A.; Guéant, J.-L.; Miller, J.W.; Molloy, A.M.; Nexo, E.; Stabler, S.; Toh, B.-H.; et al. Vitamin B12 Deficiency. *Nat. Rev. Dis. Primers* **2017**, *3*, 17040. [CrossRef]
12. Sukumar, N.; Adaikalakoteswari, A.; Venkataraman, H.; Maheswaran, H.; Saravana, P. Vitamin B12 Status in Women of Childbearing Age in the UK and Its Relationship with National Nutrient Intake Guidelines: Results From Two National Diet and Nutrition Surveys. *BMJ Open* **2016**, *6*, e011247. [CrossRef]
13. Quay, T.A.; Schroder, T.H.; Jeruszka-Bielak, M.; Li, W.; Devlin, A.M.; Barr, S.I.; Lamers, Y. High Prevalence of Suboptimal Vitamin B12 Status in Young Adult Women of South Asian and European Ethnicity. *Appl. Physiol. Nutr. Metab.* **2015**, *40*, 1279–1286. [CrossRef] [PubMed]
14. Sukumar, N.; Rafnsson, S.B.; Kandala, N.B.; Bhopal, R.; Yajnik, C.S.; Saravanan, P. Prevalence of Vitamin B-12 Insufficiency During Pregnancy and Its Effect on Offspring Birth Weight: A Systematic Review and Meta-Analysis. *Am. J. Clin. Nutr.* **2016**, *103*, 1232–1251. [CrossRef] [PubMed]
15. El-Khateeb, M.; Khader, Y.; Batieha, A.; Jaddou, H.; Hyassat, D.; Belbisi, A.; Ajlouni, K. Vitamin B12 Deficiency in Jordan: A Population-Based Study. *Ann. Nutr. Metab.* **2014**, *64*, 101–105. [CrossRef] [PubMed]
16. Alharbi, T.J.; Tourkmani, A.M.; Abdelhay, O.; Alkhashan, H.I.; Al-Asmari, A.K.; Bin Rsheed, A.M.; Abuhaimed, S.N.; Mohammed, N.; AlRasheed, A.N.; AlHarbi, N.G. The Association of Metformin Use with Vitamin B12 Deficiency and Peripheral Neuropathy in Saudi Individuals With Type 2 Diabetes Mellitus. *PLoS ONE* **2018**, *13*, e0204420. [CrossRef] [PubMed]
17. Sun, Y.; Sun, M.; Liu, B.; Du, Y.; Rong, S.; Xu, G.; Snetselaar, L.G.; Bao, W. Inverse Association Between Serum Vitamin B12 Concentration and Obesity Among Adults in the United States. *Front. Endocrinol.* **2019**, *10*, 414. [CrossRef]

18. Knight, B.A.; Shields, B.M.; Brook, A.; Hill, A.; Bhat, D.S.; Hattersley, A.T.; Yajnik, C.S. Lower Circulating B12 is Associated with Higher Obesity and Insulin Resistance During Pregnancy in a Non-Diabetic White British Population. *PLoS ONE* **2015**, *10*, e0135268. [CrossRef]
19. Krishnaveni, G.V.; Hill, J.C.; Veena, S.R.; Bhat, D.S.; Wills, A.K.; Karat, C.L.; Yajnik, C.S.; Fall, C.H. Low Plasma Vitamin B12 in Pregnancy is Associated with Gestational 'Diabesity' and Later Diabetes. *Diabetologia* **2009**, *52*, 2350–2358. [CrossRef]
20. Saraswathy, K.N.; Joshi, S.; Yadav, S.; Garg, P.R. Metabolic Distress in Lipid and One Carbon Metabolic Pathway Through Low Vitamin B-12: A Population Based Study from North India. *Lipids Health Dis.* **2018**, *17*, 96. [CrossRef]
21. Boachie, J.; Adaikalakoteswari, A.; Samavat, J.; Saravanan, P. Low Vitamin B12 and Lipid Metabolism: Evidence from Pre-Clinical and Clinical Studies. *Nutrients* **2020**, *12*, 1925. [CrossRef]
22. Mahalle, N.; Kulkarni, M.V.; Garg, M.K.; Naik, S.S. Vitamin B12 Deficiency and Hyperhomocysteinemia as Correlates of Cardiovascular Risk Factors in Indian Subjects with Coronary Artery Disease. *J. Cardiol.* **2013**, *61*, 289–294. [CrossRef]
23. Adaikalakoteswari, A.; Finer, S.; Voyias, P.D.; McCarthy, C.M.; Vatish, M.; Moore, J.; Smart-Halajko, M.; Bawazeer, N.; Al-Daghri, N.M.; McTernan, P.G.; et al. Vitamin B12 Insufficiency Induces Cholesterol Biosynthesis by Limiting S-Adenosylmethionine and Modulating the Methylation of SREBF1 and LDLR Genes. *Clin. Epigenetics* **2015**, *7*, 14. [CrossRef] [PubMed]
24. Sukumar, N.; Venkataraman, H.; Wilson, S.; Goljan, I.; Selvamoni, S.; Patel, V.; Saravanan, P. Vitamin B12 Status Among Pregnant Women in the UK and Its Association with Obesity and Gestational Diabetes. *Nutrients* **2016**, *8*, 768. [CrossRef] [PubMed]
25. Stewart, C.P.; Christian, P.; Schulze, K.J.; Arguello, M.; LeClerq, S.C.; Khatry, S.K.; West, K.P., Jr. Low Maternal Vitamin B-12 Status is Associated with Offspring Insulin Resistance Regardless of Antenatal Micronutrient Supplementation in Rural Nepal. *J. Nutr.* **2011**, *141*, 1912–1917. [CrossRef] [PubMed]
26. Bailey, L.B.; Stover, P.J.; McNulty, H.; Fenech, M.F.; Gregory, J.F., 3rd; Mills, J.L.; Pfeiffer, C.M.; Fazili, Z.; Zhang, M.; Ueland, P.M.; et al. Biomarkers of Nutrition for Development-Folate Review. *J. Nutr.* **2015**, *145*, 1636S–1680S. [CrossRef]
27. Keser, I.; Ilich, J.Z.; Vrkić, N.; Giljević, Z.; Colić Barić, I. Folic Acid and Vitamin B(12) Supplementation Lowers Plasma Homocysteine but has no Effect on Serum Bone Turnover Markers in Elderly Women: A Randomized, Double-Blind, Placebo-Controlled Trial. *Nutr. Res.* **2013**, *33*, 211–219. [CrossRef]
28. Obeid, R.; Herrmann, W. Homocysteine and Lipids: S-Adenosyl Methionine as a Key Intermediate. *FEBS Lett.* **2009**, *583*, 1215–1225. [CrossRef]
29. Rafnsson, S.B.; Saravanan, P.; Bhopal, R.S.; Yajnik, C.S. Is a Low Blood Level of Vitamin B12 a Cardiovascular and Diabetes Risk Factor? A Systematic Review of Cohort Studies. *Eur. J. Nutr.* **2011**, *50*, 97–106. [CrossRef]
30. Kumar, K.A.; Lalitha, A.; Pavithra, D.; Padmavathi, I.J.; Ganeshan, M.; Rao, K.R.; Venu, L.; Balakrishna, N.; Shanker, N.H.; Reddy, S.U.; et al. Maternal Dietary Folate and/or Vitamin B12 Restrictions Alter Body Composition (Adiposity) and Lipid Metabolism in Wistar Rat Offspring. *J. Nutr. Biochem.* **2013**, *24*, 25–31. [CrossRef]
31. Al-Rubeaan, K.; Bawazeer, N.; Al Farsi, Y.; Youssef, A.M.; Al-Yahya, A.A.; AlQumaidi, H.; Al-Malki, B.M.; Naji, K.A.; Al-Shehri, K.; Al Rumaih, F.I. Prevalence of Metabolic Syndrome in Saudi Arabia—A Cross Sectional Study. *BMC Endocr. Disord.* **2018**, *18*, 16. [CrossRef]
32. Al-Rifai, R.H.; Majeed, M.I.; Tariq, M.R.; Irfan, A. Type 2 Diabetes and Pre-Diabetes Mellitus: A Systematic Review and Meta-Analysis of Prevalence Studies in Women of Childbearing Age in the Middle East and North Africa, 2000-2018. *Syst. Rev.* **2019**, *8*, 268. [CrossRef]
33. Adaikalakoteswari, A.; Jayashri, R.; Sukumar, N.; Venkataraman, H.; Pradeepa, R.; Gokulakrishnan, K.; Anjana, R.M.; McTernan, P.G.; Tripathi, G.; Patel, V.; et al. Vitamin B12 Deficiency is Associated with Adverse Lipid Profile in Europeans and Indians With Type 2 Diabetes. *Cardiovasc. Diabetol.* **2014**, *13*, 129. [CrossRef] [PubMed]
34. Friedewald, W.T.; Levy, R.I.; Fredrickson, D.S. Estimation of the Concentration of Low-Density Lipoprotein Cholesterol in Plasma, Without Use of the Preparative Ultracentrifuge. *Clin. Chem.* **1972**, *18*, 499–502. [CrossRef] [PubMed]

35. Grundy, S.M.; Cleeman, J.I.; Daniels, S.R.; Donato, K.A.; Eckel, R.H.; Franklin, B.A.; Gordon, D.J.; Krauss, R.M.; Savage, P.J.; Smith, S.C., Jr.; et al. Diagnosis and Management of the Metabolic Syndrome: An American Heart Association/National Heart, Lung, and Blood Institute Scientific Statement. *Circulation* **2005**, *112*, 2735–2752. [CrossRef] [PubMed]
36. Saely, C.H.; Koch, L.; Schmid, F.; Marte, T.; Aczel, S.; Langer, P.; Hoefle, G.; Drexel, H. Adult Treatment Panel III 2001 but not International Diabetes Federation 2005 Criteria of the Metabolic Syndrome Predict Clinical Cardiovascular Events in Subjects Who Underwent Coronary Angiography. *Diabetes Care* **2006**, *29*, 901–907. [CrossRef]
37. Jellinger, P.S.; Handelsman, Y.; Rosenblit, P.D.; Bloomgarden, Z.T.; Fonseca, V.A.; Garber, A.J.; Grunberger, G.; Guerin, C.K.; Bell, D.S.H.; Mechanick, J.I.; et al. American Association of Clinical Endocrinologists and American College of Endocrinology Guidelines for Management of Dyslipidemia and Prevention of Cardiovascular Disease. *Endocr. Pract.* **2017**, *23*, 1–87. [CrossRef]
38. Stone, N.J.; Robinson, J.J.; Lichtenstein, A.H.; Merz, C.N.B.; Blum, C.B.; Eckel, R.H.; Goldberg, A.C.; Gordon, D.; Levy, D.; Lloyd-Jones, D.M.; et al. 2013 ACC/AHA Guideline on the Treatment of Blood Cholesterol to Reduce Atherosclerotic Cardiovascular Risk in Adults: A Report of the American College of Cardiology/American Heart Association Task Force on Practice Guidelines. *J. Am. Coll. Cardiol.* **2014**, *63*, 2889–2934. [CrossRef]
39. Genuth, S.; Alberti, K.G.; Bennett, P.; Buse, J.; Defronzo, R.; Kahn, R.; Kitzmiller, J.; Knowler, W.C.; Lebovitz, H.; Lernmark, A.; et al. Follow-Up Report on the Diagnosis of Diabetes Mellitus. *Diabetes Care* **2003**, *26*, 3160–3168. [CrossRef]
40. Hunt, A.; Harrington, D.; Robinson, S. Vitamin B12 Deficiency. *BMJ* **2014**, *349*, 5226. [CrossRef]
41. Alkhalaf, M.; Edwards, C.; Combet, E. Validation of a Food Frequency Questionnaire Specific for Salt Intake in Saudi Arabian Adults Using Urinary Biomarker and Repeated Multiple Pass 24-Hour Dietary Recall. *Proc. Nutr. Soc.* **2015**, *74*, E337. [CrossRef]
42. Roe, M.; Pinchen, H.; Church, S.; Finglas, P. McCance and Widdowson's The Composition of Foods Seventh Summary Edition and Updated Composition of Foods Integrated Dataset. *Nutr. Bull.* **2015**, *40*, 36–39. [CrossRef]
43. Mearns, G.J.; Rush, E.C. Screening for Inadequate Dietary Vitamin B-12 Intake in South Asian Women Using a Nutrient-Specific, Semi-Quantitative Food Frequency Questionnaire. *Asia Pac. J. Clin. Nutr.* **2017**, *26*, 1119. [CrossRef] [PubMed]
44. Bray, G.A. Clinical Evaluation of the Obese Patient. *Best Pract. Res. Clin. Endocrinol. Metab.* **1999**, *13*, 71–92. [CrossRef] [PubMed]
45. World Health Organizaion. Obesity and Overweight. World Health Organization, 2018. Available online: http://www.who.int/news-room/fact-sheets/detail/obesity-and-overweight (accessed on 15 January 2020).
46. Al-Musharaf, S.; Fouda, M.A.; Turkestani, I.Z.; Al-Ajlan, A.; Sabico, S.; Alnaami, A.M.; Wani, K.; Hussain, S.D.; Alraqebah, B.; Al-Serehi, A.; et al. Vitamin D Deficiency Prevalence and Predictors in Early Pregnancy Among Arab Women. *Nutrients* **2018**, *10*, 489. [CrossRef] [PubMed]
47. Alkahtani, S.A. Convergent Validity: Agreement Between Accelerometry and the Global Physical Activity Questionnaire in College-Age Saudi Men. *BMC Res. Notes* **2016**, *9*, 436. [CrossRef]
48. World Health Organization. Global Physical Activity Questionnaire (GPAQ) Analysis Guide: World Health Organization. Available online: http://www.who.int/chp/steps/resources/GPAQ_Analysis_Guide.pdf (accessed on 12 May 2020).
49. Vogiatzoglou, A.; Smith, A.D.; Nurk, E.; Berstad, P.; Drevon, C.A.; Ueland, P.M.; Vollset, S.E.; Tell, G.S.; Refsum, H. Dietary Sources of Vitamin B-12 and Their Association with Plasma Vitamin B-12 Concentrations in the General Population: The Hordaland Homocysteine Study. *Am. J. Clin. Nutr.* **2009**, *89*, 1078–1087. [CrossRef]
50. Aroda, V.R.; Edelstein, S.L.; Goldberg, R.B.; Knowler, W.C.; Marcovina, S.M.; Orchard, T.J.; Bray, G.A.; Schade, D.S.; Temprosa, M.G.; White, N.H.; et al. Long-term Metformin Use and Vitamin B12 Deficiency in the Diabetes Prevention Program Outcomes Study. *J. Clin. Endocrinol. Metab.* **2016**, *101*, 1754–1761. [CrossRef]
51. Ingelsson, E.; Schaefer, E.J.; Contois, J.H.; McNamara, J.R.; Sullivan, L.; Keyes, M.J.; Pencina, M.J.; Schoonmaker, C.; Wilson, P.W.; D'Agostino, R.B.; et al. Clinical Utility of Different Lipid Measures for Prediction of Coronary Heart Disease in Men and Women. *JAMA* **2007**, *298*, 776–785. [CrossRef]

52. Russo, G.T.; Giandalia, A.; Romeo, E.L.; Marotta, M.; Alibrandi, A.; De Francesco, C.; Horvath, K.V.; Asztalos, B.F.; Cucinotta, D. Lipid and non-lipid cardiovascular risk factors in postmenopausal type 2 diabetic women with and without coronary heart disease. *J. Endocrinol. Investig.* **2014**, *37*, 261–268. [CrossRef]
53. Kim, H.-N.; Eun, Y.-M.; Song, S.-W. Serum Folate and Vitamin B 12 Levels are not Associated with the Incidence Risk of Atherosclerotic Events Over 12 Years: The Korean Genome and Epidemiology Study. *Nutr. Res.* **2019**, *63*, 34–41. [CrossRef]
54. Gorban de Lapertosa, S.; Alvariñas, J.; Elgart, J.F.; Salzberg, S.; Gagliardino, J.J.; EduGest Group. The Triad Macrosomia, Obesity, and Hypertriglyceridemia in Gestational Diabetes. *Diabetes Metab. Res. Rev.* **2020**, *36*, e03302. [CrossRef]
55. Strain, J.J.; Dowey, L.; Ward, M.; Pentieva, K.; McNulty, H. B-Vitamins, Homocysteine Metabolism and CVD. *Proc. Nutr. Soc.* **2004**, *63*, 597–603. [CrossRef] [PubMed]
56. Rosenberg, I.H. Metabolic Programming of Offspring by Vitamin B12/folate Imbalance During Pregnancy. *Diabetologia* **2008**, *51*, 6–7. [CrossRef] [PubMed]
57. Brindle, N.P.; Zammit, V.A.; Pogson, C.I. Regulation of Carnitine Palmitoyltransferase Activity by malonyl-CoA in Mitochondria from Sheep Liver, a Tissue With a Low Capacity for Fatty Acid Synthesis. *Biochem. J.* **1985**, *232*, 177–182. [CrossRef] [PubMed]
58. Carmel, R. Biomarkers of Cobalamin (Vitamin B-12) Status in the Epidemiologic Setting: A Critical Overview of Context, Applications, and Performance Characteristics of Cobalamin, Methylmalonic Acid, and Holotranscobalamin II. *Am. J. Clin. Nutr.* **2011**, *94*, 348S–358S. [CrossRef] [PubMed]

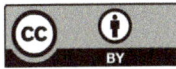

© 2020 by the authors. Licensee MDPI, Basel, Switzerland. This article is an open access article distributed under the terms and conditions of the Creative Commons Attribution (CC BY) license (http://creativecommons.org/licenses/by/4.0/).

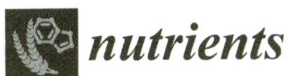

Article

A Randomized Placebo-Controlled Clinical Trial to Evaluate the Medium-Term Effects of Oat Fibers on Human Health: The Beta-Glucan Effects on Lipid Profile, Glycemia and inTestinal Health (BELT) Study

Arrigo F.G. Cicero [1,*,†], Federica Fogacci [1,†], Maddalena Veronesi [1], Enrico Strocchi [1], Elisa Grandi [1], Elisabetta Rizzoli [1], Andrea Poli [2], Franca Marangoni [2,‡] and Claudio Borghi [1,‡]

1. Atherosclerosis and Hypertension Research Group, Medical and Surgical Sciences Department, Sant'Orsola-Malpighi University Hospital, Building 2-IV Floor, Via Albertoni 15, 40138 Bologna, Italy; federicafogacci@gmail.com (F.F.); maddalena.veronesi@unibo.it (M.V.); enrico.strocchi@unibo.it (E.S.); elisa.grandi@unibo.it (E.G.); elisabetta.rizzoli@unibo.it (E.R.); claudio.borghi@unibo.it (C.B.)
2. Nutrition Foundation of Italy, Viale Tunisia 38, 20124 Milan, Italy; poli@nutrition-foundation.it (A.P.); marangoni@nutrition-foundation.it (F.M.)
* Correspondence: arrigo.cicero@unibo.it
† Are co-first authors.
‡ Are co-last authors.

Received: 6 February 2020; Accepted: 28 February 2020; Published: 3 March 2020

Abstract: The Beta-glucan Effects on Lipid profile, glycemia and inTestinal health (BELT) Study investigated the effect of 3 g/day oat beta-glucans on plasma lipids, fasting glucose and self-perceived intestinal well-being. The Study was an 8-week, double-blind, placebo-controlled, cross-over randomized clinical trial, enrolling a sample of 83 Italian free-living subjects, adherent to Mediterranean diet, with a moderate hypercholesterolemia and a low cardiovascular risk profile. Beta-glucans reduced mean LDL-Cholesterol (LDL-C) levels from baseline by 12.2% (95%CI: −15.4 to −3.8) after 4 weeks of supplementation and by 15.1% (95%CI: −17.8 to −5.9) after 8 weeks of supplementation ($p < 0.01$ for both comparison and versus placebo). Between baseline and 4 weeks Total Cholesterol (TC) levels showed an average reduction of 6.5% (95%CI: −10.9 to −1.9) in the beta-glucan sequence; while non-HDL-C plasma concentrations decreased by 11.8% (95%CI: −14.6 to −4.5). Moreover, after 8 weeks of beta-glucan supplementation TC was reduced by 8.9% (95%CI: −12.6 to −2.3) and non-HDL-C levels by 12.1% (95%CI: −15.6 to −5.3). Decreses in TC and non HDL-C were significant also versus placebo (respectively $p < 0.05$ and $p < 0.01$ to both follow-up visits). Fasting plasma glucose and self-perceived intestinal well-being were not affected by both beta-glucan and placebo supplementation.

Keywords: beta-glucan; fiber; lipid profile; cholesterol; intestinal function

---

1. Introduction

The consumption of dietary supplements to control plasma cholesterol levels has become widespread in recent years, alongside the publication of several systematic reviews and meta-analyses showing the cholesterol lowering effect of some of these products, including fibers [1–3].

A comprehensive meta-analysis of 58 clinical trials and 3974 subjects has recently showed that oat beta-glucan significantly affects the serum concentrations of low-density lipoprotein cholesterol (LDL-C), non-high-density lipoprotein cholesterol (non-HDL-C) and apolipoprotein-B (apo-B), concluding that the inclusion of oat-containing foods in the diet may be a valid strategy to prevent the onset of cardiovascular disease [2]. In particular, another meta-analysis presented a dose-response curve between fibre intakes and the reduction of total serum cholesterol, estimating a mean reduction for total cholesterol (TC) and LDL-C levels of 0.045 mmol/L and 0.057 mmol/L respectively, for each gram of dietary fiber [1]. These effects can theoretically play a major preventive role among the general population, since each 1% reduction in TC or LDL-C corresponds to an equivalent 1% decrease in the risk of developing a coronary heart disease event over time [3].

The mechanisms underlying the lipid-lowering properties of dietary fiber are still not fully understood [4]. The ability of soluble dietary fiber to form viscous solutions that prolong gastric emptying, and inhibit the transport of triglycerides and cholesterol across the intestine is a plausible explanation of their capacity to reduce LDL-C levels [5]. The consequences of the increased viscosity of the luminal contents manifest via the amplification of the thickness of the water layer and in the decrease of cholesterol uptake from the intestinal lumen [6].

The contribution of beta-glucans from oat and barley to the maintenance of normal blood cholesterol levels and their efficacy in the reduction of blood cholesterol levels at a dosage of 3 g per day was formally recognized by the European Food Safety Authority (EFSA) following specific applications and health claims that were authorized in the European Union (Commission Regulation (EU) 432/2012) [7]. However, the available clinical trials investigated the short-term lipid-lowering effect of beta-glucan administration on relatively small population samples and rarely involved European subjects [8,9]

In this context, we deemed interesting to evaluate the effect of a proprietary formulation of beta-glucans, at the dosage of 3 g/day on fasting plasma lipids and glucose, as well as its tolerability, in an Italian sample of subjects with mild hypercholesterolemia.

2. Materials and Methods

2.1. Study Design and Participants

The Beta-glucan Effects on Lipid profile, glycaemia and inTestinal health (BELT) Study was a medium-term, double-blind, placebo-controlled, cross-over randomized clinical trial, which enrolled a sample of Italian free-living subjects with moderate hypercholesterolemia recruited from the Lipid clinic of the S. Orsola-Malpighi University Hospital, Bologna, Italy.

Participants were required to be aged between 20 and 65 years, with moderately high levels of TC (TC ≥ 5.17 mmol/L and ≤ 6.2 mmol/L) and LDL-C (LDL-C ≥ 3.36 mmol/L and ≤ 4.91 mmol/L) and an estimated 10-year cardiovascular risk <10%, as per the country-specific risk charts from the CUORE project [10]. Exclusion criteria included having previously experienced any vascular event, suffering from type 1 or type 2 diabetes, massive hypertriglyceridemia (TG > 4.52 mmol/L), alcoholism, obesity (body mass index (BMI) > 30 kg/m^2), liver failure, renal failure (estimated glomerular filtration rate (eGFR) < 0.5 mL/s), irritable bowel syndrome, inflammatory bowel diseases and food allergies, as well as having been treated in the previous 2 months with fiber based dietary supplements and/or probiotics and/or lipid-lowering drugs or any other drugs potentially able to affect the lipid metabolism.

Participants were adhering to a standardized diet for four weeks before being randomized to receive adequate supplies of either the beta-glucan supplement or placebo, in order to complete the one of two 2-month treatment sequences. The crossover to the second treatment was preceded by a 4-week wash-out period. Finally, participants were asked to return for follow-up visits two and four weeks after stopping supplementation. The study timeline is described in detail in Figure 1.

At enrollment, subjects were instructed to follow the general indications of a Mediterranean diet, avoiding an excessive intake of diary and red meat derived products.

Once every two visits, subjects were provided with a food diary to record their 3-day intake (two week-days and one week-end day), which they were requested to complete and return during their subsequent visit. In particular, the food diaries were collected and the diets analyzed at the beginning and at the end of each treatment phase.

The analysis of diet composition was performed using a dedicated software (MètaDieta®) based on a large food database that is frequently updated with values from the main official Italian databases (INRAN/IEO 2008 revision/ADI). Data were handled in compliance with the company procedure IOA87.

The study was conducted in accordance with the Good Clinical Practices and fully complied with the ethical guidelines of the Declaration of Helsinki. All subjects received an informational document describing the study and signed a consent form for study participation. The study was approved by the Bologna University Ethical Committee (Code: BELT_2016) and registered on www.clinicaltrial.gov (ID: NCT03313713).

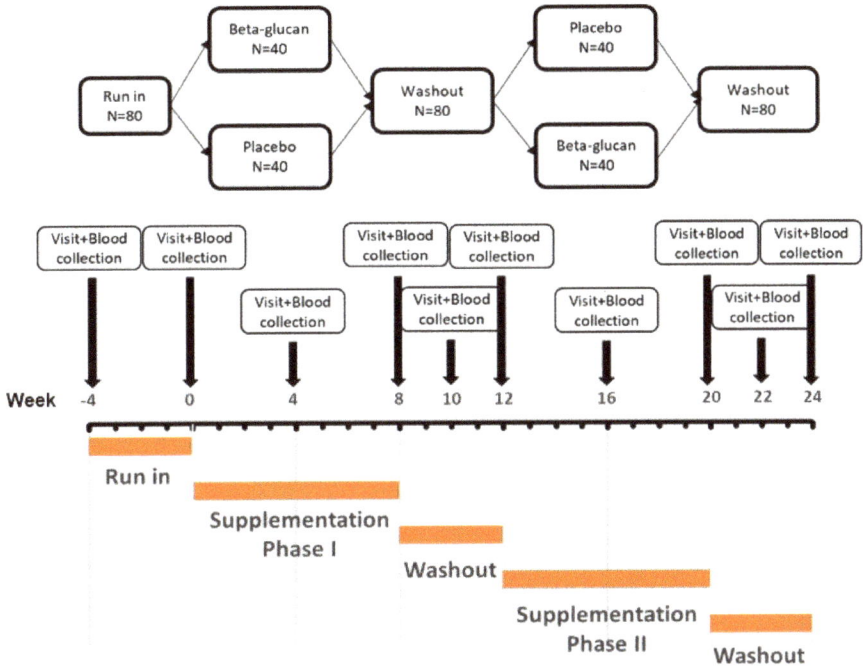

Figure 1. The flow-chart summarizes the study timeline.

2.2. Treatment

At visit at the beginning of supplementation the enrolled subjects were provided with boxes containing 28 white sachets of 15 g each; the same amount of product was provided after four weeks and at the beginning and after four weeks of the second supplementation phase. The sachets contained either 3 g oat beta-glucan (The Oatwell™ based Beta Heart®, Herbalife) or an oat-based isocaloric placebo without beta-glucan. The tested products had a similar macronutrient composition (Total energy: 50 kcal; Lipids: 1.4 g; Carbohydrates: 4 g; Proteins: 2 g) and were indistinguishable in color and taste. In particular, the Oatwell™ composition per 100 gr included 22 gr of beta-glucan soluble fiber characterized by very high molecular weight polysaccharides (>2000 kDa) and high viscosity (Table 1) [11].

Randomization was performed centrally, by computer-generated codes, and blocks were stratified by sex and age. The study staff and the investigators were blinded to the group assignment, as well as all the enrolled volunteers.

For the entire duration of the study, the subjects were instructed to take the dietary supplement regularly, dissolving the contents of one sachet in a glass of water every day in the morning.

All unused sachets were retrieved for inventory, and product compliance was assessed by counting the number of the sachets returned at the time of specific clinic visits [12]. The acceptability of the food supplements was assessed by a 10-point visual analogue score (VAS).

Table 1. Nutritional composition per 100 g of OatWell® 22.

Total dietary fiber	44 g
- Glucan soluble fiber	22 g
Carbohydrate	22 g
Protein	20 g
Total lipids	5 g
- Saturated FA	1 g
- Polyunsaturated FA	2 g
- Monounsaturated FA	2 g
Water	5 g
Minerals	
- Sodium (Na)	3 mg
- Magnesium (Mg)	250 mg
- Calcium (Ca)	120 mg
- Potassium (K)	700 mg
- Iron (Fe)	9 mg
- Zinc (Zn)	6 mg

2.3. Assessments

2.3.1. Clinical Data and Anthropometric Measurements

Subjects' personal history was evaluated taking particular attention to cardiovascular and metabolic diseases, dietary and smoking habits assessment (both evaluated with validated semi-quantitative questionnaires) [13], physical activity, and pharmacological treatments.

Waist circumference (WC) was measured at the end of a normal expiration, in a horizontal plane at the midpoint between the inferior margin of the last rib and the superior iliac crest. Height and weight were measured to the nearest 0.1 cm and 0.1 kg, respectively, with subjects standing erect with eyes directed straight wearing light clothes and with bare feet. BMI was calculated as body weight in kilograms, divided by height squared in meters (kg/m^2).

2.3.2. Blood Pressure Measurements

Systolic and diastolic blood pressure measurements were performed in each subject, supine and at rest, using a validated oscillometric device, with a cuff of the appropriate size applied on the right upper arm. To improve detection accuracy, three blood pressure (BP) readings were sequentially obtained at 1-min intervals. The first one was then discarded, and the average between the second and the third was recorded [14].

2.3.3. Laboratory Data

The biochemical analyses were carried out on venous blood, withdrawn after overnight fasting (at least 12 h). Plasma was obtained by addition of disodium ethylenediaminetetraacetate (Na_2EDTA) (1 mg/mL) and blood centrifugation at 3000 RPM for 15 min at room temperature.

Trained personnel performed laboratory analyses according to standardized methods [15], immediately after centrifugation, to assess TC, HDL-C, TG, Apo-B, apolipoprotein A1 (Apo-A1), fasting plasma glucose (FPG), creatinine, estimated glomerular filtration rate (eGFR) and liver transaminases. LDL-C was obtained by the Friedewald formula. Non-HDL-C resulted from the difference between TC and HDL-C.

2.3.4. Safety and Tolerability

Safety and tolerability were evaluated through continuous monitoring in order to detect any adverse event, clinical safety, laboratory findings, vital sign measurements, and physical examinations. A blinded, independent expert clinical event committee was appointed by the principal investigator in order to categorize the adverse events that could possibly be experienced during the trial as not related, unlikely related, possibly related, probably related, or definitely related to the study treatment.

Even if the fiber amount supplemented was low to modify the bowel function, an *ad-hoc* semi-quantitative questionnaire (Intestinal function assessment (Supplementary Material)) was administered at each visit, in order to collect information regarding possible changes in self-perceived intestinal well-being during the different phases of the study. The questionnaire evaluated the number of daily evacuations, the stool consistency and the personal perception of discomfort, swelling, stool expulsion ease and complete expulsion [16].

2.3.5. Statistical Analyses

Sample size was calculated for the change in LDL-C. Considering a type I error of 0.05, a power of 0.80 and expecting a LDL-C reduction of 7–10% with beta-glucans and 0–3% with placebo, expecting a 20% dropout rate, we calculated to enroll 80 subjects.

Data were analyzed using intention to treat by means of the Statistical Package for Social Sciences (SPSS) version 22.0 (IBM Corporation, Armonk, NY, USA) for Windows.

A full descriptive analysis of the collected parameters was carried out as per protocol. Categorical variables were expressed as absolute number and percentage and compared with the Fisher corrected chi-square test or the Wilcoxon-Rank test, based on whether they were nominal or ordinal. Continuous variables were expressed as mean ± standard deviation (SD) or mean and standard error (SEM), and compared by analysis of variance (ANOVA) followed by post-hoc Tukey test or by Kruskal-Wallis non parametric analysis of variance followed by Dunn's pairwise test, depending on their statistical distribution (if it was normal or not). To verify the basic assumption of cross-over design, the presence of a carryover effect was excluded.

The minimum level of statistical significance was set to $p < 0.05$ two-tailed. The Dixon's Q test was always carried out to exclude the extreme values.

Efficacy analyses were performed considering the intention-to-treat (ITT) population, i.e., all subjects with at least one post-baseline control. A sensitivity analysis of the primary variable was also planned in the per-protocol population, i.e., all subjects without major protocol violations.

The primay efficacy outcome analysis was also repeated by gender, age group (20–40 vs. 40–65 years old) and weight group (body mass index < 27 kg/m^2 vs. ≥ 27 kg/m^2).

Safety results were reported in all subjects who had assumed at least one dose of one study supplement.

3. Results

A total of 95 volunteers were screened, and 83 subjects underwent randomization from April through September 2017.

Subjects' characteristics at the screening visit are summarized in Table 2.

All enrolled subjects (men: 35, women: 48) successfully completed the trial according to the study design. The final distribution between men and women, when considering the treatment sequences, did not show any significant differences ($p > 0.05$). Furthermore, the study groups were well matched for all the considered variables at baseline.

Table 2. Pre-diet standardization parameters, expressed as mean ± SD.

Parameters	Pre-Diet Standardization (N = 83)
Age (years)	52.3 ± 4.4
Weight (kg)	74.5 ± 17.4
Waist (cm)	91.3 ± 14.6
Systolic blood pressure (mmHg)	128.3 ± 15.3
Diastolic blood pressure (mmHg)	81 ± 9.6
Total cholesterol (mmol/L)	5.75 ± 0.49
Triglycerides (mmol/L)	1.51 ± 0.80
HDL-cholesterol (mmol/L)	1.28 ± 0.29
Non-HDL-cholesterol (mmol/L)	4.48 ± 0.49
LDL-cholesterol (mmol/L)	3.78 ± 0.42
VLDL-cholesterol (mmol/L)	0.33 (0.32)
Apolipoprotein-A1 (mg/dL)	149.3 ± 22.9
Apolipoprotein -B (mg/dL)	100.8 ± 18.5
Fasting plasma glucose (mmol/L)	4.97 ± 0.73
Aspartate aminotransferase (µkat/L)	0.38 ± 0.12
Alanine aminotransferase (µkat/L)	0.39 ± 0.24

HDL = High-Density Lipoprotein; LDL = Low-Density Lipoprotein; VLDL = Very-Low-Density Lipoprotein.

No statistically significant changes were observed in the dietary habits of the enrolled subjects from randomization until the end of the study, nor in total energy and macronutrient intake (Table 3).

Table 3. Diet composition and total fiber intake (g/day) at the enrollment. Values are reported as mean ± SD or mean and variation range.

Parameters	Diet Composition
Total Energy (kcal/day)	1388.7 ± 245.7
Alcohol (% of total energy)	4.4 (0.1–10.4)
Lipids (% of total energy)	32.9 ± 4.9
Saturated Fatty Acids (% of total energy)	7.9 ± 2.4
Monounsaturated Fatty Acids (% of total energy)	12.4 ± 3.1
Poliunsaturated Fatty Acids (% of total energy)	4.4 ± 1.1
Proteins (% of total energy)	18.3 ± 5
Animal Proteins (% of total energy)	10.2 ± 6
Vegetal Proteins (% of total energy)	5.1 ± 2.1
Carbohydrates (% of total energy)	50.4 ± 5.9
Soluble Charbohydrates (% of total energy)	15.9 ± 3.7
Starch (% of total energy)	25.3 ± 4.5
Total dietary fibers (% of total energy)	2.2 ± 0.9
Cholesterol (mg/day)	148.4 ± 22.3

During the placebo phase, the subjects did not experience any statistically significant change in the evaluated parameters (Table 4 and Table S1 (Supplementary Materials)).

On the contrary, the active supplementation reduced mean LDL-C levels from baseline by 12.2% (95%CI: −15.4 to −3.8) after 4 weeks and by 15.1% (95%CI: −17.8 to −5.9) after 8 weeks ($p < 0.01$ for both comparison), which corresponded to an absolute decrease of 0.59 mmol/L (95%CI: −0.8 to −0.39) at the end of the intervention period (Table S2 (Supplementary Materials)). Repeating the analysis by gender and predefined age and body mass index groups, after 8 weeks we observed a slight but significantly higher LDL-lowering effect of beta-glucans effect in women than in men (women: 16.3% (95%CI: −17.8 to −6.7) vs. men: 14.9% (95%CI: −14.1 to −5.9); $p = 0.04$), in younger subjects (16.4% (95%CI: −17.5 to −8.3) vs. older 14.7% (95%CI: −17.1 to −5.2)) while no difference has been detected as regards body mass index classes ($p > 0.05$).

Table 4. Anthropometric, hemodynamic, and blood chemistry parameters from the baseline/end of wash-out to the end of the placebo sequence, expressed as mean ± SD.

Parameters	Baseline	Treatment Period		Wash-Out Period	
		4 Weeks	8 Weeks	2 Weeks	4 Weeks
Weight (kg)	73.8 ± 17.2	73.8 ± 17.1	73.7 ± 17.1	73.8 ± 17.9	74 ± 17.2
Waist (cm)	90.9 ± 14.4	90.8 ± 14.3	90.6 ± 14	90.6 ± 14.9	90.7 ± 14.1
Systolic blood pressure (mmHg)	120.9 ± 15.8	120.9 ± 15.2	120.3 ± 15.8	120.2 ± 16.7	121.1 ± 15.1
Diastolic blood pressure (mmHg)	78.5 ± 8.6	78.8 ± 8.6	79.2 ± 9.9	78.1 ± 8.4	78 ± 9.1
Heart rate (bpm)	71.9 ± 10.6	66.3 ± 4.7	70.78 ± 12.9	72.6 ± 10.2	70.2 ± 9.6
Total cholesterol (mmol/L)	5.75 ± 0.77	5.84 ± 0.73	5.75 ± 0.75	5.79 ± 0.81	5.85 ± 0.87
Triglycerides (mmol/L)	1.48 ± 0.70	1.46 ± 0.88	1.4 ± 0.78	1.59 ± 0.81	1.5 ± 0.76
HDL-cholesterol (mmol/L)	1.31 ± 0.29	1.33 ± 0.29	1.31 ± 0.3	1.26 ± 0.3	1.34 ± 0.28
LDL-cholesterol (mmol/L)	3.76 ± 0.75	3.84 ± 0.65	3.8 ± 0.65	3.81 ± 0.8	3.83 ± 0.80
Non HDL-cholesterol (mmol/L)	4.44 ± 0.71	4.51 ± 0.73	4.44 ± 0.72	4.53 ± 0.75	4.51 ± 0.83
Apolipoprotein A1 (mg/dL)	157.3 ± 32.5	151.2 ± 25.7	151.6 ± 26.5	148.4 ± 25.7	161 ± 29.2
Apolipoprotein B (mg/dL)	101.4 ± 22.7	101.6 ± 15.3	99.8 ± 17.6	102.9 ± 14.4	100.3 ± 17.1
VLDL-cholesterol (mmol/L)	0.68 ± 0.32	0.71 ± 0.65	0.68 ± 0.62	0.73 ± 0.37	0.69 ± 0.35
Fasting plasma glucose (mmol/L)	5.01 ± 0.56	5.06 ± 0.50	5.02 ± 0.49	4.99 ± 0.51	5.09 ± 0.59
Aspartate aminotransferase (μkat/L)	0.36 ± 0.09	0.37 ± 0.11	0.37 ± 0.12	0.36 ± 0.10	0.35 ± 0.08
Alanine aminotransferase (μkat/L)	0.36 ± 0.17	0.4 ± 0.27	0.44 ± 0.37	0.4 ± 0.18	0.41 ± 0.20

HDL = High-density lipoprotein; LDL = Low-density lipoprotein; VLDL = Very-low-density lipoprotein.

Considering the first-ranked secondary endpoints, the mean percentage change in TC levels between baseline and 4 weeks was a reduction of 6.5% (95%CI: −10.9 to −1.9) in the beta-glucan sequence, while non-HDL-C plasma concentrations decreased by 11.8% (95%CI: −14.6 to −4.5). Moreover, after 8 weeks of treatment, beta-glucan reduced TC by 8.9% (95%CI: −12.6 to −2.3), corresponding to an absolute decrease of 0.52 mmol/L (95%CI: −0.72 to −0.32), and non-HDL-C levels were reduced by 12.1% (95%CI: −15.6 to −5.3), which corresponded to 0.53 mmol/L (95%CI: −0.73 to −0.33) (Table S2 (Supplementary Materials)).

Descriptions and results of exploratory analyses of the other secondary endpoints, the effect on which were considered non-significant, are provided in Table 5.

Table 5. Changes in anthropometric, hemodynamic, and blood chemistry parameters from the baseline/end of washout to the end of the supplementation with beta-glucan, expressed as mean ± SD.

Parameters	Baseline	Treatment Period		Wash-Out Period	
		4 Weeks	8 Weeks	2 Weeks	4 Weeks
Weight (kg)	73.9 ± 17.6	73.8 ± 17.7	73.4 ± 17.6	73.9 ± 14.6	73.6 ± 17.7
Waist (cm)	90.3 ± 14.2	90.2 ± 14.0	89.9 ± 13.7	88.5 ± 13.7	90.3 ± 13.8
Systolic blood pressure (mmHg)	124.3 ± 16.0	121.1 ± 14.1	119.5 ± 15.2	122.2 ± 16.5	120.7 ± 14.2
Diastolic blood pressure (mmHg)	80.4 ± 9.6	78.6 ± 8.8	79.4 ± 9	80.4 ± 8.9	78.4 ± 9.4
Heart rate (bpm)	72.1 ± 11.5	68 ± 1.4	72.3 ± 12.9	72.1 ± 11.8	72 ± 8.2
Total cholesterol (mmol/L)	5.77 ± 0.68	5.38 ± 0.58 *,°	5.24 ± 0.57 *,°	5.76 ± 0.71	5.81 ± 0.76
Triglycerides (mmol/L)	1.48 ± 0.81	1.6 ± 0.89	1.62 ± 1.10	1.46 ± 0.80	1.52 ± 0.72
HDL-cholesterol (mmol/L)	1.29 ± 0.33	1.32 ± 0.29	1.3 ± 0.29	1.28 ± 0.32	1.33 ± 0.29
LDL-cholesterol (mmol/L)	3.8 ± 0.64	3.33 ± 0.60 *,§	3.21 ± 0.65 *,§	3.82 ± 0.64	3.78 ± 0.74
Non HDL-cholesterol (mmol/L)	4.48 ± 0.67	4.07 ± 0.60 *,§	3.95 ± 0.62 *,§	4.49 ± 0.66	4.48 ± 0.73
Apolipoprotein A1 (mg/dL)	151.7 ± 27.2	149.1 ± 27.5	147.33 ± 26.9	150.1 ± 25.7	166.8 ± 27.6
Apolipoprotein B (mg/dL)	99.2 ± 16.7	101.5 ± 16	100.1 ± 15.4	96.9 ± 14.6	102.8 ± 14.4
VLDL-cholesterol (mmol/L)	0.66 ± 0.32	0.73 ± 0.41	0.81 ± 0.83	0.67 ± 0.36	0.7 ± 0.33
Fasting plasma glucose (mmol/L)	4.78 ± 0.55	5.05 ± 0.48	5.02 ± 0.52	4.97 ± 0.51	5.07 ± 0.52
Aspartate aminotransferase (μkat/L)	0.38 ± 0.10	0.38 ± 0.11	0.37 ± 0.1	0.37 ± 0.10	0.36 ± 0.10
Alanine aminotransferase (μkat/L)	0.37 ± 0.18	0.42 ± 0.21	0.42 ± 0.22	0.36 ± 0.18	0.42 ± 0.20

* $p < 0.05$ versus baseline; ° $p < 0.05$ versus placebo; § $p < 0.01$ versus placebo. HDL = High-Density Lipoprotein; LDL = Low-Density Lipoprotein; VLDL = Very-Low-Density Lipoprotein.

After treatment discontinuation, both TC and LDL-C rapidly reversed to basal values. Lipid plasma levels assessed after 2 weeks of washout were comparable with those measured at baseline and not significantly different from those observed at the end of the wash-out period (Table 5).

The compliance with the treatment was almost complete (89%) during both treatment periods.

The tolerability profile of the beta-glucan supplement used was rated as acceptable by most subjects. During supplementation with beta-glucan, three subjects experienced moderate abdominal discomfort (reported as reversible abdominal cramps and diarrhoea) and one subjects experienced dysphagia. No one experienced adverse events regarding laboratory parameters during the trial. No volunteer discontinued the trial because of adverse events that occurred during the treatment and no effects reported in conjunction with use of the placebo.

In particular, the tested products did not exert any significant unvafourable effect on the self-perceived intestinal well-being. The results of the second-ranked secondary endpoint are summarized in Table 6.

Table 6. Pre-versus post-treatment effects on intestinal function of the tested products.

Parameters	Placebo		Beta-Glucan	
	Mean	p	Mean	p
Number of defecations per week	7	0.264	7	0.730
Stool consistency	3	0.482	3	0.438
Easiness of stool expulsion	4	0.610	3	0.699
Perception of total expulsion	3	0.691	4	0.583
Abdominal discomfort intensity	2	0.744	2	0.923
Abdominal swelling perception	3	0.749	3	0.760

4. Discussion

Beta-glucans (1-3,1-4 beta-D-glucans) are polysaccharides naturally occurring in the cell wall of grains and cereals, especially barley and oats [17]. In our double-blind, placebo-controlled, cross-over randomized clinical trial, 3 g/day of oat beta-glucan were shown to safely reduce LDL-C, TC and non-HDL-C in a large sample of adults characterized by mild hypercholesterolemia and with a low cardiovascular risk profile. The trial failed to detect any significant change in FPG. On the other hand, no significant adverse effects have been assessed on the self-perceived intestinal wellbeing and of both the beta-glucan supplement and the placebo were considered accettable.

The observed effect on TC and LDL-C are larger (0.53 and 0.59 mml/L, on average, corresponding to 15.1% and 8.9% of baseline values respectively) than expected, based on the most recent meta-analysis and EFSA opinion, which estimate respectively a mean change in LDL-C of 0.3 mmol/L and 0.21 mmol/L (about 7–10% of baseline concentratios) [7,18]. The reasons of such better performance are not easily explained, but it should be considered the possibility that the tested formulation, to be dissolved in fluids before consumption, might have specific pharmaceutic properties able to enhance the efficacy of the fibers in binding cholesterol and/or its metabolites (i.e., bile salts) and/or dietary fat. However, the supply of oat beta-glucan in the form of beverages (where nutrients are in contact with free water) has been found to have, in general, a more regular effect on cholesterol reduction compared to more complex matrices [19]. Moreover, the beta-glucan used for the BELT study consists of very high molecular weight beta-glucan, which has been proved to be more effective in cholesterol lowering then that with medium and low molecular weight [11,20].

Furthermore, the observed effect might also be due to the characteristics of the considered population sample. In this regard, a reliable meta-regression analysis recently demonstrated a significant inverse association between baseline LDL-C levels and the extent of LDL-C reduction after supplementation with oat beta-glucan [2]. These results are of particular interest, also considering that the observed effect is larger than the one expected after the administration of most available lipid-lowering nutraceuticals [21,22].

Similarly, the lack of any significant effect on FPG in the trial might be due to the characteristics of the enrolled subjects, being all euglycemic. Actually, a recent meta-analysis found that oat beta-glucan intake was more effective in people with type 2 diabetes [23].

The lack of changes in metabolic parameters during supplementation with placebo may be attributed to both the enrollment in the setting of a lipid clinic (and consequently, presumably, of subject *a priori* more attentive to a healthy lifestyle) and to the run-in stabilization diet period preceding the treatment phase, during which possible dietary mistakes were corrected before the start of the trial. Thus, the results obtained with beta-glucan supplementation are more representative of what would be observed in a setting of clinical practice.

At the same time, the lack of effects of beta-glucans on intestinal function parameters in our study should be related to the Mediterranean diet pattern of the enrolled subjects and the exclusion from the enrolment of subjects affected by irritable bowel syndrome, inflammatory bowel diseases and food allergies, but also because of the low amount of supplemented fibers.

The observed results are largely supported by the mechanisms of action by wich beta-glucans can improve cholesterolemia. The LDL-C lowering effect of beta-glucans has mainly related to the their ability to act as dietary fibers, consequently entrapping bile acid micelles, impairing their ability to interact with luminal membrane transporters on the intestinal epitelium, thereby increasing the fecal cholesterol output. [24] The following decrease in bile acid level up-regulates the 7-alpha-hydroxylase expression in the liver, thus further contributing to LDL-C decrease. [11] This seems to be more evident with high molecular weight and high viscosity of the fibers [25], as the one we tested in our trial. More recent literature suggesta that a part of the LDL-C reducing effect of beta-glucans could be mediated by modulation of microbiota [26]. A part of the beta-glucans effects (i.e., the antinflammatory and immunomodulatory ones) seems to be dependent by the contact of beta-glucans with dectin-1 [27], but this could be less relevant for th metabolic activities.

The BELT Study has some relevant limitations. For instance, the observational period was not long enough to assess any adaptation phenomena possibly occurring by changes in the gut microbiota composition. For this reason, further longer-term clinical studies are needed to confirm if the dietary intake of beta-glucan enriched foods is able to maintain the observed positive metabolic effect over the time.

Secondly, we did not evaluate any marker of intestinal absorption during the study, since the aim of this study was a clinical and not a pharmacological evaluation of the effects of supplementation with beta-glucan-enriched dietary supplement in moderately hypercholesterolemic subjects.

However, the BELT Study is the first placebo-controlled clinical trial testing the effect of oat beta-glucan supplementation on a large sample of a South European population strictly adherent to the Mediterranean diet. This is of particular interest because the high fiber content of the Mediterranean diet might have theoretically reduced the effect of beta-glucan supplementation on serum lipids [28], while this actually did not occur. Moreover, the observation that both total and LDL-C concentrations tend to return to basal values after weeks of wash-out, highlights the importance of a regular and constant supplementation with beta-glucan to achieve clinically relevant results in the long term. Finally, the profile of tolerability of the product might suggest that compliance to long term treatment with beta-glucan formulation might be good.

5. Conclusions

In conclusion, the BELT study confirms the medium-term efficacy of supplementation with 3 g/day of beta-glucan in reducing LDL-C, TC and non-HDL-C in mild hypercholesterolemic subjects, even in the context of a Mediterranean setting.

Supplementary Materials: The following are available online at http://www.mdpi.com/2072-6643/12/3/686/s1, Table S1: Changes in the collected parameters during supplementation with placebo in the overall study population, Table S2: Changes in the collected parameters during supplementation with beta-glucan in the overall study population.

Author Contributions: Conceptualization, A.P. and F.M. methodology, A.F.G.C. and F.M. formal analysis, A.F.G.C. and F.M.; investigation, A.F.G.C., F.F., M.V., E.S., E.G. and E.R. resources, F.M. and A.P. data curation, A.F.G.C., F.F. and F.M. writing-original draft preparation, A.F.G.C., F.F. and F.M. writing-review and editing, A.P. and C.B.

supervision, A.P. and C.B. project administration, A.F.G.C. and C.B. funding acquisition, F.M. and A.P. All authors have read and agree to the published version of the manuscript.

Funding: The BELT study has been supported by a research grant from NFI to S. Orsola-Malpighi University Hospital. The NFI grant has been partially covered by an unrestricted contribution received from Herbalife Nutrition. Herbalife Nutrition had no role in the design of the study, in the collection, analyses of the data, in the preparation or approval of this manuscript.

Conflicts of Interest: The authors declare no conflict of interest. The funders had no role in the design of the study; in the collection, analyses, or interpretation of data; in the writing of the manuscript, or in the decision to publish the results.

References

1. Brown, L.; Rosner, B.; Willett, W.W.; Sacks, F.M. Cholesterol-lowering effects of dietary fiber: A meta-analysis. *Am. J. Clin. Nutr.* **1999**, *69*, 30–42. [CrossRef]
2. Ho, H.V.; Sievenpiper, J.L.; Zurbau, A.; Blanco Mejia, S.; Jovanovski, E.; Au-Yeung, F.; Jenkins, A.L.; Vuksan, V. The effect of oat β-glucan on LDL-cholesterol, non-HDL-cholesterol and apoB for CVD risk reduction: A systematic review and meta-analysis of randomised-controlled trials. *Br. J. Nutr.* **2016**, *116*, 1369–1382. [CrossRef]
3. Poli, A.; Barbagallo, C.M.; Cicero, A.F.G.; Corsini, A.; Manzato, E.; Trimarco, B.; Bernini, F.; Visioli, F.; Bianchi, A.; Canzone, G.; et al. Nutraceuticals and functional foods for the control of plasma cholesterol levels. An intersociety position paper. *Pharmacol. Res.* **2018**, *134*, 51–60. [CrossRef]
4. Sima, P.; Vannucci, L.; Vetvicka, V. β-glucans and cholesterol (Review). *Int J. Mol. Med.* **2018**, *41*, 1799–1808. [CrossRef]
5. Jenkins, D.J.; Kendall, C.W.; Axelsen, M.; Augustin, L.S.; Vuksan, V. Viscous and nonviscous fibres, nonabsorbable and low glycaemic index carbohydrates, blood lipids and coronary heart disease. *Curr. Opin. Lipidol.* **2000**, *11*, 49–56. [CrossRef]
6. Gee, J.M.; Blackburn, N.A.; Johnson, I.T. The influence of guar gum on intestinal cholesterol transport in the rat. *Br. J. Nutr.* **1983**, *50*, 215–224. [CrossRef]
7. Kinner, M.; Nitschko, S.; Sommeregger, J.; Petrasch, A.; Linsberger-Martin, G.; Grausgruber, H.; Berghofer, E.; Siebenhandl-Ehn, S. Naked barley-Optimized recipe for pure barley bread with sufficient beta-glucan according to the EFSA health claims. *J. Cereal Sci.* **2011**, *53*, 225–230. [CrossRef]
8. Karmally, W.; Montez, M.G.; Palmas, W.; Martinez, W.; Branstetter, A.; Ramakrishnan, R.; Holleran, S.F.; Haffner, S.M.; Ginsberg, H.N. Cholesterol-lowering benefits of oat-containing cereal in Hispanic americans. *J. Am. Diet. Assoc.* **2005**, *105*, 967–970. [CrossRef]
9. Leadbetter, J.; Ball, M.J.; Mann, J.I. Effects of increasing quantities of oat bran in hypercholesterolemic people. *Am. J. Clin. Nutr.* **1991**, *54*, 841–845. [CrossRef]
10. Fornari, C.; Donfrancesco, C.; Riva, M.A.; Palmieri, L.; Panico, S.; Vanuzzo, D.; Ferrario, M.M.; Pilotto, L.; Giampaoli, S.; Cesana, G. Social status and cardiovasculardisease: A Mediterranean case. Results from the Italian Progetto CUORE cohort study. *BMC Public Health* **2010**, *10*, 574. [CrossRef]
11. Wolever, T.M.S.; Tosh, S.M.; Gibbs, A.L.; Brand-Miller, J.; Duncan, A.M.; Hart, V.; Lamarche, B.; Thomson, B.A.; Duss, R.; Wood, P.J. Physicochemical properties of oat b-glucan influence its ability to reduce serum LDL cholesterol in humans: A randomied clinical trial. *Am. J. Clin. Nutr.* **2010**, *92*, 723–732. [CrossRef] [PubMed]
12. Cicero, A.F.G.; Fogacci, F.; Rosticci, M.; Parini, A.; Giovannini, M.; Veronesi, M.; D'Addato, S.; Borghi, C. Effect of a short-term dietary supplementation with phytosterols, red yeast rice or both on lipid pattern in moderately hypercholesterolemic subjects: A three-arm, double-blind, randomized clinical trial. *Nutr. Metab.* **2017**, *14*, 61. [CrossRef] [PubMed]
13. Cicero, A.F.G.; Caliceti, C.; Fogacci, F.; Giovannini, M.; Calabria, D.; Colletti, A.; Veronesi, M.; Roda, A.; Borghi, C. Effect of apple polyphenols on vascular oxidative stress and endothelium function: A translational study. *Mol. Nutr. Food Res.* **2017**, *61*. [CrossRef]

14. Williams, B.; Mancia, G.; Spiering, W.; Agabiti Rosei, E.; Azizi, M.; Burnier, M.; Clement, D.L.; Coca, A.; de Simone, G.; Dominiczak, A.; et al. Authors/Task Force Members. 2018 ESC/ESH Guidelines for the management of arterial hypertension: The Task Force for the management of arterial hypertension of the European Society of Cardiology and the European Society of Hypertension: The Task Force for the management of arterial hypertension of the European Society of Cardiology and the European Society of Hypertension. *J. Hypertens* **2018**, *36*, 1953–2041. [CrossRef]
15. Cicero, A.F.G.; Fogacci, F.; Giovannini, M.; Grandi, E.; Rosticci, M.; D'Addato, S.; Borghi, C. Serum uric acid predicts incident metabolic syndrome in the elderly in an analysis of the Brisighella Heart Study. *Sci. Rep.* **2018**, *8*, 11529. [CrossRef]
16. Frank, L.; Kleinman, L.; Farup, C.; Taylor, L.; Miner, P., Jr. Psychometric validation of a constipation symptom assessment questionnaire. *Scand. J. Gastroenterol.* **1999**, *34*, 870–877. [CrossRef]
17. Theuwissen, E.; Plat, J.; Mensink, R.P. Consumption of oat beta-glucan with or without plant stanols did not influence inflammatory markers in hypercholesterolemic subjects. *Mol. Nutr. Food Res.* **2009**, *53*, 370–376. [CrossRef]
18. Whitehead, A.; Beck, E.J.; Tosh, S.; Wolever, T.M. Cholesterol-lowering effects of oat β-glucan: A meta-analysis of randomized controlled trials. *Am. J. Clin. Nutr.* **2014**, *100*, 1413–1421. [CrossRef]
19. Grundy, M.M.; Fardet, A.; Tosh, S.M.; Rich, G.T.; Wilde, P.J. Processing of oat: The impact on oat's cholesterol lowering effect. *Food Funct.* **2018**, *9*, 1328–1343. [CrossRef]
20. Wang, Y.; Harding, S.V.; Eck, P.; Thandapilly, S.J.; Gamel, T.H.; Abdel-Aal, E.S.M.; Crow, G.H.; Tosh, S.M.; Jones, P.J.; Ames, N.P. High-Molecular-Weight β-Glucan Decreases Serum Cholesterol Differentially Based on the CYP7A1 rs3808607 Polymorphism in Mildly Hypercholesterolemic Adults. *J. Nutr.* **2016**, *146*, 720–727. [CrossRef]
21. He, L.X.; Zhao, J.; Huang, Y.S.; Li, Y. The difference between oats and beta-glucan extract intake in the management of HbA1c, fasting glucose and insulin sensitivity: A meta-analysis of randomized controlled trials. *Food Funct.* **2016**, *7*, 1413–1428. [CrossRef]
22. Patti, A.M.; Al-Rasadi, K.; Giglio, R.V.; Nikolic, D.; Mannina, C.; Castellino, G.; Chianetta, R.; Banach, M.; Cicero, A.F.G.; Lippi, G.; et al. Natural approaches in metabolic syndrome management. *Arch. Med. Sci.* **2018**, *14*, 422–441. [CrossRef]
23. Cicero, A.F.G.; Colletti, A.; Bajraktari, G.; Descamps, O.; Djuric, D.M.; Ezhov, M.; Fras, Z.; Katsiki, N.; Langlois, M.; Latkovskis, G.; et al. Lipid-lowering nutraceuticals in clinical practice: Position paper from an International Lipid Expert Panel. *Nutr. Rev.* **2017**, *75*, 731–767. [CrossRef]
24. Lia, A.; Hallmans, G.; Sandberg, A.S.; Sundberg, B.; Aman, P.; Andersson, H. Oat beta-glucan increases bile acid excretion and a fiber-rich barley fraction increases cholesterol excretion in ileostomy subjects. *Am. J. Clin. Nutr.* **1995**, *62*, 1245–1251. [CrossRef]
25. Ellegård, L.; Andersson, H. Oat bran rapidly increases bile acid excretion and bile acid synthesis: An ileostomy study. *Eur J. Clin. Nutr.* **2007**, *61*, 938–945. [CrossRef]
26. Nakashima, A.; Yamada, K.; Iwata, O.; Sugimoto, R.; Atsuji, K.; Ogawa, T.; Ishibashi-Ohgo, N.; Suzuki, K. β-Glucan in Foods and Its Physiological Functions. *J. Nutr. Sci. Vitaminol.* **2018**, *64*, 8–17. [CrossRef]
27. Sahasrabudhe, N.M.; Tian, L.; van den Berg, M.; Bruggeman, G.; Bruininx, E.; Schols, H.A.; Faas, M.M.; de Vos, P. Endo-glucanase digestion of oat beta-Glucan enhances Dectin-1 activation in human dendritic cells. *J. Funct. Foods.* **2016**, *21*, 104–112. [CrossRef]
28. Zhu, X.; Sun, X.; Wang, M.; Zhang, C.; Cao, Y.; Mo, G.; Liang, J.; Zhu, S. Quantitative assessment of the effects of beta-glucan consumption on serum lipid profile and glucose level in hypercholesterolemic subjects. *Nutr. Metab. Cardiovasc. Dis.* **2015**, *25*, 714–723. [CrossRef]

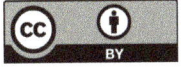

© 2020 by the authors. Licensee MDPI, Basel, Switzerland. This article is an open access article distributed under the terms and conditions of the Creative Commons Attribution (CC BY) license (http://creativecommons.org/licenses/by/4.0/).

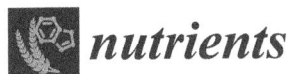

Article

The Association between Dyslipidemia, Dietary Habits and Other Lifestyle Indicators among Non-Diabetic Attendees of Primary Health Care Centers in Jeddah, Saudi Arabia

Sumia Enani [1,2,*], Suhad Bahijri [1,3], Manal Malibary [1,2], Hanan Jambi [1,2], Basmah Eldakhakhny [1,3], Jawaher Al-Ahmadi [1,4], Rajaa Al Raddadi [1,5], Ghada Ajabnoor [1,3], Anwar Boraie [1,6] and Jaakko Tuomilehto [1,7,8]

[1] Saudi Diabetes Research Group, King Fahd Medical Research Center, King Abdulaziz University, Jeddah 3270, Saudi Arabia; sb@kau.edu.sa (S.B.); mamalibary@kau.edu.sa (M.M.); hjambi@kau.edu.sa (H.J.); beldakhakhny@kau.edu.sa (B.E.); j_al_ahmadi@yahoo.com (J.A.-A.); rmsalharbi@kau.edu.sa (R.A.R.); gajabnour@kau.edu.sa (G.A.); boraiaa@ngha.med.sa (A.B.); jotuomilehto@gmail.com (J.T.)
[2] Department of Food and Nutrition, Faculty of Human Sciences and Design, King Abdulaziz University, Jeddah 3270, Saudi Arabia
[3] Department of Clinical Biochemistry, Faculty of Medicine, King Abdulaziz University, Jeddah 22252, Saudi Arabia
[4] Department of Family Medicine, Faculty of Medicine, King Abdulaziz University, Jeddah 22252, Saudi Arabia
[5] Department of Community Medicine, Faculty of Medicine, King Abdulaziz University, Jeddah 22252, Saudi Arabia
[6] King Abdullah International Medical Research Center (KAIMRC), College of Medicine, King Saud Bin Abdulaziz, University for Health Sciences (KSAU-HS), Jeddah 22384, Saudi Arabia
[7] Department of Public Health, University of Helsinki, FI-00014 Helsinki, Finland
[8] Public Health Promotion Unit, Finnish Institute for Health and Welfare, FI-00271 Helsinki, Finland
* Correspondence: senani@kau.edu.sa

Received: 12 July 2020; Accepted: 12 August 2020; Published: 13 August 2020

Abstract: Diet and other lifestyle habits have been reported to contribute to the development of dyslipidemia in various populations. Therefore, this study investigated the association between dyslipidemia and dietary and other lifestyle practices among Saudi adults. Data were collected from adults (≥20 years) not previously diagnosed with diabetes in a cross-sectional design. Demographic, anthropometric, and clinical characteristics, as well as lifestyle and dietary habits were recorded using a predesigned questionnaire. Fasting blood samples were drawn to estimate the serum lipid profile. Out of 1385 people, 858 (62%) (491 men, 367 women) had dyslipidemia. After regression analysis to adjust for age, body mass index, and waist circumference, an intake of ≥5 cups/week of Turkish coffee, or carbonated drinks was associated with increased risk of dyslipidemia in men (OR (95% CI), 2.74 (1.53, 4.89) $p = 0.001$, and 1.53 (1.04, 2.26) $p = 0.03$ respectively), while the same intake of American coffee had a protective effect (0.53 (0.30, 0.92) $p = 0.025$). Sleep duration <6 h, and smoking were also associated with increased risk in men (1.573 (1.14, 2.18) $p = 0.006$, and 1.41 (1.00, 1.99) $p = 0.043$ respectively). In women, an increased intake of fresh vegetables was associated with increased risk (2.07 (1.09, 3.94) $p = 0.026$), which could be attributed to added salad dressing. Thus, there are sex differences in response to dietary and lifestyle practices.

Keywords: dyslipidemia; serum cholesterol; serum triglycerides; serum low density lipoprotein; serum high density lipoprotein; dietary intake; lifestyle

1. Introduction

Cardiovascular diseases (CVD) are major health problems contributing to 31% of global death in 2017 according to the World Health Organization (WHO) [1]. The prevalence of CVD in Saudi Arabia in 2004 has been reported to be 5.5% [2], accounting for almost 45.7% of deaths [3]. CVD has many modifiable and non-modifiable risk factors, including certain diseases and disorders such as diabetes, hypertension, and dyslipidemia, which commonly coexist in various populations [4–6]. Indeed, dyslipidemia, defined as any abnormalities in serum lipids is considered atherogenic, and is reported to be associated with an increased risk of ischemic heart disease [7,8]. Several studies have been conducted to investigate the prevalence of dyslipidemia in Saudi Arabia in the past reporting an overall prevalence of 20–54% [9–11]. A more recent study published in 2018 on people in the eastern region of Saudi Arabia reported that the prevalence of (diagnosed and borderline) hypercholesterolemia, hypertriglyceridemia, increased low-density lipoprotein (LDL-C)-cholesterol, and decreased high density lipoprotein (HDL-C)-cholesterol were 51%, 26.9%, 38.1%, and 90.5%, respectively [12].

Many factors contribute to the development of dyslipidemia, including genetics, sex, ethnicity, increased body mass index (BMI), dietary habits, and smoking [13]. In addition, changes in sleeping patterns, and a short duration of sleep have also been associated with dyslipidemia [14]. Studies in Saudi Arabia showed that age, sex, high BMI, and waist circumference (WC), smoking, low physical activity, as well as intake of margarine were associated with dyslipidemia [10–12]. In spite of their reported importance in controlling dyslipidemia and CVD [15,16], the association of dietary as well as other lifestyle practices, including sleeping duration, with dyslipidemia were not fully investigated in previous Saudi studies. Saudi Arabia is a very large country, with each region having its own dietary and lifestyle characteristics. Therefore, we aimed to investigate such associations in more detail in inhabitants of the city of Jeddah, the largest city in the western region, and the gateway to the two holy cities of Islam, with a population of mixed ethnicities, bringing with them their own dietary habits. We hope that our results will help in the formulation of evidence-based dietary and lifestyle guidelines for people in our region to decrease the prevalence of dyslipidemia, which can be adopted in future, more comprehensive programs for the prevention of CVD.

2. Materials and Methods

2.1. Study Design and Sample Collection

Presented data in this study were obtained between July 2016 and February 2017 from a cross-sectional survey conducted in the city of Jeddah to develop a Saudi Dysglycemia Risk Score. The Committee on the Ethics of Human Research at the Faculty of Medicine-King Abdulaziz University, Jeddah approved the study (Reference No. 338-10). A full explanation of the sampling methodology has been outlined in an earlier publication [17] and is summarized here as follows: adults (age ≥ 20 years), not previously diagnosed with diabetes, were recruited from attendees of primary health care centers (PHCC) in Jeddah, Saudi Arabia. An informed consent form was signed by consenting volunteers. Demographic, dietary, and lifestyle variables, as well as medical history, and family history of chronic diseases were collected from recruits using a predesigned questionnaire in the Arabic language which was based on validated questionnaires used in previous risk score studies [18–22] including an Arabic one [23]. The questionnaire was completed during a face to face interview by trained medical students. Anthropometric and clinical measurements (weight, height, WC, and blood pressure (BP)) were measured using standardized equipment and techniques as previously explained [17]. Weight and fat percentage were measured using a portable calibrated scale (Omron BF511; OMRON Healthcare, Kyoto, Japan). Weight and height were used to calculate BMI. A value less than 18.5 indicates underweight, while a value of 18.5–<25 kg/m^2 indicates healthy normal weight, 25–<30 indicates overweight, and ≥30 indicates obesity. Using WC to indicate abdominal adiposity the first cut-off value for increased risk was defined as >94 cm for men, >80 cm for women, and the second cut-off value as >102 cm for men, >88 cm for women [24,25].

The section on dietary practices consisted of food frequency questions including 17 questions covering intake of fruits, vegetables, red meat, whole grain bread/cereals, and various commonly consumed beverages including fruit juices (fresh and otherwise), carbonated beverages, energy drinks, different types of coffee such as Arabic, American, Turkish, and cappuccino, and various teas such as red, green, cinnamon, and hibiscus tea. Participants were asked to specify whether they consumed each item more than once daily, once daily, 5–6 portions per week, 1–4 portions per week, or not at all. Food models representing portion sizes of relevant food items were presented to all participants to help in making the correct decisions.

Fasting blood samples were taken, and serum was separated and stored at −80 °C for the estimation of the lipid profile. A flow chart outlining steps in data collection is presented in Supplementary Figure S1.

2.2. Biochemical Assays

Serum samples were sent regularly every 10 to 12 weeks to a collaborating laboratory at the National Guard Hospital in Jeddah which is accredited by the College of American Pathologist. Total cholesterol (TC), HDL-C and triglycerides (TG) levels were measured by spectrophotometric methods using Architect c8000 auto-analyzer (Abbott Park, IL, USA). LDL-C was calculated using the Friedewald equation [26].

2.3. Diagnosis of Dyslipidemia

Dyslipidemia was defined as LDL-C ≥ 3.37 mmol/L, HDL-C < 1.04 mmol/L for men and < 1.3 mmol/L for women, TC ≥ 5.18 mmol/L, TG ≥ 1.7 mmol/L or treatment with lipid-lowering drugs with all lipid levels in the normal range [27,28].

2.4. Statistical Analysis

IBM SPSS statistics version 20.0 for Windows was used to enter and analyze collected data. The baseline characteristics of the study population were calculated statistically and described as mean, standard deviations (SD), and frequencies.

Demographic, lifestyle, and clinical factors of people with high levels of TC, LDL-C, and TG, and/or low level of HDL-C, as well as dyslipidemia in general, were analyzed by comparing to those with normal lipid levels. Factors with continuous variables were analyzed using an independent t-test to compare two groups, while those with categorical variables were analyzed using the Chi-square test or Fisher's exact test, as appropriate. Unadjusted and adjusted logistic regression models were used for assessing the association between demographic, lifestyle, and dietary variables, and outcome variables: specific and general types of dyslipidemia. Stepwise regression analysis was performed to determine the dietary factors that had an influence on dyslipidemia. Independent factors included age, BMI, and WC. Only related independent variables, where $p < 0.15$ after an initial logistic regression between the dependent and independent variable was used in the corresponding stepwise regression model to avoid excluding important covariates from the final model and to include predictors that are serious or have high potential effect [29]. Values of $p < 0.05$ (two-sided test) were accepted as statistically significant.

3. Results

A total of 1477 adults were recruited by the end of February 2017 (Supplementary Figure S1). Complete data were obtained for 1385 people. Missing data were mainly due to missing, hemolysed, broken, or unlabeled blood samples. This was completely random and is not expected to affect validity. Following biochemical measurements, a total of 527 people (38%) (287 men, and 240 women) were found to be normolipidemic, and 858 (62%) (491 men, and 367 women) had dyslipidemia. Thus, there was no association between sex and dyslipidemia in general. The most prevalent type of dyslipidemia was high LDL-C found in 567 people (40.9%) (341 men and 226 men), followed by high

TC in 480 people (34.7%) (277 men and 203 women), and low HDL-C in 338 people (24.4%) (171 men and 167 women) and the least prevalent type of dyslipidemia was high TG levels in 301 people (21.7%) (218 men and 83 women). Therefore, increased LDL-C and TG were significantly more common in men ($p < 0.05$ and $p < 0.001$ respectively) whereas low HDL-C was significantly more common in women ($p < 0.05$).

3.1. Association between Dyslipidemia with Anthropometric Measurements

Demographic, clinical, and anthropometric characteristics of the study groups for men and women are presented in Supplementary Table S1. There was a significant difference in demographic and anthropometric measurements between the normolipidemic and dyslipidemic groups, with the dyslipidemia group having a significantly higher means of age, BMI, weight, body fat percentage, neck, waist and hip circumferences, and waist to hip and waist to height ratios (all $p < 0.001$, Supplementary Table S1). In addition, men and women with dyslipidemia also had significantly higher means of systolic and diastolic Bp and significantly higher means of TC, TG, LDL-C, and lower HDL-C compared with people with normolipidemia (Supplementary Table S1). Comparing the distribution of various characteristics between the normolipidemic and the dyslipidemic groups of men and women, age, BMI, and WC were found to be significantly and directly associated with dyslipidemia ($p < 0.001$ at least, Supplementary Table S2) and all its types ($p < 0.015$ at least, Supplementary Table S2). Dyslipidemia was detected in 75% of participants over 30 years of age compared with 48.8% of those <30 years. Moreover, dyslipidemia was present in 74.8% and 72% of obese men and women compared with 53.5% and 43.7% of normal weight and 29.2% and 32% underweight men and women respectively (Supplementary Table S2a,b).

3.2. Patterns of Food Intake in Studied Men and Women

Recorded frequencies of the questionnaire were recategorized to no intake, 1–4 and 5 or more portions per week due to small numbers in some categories. The difference in the recorded pattern of food intake between men and women is shown in Table 1. Women reported eating more fresh and cooked vegetables than men, whereas men had a higher intake of red meat ($p < 0.001$ at least, Table 1). In addition, men reported drinking more fresh and non-fresh juice, soft drinks, energy drinks, red tea, and American coffee compared with women ($p < 0.01$ at least, Table 1) whereas women reported drinking more green tea, Arabic coffee, and cinnamon drink compared with men ($p < 0.05$ at least, Table 1). There were no sex-differences in the consumption of fruits, whole grain products, Turkish coffee, and hibiscus drink (Table 1).

The association between diet and dyslipidemia was analyzed in each sex group separately due to the sex differences in both the prevalence of some types of dyslipidemia as well as food intake patterns.

3.2.1. Association between Food Intake and Dyslipidemia in Men

Comparing dietary habits in men between the two groups, a high intake of Turkish coffee was significantly associated with dyslipidemia ($p < 0.001$, Table 2). On the other hand, people with a moderate intake of 1–4 portions/week of American coffee had a lower prevalence of dyslipidemia ($p = 0.027$, Table 2). Dyslipidemia was detected in 79% of people drinking five or more portions a week Turkish coffee and in 65% of people who did not drink American coffee (Table 2). Turkish coffee consumption was associated in particular with low HDL-C and high TC ($p = 0.036$ and $p = 0.018$, respectively, Table 2). This association had a U-shape association as low HDL-C was detected in 22% in people with no intake, in 15% of those with an intake of 1–4 portions per week and in 29% in those with a weekly intake of five or more portions of Turkish coffee (Table 2). A similar U-shaped association was found between American coffee consumption and TC (Table 2).

Table 1. Food intake pattern by sex.

	Men	Women	χ^2 (p-Value)
	N (N%)	N (N%)	
Fruit (portion)			
No intake	111 (14.0%)	72 (11.8%)	1.727
1–4/week	399 (50.4%)	323 (52.8%)	$p = 0.422$
5 or more/week	281 (35.5%)	217 (35.5%)	
Fresh vegetable (portion)			
No intake	115 (14.5%)	53 (8.7%)	**15.259**
1–4/week	310 (39.2%)	225 (36.8%)	**$p < 0.001$**
5 or more/week	366 (46.3%)	334 (54.6%)	
Cooked vegetable (portion)			
No intake	164 (20.7%)	67 (10.9%)	**27.975**
1–4/week	356 (45.0%)	278 (45.4%)	**$p < 0.001$**
5 or more/week	271 (34.3%)	267 (43.6%)	
Whole grains (portion)			
No intake	113 (14.3%)	93 (15.2%)	3.187
1–4/week	146 (18.5%)	91 (14.9%)	$p = 0.203$
5 or more/week	532 (67.3%)	428 (69.9%)	
Red meat (portion)			
No intake	58 (7.3%)	139 (22.7%)	**77.64**
1–4/week	453 (57.3%)	335 (54.7%)	**$p < 0.001$**
5 or more/week	280 (35.4%)	138 (22.5%)	
Fresh juice (portion)			
No intake	182 (23.0%)	186 (30.4%)	**10.039**
1–4/week	412 (52.1%)	281 (45.9%)	**$p = 0.007$**
5 or more/week	197 (24.9%)	145 (23.7%)	
Non fresh juice (portion)			
No intake	252 (31.9%)	259 (42.3%)	**20.572**
1–4/week	253 (32.0%)	191 (31.2%)	**$p < 0.001$**
5 or more/week	286 (36.2%)	162 (26.5%)	
Soft drinks (portion)			
No intake	247 (31.2%)	298 (48.7%)	**56.848**
1–4/week	233 (29.5%)	175 (28.6%)	**$p < 0.001$**
5 or more/week	311 (39.3%)	139 (22.7%)	
Red tea (portion)			
No intake	166 (21.0%)	182 (29.7%)	**14.346**
1–4/week	201 (25.4%)	133 (21.7%)	**$p = 0.001$**
5 or more/week	424 (53.6%)	297 (48.5%)	
Green tea (portion)			
No intake	464 (58.7%)	323 (52.8%)	**7.39**
1–4/week	168 (21.2%)	130 (21.2%)	**$p = 0.025$**
5 or more/week	159 (20.1%)	159 (26.0%)	
Arabic coffee (portion)			
No intake	347 (43.9%)	232 (37.9%)	**10.33**
1–4/week	214 (27.1%)	153 (25.0%)	**$p = 0.006$**
5 or more/week	230 (29.1%)	227 (37.1%)	
Turkish coffee (portion)			
No intake	565 (71.4%)	440 (71.9%)	0.112
1–4/week	124 (15.7%)	92 (15.0%)	$p = 0.946$
5 or more/week	102 (12.9%)	80 (13.1%)	

Table 1. Cont.

	Men N (N%)	Women N (N%)	χ² (p-Value)
American coffee (portion)			
No intake	626 (79.1%)	531 (86.8%)	14.183
1–4/week	81 (10.2%)	43 (7.0%)	$p = 0.001$
5 or more/week	84 (10.6%)	38 (6.2%)	
Cappuccino (portion)			
No intake	536 (67.8%)	368 (60.1%)	9.881
1–4/week	157 (19.8%)	139 (22.7%)	$p = 0.007$
5 or more/week	98 (12.4%)	105 (17.2%)	
Energy drinks (portion)			
No intake	623 (78.8%)	545 (89.1%)	26.237
1–4/week	115 (14.5%)	45 (7.4%)	$p < 0.001$
5 or more/week	53 (6.7%)	22 (3.6%)	
Hibiscus drinks (portion)			
No intake	719 (90.9%)	556 (90.8%)	0.57
1–4/week	58 (7.3%)	42 (6.9%)	$p = 0.752$
5 or more/week	14 (1.8%)	14 (2.3%)	
Cinnamon drink (portion)			
No intake	707 (89.4%)	478 (78.1%)	37.241
1–4/week	52 (6.6%)	100 (16.3%)	$p < 0.001$
5 or more/week	32 (4.0%)	34 (5.6%)	

Data is shown as frequency and percentages of all people in the sex group. χ² is the Chi-square test value followed by its p-value. Significant differences between groups are shown in bold font.

After adjusting for age, BMI, and WC the weekly intake of five or more portions of Turkish coffee was associated in men with a 2.77 increased odds for having dyslipidemia compared with those with no intake ($p < 0.001$, Table 3), while a moderate and high intake of American coffee was associated with 0.55 and 0.55 decreased odds for having dyslipidemia compared with those with no intake ($p = 0.037$ and $p = 0.031$, respectively; Table 3). After performing the multivariable regression analysis for each type of dyslipidemia separately and adjusting for age, BMI, and WC, there was no longer a significant effect of Turkish coffee on any type; however, the effect of American coffee appeared only for moderate consumption (1–4 portions/week) which was only significant for high TC (OR = 0.50; 95% CI: 0.27, 0.94; $p = 0.038$) (data not shown).

There was no significant association between the consumption of carbonated drinks and dyslipidemia when analyzed by Chi-square test. However, the regression analysis showed that the weekly intake of five or more portions of carbonated drinks was associated with a 1.56 increased odds for having dyslipidemia in general (but not specific types of dyslipidemia) in men compared with those with no intake after adjusting for age, BMI, and WC (OR = 1.53 (CI: 1.04, 2.26) $p = 0.03$, data not shown).

There was a U-shaped association between some other dietary variables and dyslipidemia when analyzed by the Chi-square test. For example, fruits, fresh and cooked vegetables, and red tea consumption had a U-shaped relationship with low HDL-C in men. However, these food types were not predictors of dyslipidemia when analyzed using regression, adjusting for age and BMI (Table 3).

Table 2. Comparison of dietary habits between normolipidemic and dyslipidemic men groups presented as number of men (%) for overall dyslipidemia, and abnormalities in different lipid parameters.

Variable	General Dyslipidemia		LDL-C			HDL-C			TC			TG		
	No (n = 287) N (%)	Yes (n = 491) N (%)	Normal (n = 437) N (%)	High (n = 341) N (%)		Normal (n = 607) N (%)	Low (n = 171) N (%)		Normal (n = 501) N (%)	High (n = 277) N (%)		Normal (n = 560) N (%)	High (n = 218) N (%)	
Fruit (portion)														
No intake	39 (35.8)	70 (64.2)	60 (55.0)	49 (45.0)		84 (77.1)	25 (22.9)		66 (60.6)	43 (39.4)		71 (65.1)	38 (34.9)	
1–4/week	154 (39.1)	240 (60.9)	217 (55.1)	177 (44.9)		328 (83.2)	66 (16.8)		256 (65.0)	138 (35.0)		290 (73.6)	104 (26.4)	
5 or more/week	94 (34.2)	181 (65.8)	160 (58.2)	115 (41.8)		195 (70.9)	80 (29.1)		179 (65.1)	96 (34.9)		199 (72.4)	76 (27.6)	
X² (p-value)	1.74 (p = 0.419)		0.7 (p = 0.705)			14.448 (p = 0.001)			0.818 (p = 0.664)			3.066 (p = 0.216)		
Fresh vegetable (portion)														
No intake	43 (37.7)	71 (62.3)	68 (59.6)	46 (40.4)		91 (79.8)	23 (20.2)		72 (63.2)	42 (36.8)		78 (68.4)	36 (31.6)	
1–4/week	120 (39.3)	185 (60.7)	160 (52.5)	145 (47.5)		254 (83.3)	51 (16.7)		195 (63.9)	110 (36.1)		236 (77.4)	69 (22.6)	
5 or more/week	124 (34.5)	235 (65.5)	209 (58.2)	150 (41.8)		262 (73.0)	97 (27.0)		234 (65.2)	125 (34.8)		246 (68.5)	113 (31.5)	
X² (p-value)	1.674 (p = 0.433)		2.878 (p = 0.237)			10.452 (p = 0.005)			0.201 (p = 0.905)			7.247 (p = 0.027)		
Cooked vegetable (portion)														
No intake	66 (41.3)	94 (58.8)	97 (60.6)	63 (39.4)		128 (80.0)	32 (20.0)		111 (69.4)	49 (30.6)		126 (78.8)	34 (21.3)	
1–4/week	128 (36.4)	224 (63.4)	187 (53.1)	165 (46.9)		291 (82.7)	61 (17.3)		212 (60.2)	140 (39.8)		245 (69.6)	107 (30.4)	
5 or more/week	93 (35.8)	173 (65.0)	153 (57.5)	113 (42.5)		188 (70.7)	78 (29.3)		178 (66.9)	88 (33.1)		189 (71.1)	77 (28.9)	
X² (p-value)	1.773 (p = 0.412)		2.812 (p = 0.245)			13.17 (p = 0.001)			5.136 (p = 0.077)			4.736 (p = 0.077)		
Whole grains (portion)														
No intake	40 (36.4)	70 (63.6)	64 (58.2)	46 (41.8)		81 (73.6)	29 (26.4)		69 (62.7)	41 (37.3)		79 (71.8)	31 (28.2)	
1–4/week	54 (37.5)	90 (62.5)	77 (53.5)	67 (46.5)		118 (81.9)	26 (18.1)		8(61.1)	56 (38.9)		105 (72.9)	39 (27.1)	
5 or more/week	193 (36.8)	331 (63.2)	296 (56.5)	228 (43.5)		408 (77.9)	116 (22.1)		344 (65.6)	180 (34.4)		376 (71.8)	148 (28.2)	
X² (p-value)	0.037 (p = 0.982)		0.628 (p = 0.73)			2.533 (p = 0.282)			1.17 (p = 0.557)			0.77 (p = 0.962)		
Red meat (portion)														
No intake	19 (33.3)	38 (66.7)	33 (57.9)	24 (42.1)		41 (71.9)	16 (28.1)		35 (61.4)	22 (38.6)		43 (75.4)	14 (24.6)	
1–4/week	167 (37.5)	287 (62.5)	260 (58.4)	185 (41.6)		347 (78.0)	98 (22.0)		290 (65.2)	155 (34.8)		317 (71.2)	128 (28.8)	
5 or more/week	101 (36.6)	175 (63.4)	144 (52.2)	132 (47.8)		219 (79.3)	57 (20.7)		176 (63.8)	100 (36.2)		200 (72.5)	76 (27.5)	
X² (p-value)	0.398 (p = 0.82)		2.78 (p = 0.249)			1.517 (p = 0.468)			0.386 (p = 0.825)			0.492 (p = 0.782)		

Table 2. Cont.

Variable	General Dyslipidemia		LDL-C			HDL-C			TC			TG	
	No (n = 287) N (%)	Yes (n = 491) N (%)	Normal (n = 437) N (%)	High (n = 341) N (%)		Normal (n = 607) N (%)	Low (n = 171) N (%)		Normal (n = 501) N (%)	High (n = 277) N (%)		Normal (n = 560) N (%)	High (n = 218) N (%)
Fresh juice (portion)													
No intake	72 (40.2)	107 (59.8)	112 (62.6)	67 (37.4)		133 (74.3)	46 (25.7)		124 (69.3)	55 (30.7)		128 (71.5)	51 (28.5)
1–4/week	141 (34.8)	264 (65.2)	213 (52.6)	192 (47.4)		319 (78.8)	86 (21.2)		249 (61.5)	156 (38.5)		294 (72.6)	111 (27.4)
5 or more/week	74 (38.1)	120 (61.9)	112 (57.7)	82 (42.3)		155 (79.9)	39 (20.1)		128 (66.0)	66 (34.0)		138 (71.1)	56 (28.9)
X² (p-value)	1.735 (p = 0.42)		5.275 (p = 0.072)			1.973 (p = 0.373)			3.57 (p = 0.168)			0.164 (p = 0.921)	
Non fresh juice (portion)													
No intake	87 (34.9)	162 (65.1)	141 (56.6)	108 (43.4)		186 (74.7)	63 (25.3)		155 (62.2)	94 (37.8)		179 (71.9)	70 (28.1)
1–4/week	97 (38.8)	153 (61.2)	136 (54.4)	114 (45.6)		200 (80.0)	50 (20.0)		158 (63.2)	92 (36.8)		183 (73.2)	67 (26.8)
5 or more/week	103 (36.9)	176 (63.1)	160 (57.3)	119 (42.7)		221 (79.2)	58 (20.8)		188 (67.4)	91 (32.6)		198 (71.0)	81 (29.0)
X² (p-value)	0.779 (p = 0.671)		0.496 (p = 0.78)			2.404 (p = 0.301)			1.743 (p = 0.418)			0.327 (p = 0.849)	
Carbonated drinks (portion)													
No intake	92 (38.2)	149 (61.8)	145 (60.2)	96 (39.8)		184 (76.3)	57 (23.7)		152 (63.1)	89 (36.9)		173 (71.8)	68 (28.2)
1–4/week	88 (37.9)	144 (62.1)	126 (54.3)	106 (45.7)		187 (80.6)	45 (19.4)		155 (66.8)	77 (33.2)		171 (73.7)	61 (26.3)
5 or more/week	107 (35.1)	198 (64.9)	166 (54.4)	139 (45.6)		236 (77.4)	69 (22.6)		194 (63.6)	111 (36.4)		216 (70.8)	89 (29.2)
X² (p-value)	0.707 (p = 0.702)		2.266 (p = 0.322)			1.369 (p = 0.504)			0.857 (p = 0.615)			0.551 (p = 0.759)	
Red tea (portion)													
No intake	61 (37.2)	103 (62.8)	98 (59.8)	66 (40.2)		130 (79.3)	34 (20.7)		112 (68.3)	52 (31.7)		124 (75.6)	40 (24.4)
1–4/week	82 (41.6)	115 (58.4)	110 (55.8)	87 (44.2)		168 (85.3)	29 (14.7)		131 (66.5)	66 (33.5)		149 (75.6)	48 (24.4)
5 or more/week	144 (34.5)	273 (65.5)	229 (54.9)	188 (45.1)		309 (74.1)	108 (25.9)		258 (61.9)	159 (38.1)		287 (68.8)	130 (31.2)
X² (p-value)	2.899 (p = 0.235)		1.132 (p = 0568)			9.938 (p = 0.007)			2.626 (p = 0.269)			4.434 (p = 0.109)	
Green tea (portion)													
No intake	174 (38.2)	281 (61.8)	263 (57.8)	192 (42.2)		354 (77.8)	101 (22.2)		304 (66.8)	151 (33.2)		329 (72.3)	126 (27.7)
1–4/week	62 (37.6)	103 (62.4)	87 (52.7)	78 (47.3)		135 (81.8)	30 (18.2)		98 (59.4)	67 (40.6)		123 (74.5)	42 (25.5)
5 or more/week	51 (32.3)	107 (67.7)	87 (55.1)	71 (44.9)		118 (74.7)	40 (25.3)		99 (62.7)	59 (37.3)		108 (68.4)	50 (31.6)
X² (p-value)	1.834 (p = 0.4)		1.365 (p = 0.505)			2.426 (p = 0.297)			3.168 (p = 0.205)			1.592 (p = 0.451)	

Table 2. *Cont.*

Variable	General Dyslipidemia		LDL-C			HDL-C			TC			TG		
	No (n = 287) N (%)	Yes (n = 491) N (%)	Normal (n = 437) N (%)	High (n = 341) N (%)		Normal (n = 607) N (%)	Low (n = 171) N (%)		Normal (n = 501) N (%)	High (n = 277) N (%)		Normal (n = 560) N (%)	High (n = 218) N (%)	
Arabic coffee (portion)														
No intake	124 (36.3)	218 (63.7)	197 (57.6)	145 (42.4)		261 (76.3)	81 (23.7)		218 (63.7)	124 (36.3)		236 (69.0)	106 (31.0)	
1–4/week	84 (40.0)	126 (60.0)	112 (53.3)	98 (46.7)		176 (83.8)	34 (16.2)		139 (66.2)	71 (33.8)		163 (77.6)	47 (22.4)	
5 or more/week	79 (35.0)	147 (65.0)	128 (56.6)	98 (43.4)		170 (75.2)	56 (24.8)		144 (63.7)	82 (36.3)		161 (71.2)	65 (28.8)	
X² (*p*-value)	1.294 (*p* = 0.524)		0.991 (*p* = 0.609)			5.716 (*p* = 0.057)			0.404 (*p* = 0.817)			4.872 (*p* = 0.087)		
Turkish coffee (portion)														
No intake	212 (38.0)	346 (62.0)	317 (56.8)	241 (43.2)		434 (77.8)	124 (22.2)		361 (64.7)	197 (35.3)		401 (71.9)	157 (28.1)	
1–4/week	54 (44.6)	67 (55.4)	72 (59.5)	49 (40.5)		103 (85.1)	18 (14.9)		87 (71.9)	34 (28.1)		94 (77.7)	27 (22.3)	
5 or more/week	21 (21.2)	78 (78.8)	48 (48.5)	51 (51.5)		70 (70.7)	29 (29.3)		53 (53.5)	46 (46.5)		65 (65.7)	34 (34.3)	
X² (*p*-value)	13.856 (*p* ≤ 0.001)		3.014 (*p* = 0.222)			6.667 (*p* = 0.036)			8.087 (*p* = 0.018)			3.92 (*p* = 0.141)		
American coffee (portion)														
No intake	215 (34.8)	402 (65.2)	341 (55.3)	276 (44.7)		472 (76.5)	145 (23.5)		393 (63.7)	224 (36.3)		435 (70.5)	182 (29.5)	
1–4/week	40 (50.0)	40 (50.0)	53 (66.3)	27 (33.8)		69 (86.3)	11 (13.8)		63 (78.8)	17 (21.3)		64 (80.0)	16 (20.0)	
5 or more/week	32 (39.5)	49 (60.5)	43 (53.1)	38 (46.9)		66 (81.5)	15 (18.5)		45 (55.6)	36 (44.4)		61 (75.3)	20 (24.7)	
X² (*p*-value)	7.251 (*p* = 0.027)		3.819 (*p* = 0.148)			4.558 (*p* = 0.102)			10.082 (*p* = 0.006)			3.664 (*p* = 0.16)		
Cappuccino (portion)														
No intake	195 (36.9)	333 (63.1)	298 (56.4)	230 (43.6)		404 (76.5)	124 (23.5)		342 (64.8)	186 (35.2)		380 (72.0)	148 (28.0)	
1–4/week	64 (41.6)	90 (58.4)	88 (57.1)	66 (42.9)		130 (84.4)	24 (15.6)		104 (67.5)	50 (32.5)		114 (74.0)	40 (26.0)	
5 or more/week	28 (29.2)	68 (70.8)	51 (53.1)	45 (46.9)		73 (76.0)	23 (24.0)		55 (57.3)	41 (42.7)		66 (68.8)	30 (31.3)	
X² (*p*-value)	3.902 (*p* = 0.142)		0.436 (*p* = 0.804)			4.59 (*p* = 0.101)			2.807 (*p* = 0.246)			0.816 (*p* = 0.665)		
Energy drinks (portion)														
No intake	219 (35.7)	395 (64.3)	338 (55.0)	276 (45.0)		468 (76.2)	146 (23.8)		389 (63.4)	225 (36.6)		432 (70.4)	182 (29.6)	
1–4/week	45 (39.8)	68 (60.2)	65 (57.5)	48 (42.5)		96 (85.0)	17 (15.0)		74 (65.5)	39 (34.5)		86 (76.1)	27 (23.9)	
5 or more/week	23 (45.1)	28 (54.9)	34 (66.7)	17 (33.3)		43 (84.3)	8 (15.7)		38 (74.5)	13 (25.5)		42 (82.4)	9 (17.6)	
X² (*p*-value)	2.287 (*p* = 0.319)		2.68 (*p* = 0.262)			5.506 (*p* = 0.064)			2.624 (*p* = 0.269)			4.475 (*p* = 0.107)		

Table 2. Cont.

Variable	General Dyslipidemia		LDL-C			HDL-C			TC			TG	
	No (n = 287) N (%)	Yes (n = 491) N (%)	Normal (n = 437) N (%)	High (n = 341) N (%)		Normal (n = 607) N (%)	Low (n = 171) N (%)		Normal (n = 501) N (%)	High (n = 277) N (%)		Normal (n = 560) N (%)	High (n = 218) N (%)
Hibiscus drinks (portion)													
No intake	271 (38.4)	435 (61.6)	406 (57.5)	300 (42.5)		557 (78.9)	149 (21.1)		460 (65.2)	246 (34.8)		516 (73.1)	190 (26.9)
1–4/week	12 (20.7)	46 (79.3)	24 (41.4)	34 (58.6)		40 (69.0)	18 (31.0)		34 (58.6)	24 (41.4)		36 (62.1)	22 (37.9)
5 or more/week	4 (28.6)	10 (71.4)	7 (50.0)	7 (50.0)		10 (71.4)	4 (28.6)		7 (50.0)	7 (50.0)		8 (57.1)	6 (42.9)
χ^2 (p-value)	**7.633 (p = 0.022)**		5.883 (p = 0.053)			3.443 (p = 0.179)			2.287 (p = 0.319)			4.782 (p = 0.092)	
Cinnamon drink (portion)													
No intake	268 (38.6)	426 (61.4)	398 (57.3)	296 (42.7)		549 (79.1)	145 (20.9)		457 (65.9)	237 (34.1)		511 (73.6)	183 (26.4)
1–4/week	11 (21.2)	41 (78.8)	22 (42.3)	30 (57.7)		36 (69.2)	16 (30.8)		24 (46.2)	28 (53.8)		29 (55.8)	23 (44.2)
5 or more/week	8 (25.0)	24 (75.0)	17 (53.1)	15 (46.9)		22 (68.8)	10 (31.3)		20 (62.5)	12 (37.5)		20 (62.5)	12 (37.5)
χ^2 (p-value)	**8.363 (p = 0.015)**		4.571 (p = 0.102)			4.424 (p = 0.109)			**8.238 (p = 0.016)**			**9.139 (p = 0.01)**	

Data are shown as frequency and percentages. χ^2 is the Chi-square test value followed by its p-value. Significant differences between groups are shown in bold font LDL-C, low-density lipoprotein cholesterol; HDL-C, high-density lipoprotein cholesterol; TC, total cholesterol; TG, triglycerides.

Table 3. Unadjusted and adjusted Odds Ratios (OR) with its 95% Confidence Interval (CI) for dietary and lifestyle predictors of dyslipidemia in men.

Covariate	Unadjusted OR (95% CI) P	Adjusted for Age, BMI and WC OR (95% CI) P
Turkish coffee intake		
p for trend	$p < 0.001$	$p = 0.001$
No intake (reference)		
1–4 /week	0.955 (0.604, 1.512) $p = 0.846$	0.929 (0.573, 1.507) $p = 0.766$
5 or more /week	**2.783 (1.566, 4.944) $p < 0.001$**	**2.737 (1.532, 4.889) $p = 0.001$**
American coffee intake		
p for trend	$p = 0.005$	$p = 0.025$
No intake (reference)		
1–4 /week	**0.469 (0.273, 0.805) $p = 0.006$**	0.577 (0.326, 1.021) $p = 0.059$
5 or more /week	**0.544 (0.318, 0.933) $p = 0.027$**	**0.525 (0.298, 0.923) $p = 0.025$**
Carbonated drinks intake		
p for trend	$p > 0.15$	$p = 0.093$
No intake (reference)		
1–4 /week		1.226 (0.815, 1.842) $p = 0.326$
5 or more /week		**1.533 (1.041, 2.257) $p = 0.03$**
Sleep duration		
p for trend	$p = 0.011$	$p = 0.012$
6–8 h (reference)		
<6 h	**1.566 (1.155, 2.123) $p = 0.004$**	**1.573 (1.137, 2.175) $p = 0.006$**
>8 h	1.545 (0.795, 3.003) $p = 0.2$	1.844 (0.88, 3.864) $p = 0.105$
Smoking		
p for trend	$p > 0.15$	$p = 0.073$
Non-smokers (reference)		
Smokers		**1.41 (1.001, 1.986) $p = 0.043$**
Previous smokers		0.755 (0.381, 1.497) $p = 0.422$

Variables having a $p > 0.15$ in the initial logistic regression analysis between the dependent and independent variables were not included in the stepwise regression model. Significant differences between groups are shown in bold font.

3.2.2. Association between Food Intake and Dyslipidemia in Women

Comparing dietary habits in women between the two groups of normolipidemia and dyslipidemia, a high intake of the cinnamon drink was significantly associated with dyslipidemia in general ($p = 0.027$) and high LDL-C ($p = 0.036$) and TC in specific ($p = 0.002$) (Table 4). Dyslipidemia was present in 77% of women drinking five or more portions a week cinnamon drink compared to 58% in women who do not. The weekly intake of five or more portions of the cinnamon drink was associated with 2.6 times increased odds for having dyslipidemia in women compared with those with no intake. However, after adjusting for age, BMI, and WC, these odds became insignificant (Table 5). The adjustment for age and BMI regression analysis for each type of dyslipidemia separately showed that the weekly intake of five or more portions of the cinnamon drink was associated with a 2.57 times increased odds for having high TC in women compared with those with no intake (OR = 2.57; 95% CI: 1.22, 5.42; $p = 0.02$), but this was not significant after adjustment for age, BMI, and WC.

Table 4. Comparison of dietary habits between normolipidemic and dyslipidemic women groups presented as the number of women and (% of the group) for overall dyslipidemia, and abnormalities in different lipid fractions.

Variable	General Dyslipidemia		LDL-C			HDL-C			TC			TG		
	No (n = 240)	Yes (n = 367)	Normal (n = 381)	High (n = 226)		Normal (n = 440)	Low (n = 167)		Normal (n = 404)	High (n = 203)		Normal (n = 524)	High (n = 82)	
	N (%)	N (%)	N (%)	N (%)		N (%)	N (%)		N (%)	N (%)		N (%)	N (%)	
Fruit (portion)														
No intake	33 (47.1)	37 (52.9)	47 (67.1)	23 (32.9)		56 (80.0)	14 (20.0)		53 (75.7)	17 (24.3)		61 (87.1)	9 (12.9)	
1–4/week	123 (38.2)	199 (61.8)	209 (64.9)	113 (35.1)		219 (68.0)	103 (32.0)		221 (68.6)	101 (31.4)		284 (88.2)	38 (11.8)	
5 or more/week	84 (39.1)	131 (60.9)	125 (58.1)	90 (41.9)		165 (76.7)	50 (23.3)		130 (60.5)	85 (39.5)		179 (83.3)	36 (16.7)	
X² (p-value)	1.955 (p = 0.372)		3.174 (p = 0.204)			7.168 (p = 0.028)			6.846 (p = 0.033)			2.713 (p = 0.258)		
Fresh vegetable (portion)														
No intake	33 (62.3)	20 (37.7)	42 (79.2)	11 (20.8)		44 (83.0)	9 (17.0)		45 (84.9)	8 (15.1)		50 (94.3)	3 (5.7)	
1–4/week	79 (35.3)	145 (64.7)	137 (61.2)	87 (38.8)		152 (67.9)	72 (32.1)		150 (67.0)	74 (33.0)		194 (86.6)	30 (13.4)	
5 or more/week	128 (28.8)	202 (61.2)	202 (61.2)	128 (38.8)		244 (73.9)	86 (26.1)		209 (63.3)	121 (36.7)		280 (84.8)	50 (15.2)	
X² (p-value)	13.237 (p < 0.001)		6.747 (p = 0.034)			5.704 (p = 0.058)			9.574 (p = 0.008)			3.509 (p = 0.173)		
Cooked vegetable (portion)														
No intake	32 (48.5)	34 (51.5)	42 (63.6)	24 (36.4)		53 (80.3)	13 (19.7)		51 (77.3)	15 (22.7)		58 (87.9)	8 (12.1)	
1–4/week	100 (36.1)	177 (63.9)	172 (62.1)	105 (37.9)		195 (70.4)	82 (29.6)		176 (63.5)	101 (36.5)		237 (85.6)	40 (14.4)	
5 or more/week	108 (40.9)	156 (59.1)	167 (63.3)	97 (36.7)		192 (72.7)	72 (27.3)		177 (67.0)	87 (33.0)		229 (86.7)	35 (13.3)	
X² (p-value)	3.786 (p = 0.151)		0.102 (p = 0.95)			2.636 (p = 0.268)			4.567 (p = 0.102)			0.311 (p = 0.856)		
Whole grains (portion)														
No intake	40 (44.0)	51 (56.0)	61 (67.0)	30 (33.0)		64 (70.3)	27 (29.7)		66 (72.5)	25 (27.5)		81 (89.0)	10 (11.0)	
1–4/week	34 (37.4)	57 (62.6)	54 (59.3)	37 (40.7)		65 (71.4)	26 (28.6)		57 (62.6)	34 (37.4)		76 (83.5)	15 (16.5)	
5 or more/week	166 (39.1)	259 (60.9)	266 (62.6)	159 (37.4)		311 (73.2)	114 (26.8)		281 (66.1)	144 (33.9)		367 (86.4)	58 (13.6)	
X² (p-value)	0.964 (p = 0.618)		1.172 (p = 0.557)			0.365 (p = 0.833)			2.122 (p = 0.346)			1.165 (p = 0.559)		
Red meat (portion)														
No intake	65 (46.8)	74 (53.2)	92 (66.2)	47 (33.8)		105 (75.5)	34 (24.5)		95 (68.3)	44 (31.9)		122 (87.8)	17 (12.2)	
1–4/week	113 (33.7)	222 (66.3)	204 (60.9)	131 (39.1)		231 (69.0)	104 (31.0)		217 (64.8)	118 (35.2)		287 (85.7)	48 (14.3)	
5 or more/week	62 (46.6)	71 (53.4)	85 (63.9)	48 (36.1)		104 (78.2)	29 (21.8)		92 (69.2)	41 (30.8)		115 (86.5)	18 (13.5)	
X² (p-value)	10.547 (p = 0.005)		1.272 (p = 0.529)			4.918 (p = 0.086)			1.086 (p = 0.581)			0.369 (p = 0.831)		

Table 4. Cont.

Variable	General Dyslipidemia		LDL-C			HDL-C			TC			TG		
	No (n = 240) N (%)	Yes (n = 367) N (%)	Normal (n = 381) N (%)	High (n = 226) N (%)		Normal (n = 440) N (%)	Low (n = 167) N (%)		Normal (n = 404) N (%)	High (n = 203) N (%)		Normal (n = 524) N (%)	High (n = 82) N (%)	
Fresh juice (portion)														
No intake	78 (42.2)	107 (57.8)	118 (63.8)	67 (36.2)		134 (72.4)	51 (27.6)		127 (68.6)	58 (31.4)		167 (90.3)	18 (9.7)	
1–4/week	103 (36.9)	176 (63.1)	174 (62.4)	105 (37.6)		198 (71.0)	81 (29.0)		181 (64.9)	98 (35.1)		236 (84.6)	43 (15.4)	
5 or more/week	59 (41.3)	84 (58.7)	89 (62.2)	54 (37.8)		108 (75.5)	35 (24.5)		96 (67.1)	47 (32.9)		121 (84.6)	22 (15.4)	
X² (p-value)	1.511 (p = 0.47)		0.118 (p = 0.943)			0.985 (p = 0.611)			0.74 (p = 0.691)			3.507 (p = 0.173)		
Non fresh juice (portion)														
No intake	93 (36.0)	165 (64.0)	158 (61.2)	100 (38.8)		183 (70.9)	75 (29.1)		160 (62.0)	98 (38.0)		220 (85.3)	38 (14.7)	
1–4/week	74 (38.9)	116 (61.1)	123 (64.7)	67 (35.3)		136 (71.6)	54 (28.4)		134 (70.5)	56 (29.5)		164 (86.3)	26 (13.7)	
5 or more/week	73 (45.9)	86 (54.1)	100 (62.9)	59 (37.1)		121 (76.1)	38 (23.9)		110 (69.2)	49 (30.8)		140 (88.1)	19 (11.9)	
X² (p-value)	4.046 (p = 0.132)		0.574 (p = 0.751)			1.433 (p = 0.488)			4.228 (p = 0.121)			0.644 (p = 0.725)		
Carbonated drinks (portion)														
No intake	113 (38.2)	183 (61.8)	182 (61.5)	114 (38.5)		207 (69.9)	89 (30.1)		193 (65.2)	103 (34.8)		248 (83.8)	48 (16.2)	
1–4/week	68 (39.1)	106 (60.9)	108 (62.1)	66 (37.9)		130 (74.7)	44 (25.3)		115 (66.1)	59 (33.9)		156 (89.7)	18 (10.3)	
5 or more/week	59 (43.1)	78 (56.9)	91 (66.4)	46 (33.6)		103 (75.2)	34 (24.8)		96 (70.1)	41 (29.9)		120 (87.6)	17 (12.4)	
X² (p-value)	0.958 (p = 0.619)		1.028 (p = 0.598)			1.9 (p = 0.387)			1.022 (p = 0.6)			3.44 (p = 0.179)		
Red tea (portion)														
No intake	79 (43.4)	103 (56.6)	125 (68.7)	57 (31.3)		129 (70.9)	53 (29.1)		136 (74.7)	46 (25.3)		161 (88.5)	21 (11.5)	
1–4/week	42 (32.1)	89 (67.9)	75 (57.3)	56 (42.7)		91 (69.5)	40 (30.5)		77 (58.8)	54 (41.2)		110 (84.0)	21 (16.0)	
5 or more/week	119 (40.5)	175 (59.5)	181 (61.6)	113 (38.4)		220 (74.8)	74 (25.2)		191 (65.0)	103 (35.0)		253 (86.1)	41 (13.9)	
X² (p-value)	4.311 (p = 0.116)		4.611 (p = 0.1)			1.645 (p = 0.439)			9.351 (p = 0.009)			1.338 (p = 0.512)		
Green tea (portion)														
No intake	134 (41.9)	186 (58.1)	215 (67.2)	105 (32.8)		227 (70.9)	93 (29.1)		226 (70.6)	94 (29.4)		281 (87.8)	39 (12.2)	
1–4/week	50 (38.5)	80 (61.5)	75 (57.7)	55 (42.3)		94 (72.3)	36 (27.7)		85 (65.4)	45 (34.6)		108 (83.1)	22 (16.9)	
5 or more/week	56 (35.7)	101 (64.3)	91 (58.0)	66 (42.0)		119 (75.8)	38 (24.2)		93 (59.2)	64 (40.8)		135 (86.0)	22 (14.0)	
X² (p-value)	1.777 (p = 0.411)		5.659 (p = 0.059)			1.249 (p = 0.535)			6.24 (p = 0.044)			1.777 (p = 0.411)		

Table 4. Cont.

Variable	General Dyslipidemia		LDL-C			HDL-C			TC			TG	
	No (n = 240)	Yes (n = 367)	Normal (n = 381)	High (n = 226)		Normal (n = 440)	Low (n = 167)		Normal (n = 404)	High (n = 203)		Normal (n = 524)	High (n = 82)
	N (%)	N (%)	N (%)	N (%)		N (%)	N (%)		N (%)	N (%)		N (%)	N (%)
Arabic coffee (portion)													
No intake	93 (40.4)	137 (59.6)	148 (64.3)	82 (35.7)		161 (70.0)	69 (30.0)		159 (69.1)	71 (30.9)		199 (86.5)	31 (13.5)
1–4/week	57 (37.3)	96 (62.7)	98 (64.1)	55 (35.9)		104 (68.0)	49 (32.0)		104 (68.0)	49 (32.0)		130 (85.0)	23 (15.0)
5 or more/week	90 (40.2)	134 (59.8)	135 (60.3)	89 (39.7)		175 (78.1)	49 (21.9)		141 (62.9)	83 (37.1)		195 (87.1)	29 (12.9)
X² (p-value)	0.449 (p = 0.799)		0.953 (p = 0.621)			5.846 (p = 0.054)			2.134 (p = 0.344)			0.347 (p = 0.841)	
Turkish coffee (portion)													
No intake	170 (39.1)	265 (60.9)	280 (64.4)	155 (35.6)		310 (71.3)	125 (28.7)		284 (65.3)	151 (34.7)		378 (86.9)	57 (13.1)
1–4/week	31 (33.7)	61 (66.3)	52 (56.5)	40 (43.5)		65 (70.7)	27 (29.3)		64 (69.6)	28 (30.4)		77 (83.7)	15 (16.3)
5 or more/week	39 (48.8)	41 (51.2)	49 (61.3)	31 (38.8)		65 (81.3)	15 (18.8)		56 (70.0)	24 (30.0)		69 (86.3)	11 (13.8)
X² (p-value)	4.192 (p = 0.123)		2.091 (p = 0.351)			3.562 (p = 0.168)			1.115 (p = 0.573)			0.66 (p = 0.719)	
American coffee (portion)													
No intake	212 (40.2)	315 (59.8)	332 (63.0)	195 (37.0)		382 (72.5)	145 (27.5)		353 (67.0)	174 (33.0)		460 (87.3)	67 (12.7)
1–4/week	12 (27.9)	31 (72.1)	27 (62.8)	16 (37.2)		27 (62.8)	16 (37.2)		30 (69.8)	13 (30.2)		34 (79.1)	9 (20.9)
5 or more/week	16 (43.2)	21 (56.8)	22 (59.5)	15 (40.5)		31 (83.8)	6 (16.2)		21 (56.8)	16 (43.2)		30 (81.1)	7 (18.9)
X² (p-value)	2.751 (p = 0.253)		0.185 (p = 0.912)			4.395 (p = 0.111)			1.839 (p = 0.300)			3.192 (p = 0.203)	
Cappuccino (portion)													
No intake	140 (38.6)	223 (61.4)	216 (59.5)	147 (40.5)		255 (70.2)	108 (29.8)		238 (65.6)	125 (34.4)		306 (84.3)	57 (15.7)
1–4/week	60 (43.2)	79 (56.8)	99 (71.2)	40 (28.8)		104 (74.8)	35 (25.2)		98 (70.5)	41 (29.5)		123 (88.5)	16 (11.5)
5 or more/week	40 (38.1)	65 (61.9)	66 (62.9)	39 (37.1)		81 (77.1)	24 (22.9)		68 (64.8)	37 (35.2)		95 (90.5)	10 (9.5)
X² (p-value)	1 (p = 0.607)		5.907 (p = 0.052)			2.433 (p = 0.296)			1.285 (p = 0.526)			3.349 (p = 0.187)	
Energy drinks (portion)													
No intake	212 (39.3)	328 (60.7)	334 (61.9)	206 (38.1)		388 (71.9)	152 (28.1)		356 (65.9)	184 (34.1)		464 (85.9)	76 (24.1)
1–4/week	15 (33.3)	30 (66.7)	31 (68.9)	14 (31.1)		32 (71.1)	13 (28.9)		30 (66.7)	15 (33.3)		40 (88.9)	5 (11.1)
5 or more/week	13 (59.1)	9 (40.9)	16 (72.7)	6 (27.3)		20 (90.9)	2 (9.1)		18 (81.8)	4 (18.2)		20 (90.0)	2 (9.1)
X² (p-value)	2.261 (p = 0.119)		1.849 (p = 0.397)			3.896 (p = 0.143)			2.399 (p = 0.301)			0.715 (p = 0.699)	

Table 4. Cont.

Variable	General Dyslipidemia		LDL-C			HDL-C			TC			TG	
	No (n = 240)	Yes (n = 367)	Normal (n = 381)	High (n = 226)		Normal (n = 440)	Low (n = 167)		Normal (n = 404)	High (n = 203)		Normal (n = 524)	High (n = 82)
	N (%)	N (%)	N (%)	N (%)		N (%)	N (%)		N (%)	N (%)		N (%)	N (%)
Hibiscus drinks (portion)													
No intake	220 (39.9)	331 (60.1)	352 (63.9)	199 (36.1)		396 (71.9)	155 (28.1)		374 (67.9)	177 (32.1)		474 (86.0)	77 (14.0)
1–4/week	15 (35.7)	27 (64.3)	21 (50.0)	21 (50.0)		32 (76.2)	10 (23.8)		24 (57.1)	18 (42.9)		38 (90.5)	4 (9.5)
5 or more/week	5 (35.7)	9 (64.3)	8 (57.1)	6 (42.9)		12 (85.7)	2 (14.3)		6 (42.9)	8 (57.1)		12 (85.7)	2 (14.3)
χ^2 (p-value)	0.377 (p = 0.828)		3.413 (p = 0.182)			1.622 (p = 0.444)			5.636 (p = 0.06)			0.659 (p = 0.719)	
Cinnamon drink (portion)													
No intake	200 (42.2)	274 (57.8)	310 (65.4)	164 (34.6)		348 (73.4)	126 (26.6)		328 (69.2)	146 (30.8)		412 (86.9)	62 (13.1)
1–4/week	32 (32.30)	67 (67.7)	54 (54.5)	45 (45.5)		70 (70.7)	29 (29.3)		62 (62.6)	37 (37.4)		85 (85.9)	14 (14.1)
5 or more/week	8 (23.5)	26 (76.5)	17 (50.0)	17 (50.0)		22 (64.7)	12 (35.3)		14 (41.2)	20 (58.8)		27 (79.4)	7 (20.6)
χ^2 (p-value)	**7.199 (p = 0.027)**		**6.642 (p = 0.036)**			1.395 (p = 0.498)			**12.013 (p = 0.002)**			1.537 (p = 0.464)	

Data are shown as frequency and percentages. χ^2 is the Chi-square test value followed by its p-value. Significant differences between groups are shown in bold font. LDL-C, low-density lipoprotein cholesterol; HDL-C, high-density lipoprotein cholesterol; TC, total cholesterol; TG, triglycerides.

Table 5. Unadjusted and adjusted Odds Ratio (OR) with its 95% Confidence Interval (CI) for the predictors of dyslipidemia in women.

Covariate	Unadjusted	Adjusted for Age, BMI and WC
	OR (95% CI) P	OR (95% CI) P
Fresh vegetables intake		
p for trend	*p* = 0.007	*p* = 0.024
No intake (reference)		
1–4/week	**2.683 (1.416, 5.085)** *p* = **0.002**	**2.499 (1.285, 4.859)** *p* = **0.007**
5 or more/week	**2.489 (1.34, 4.624)** *p* = **0.004**	**2.072 (1.089, 3.941)** *p* = **0.026**
Cinnamon drink intake		
p for trend	*p* = 0.027	*p* > 0.15
No intake (reference)		
1–4/week	1.395 (0.873, 2.228) *p* = 0.163	
5 or more/week	**2.613 (1.142, 5.978)** *p* = **0.023**	

Variables having a $p > 0.15$ in the initial logistic regression analysis between the dependent and independent variables were not included in the stepwise regression model. Significant differences between groups are shown in bold font.

Moderate and high intakes of fresh vegetables were also found to be significantly associated with dyslipidemia ($p < 0.001$; Table 4) and mainly high LDL-C and TC ($p = 0.034$ and $p = 0.008$ respectively, Table 4). Dyslipidemia was diagnosed in 61% and 65% of women who ate either five or more portions of fresh vegetables/week or 1–4 times per week respectively compared to 38% of women who did not. This was associated with 2.50 and 2.07 times increased odds of having dyslipidemia, respectively, compared with those with no intake after adjusting for age, BMI, and WC (OR = 0.50 (95% CI: 1.29, 4.86) $p = 0.007$ and OR = 2.07 (95% CI: 1.09, 3.94) $p = 0.026$ respectively; Table 5).

Following the finding of this interesting results, further analysis was performed to identify the characteristics of females with high intake of fresh vegetables. Women who reported to have an intake of 1–4 and 5 or more portions per week were significantly older than those who reported no intake ($p < 0.01$ at least). They also had a significantly higher mean weight and neck circumference ($p < 0.05$ at least). In addition, a higher proportion of these women were previously diagnosed with dyslipidemia and taking medication, however, this was not statistically significant (Supplementary Table S3).

There was no effect of other food types on dyslipidemia in women when analyzed using regression analysis after adjusting for age, BMI, and WC.

3.3. Association between Lifestyle Characteristics and Dyslipidemia in Men and Women

After analyzing sex groups separately, only short and long sleep durations were associated with general dyslipidemia in men only (Supplementary Table S2a, $p = 0.012$). Dyslipidemia was detected in 68.5% and 68.2% of men who reported sleeping either <6 h/day, or >8 h/day respectively compared with 58.1% of people who slept 6–8 h per day. This association was particularly evident for increased TC ($p < 0.029$). There was no association between sleep duration and dyslipidemia in women.

There was no association between physical activity or daily sitting duration and dyslipidemia in general (Supplementary Table S2a,b). However, low physical activity was associated with high TC and TG in men ($p = 0.024$ and $p = 0.048$ respectively; Supplementary Table S2a). High TC and TG were detected in 39.1% and 30.9% of men reporting low physical activity compared with 31.3% and 24.5%, respectively, in men who were more physically active. In women, low physical activity was associated with low HDL-C only ($p = 0.024$; Supplementary Table S2b). Low HDL-C was detected in 41% of women reporting low physical activity compared with 32% of women who were more physically active. On the other hand, very short sitting duration (<4 h per day) was associated with decreased HDL-C in women as it was found in 36.3% of women reporting sitting for <4 h per day compared with 20–26% of those sitting for more than 4 h ($p = 0.031$, Supplementary Table S2b).

Smoking was not associated with dyslipidemia in general (Supplementary Table S2a,b). However, it was associated with high TG in men ($p = 0.011$; Supplementary Table S2a). High TG was detected in 34.2% of men who smoke compared with 25.7% of non-smoking men. In women, smoking was associated with low HDL-C ($p = 0.035$; Supplementary Table S2b). Low HDL-C was detected in 50% of women who smoked compared with 36.1% of who were non-smokers.

After adjusting for age, BMI, and WC, only sleep duration and smoking were predictors for dyslipidemia in men (Table 3). Having <6 h of sleep per day was associated with increased odds of having general dyslipidemia compared with those sleeping 6–8 h (OR = 1.57 (CI: 1.14, 2.18) $p = 0.006$; Table 3). In addition, smoking was associated with increased odds of having general dyslipidemia compared with those who did not smoke (OR = 1.42 (CI: 1.00, 1.98) $p = 0.043$; Table 3).

Lifestyle characteristics were not predictors for dyslipidemia in women after adjusting for age, BMI, and WC.

4. Discussion

In this study, we investigated the association between dyslipidemia, dietary, and other lifestyle practices among Saudi adults not previously diagnosed with diabetes. Dyslipidemia was found to be associated with increased age, BMI, and WC in men and women. However, notable differences between sexes in the association of dyslipidemia with dietary and other lifestyle practices were noted. In men, an increased risk of dyslipidemia was found to be associated with high consumption of Turkish coffee, and carbonated drinks, short (<6 h) and long (>8 h) sleep duration, and smoking, while high consumption of American coffee was associated with decreased risk after adjusting for age, BMI and WC. However, only increased consumption of fresh vegetables was associated with an increased risk of dyslipidemia in women after adjusting for confounding factors.

The prevalence of dyslipidemia among Saudi adults in our study was 62% which is higher than previously reported [10,11]. The difference could be due to the variations in dietary, and lifestyle practices between regions of the Kingdom as well ethnic origin of studied populations since ethnicity among Saudi nationals can vary to some extent and influence genetic and lifestyle factors. Our study was conducted in the city of Jeddah in the Western Region of the Kingdom, while the previous study [10,11] included people from all the regions in Saudi Arabia. Another reason could be the variation in defining dyslipidemia and all its types. In this study, the used dyslipidemia definition was more comprehensive as it included laboratory-measured high TG, high fasting serum cholesterol, low fasting plasma HDL-C and/or high fasting plasma LDL-C levels, as well as treatment with hyperlipidemic drugs [27,28].

The most prevalent type of dyslipidemia in this study was high LDL-C which was detected in 40.9% of studied Saudi adults. This was followed by high TC in 34.7%, low HDL-C in 24.4%, and least of all high TG levels in 21.7% of the study population. A comparably high prevalence of high LDL-C and hypercholesterolemia in a Saudi population was reported in previous large community-based national cross-sectional studies [9–11]. However, one of these studies [9] reported a much higher prevalence for hypertriglyceridemia despite using similar definition. This could be caused by the difference in the age range of participants as the previous study [9] included people aged 30–70 years, whereas the current study included adults ≥18 years of age.

As reported in previous studies on Saudi and other populations [9–11,30,31] older age, increased BMI and WC were associated with a higher prevalence of dyslipidemia in general, and all its types. The prevalence of high TG in the current study was lower than previously reported [11] being 11.4% for young adults aged 30 years or under compared to with 32% in the older adults aged more than 30 years. This difference in prevalence is due to the variation in the cut-off point to determine hypertriglyceridemia as it was ≥ 1.7 mmol/L in our study as well as in that of Al-Amri et al. [32] whereas ≥ 1.27 mmol/L was adopted in the previous study [11]. The cut-off point in this previous study allowed a wider range of the population to be diagnosed with hypertriglyceridemia, and therefore a higher prevalence was reported.

In our study sex had no effect on the prevalence of dyslipidemia in general but both hypertriglyceridemia and high LDL-C were more prevalent in men than women. Similar sex-differences were reported previously [9,11]. This could be due to the higher proportion of smokers, and the higher prevalence of low sleep duration (<6 h) among men. These lifestyle factors were associated with both hypertriglyceridemia and elevated LDL-C in this study. On the other hand, low HDL-C was more prevalent among women, which is different from that previously reported [11]. Similar sex differences in the prevalence of low HDL-C was previously found in Iranian population [33], which reported a much higher prevalence in both men and women compared with that found in our study.

Emerging evidence collected from self-reported data indicated that both short and long sleep duration are associated with adverse health consequences including obesity hypertension, diabetes mellitus, and CVDs, showing a curvilinear relationship between habitual sleep duration and these conditions [34–36]. In line with this, in our study in men but not in women, both short (<6 h) and long (>8 h) sleep durations were associated with dyslipidemia, particularly with elevated LDL-C and TG levels. In contrast, a recent systemic review, meta-analysis, and meta-regression suggested that a causal relationship existed between short sleep durations and adverse health outcomes including increased risk of diabetes, hypertension, and CVD [14]. However, there was insufficient data to draw a conclusion regarding the association between short sleep duration and dyslipidemia [14,34]. On the other hand, another systematic review indicated that long sleep may have more adverse health effect than short sleep [37]. Findings from cross-sectional data for the middle-aged and older Chinese population partly supported our finding that both short and long sleep durations were associated with dyslipidemia; since their cohort data suggested that long sleep duration (>9 h) only was associated with dyslipidemia [35].

In experimental studies, sleep debt has shown to induce alterations in the endocrine functions, so that sleep debt for 4 h resulted in raising evening cortisol concentrations, suggesting that it results in the disturbance of the negative-feedback regulation of the hypothalamus-pituitary-adrenal axis [37,38]. A previous cross-sectional study reported that excess cortisol secretion was linked to increased TG concentrations in South Asians [39]. The association between sleep duration, cortisol secretion, and dyslipidemia needs to be further investigated [40]. Even though the cortisol level was not measured in our study, dysregulated cortisol secretion might be the cause for the observed association between short sleep duration and dyslipidemia.

High consumption of Turkish coffee in this study was associated with dyslipidemia in men only. This is consistent with findings from previous clinical studies [41]. In contrast, we found that high consumption of American coffee was associated with decreased risk of dyslipidemia in men also, which contradicts findings in a clinical cohort study reporting that abstention from filtered coffee for 3 weeks resulted in a decrease in TC [42]. In an attempt to explain the different findings, a previous review suggested that brewing and preparation techniques influence this association as the long contact of beans with hot water in unfiltered coffee results in the formation of cholesterol elevating compounds, such as cafestol and kahweol, and that up to 90% of these diterpenes may be carried by floating coffee bean particles [43]. The same review suggested that the predicted rise in serum cholesterol levels with consumption of five cups of Turkish coffee per day is 0.25 mmol/L whereas filtered coffee is not predicted to increase serum cholesterol levels. In addition to diterpene alcohols, other compounds are found in the complex coffee beverage [43]. Moreover, a previous meta-regression analysis revealed that coffee consumption, particularly unfiltered coffee, is related to increased LDL-C, TC, and TG in a dose dose-dependent manner [42]. Coffee also contains antioxidant and anti-inflammatory compounds such as chlorogenic acid [43]. This might explain the observed U-shaped relationship between coffee consumption and low HDL-C and high TC in the current study. The observation that Turkish coffee was related to increased dyslipidemia in men but not women in the current study cannot be explained by variation in consumption patterns between sexes since these were comparable. Similar to our findings, a previous Norwegian study reported that unfiltered coffee consumption was associated with elevated cholesterol levels in men but not women [44].

In the current study fruit and vegetable intake were associated with dyslipidemia in men in a U-shaped manner. However, following adjustment for age, BMI, and WC consumption of fruits and vegetables lost their association with dyslipidemia in men. This suggests that this association could be caused by the high intake of total food in general and thus confounded by other constituents of diet. On the other hand, the consumption of fruit and fresh vegetables was associated with an increased risk of dyslipidemia, particularly elevated TC, in women, thus contradicting the previously reported beneficial effects of fruits and vegetables on serum lipids [45]. However, following adjustment for age, BMI, and WC, only the consumption of fresh vegetables retained its association with dyslipidemia. This could be a chance finding given several statistical comparisons, or due to the residual confounding since we did not collect data on all possible factors that may be associated with dyslipidemia. Following this unexpected finding, further statistical analysis was carried out, and the mean neck circumference (NC) was found to be higher in women reporting medium and high intake of fresh vegetables. In a systemic review and meta-analysis, positive associations between NC, high TC, and LDL-C, and low HDL-C concentrations were found, and subjects with higher NC had approximately two-fold higher risk for hypertriglyceridemia compared to those with lower NC [46]. NC was not adjusted for in our study, hence its increased mean in women consuming fresh vegetables could contribute to the noted association. Another reason could be that women who knew about their dyslipidemia or were trying to lose weight had modified their diet to include more fresh vegetables, i.e., representing reverse causation. Indeed, the mean weight of women ingesting fresh vegetables was significantly higher than the mean of those reporting no intake, and a higher percentage were on lipid-lowering therapy, but the difference to those reporting no intake did not reach statistical significance. Also, the addition of salad dressings to fresh vegetable salads is a very common dietary practice. Salad dressings often contain around 40% of fat, and a considerable amount of high fructose corn syrup, which has been proven to increase lipid synthesis and is associated with dyslipidemia [47]. Furthermore, mayonnaise is a major ingredient as a salad dressing alone or as part of other popular dressings (e.g., thousand islands), and studies have found that the use of palm oil, a cheaper oil comparatively, in its preparation caused an increase in total and LDL-C compared to the use of soybean oil, which is a more expensive type [48]. Therefore, the consumption of dressing can distort potential beneficial influences of vegetable consumption on serum lipids.

Studies with more detailed dietary assessment methods such as food diaries that provide information about consumed additives to vegetables are required to get a clear picture of the influence of vegetable consumption on serum lipids in Saudis.

It was interesting to note that in men, smoking and high consumption of carbonated drinks were significantly associated with dyslipidemia only following adjustment for age, BMI, and WC. Both cigarette smoking and dyslipidemia are well-established major risk factors for cardiovascular disease. Studies on different populations reported an increased risk of dyslipidemia in smokers [1–3]. A Korean cross-sectional study [49] conducted in adults aged ≥19 years reported that there was an increased risk of low HDL-C, high TG and high LDL-C in male smokers compared with non-smokers. On the other hand, female smokers were found to have a significantly increased risk for high TC, high TG, and high LDL-C compared with non-smokers. These results emphasize the sex difference in response to the same lifestyle factors as noted in our study. A Tunisian study [50] reported an increased risk of high triglyceridemia, and low HDL-C in smokers in a dose-response manner. Our study did not investigate the amount or type of smoking, however it was noted that a higher percentage of smokers had hypertriglyceridemia. Similar findings were reported in a Chinese study of elderly adults [51] that concluded that smoking was an independent risk factor for dyslipidemia and that it had a bigger effect than other studied factors including alcohol intake, BMI, and age.

High consumption of carbonated drinks was a predictor of dyslipidemia in men. A prospective study reported that daily consumption of carbonated drinks was associated with increased risk of hypertriglyceridemia and low HDL-C. In a cross-sectional study performed in Oslo, Norway, the consumption of colas but not other carbonated drinks was associated with low serum HDL-C, as well as high TG and LDL-C [52]. The association between high carbonated drink intake and dyslipidemia could be attributed to the high sucrose content in these drinks as it was reported to be linked to hypertriglyceridemia previously [53]. The questionnaire that was used in this study did not provide specific data about the type of carbonated drink. Future work should include more details on type of drinks, and whether it was sugar-free or not.

A number of lifestyle practices showed an association initially, but this association was lost after adjustment for confounding factors. These practices include decreased physical activity and sitting duration. Physical activity and sedentary behavior are common factors reported to be associated with serum lipid levels [54,55]. A previous review on the effect of aerobic exercise on serum lipids recommended that clinicians should rely more on physical activity and less on lipid lowering drugs to modify lipid variables, thus to reduce the risk of myocardial infractions and CVD [56]. Low physical activity was found to be associated with dyslipidemia and particularly with high TC and TG in men, but it was not a significant predictive factor. However, the questionnaire used in our study did not provide detailed information about the type, timing, and intensity of physical activity. People tend to start exercising in an attempt to control weight, and various ill-health conditions, which could explain the loss of association following adjustment for BMI and WC in our study. Specific specialized questionnaires should be used in future work to provide more detailed information about physical activity, which would aid in providing more information about the association between physical activity and dyslipidemia in the Saudi population.

Very short sitting duration (for less than 4 h) was associated with a decreased level of HDL-C in women in the current study. Short sitting duration might be associated with stress at work. Indeed, it has been observed in individuals whose career requires high labor work and low sitting hours and provides low salaries [57]. A previous cross-sectional study on women employees of a retail company in Japan reported that employees with effort-reward imbalance had a 4.4-fold higher risk of low HDL-C compared with employees who have balanced effort-reward [57]. This suggests that the stress in careers or other work-related factors could distort the relationship between physical activity and dyslipidemia and might explain the observed relationship between low sitting duration and unfavorable HDL-C profile noted in our study.

Another unexpected finding in this study was that cinnamon drink consumption was associated with increased risk of dyslipidemia, particularly elevated TC, in women before adjustment for confounding factors. This was not observed in men probably due to the higher intake of cinnamon drink in women. In contrast, a previous systematic review and meta-analysis suggested that cinnamon supplementation has an anti-lipidemic effect especially on plasma cholesterol and TG in a duration-dependent but not dose-dependent manner [58]. After adjusting for age, BMI, and WC the association ceased to exist in our study. The inverse association between cinnamon drink consumption and dyslipidemia observed might be due to the addition of sugar to the drink which is a common practice among Saudis. Another possible explanation could be due to changes in the diet by individuals who have been recently diagnosed with dyslipidemia or hyperglycemia. The current study had a cross-sectional design, which is the main limitation since it did not provide information on the duration of the recorded dietary pattern. Cinnamon drink is commonly ingested by Saudi individuals who are diagnosed with dysglycemia due to the common belief that cinnamon lowers blood sugar. Since dysglycemia occurs more in individuals with dyslipidemia particularly high LDL-C [32], changes in dietary habits such as increasing consumption of cinnamon drink or fresh vegetables in individuals diagnosed with dysglycemia or dyslipidemia can result in biased observations regarding the effect of these food types on serum lipids. In order to obtain a clear picture, future studies should include information on the duration of the recorded dietary habits, and whether dietary practices have been changed due to medical advice.

There are limitations to our study. First, its cross-sectional design did not allow for inferences about cause and effect and can suggest associations only. In addition, collected data was based on a questionnaire providing self-reported dietary and lifestyle data, hence errors of reporting are expected. However, conducting face to face interviews by trained data collectors is believed to minimize such errors. In addition, our study had a relatively small sample size, but it was enough to detect several associations.

In spite of the limitation, our study has many points of strength. The first being that bias was avoided by a random selection of PHC and included volunteers. Secondly, standardized methods for data collections by well-trained data collectors were used. Moreover, a comprehensive definition was used to diagnose dyslipidemia, and all collected samples were analyzed in one accredited lab to avoid variations leading to misclassification.

5. Conclusions

In this studied population, there was a high prevalence of dyslipidemia among men and women which was found to be associated with increased age, BMI, and WC. Dyslipidemia was associated with several lifestyle and dietary factors, which was sex-specific. After adjusting for age, BMI, and WC, short (<6 h), and long (>8 h) sleep duration, and high consumption of Turkish coffee and carbonated drinks were associated with increased risk of dyslipidemia in men, while high consumption of American coffee was associated with a decreased risk. However, in women, only increased consumption of fresh vegetables was associated with an increased risk of dyslipidemia after adjusting for confounding factors.

This highlights the necessity of the adjustment of these modifiable risk factors since individuals with dyslipidemia are at increased risk of developing CVD. More detailed cohort studies are needed to reach firmer conclusions and lead to prevention recommendations. Nevertheless, results from this study provide useful information for the planning of future preventive actions against CVD.

Supplementary Materials: The following are available online at http://www.mdpi.com/2072-6643/12/8/2441/s1, Figure S1: Recruitment flow diagram, Table S1: Demographic, anthropometric, clinical and biochemical characteristics of studied groups, Table S2: Comparison of demographic, anthropometric, and lifestyle characteristics of normolipidemia vs. dyslipidemia groups presented as number of people (%) for overall dyslipidemia, and abnormalities in different lipid parameters in men (a) and women (b), Table S3: Anthropometric and clinical characteristics of vegetable intake groups in women.

Author Contributions: Conceptualization, all authors; methodology, S.B., H.J., R.A.R., G.A., J.A.-A., A.B., and J.T.; software, H.J., R.A.R., G.A., J.A.-A., and S.E.; validation, S.B., H.J., R.A.R., G.A., J.A.-A., and J.T.; formal analysis, S.E., S.B., and H.J.; investigation, S.B., H.J., R.A.R., G.A., J.A.-A., A.B., and J.T.; resources, S.B., H.J., R.A.R., G.A., J.A.-A., and A.B.; data curation, S.B., H.J., R.A.R., G.A., and J.A.-A.; writing—original draft preparation, S.B., S.E., B.E., and M.M.; writing—review and editing, all authors; visualization, S.B., S.E., and J.T.; supervision, S.B., H.J., R.A.R., G.A., and J.A.-A.; project administration, S.B. and G.A.; funding acquisition, S.B., G.A., and J.T. All authors have read and agreed to the published version of the manuscript.

Funding: This research was funded by King Abdulaziz University, grant number (2-140-1434-HiCi).

Acknowledgments: We thank the Deanship of Research in King AbdulAziz University in the highly cited program for supporting this work. We also thank Lubna Al-Shaikh for cleaning the data.

Conflicts of Interest: The authors declare no conflict of interest.

Abbreviations

BMI, body mass index; BP, blood pressure; CVD, cardiovascular disease; HDL-C, high density lipoprotein cholesterol; LDL-C, low density lipoprotein cholesterol; PHCC, primary health care centers; SD, standard deviation; TC, total cholesterol; TG, triglycerides; WC, waist circumference; WHO, World Health Organization.

References

1. World Health Organization. Cardiovascular Diseases (CVDs). Available online: https://www.who.int/news-room/fact-sheets/detail/cardiovascular-diseases-(cvds) (accessed on 17 June 2020).
2. Al-Nozha, M.; Arafah, M.; Al-Mazrou, Y.; Al-Maatouq, M.; Khan, N.; Khalil, M.; Al-Khadra, A.; Al-Marzouki, K.; Abdullah, M.; Al-Harthi, S. Coronary artery disease in Saudi Arabia. *Saudi Med. J.* **2004**, *25*, 1165–1171.

3. World Health Organization; United Nations Development Programme. Prevention and Control of Noncommunicable Diseases in the Kingdom of Saudi Arabia: The Case for Investment. Available online: https://www.sa.undp.org/content/saudi_arabia/en/home/library/poverty/prevention-and-control-of-noncommunicable-diseases-in-the-kingdo.html (accessed on 17 June 2020).
4. Ahmed, A.M.; Hersi, A.; Mashhoud, W.; Arafah, M.R.; Abreu, P.C.; Al Rowaily, M.A.; Al-Mallah, M. Cardiovascular risk factors burden in Saudi Arabia: The Africa Middle East cardiovascular epidemiological (ACE) study. *J. Saudi Heart Assoc.* **2017**, *29*, 235–243. [CrossRef] [PubMed]
5. Tietge, U.J. Hyperlipidemia and cardiovascular disease: Inflammation, dyslipidemia, and atherosclerosis. *Curr. Opin. Lipidol.* **2014**, *25*, 94–95. [CrossRef] [PubMed]
6. World Heart Federation. Cardiovascular Risk Factors. Available online: https://www.world-heart-federation.org/resources/risk-factors/ (accessed on 17 June 2020).
7. Barter, P.; Gotto, A.M.; LaRosa, J.C.; Maroni, J.; Szarek, M.; Grundy, S.M.; Kastelein, J.J.P.; Bittner, V.; Fruchart, J.-C. HDL Cholesterol, Very Low Levels of LDL Cholesterol, and Cardiovascular Events. *N. Engl. J. Med.* **2007**, *357*, 1301–1310. [CrossRef] [PubMed]
8. Chang, W.-T.; Yin, W.-H.; Lin, F.-J.; Tseng, W.-K.; Wu, Y.-W.; Li, Y.-H.; Yeh, H.-I.; Chen, J.-W.; Wu, C.-C. Non-High-Density-Lipoprotein Cholesterol is an Important Residual Risk Factor in the Secondary Prevention for Patients With Established Atherosclerotic Cardiovascular Diseases. *Circulation* **2016**, *134*, A16414.
9. Al-Nozha, M.; Arafah, M.; Al-Maatouq, M.; Khalil, M.; Khan, N.; Al-Marzouki, K.; Al-Mazrou, Y.; Abdullah, M.; Al-Khadra, A.; Al-Harthi, S.; et al. Hyperlipidemia in Saudi Arabia. *Saudi Med. J.* **2008**, *29*, 282–287. [PubMed]
10. Basulaiman, M.; El Bcheraoui, C.; Tuffaha, M.; Robinson, M.; Daoud, F.; Jaber, S.; Mikhitarian, S.; Wilson, S.; Memish, Z.A.; Al Saeedi, M.; et al. Hypercholesterolemia and its associated risk factors—Kingdom of Saudi Arabia, 2013. *Ann. Epidemiol.* **2014**, *24*, 801–808. [CrossRef] [PubMed]
11. Alkaabba, A.; Al-Hamdan, N.; Tahir, A.; Abdalla, A.; Hussein, G.; Saeed, A.; Hamza, M.A. Prevalence and Correlates of Dyslipidemia among Adults in Saudi Arabia: Results from a National Survey. *Open J. Endocr. Metab. Dis.* **2012**, *2*, 89. [CrossRef]
12. Al-Hassan, Y.; Fabella, E.; Estrella, E.; Aatif, M. Prevalence and Determinants of Dyslipidemia: Data from a Saudi University Clinic. *Open Public Health J.* **2018**, *11*, 416–424. [CrossRef]
13. Opoku, S.; Gan, Y.; Fu, W.; Chen, D.; Addo-Yobo, E.; Trofimovitch, D.; Yue, W.; Yan, F.; Wang, Z.; Lu, Z. Prevalence and risk factors for dyslipidemia among adults in rural and urban China: Findings from the China National Stroke Screening and prevention project (CNSSPP). *BMC Public Health* **2019**, *19*, 1500. [CrossRef]
14. Itani, O.; Jike, M.; Watanabe, N.; Kaneita, Y. Short sleep duration and health outcomes: A systematic review, meta-analysis, and meta-regression. *Sleep Med.* **2017**, *32*, 246–256. [CrossRef] [PubMed]
15. Darnton-Hill, I.; Nishida, C.; James, W. A life course approach to diet, nutrition and the prevention of chronic diseases. *Public Health Nutr.* **2004**, *7*, 101–121. [CrossRef] [PubMed]
16. Ziegler, O.; Got, I.; Jan, P.; Drouin, P. Diet therapy of hypercholesterolemia. From theory to practice. In Proceedings of Annales de cardiologie et d'angeiologie. *Ann. Cardiol. Angeiol. (Paris)* **1989**, *38*, 249–253. [PubMed]
17. Bahijri, S.; Al-Raddadi, R.; Ajabnoor, G.; Jambi, H.; Al Ahmadi, J.; Borai, A.; Barengo, N.C.; Tuomilehto, J. Dysglycemia risk score in Saudi Arabia: A tool to identify people at high future risk of developing type 2 diabetes. *J. Diabetes Investig.* **2020**, *11*, 844–855. [CrossRef]
18. Lindström, J.; Tuomilehto, J. The diabetes risk score: A practical tool to predict type 2 diabetes risk. *Diabetes Care* **2003**, *26*, 725–731. [CrossRef]
19. Saaristo, T.; Peltonen, M.; Keinänen-Kiukaanniemi, S.; Vanhala, M.; Saltevo, J.; Niskanen, L.; Oksa, H.; Korpi-Hyövälti, E.; Tuomilehto, J. National type 2 diabetes prevention programme in Finland: FIN-D2D. *Int. J. Circumpolar Health* **2007**, *66*, 101–112. [CrossRef]
20. Kaczorowski, J.; Robinson, C.; Nerenberg, K. Development of the CANRISK questionnaire to screen for prediabetes and undiagnosed type 2 diabetes. *Can. J. Diabetes* **2009**, *33*, 381–385. [CrossRef]
21. Makrilakis, K.; Liatis, S.; Grammatikou, S.; Perrea, D.; Stathi, C.; Tsiligros, P.; Katsilambros, N. Validation of the Finnish diabetes risk score (FINDRISC) questionnaire for screening for undiagnosed type 2 diabetes, dysglycaemia and the metabolic syndrome in Greece. *Diabetes Metab.* **2011**, *37*, 144–151. [CrossRef]

22. Franciosi, M.; De Berardis, G.; Rossi, M.C.; Sacco, M.; Belfiglio, M.; Pellegrini, F.; Tognoni, G.; Valentini, M.; Nicolucci, A. Use of the diabetes risk score for opportunistic screening of undiagnosed diabetes and impaired glucose tolerance: The IGLOO (Impaired Glucose Tolerance and Long-Term Outcomes Observational) study. *Diabetes Care* **2005**, *28*, 1187–1194. [CrossRef]
23. Al-Lawati, J.; Tuomilehto, J. Diabetes risk score in Oman: A tool to identify prevalent type 2 diabetes among Arabs of the Middle East. *Diabetes Res. Clin. Pract.* **2007**, *77*, 438–444. [CrossRef]
24. Karter, A.; D'Agostino, R., Jr.; Mayer-Davis, E.; Wagenknecht, L.; Hanley, A.; Hamman, R.; Bergman, R.; Saad, M.; Haffner, S. Abdominal obesity predicts declining insulin sensitivity in non-obese normoglycaemics: The Insulin Resistance Atherosclerosis Study (IRAS). *Diabetes Obes. Metab.* **2005**, *7*, 230–238. [CrossRef] [PubMed]
25. Zhu, S.; Wang, Z.; Heshka, S.; Heo, M.; Faith, M.; Heymsfield, S. Waist circumference and obesity-associated risk factors among whites in the third National Health and Nutrition Examination Survey: Clinical action thresholds. *Am. J. Clin. Nutr.* **2002**, *76*, 743. [CrossRef] [PubMed]
26. Friedewald, W.; Levy, R.; Fredrickson, D. Estimation of the concentration of low-density lipoprotein cholesterol in plasma, without use of the preparative ultracentrifuge. *Clin. Chem.* **1972**, *18*, 499–502. [CrossRef] [PubMed]
27. Alberti, K.; Eckel, R.H.; Grundy, S.M.; Zimmet, P.Z.; Cleeman, J.I.; Donato, K.A.; Fruchart, J.-C.; James, W.P.T.; Loria, C.M.; Smith, S., Jr. Harmonizing the metabolic syndrome: A joint interim statement of the international diabetes federation task force on epidemiology and prevention; national heart, lung, and blood institute; American heart association; world heart federation; international atherosclerosis society; and international association for the study of obesity. *Circulation* **2009**, *120*, 1640–1645. [PubMed]
28. National Cholesterol Education Program. *Third Report of the National Cholesterol Education Program (Ncep) Expert Panel on Detection, Evaluation, and Treatment of High Blood Cholesterol in Adults (Adult Treatment Panel Iii)*; National Cholesterol Education Program, National Heart, Lung, and Blood: Bethesda, MD, USA, 2002.
29. Field, A. *Discovering Statistics Using IBM SPSS Statistics*; SAGE: London, UK, 2013.
30. Erem, C.; Hacihasanoglu, A.; Deger, O.; Kocak, M.; Topbas, M. Prevalence of dyslipidemia and associated risk factors among Turkish adults: Trabzon lipid study. *Endocrine* **2008**, *34*, 36–51. [CrossRef] [PubMed]
31. Polychronopoulos, E.; Panagiotakos, D.B.; Polystipioti, A. Diet, lifestyle factors and hypercholesterolemia in elderly men and women from Cyprus. *Lipids Health Dis.* **2005**, *4*, 17. [CrossRef]
32. Al Amri, T.; Bahijri, S.; Al-Raddadi, R.; Ajabnoor, G.; Al Ahmadi, J.; Jambi, H.; Borai, A.; Tuomilehto, J. The Association Between Prediabetes and Dyslipidemia Among Attendants of Primary Care Health Centers in Jeddah, Saudi Arabia. *Diabetes Metab. Syndr. Obes. Targets Ther.* **2019**, *12*, 2735–2743. [CrossRef]
33. Sharifi, F.; Mousavinasab, S.; Soruri, R.; Saeini, M.; Dinmohammadi, M. High prevalence of low high-density lipoprotein cholesterol concentrations and other dyslipidemic phenotypes in an Iranian population. *Metab. Syndr. Relat. Disord.* **2008**, *6*, 187–195. [CrossRef]
34. Jike, M.; Itani, O.; Watanabe, N.; Buysse, D.J.; Kaneita, Y. Long sleep duration and health outcomes: A systematic review, meta-analysis and meta-regression. *Sleep Med. Rev.* **2018**, *39*, 25–36. [CrossRef]
35. Wang, D.; Chen, J.; Zhou, Y.; Ma, J.; Zhou, M.; Xiao, L.; He, M.; Zhang, X.; Guo, H.; Yuan, J.; et al. Association between sleep duration, sleep quality and hyperlipidemia in middle-aged and older Chinese: The Dongfeng–Tongji Cohort Study. *Eur. J. Prev. Cardiol.* **2019**, *26*, 1288–1297. [CrossRef]
36. Bin, Y.S.; Marshall, N.S.; Glozier, N. Sleeping at the limits: The changing prevalence of short and long sleep durations in 10 countries. *Am. J. Epidemiol.* **2013**, *177*, 826–833. [CrossRef]
37. Spiegel, K.; Leproult, R.; Van Cauter, E. Impact of sleep debt on metabolic and endocrine function. *Lancet* **1999**, *354*, 1435–1439. [CrossRef]
38. Bahijri, S.; Borai, A.; Ajabnoor, G.; Khaliq, A.A.; AlQassas, I.; Al-Shehri, D.; Chrousos, G. Relative metabolic stability, but disrupted circadian cortisol secretion during the fasting month of Ramadan. *PLoS ONE* **2013**, *8*, e60917. [CrossRef] [PubMed]
39. Ward, A.M.V.; Fall, C.H.D.; Stein, C.E.; Kumaran, K.; Veena, S.R.; Wood, P.J.; Syddall, H.E.; Phillips, D.I.W. Cortisol and the metabolic syndrome in South Asians. *Clin. Endocrinol.* **2003**, *58*, 500–505. [CrossRef]
40. Whitworth, J.A.; Williamson, P.M.; Mangos, G.; Kelly, J.J. Cardiovascular consequences of cortisol excess. *Vasc. Health Risk Manag.* **2005**, *1*, 291–299. [CrossRef] [PubMed]
41. Strandhagen, E.; Thelle, D.S. Filtered coffee raises serum cholesterol: Results from a controlled study. *Eur. J. Clin. Nutr.* **2003**, *57*, 1164–1168. [CrossRef] [PubMed]

42. Cai, L.; Ma, D.; Zhang, Y.; Liu, Z.; Wang, P. The effect of coffee consumption on serum lipids: A meta-analysis of randomized controlled trials. *Eur. J. Clin. Nutr.* **2012**, *66*, 872–877. [CrossRef] [PubMed]
43. Urgert, R.; Katan, M.B. The cholesterol-raising factor from coffee beans. *Annu. Rev. Nutr.* **1997**, *17*, 305–324. [CrossRef]
44. Nystad, T.; Melhus, M.; Brustad, M.; Lund, E. The effect of coffee consumption on serum total cholesterol in the Sami and Norwegian populations. *Public Health Nutr.* **2010**, *13*, 1818–1825. [CrossRef]
45. Jacobson, T.A.; Maki, K.C.; Orringer, C.E.; Jones, P.H.; Kris-Etherton, P.; Sikand, G.; La Forge, R.; Daniels, S.R.; Wilson, D.P.; Morris, P.B.; et al. National Lipid Association Recommendations for Patient-Centered Management of Dyslipidemia: Part 2. *J. Clin. Lipidol.* **2015**, *9*, S1–S122.e121. [CrossRef]
46. Namazi, N.; Larijani, B.; Surkan, P.J.; Azadbakht, L. The association of neck circumference with risk of metabolic syndrome and its components in adults: A systematic review and meta-analysis. *Nutr. Metab. Cardiovasc. Dis. NMCD* **2018**, *28*, 657–674. [CrossRef]
47. Ferder, L.; Ferder, M.D.; Inserra, F. The role of high-fructose corn syrup in metabolic syndrome and hypertension. *Curr. Hypertens. Rep.* **2010**, *12*, 105–112. [CrossRef] [PubMed]
48. Karupaiah, T.; Chuah, K.A.; Chinna, K.; Matsuoka, R.; Masuda, Y.; Sundram, K.; Sugano, M. Comparing effects of soybean oil- and palm olein-based mayonnaise consumption on the plasma lipid and lipoprotein profiles in human subjects: A double-blind randomized controlled trial with cross-over design. *Lipids Health Dis.* **2016**, *15*, 131. [CrossRef] [PubMed]
49. Shin, D.Y.; Jang, Y.K.; Lee, J.H.; Wee, J.H.; Chun, D.H. Relationship with Smoking and Dyslipidemia in Korean Adults. *J. Korean Soc. Res. Nicotine Tob.* **2017**, *8*, 73–79. [CrossRef]
50. Mouhamed, D.H.; Ezzaher, A.; Neffati, F.; Gaha, L.; Douki, W.; Najjar, M. Association between cigarette smoking and dyslipidemia. *Immuno-analyse Biol. Spécialisée* **2013**, *28*, 195–200. [CrossRef]
51. Tan, X.; Jiao, G.; Ren, Y.; Gao, X.; Ding, Y.; Wang, X.; Xu, H. Relationship between smoking and dyslipidemia in western Chinese elderly males. *J. Clin. Lab. Anal.* **2008**, *22*, 159–163. [CrossRef]
52. Høstmark, A.T.; Tomten, S.E. Cola intake and serum lipids in the Oslo Health Study. *Appl. Physiol. Nutr. Metab.* **2009**, *34*, 901–906. [CrossRef]
53. Dunnigan, M.; Fyfe, T.; McKiddie, M.; Crosbie, S. The effects of isocaloric exchange of dietary starch and sucrose on glucose tolerance, plasma insulin and serum lipids in man. *Clin. Sci.* **1970**, *38*, 1–9. [CrossRef]
54. Crichton, G.E.; Alkerwi, A.a. Physical activity, sedentary behavior time and lipid levels in the Observation of Cardiovascular Risk Factors in Luxembourg study. *Lipids Health Dis.* **2015**, *14*, 87. [CrossRef]
55. Leclerc, S.; Allard, C.; Talbot, J.; Gauvin, R.; Bouchard, C. High density lipoprotein cholesterol, habitual physical activity and physical fitness. *Atherosclerosis* **1985**, *57*, 43–51. [CrossRef]
56. Wang, Y.; Xu, D. Effects of aerobic exercise on lipids and lipoproteins. *Lipids Health Dis.* **2017**, *16*. [CrossRef] [PubMed]
57. Kobayashi, Y.; Hirose, T.; Tada, Y.; Tsutsumi, A.; Kawakami, N. Relationship between Two Job Stress Models and Coronary Risk Factors among Japanese Part-Time Female Employees of a Retail Company. *J. Occup. Health* **2005**, *47*, 201–210. [CrossRef] [PubMed]
58. Maierean, S.M.; Serban, M.-C.; Sahebkar, A.; Ursoniu, S.; Serban, A.; Penson, P.; Banach, M. The effects of cinnamon supplementation on blood lipid concentrations: A systematic review and meta-analysis. *J. Clin. Lipidol.* **2017**, *11*, 1393–1406. [CrossRef] [PubMed]

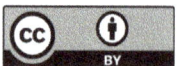

© 2020 by the authors. Licensee MDPI, Basel, Switzerland. This article is an open access article distributed under the terms and conditions of the Creative Commons Attribution (CC BY) license (http://creativecommons.org/licenses/by/4.0/).

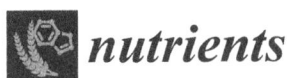

Article

A Randomized, Double-Blinded, Placebo-Controlled, Clinical Study of the Effects of a Nutraceutical Combination (LEVELIP DUO®) on LDL Cholesterol Levels and Lipid Pattern in Subjects with Sub-Optimal Blood Cholesterol Levels (NATCOL Study)

Arrigo F.G. Cicero *, Sergio D'Addato and Claudio Borghi

Medical an Surgery Sciences Department, Dyslipidemia and Atherosclerosis Research Unit, Alma Mater Studiorum University of Bologna, 40138 Bologna, Italy; sergio.daddato@unibo.it (S.D.); claudio.borghi@unibo.it (C.B.)
* Correspondence: arrigo.cicero@unibo.it; Tel.: +39-512142224

Received: 8 September 2020; Accepted: 11 October 2020; Published: 14 October 2020

Abstract: Phytosterols and red yeast rice are largely studied cholesterol-lowering nutraceuticals, respectively inhibiting the bowel absorption and liver synthesis of cholesterol. Our aim was to test the effect of combined nutraceutical-containing phytosterols and red yeast rice vs. a placebo on the lipid profile. We performed a parallel arms, double-blind, placebo-controlled clinical trial, randomizing 88 moderately hypercholesterolemic subjects to treatment with a combined nutraceutical containing phytosterols (800 mg) and red yeast rice, standardized to contain 5 mg of monacolins from *Monascus purpureus*, with added niacin (27 mg) and policosanols (10 mg) (LEVELIP DUO®), or placebo. The mean LDL-Cholesterol (LDL-C) change at Week 8 was -32.5 ± 30.2 mg/dL (-19.8%) in the combined nutraceutical group and 2.5 ± 19.4 mg/dL (2.3%) in the placebo group. The estimated between-group difference of -39.2 mg/dL (95% CI: -48.6; -29.8) indicates a statistically significant difference between treatments in favor of the combined nutraceutical ($p < 0.0001$). Total Cholesterol (TC), non-HDL cholesterol (non-HDL-C), Apolipoprotein B, TC/HDL-C and LDL-C/HDL-C improved in a similar way in the combined nutraceutical group only. No significant changes in other clinical and laboratory parameters were observed. In conclusion, the tested combined nutraceutical was well tolerated, while significantly reducing the plasma levels of LDL-C, TC, non-HDL-C, ApoB, TC/HDL-C and LDL-C/HDL-C ratios in mildly hypercholesterolemic patients. Trial registration (ClinicalTrials.gov): NCT03739242.

Keywords: monacolins; LDL-cholesterol; phytosterols; red yeast rice; nutraceuticals; clinical trial; endothelial function

1. Introduction

Hypercholesterolemia is a largely prevalent cardiovascular disease risk factor in the general population, and its early reduction seems to be an effective preventive strategy [1]. However, pharmacologically treating moderately hypercholesterolemic subjects without other cardiovascular risk factors in the primary prevention for cardiovascular disease is still debated [2]. In fact, the guidelines suggest managing these subjects with a more conservative approach, stressing the need for a therapeutic lifestyle promotion, eventually added with lipid-lowering nutraceuticals and/or functional foods [1,3].

In the last few decades, a relatively large number of nutraceuticals and functional foods has been studied for their ability to decrease cholesterolemia in humans [4]. The most clinically studied include soluble fibers, phytosterols, soy proteins, monacolins from red yeast rice, berberine, and garlic and artichoke extracts [5]. In particular, the most recent guidelines for dyslipidaemia management from the European Atherosclerosis Society and from the European Cardiology Society suggest increasing the amounts of fiber and omega 3 polyunsaturated fatty acids in the diet, while adding phytosterols and monacolins as dietary supplements, when a lifestyle intervention is needed to reduce cholesterolemia [6].

Plant sterols and stanols (phytosterols) are natural constituents of the plant cell membrane [7]. From a chemical point of view, they are very similar to cholesterol, with minor differences in the relative positions of ethyl and methyl groups. Based on this similarity, phytosterols may compete with dietary and biliary cholesterol for micellar solubilization in the intestinal lumen, impairing intestinal cholesterol absorption [8]. Moreover, several clinical trials have consistently shown that an intake of 2–3 g/day of plant sterols is associated with a significant lowering (between 4% and 15%) of low-density lipoprotein-cholesterol (LDL-C) [9,10]. The variability in the observed LDL-reduction is mainly related to genetic factors [11]. Based on the available data, the European Food Safety Agency (EFSA) accepted a health claim for the phytosterols' LDL-C-lowering effect [12].

Red yeast rice is a nutraceutical obtained by the fermentation of rice (*Oryza sativa*) as result of a yeast (in general *Monascus purpureus*), whose typical red coloration is due to the presence of some specific pigments, by-products of the fermentative metabolism process [13]. Monascus yeast produces a family of substances called monacolins, including monacolin K. Monacolins act as reversible inhibitors of the 3-hydroxy-3-methyl-glutaryl-coenzyme A reductase, the key enzyme in cholesterol biosynthesis [14].

A recent meta-analysis of 20 randomized clinical trials, including 6663 subjects, showed that, after 2–24 months of treatment, red yeast rice (RYR) reduced LDL-C on average by 39.4 mg/dL compared to placebo, which was comparable to the reduction achieved with regular-dosed statins (pravastatin 40 mg, simvastatin 10 mg, lovastatin 20 mg) [15]. Based on these data, the EFSA has expressed a scientific opinion supporting the health claims for the relationship between the administration of RYR and the control of plasma LDL-C levels [16]. Even if recently the same EFSA raised some concerns about RYR's safety [17], a recent large metanalysis of 53 randomized clinical trials, including 8535 subjects, has shown that monacolin K administration is not associated with an increased risk of Statin Associated Muscle Symptoms (SAMS) (odds ratio (OR) = 0.94, 95% confidence interval (CI) 0.53, 1.65) for daily doses of monacolin K of between 3 and 10 mg [18].

In this context, the primary objective of the study was to evaluate the effects of LEVELIP DUO® on LDL-C blood levels in subjects with sub-optimal blood cholesterol levels over an 8-week period. The secondary objective was the evaluation of effects of the tested combined nutraceuticals on other lipoproteins and on the estimated cardiovascular risk.

2. Materials and Methods

This parallel-armed, double-blind, randomized clinical trial was carried out in 90 moderately hypercholesterolemic subjects, non-smokers, pharmacologically untreated, in primary prevention for cardiovascular diseases, consecutively enrolled in the ambulatory service of cardiovascular disease prevention in the Medical and Surgical Sciences Department of the University of Bologna.

The inclusion criteria were age between 30 and 75, and LDL-C level between 115 and 190 mg/dL, confirmed in at least two sequential checks prior to signing the consent form.

The exclusion criteria were as follows:

- Personal history of cardiovascular disease or risk equivalents;
- Triglycerides (TG) ≥400 mg/dL;
- Obesity (Body Mass Index > 32 kg/m^2);
- Assumption of lipid-lowering drugs or supplements affecting lipid metabolism;

- Uncontrolled diabetes mellitus;
- Known thyroid, liver, renal or muscle diseases.

The study was fully conducted in accordance with the Declaration of Helsinki, its protocol was approved by the Ethical Committee of the University of Bologna, and informed consent was obtained from all patients before inclusion in the study (Clinical trial.gov ID NCT03739242).

The study design has been detailed in Figure 1.

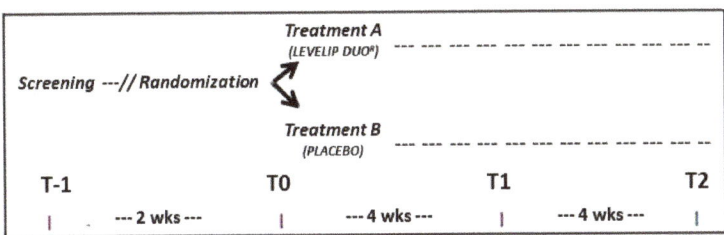

Figure 1. Study design.

At the enrollment visit (T-1, Day-14), patients were given standard behavioral and qualitative (not quantitative) dietary suggestions to correct unhealthy habits. Standard diet advice was given by a dietitian and/or specialist doctor. A dietitian and/or specialist doctor periodically provided instructions on dietary intake recording procedures as part of a behavior modification program, and then later used the subject's food diaries for counseling. In particular, the subjects were instructed to follow the general structure of a Mediterranean diet, avoid excessive intakes of dairy products and red meat-derived products during the study, and maintain overall constant dietary habits [19]. Individuals were also generically encouraged to increase their physical activity by walking briskly for 20 to 30 min, 3 to 5 times per week, or by cycling [20].

After 2 weeks of diet and physical activity (Randomization visit, T0), if the LDL-C and TG values were confirmed, the patients were randomly allocated to a treatment with LEVELIP DUO® or placebo, one tablet after dinner. LEVELIP DUO® is a registered combination of phytosterols (800 mg) and other registered ingredients including red yeast rice standardized to contain 5 mg monacolins from *Monascus purpureusi*, with niacin (27 mg) and policosanols (10 mg) (Dif1/Stat®) [21,22]. The red yeast rice extract used was certified to be highly purified in monacolins, without chromatographically detectable levels of dehydromonacolins, decalin derivatives and contaminants. The phytosterol dose was chosen based on the minimal efficacious dose identified by the meta-analysis of randomized clinical trials, performed by Demonty et al. [23].

The active products and placebo were administered as indistinguishable tablets (kindly provided by Menarini IFR, Firenze, Italy). The treatment then continued for 8 weeks. Clinical and laboratory data have been obtained at the baseline (T0), after 4 weeks (T1) and at the end of the trial (8 weeks, T2).

A computer-generated randomization list produced by the trial statistician randomized patients to one of the two treatment groups (LEVELIP DUO® or placebo) in a 1:1 ratio. A paper-based randomization procedure assigned a randomization number to the patient, which has been used to link the patient to a treatment arm and specified a unique kit number for the package of treatment to be dispensed to the patient. The randomization numbers were generated using a procedure to ensure that treatment assignment is unbiased.

Throughout the study, we instructed patients to take the first dose on the day after they were given the study product in a blinded box. At the end of the study, all unused products were retrieved for inventory. Product compliance was assessed by counting the number of product doses returned at the times of specified clinic visits.

At each visit, enrolled patients were interviewed about eventual changes in lifestyle and possible adverse events raised in the previous weeks. Then, anthropometric measurement and vital signs were recorded, and a plasma sample was obtained after a 12-h overnight fast. Venous blood samples were drawn by a nurse from all patients between 8:00 a.m. and 9:00 a.m. The serum used was centrifuged at 3000 g for 15 min at ambient temperature. Immediately after centrifugation, the samples were frozen and stored at −80 °C for no more than 3 months. The following parameters were evaluated via standardized methods [24,25]: total cholesterol (TC), HDL-C, TG, apolipoprotein B100 (apoB), glucose, creatinine, serum uric acid, liver transaminases, gamma-glutamyl transferase, and creatinine phosphokinase (CPK). All measurements were performed by trained personnel in the Lipid Clinic laboratory of the Medicine and Surgery Sciences Department, by the S. Orsola-Malpighi University Hospital. Since hypertriglyceridemia was an exclusion criterion, the LDL-C level was estimated by the application of the Friedewald's formula (LDL-C = TC − HDL-C − TG/5).

As post-hoc analysis, the cardiovascular disease risk was estimated with a validated nation-specific algorithm (Progetto CUORE) [26].

Considering the primary endpoint of the study as the reduction from baseline to week 8 in LDL cholesterol level, and the data available from literature [27], a reduction in LDL level of approximately 10% is expected after the intake of the nutraceutical. Therefore, assuming a baseline LDL level of 145 ± 19 mg/dL, a power of 90% and a 5% two-sided alpha level to detect a difference in mean change in LDL from baseline to week 8 equal to 15 mg/dL between the nutraceutical and the placebo group, the total number of patients to be evaluated should be 35 per treatment arm in a 1:1 ratio (NQuery Advisor, 7.0). Allowing for an approximate 20% dropout rate, at least 88 patients should be randomized—44 patients in each treatment group.

Statistical tables, figures, listings and analyses were produced using SAS® for Windows release 9.4 (64-bit) or later (SAS Institute Inc., Cary, NC, USA). For each secondary efficacy variable, an ANCOVA model was used to estimate the treatment's effect on the changes from baseline at week 8, considering the planned treatment group as the factor and the baseline value of the parameter as the continuous covariate. The results are reported as Least Squares Means together with associated two-tailed 95% CI. The difference in Least Squares Means between the nutraceutical combination group and placebo group was estimated with two-tailed 95% CI and p value. If the assumption of the normality of the residuals was violated, the ANCOVA model was fitted to rank transformed data. A p value less than 0.05 was considered significant for all tests.

3. Results

Enrolled patients were age- and sex-matched. We enrolled 38 men (19 randomized to the combined nutraceutical, 19 to placebo) and 47 women (24 randomized to the combined nutraceutical, 23 to placebo). The baseline characteristics of patients assigned to the different treatments (active and placebo) were similar, and no significant differences were observed regarding the studied parameters (Table 1). Patient disposition is outlined in Figure 2.

Table 1. Baseline characteristics of the enrolled subjects: non-statistically significant difference has been detected between the treatment groups (values reported as mean ± standard deviation; No significant difference between groups has been observed).

	Active Treatment	Placebo
Age (years)	51.3 ± 9.6	51.8 ± 10.7
Height (m)	1.69 ± 0.09	1.69 ± 0.10
Weight (kg)	70.3 ± 12.0	71.2 ± 14.8
Body Mass Index (kg/m^2)	24.5 ± 3.2	24.7 ± 3.1
Waist circumference (cm)	89.5 ± 10.6	91.6 ± 11.1
Systolic Blood Pressure (mmHg)	124 ± 16	124 ± 15
Diastolic Blood Pressure (mmHg)	77 ± 10	78 ± 9
Heart Rate (bpm)	70 ± 10	70 ± 9
Total cholesterol (mg/dL)	229.1 ± 27.9	232.6 ± 21.6
LDL cholesterol (mg/dL)	155.1 ± 19.9	161.5 ± 21.3
HDL cholesterol (mg/dL)	51.0 ± 13.5	49.0 ± 11.3
Non-HDL cholesterol (mg/dL)	178.1 ± 25.5	183.6 ± 22.2
Triglycerides (mg/dL)	114.9 ± 46.2	110.4 ± 46.3
Apolipoprotein B (mg/dL)	106.9 ± 13.6	110.8 ± 15.8
TC/HDL-Cholesterol	4.76 ± 1.22	4.98 ± 1.19
LDL-C/HDL-Cholesterol	3.25 ± 0.99	3.48 ± 0.93
Fasting Glucose (mg/dL)	89.1 ± 11.6	88.8 ± 11.4
Alanine aminotransferase (U/L)	22.5 ± 8.6	23.4 ± 10.3
Aspartate aminotransferase (U/L)	20.9 ± 5.6	21.7 ± 4.0
Gamma-glutamyl transferase (U/L)	22.1 ± 13.6	21.2 ± 13.1
Serum uric acid (mg/dL)	4.4 ± 1.3	4.2 ± 0.9
Serum creatinine (mg/dL)	0.94 ± 0.13	0.96 ± 0.16
Estimated GFR (ml/min/1.73 m^2)	77.3 ± 8.3	76.1 ± 11.9
Creatine phosphokinase (U/L)	110 ± 65	131 ± 77

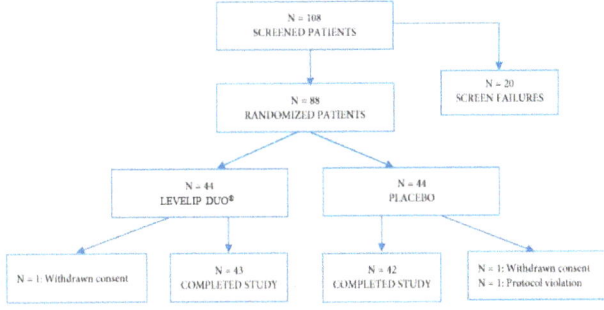

Figure 2. Patient disposition.

Overal, 85 subjects (94.4%), 43 in the active treatment group and 42 in the placebo group, were compliant (compliance levels between 80% and 120%). One patient (2.33%) in the active treatment group had compliance lower than 80%, whereas 1 patient (2.33%) in the placebo group had compliance greater than 120%.

Dietary habits remained overall unchanged during the study.

The primary variable of the study was the change from baseline at week 8 in LDL cholesterol (Figure 3).

The LDL-C levels decreased from visit to visit in the combined nutraceutical group, and, on the contrary, increased in the placebo group. The mean change at week 8 was −32.5 ± 30.2 mg/dL (−19.8%) in the combined nutraceutical group and 2.5 ± 19.4 mg/dL (2.3%) in the placebo group. The ANCOVA model results for the estimated change from baseline at week 8 in LDL-C levels, adjusting for the baseline value of LDL-C, provided Least Squares Means equal to −34.5 mg/dL (95% CI: −41.1; −27.9) for the combined nutraceutical group and 4.6 mg/dL (95% CI: −2.0; 11.3) for the placebo group. The estimated between-group difference of −39.2 mg/dL (95% CI: −48.6; −29.8) indicates a statistically significant difference between treatments in favor of the combined nutraceutical ($p < 0.0001$).

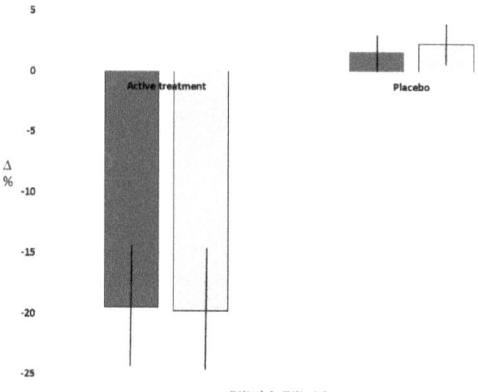

Figure 3. Plasma LDL-Cholesterol level percentage change from the baseline to 4 and 8 weeks in subjects treated with the tested combined nutraceutical or placebo.

The Least Squares Means of TC changes from baseline at week 8, adjusting for baseline value, were −33.0 mg/dL (95% CI: −40.4; −25.7) for the combined nutraceutical group and 8.2 mg/dL (95% CI: 0.8; 15.7) for the placebo group. The estimated between-group difference of −41.2 mg/dL (95% CI: −51.7; −30.7) and a $p < 0.0001$ suggest a statistically significant difference between treatments in favor of the combined nutraceutical.

The Least Squares Means of non-HDL cholesterol change from baseline at week 8, estimated adjusting for baseline value, were equal to −34.2 mg/dL (95% CI: −41.1; −27.3) in the combined nutraceutical group and 7.5 mg/dL (95% CI: 0.5; 14.5) in the placebo group. The between-group difference of −41.7 mg/dL (95% CI: −51.6; −31.8) was significantly in favor of treatment with the combined nutraceutical ($p < 0.0001$).

The Least Squares Means of Apo B change at week 8, adjusting for baseline value, were −15.2 mg/dL (95% CI: −19.6; −10.8) for the combined nutraceutical group and 2.0 mg/dL (95% CI: −2.4; 6.5) for placebo. The between-group difference of −17.3 mg/dL (95% CI: −23.5; −11.0) indicates a statistically significant difference between treatments in favor of the combined nutraceutical ($p < 0.0001$).

The Least Squares Means of the TC/HDL-C ratio change from baseline at week 8, adjusting for baseline value, were −0.8 (95% CI: −1.0; −0.6) for the combined nutraceutical group and 0.1 (95% CI: −0.1; 0.3) for placebo. The estimated between-group difference was −0.9 (95% CI: −1.2; −0.6), and a $p < 0.0001$ indicates a significantly greater change in the TC/HDL ratio in subjects treated with the combined nutraceutical.

The Least Squares Means of the LDL-C/HDL-C ratio change from baseline at week 8, adjusting for baseline value, were −0.8 (95% CI: −0.9; −0.6) for the combined nutraceutical group and 0.02 (95% CI: −0.1; 0.2) for the placebo group. The between-group difference of −0.8 (95% CI: −1.1; −0.6) was statistically significant ($p < 0.0001$).

Body weight, BMI, waist circumference, blood pressure, FPG, HDL-C, TG, GOT, GPT, gGT, SUA, eGFR and CPK did not significantly change in both groups during the study (Table 2).

During the study, no treatment-emergent adverse event was reported. The trends of hematology and clinical chemistry values did not indicate any safety concerns.

Table 2. Laboratory parameter changes during the study (values reported as mean ± standard deviation).

Variable	Active Treatment			Placebo		
	Baseline (T0)	Day 28 (T1)	Day 56 (T2)	Baseline (T0)	Day 28 (T1)	Day 56 (T2)
TC (mg/dL)	229.1 ± 27.9	196.7 ± 24.1 *°	197.1 ± 28.3 *°	232.6 ± 21.6	237.5 ± 23.6	239.8 ± 23.6
LDL-C (mg/dL)	155.1 ± 19.9	124.0 ± 22.3 *°	122.6 ± 24.7 *°	161.5 ± 21.3	163.3 ± 22.3	164.0 ± 20.4
HDL-C (mg/dL)	51.0 ± 13.5	52.0 ± 13.1	51.8 ± 12.1	49.0 ± 11.3	50.3 ± 13.9	50.1 ± 11.9
Non-HDL-C (mg/dL)	178.1 ± 25.5	144.7 ± 23.6 *°	145.3 ± 26.5 *°	183.6 ± 22.2	187.2 ± 24.3	189.6 ± 24.0
Triglycerides (mg/dL)	114.9 ± 46.2	103.7 ± 53.9	113.5 ± 46.8	110.4 ± 46.3	119.5 ± 71.9	127.9 ± 79.6
Apo B (mg/dL)	106.9 ± 13.6	88.5 ± 14.6 *°	92.1 ± 17.0 *°	110.8 ± 15.8	111.8 ± 15.9	112.4 ± 19.6
TC/HDL-C	4.76 ± 1.22	4.01 ± 1.07 *°	3.97 ± 0.92 *°	4.98 ± 1.19	5.02 ± 1.34	5.05 ± 1.28
LDL-C/HDL-C	3.25 ± 0.99	2.54 ± 0.81 *°	2.49 ± 0.74 *°	3.48 ± 0.93	3.47 ± 1.05	3.46 ± 0.95
FPG (mg/dL)	89.1 ± 11.6	88.5 ± 12.7	88.2 ± 12.5	88.8 ± 11.4	88.7 ± 12.2	87.2 ± 12.2
ALT (U/L)	22.5 ± 8.6	26.3 ± 12.6	27.1 ± 13.8	23.4 ± 10.3	27.2 ± 17.1	26.3 ± 14.6
AST (U/L)	20.9 ± 5.6	23.6 ± 7.6	21.8 ± 5.6	21.7 ± 4.0	21.7 ± 5.5	22.6 ± 4.8
γ-GT (U/L)	22.1 ± 13.6	22.9 ± 16.4	23.2 ± 17.5	21.2 ± 13.1	24.4 ± 25.8	24.3 ± 21.2
SUA (mg/dL)	4.4 ± 1.3	4.1 ± 0.9	4.1 ± 1.0	4.2 ± 0.9	4.2 ± 0.9	4.2 ± 0.9
Serum creatinine (mg/dL)	0.94 ± 0.13	0.95 ± 0.13	0.94 ± 0.11	0.96 ± 0.16	0.99 ± 0.14	0.96 ± 0.15
sGFR (mL/min/1.73 m^2)	77.3 ± 8.3	77.2 ± 7.9	77.4 ± 7.8	76.1 ± 11.9	77.2 ± 10.9	76.9 ± 9.3
CPK (U/L)	110 ± 65	125 ± 85	112 ± 61	131 ± 77	124 ± 76	124 ± 61

* $p < 0.01$ vs. baseline; ° $p < 0.01$ vs. control. TC = Total Cholesterol, ApoB = Apolipoprotein B, FPG = Fasting Plasma Glucose, ALT = Alanine Aminotranferase, AST = Aspartate Aminotranferase, gGT = γ-glutamyl transferase, SUA = Serum Uric Acid, eGFR = estimated glomerular filtration rate, CPK = creatine phosphokinase.

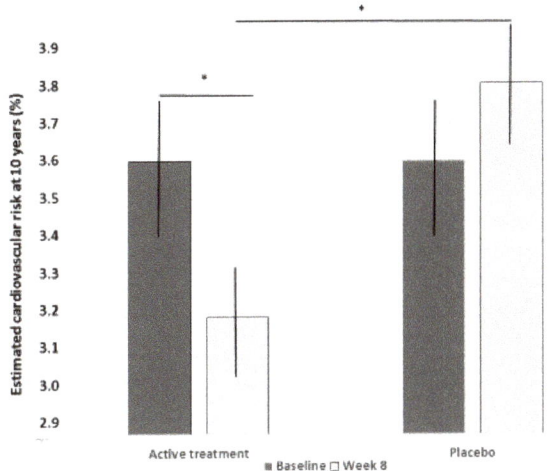

Figure 4. Change in estimated 10-year cardiovascular disease risk in the two treatment groups (post-hoc analysis; * $p < 0.05$).

4. Discussion

The Mediterranean diet remains a milestone in cardiovascular disease prevention, [28] even if its impact on LDL-cholesterolemia is limited. For this reason, the ESC/EAS guidelines [6] and the International Lipid Expert Panel (ILEP) [5] consider the use of some dietary supplements (namely, red yeast rice and phytosterols) as a support to a balanced diet in order to improve cholesterolemia control. Many trials evaluating the effect of nutraceuticals on lipid pattern are not adequately designed, being often not double-blinded and underpowered.

In our double-blind, placebo-controlled, randomized clinical trial, we observed that the LEVELIP DUO® was able in the short-term to significantly reduce the plasma levels of LDL-C, TC, non-HDL-C, and apoB, and the TC/HDL-C and LDL-C/HDL-C ratios. In particular, the estimated between-group difference in LDL-C was −39.2 mg/dL (95% CI: −48.6; −29.8). This effect was observed after 4 weeks of treatment and confirmed after 8 weeks, excluding short-term adaptation phenomena. This is compatible with the mechanism of action of the nutraceutical components of the tested product. The LDL-C reduction that was achieved is near to that 39.8 mg/dL, which is estimated to be associated in long-term trials with a corresponding 22% reduction in cardiovascular mortality and morbidity [29]. This is also in line with our observation that the estimated cardiovascular risk was significantly modified by the tested treatment, but not by the placebo. This impressive result was partly expected. In fact, it confirms what we already observed in a previous smaller pilot study, where the association of phytosterols and red yeast rice was able to increase red yeast rice's LDL-C-lowering efficacy [30]. On the other side, because the mechanisms of action of red yeast rice and phytosterols should be additive or synergistic, they represent the natural alternative to the synergistic association of statins with ezetimibe [27].

In this context, the tested combined nutraceutical was shown to be effective and well-tolerated. In 2017, the ILEP [5] classified the association of phytosterols and red yeast rice as recommendation IIa (should be considered), based on a level of evidence classified as B (Data derived from single randomized clinical trial or large non-randomized studies). Considering the results of our current trial and of our previous one [31], combined with the ESC/EAS suggestion, the class of recommendation could probably improve.

We can argue that the greater part of the observed effect of LEVELIP DUO® is be related to the contents of phytosterols and red yeast rice. However, the minor components of the products could have also minimally contributed to the final effect. In particular, EFSA approves the health claim of niacin supporting energy metabolism and macronutrient metabolism [32]. Policosanols seem to have a small impact on hypercholesterolemia, however their efficacy when consumed with red yeast rice has been observed in a large number of trials [5].

Our study has some relevant limitations. The first one is the relatively low number of subjects investigated per treatment group, while, however, the study was sufficiently powered to detect differences between treatment groups. Of course, we could have used a cross-over design, but we feared losing the volunteers' compliance to the treatment if the study duration was excessive. The second one is the lack of the measurement of markers of cholesterol absorption and synthesis, as cholesterol hyperabsorbers could have manifested a more significant LDL-C reduction than standard cholesterol absorbers [31]. Finally, the study was relatively short, so that we do not know if the observed effect could be confirmed in the long term. However, since the monacolins' and phytosterols' mechanisms of action are the same as those of statins and ezetimibe, drugs that have largely proven to maintain their efficacy over decades, we could reasonably assume that this evidence could be translated to the tested combined nutraceutical. Moreover, the study was adequately powered, so that we can be confident in the reported results.

5. Conclusions

LEVELIP DUO® was well-tolerated while significantly reducing the plasma levels of LDL-C, TC, non-HDL-C, ApoB, TC/HDL-C and LDL/HDL-C ratios in mildly hypercholesterolemic patients. Further long-term studies are needed to confirm the maintenance of this impressive effect over time.

Author Contributions: Conceptualization, A.F.G.C. and C.B.; methodology, A.F.G.C. and S.D.; investigation, A.F.G.C. and S.D.; writing—original draft preparation, A.F.G.C.; writing—review and editing, S.D. and C.B.; supervision, C.B.; project administration, C.B. All authors have read and agreed to the published version of the manuscript.

Funding: This research was funded by Menarini IFR, Firenze, Italy.

Conflicts of Interest: The authors declare no conflict of interest.

References

1. Bittner, V.A. The New 2019 ACC/AHA Guideline on the Primary Prevention of Cardiovascular Disease. *Circulation* **2019**. [CrossRef] [PubMed]
2. Michos, E.D.; McEvoy, J.W.; Blumenthal, R.S. Lipid Management for the Prevention of Atherosclerotic Cardiovascular Disease. *N. Engl. J. Med.* **2019**, *381*, 1557–1567. [CrossRef] [PubMed]

3. Ferraro, R.A.; Fischer, N.M.; Xun, H.; Michos, E.D. Nutrition and physical activity recommendations from the United States and European cardiovascular guidelines: A comparative review. *Curr. Opin. Cardiol.* **2020**, *35*, 508–516. [CrossRef] [PubMed]
4. Cicero, A.F.; Fogacci, F.; Colletti, A. Food and plant bioactives for reducing cardiometabolic disease risk: An evidence based approach. *Food Funct.* **2017**, *8*, 2076–2088. [CrossRef]
5. Cicero, A.F.; Colletti, A.; Bajraktari, G.; Descamps, O.; Djuric, D.M.; Ezhov, M.; Fras, Z.; Katsiki, N.; Langlois, M.; Latkovskis, G.; et al. Lipid-lowering nutraceuticals in clinical practice: Position paper from an International Lipid Expert Panel. *Nutr. Rev.* **2017**, *75*, 731–767. [CrossRef]
6. Authors/Task Force Members; ESC Committee for Practice Guidelines (CPG); ESC National Cardiac Societies. 2019 ESC/EAS guidelines for the management of dyslipidaemias: Lipid modification to reduce cardiovascular risk. *Atherosclerosis* **2019**, *290*, 140–205. [CrossRef]
7. Goldstein, M.R. Effects of dietary phytosterols on cholesterol metabolism and atherosclerosis. *Am. J. Med.* **2000**, *109*, 72–73. [CrossRef]
8. Cedó, L.; Farràs, M.; Lee-Rueckert, M.; Escolà-Gil, J.C. Molecular Insights into the Mechanisms Underlying the Cholesterol-Lowering Effects of Phytosterols. *Curr. Med. Chem.* **2019**, *26*, 6704–6723. [CrossRef]
9. Ras, R.T.; Geleijnse, J.M.; Trautwein, E.A. LDL-cholesterol-lowering effect of plant sterols and stanols across different dose ranges: A meta-analysis of randomised controlled studies. *Br. J. Nutr.* **2014**, *112*, 214–219. [CrossRef]
10. Han, S.; Jiao, J.; Xu, J.; Zimmermann, D.; Actis-Goretta, L.; Guan, L.; Zhao, Y.; Qin, L. Effects of plant stanol or sterol-enriched diets on lipid profiles in patients treated with statins: Systematic review and meta-analysis. *Sci. Rep.* **2016**, *6*, 31337. [CrossRef]
11. Fumeron, F.; Bard, J.M.; Lecerf, J.M. Interindividual variability in the cholesterol-lowering effect of supplementation with plant sterols or stanols. *Nutr. Rev.* **2017**, *75*, 134–145. [CrossRef] [PubMed]
12. EFSA Panel on Dietetic Products, Nutrition and Allergies (NDA). Scientific Opinion on the modification of the authorisation of a health claim related to plant sterol esters and lowering blood LDL-cholesterol; high blood LDL-cholesterol is a risk factor in the development of (coronary) heart disease pursuant to Article 14 of Regulation (EC) No 1924/2006, following a request in accordance with Article 19 of Regulation (EC) No 1924/2006. *EFSA J.* **2014**, *12*, 3577.
13. Cicero, A.F.; Fogacci, F.; Banach, M. Red Yeast Rice for Hypercholesterolemia. *Methodist Debakey Cardiovasc. J.* **2019**, *15*, 192–199. [PubMed]
14. Ma, J.; Li, Y.; Ye, Q.; Li, J.; Hua, Y.; Ju, D.; Zhang, D.; Cooper, R.; Chang, M. Constituents of red yeast rice, a traditional Chinese food and medicine. *J. Agric. Food Chem.* **2000**, *48*, 5220–5225. [CrossRef]
15. Gerards, M.C.; Terlou, R.J.; Yu, H.; Koks, C.H.; Gerdes, V.E. Traditional Chinese lipid-lowering agent red yeast rice results in significant LDL reduction but safety is uncertain—A systematic review and meta-analysis. *Atherosclerosis* **2015**, *240*, 415–423. [CrossRef]
16. EFSA. Scientific Opinion on the substantiation of health claims related to monacolin K from red yeast rice and maintenance of normal blood LDL-cholesterol concentrations (ID 1648, 1700) pursuant to Article 13 of Regulation (EC) No 1924/20061; EFSA Panel on Dietetic Products, Nutrition and Allergies (NDA), European Food Safety Authority (EFSA), Parma, Italy. *EFSA J.* **2011**, *9*, 2304.
17. EFSA. Scientific opinion on the safety of monacolins in red yeast rice. EFSA Panel on Food Additives and Nutrient Sources added to Food (ANS). European Food Safety Authority (EFSA), Parma, Italy. *EFSA J.* **2018**, *16*, 5368.
18. Fogacci, F.; Banach, M.; Mikhailidis, D.P.; Bruckert, E.; Toth, P.P.; Watts, G.F.; Reiner, Ž.; Mancini, J.; Rizzo, M.; Mitchenko, O.; et al. Safety of red yeast rice supplementation: A systematic review and meta-analysis of randomized controlled trials. *Pharmacol. Res.* **2019**, *143*, 1–16. [CrossRef]
19. Cicero, A.F.; Fogacci, F.; Bove, M.; Giovannini, M.; Borghi, C. Three-arm, placebo-controlled, randomized clinical trial evaluating the metabolic effect of a combined nutraceutical containing a bergamot standardized flavonoid extract in dyslipidemic overweight subjects. *Phytother. Res.* **2019**, *33*, 2094–2101. [CrossRef]
20. Nasi, M.; Patrizi, G.; Pizzi, C.; Landolfo, M.; Boriani, G.; Dei Cas, A.; Cicero, A.F.; Fogacci, F.; Rapezzi, C.; Sisca, G.; et al. The role of physical activity in individuals with cardiovascular risk factors: An opinion paper from Italian Society of Cardiology-Emilia Romagna-Marche and SIC-Sport. *J. Cardiovasc. Med.* **2019**, *20*, 631–639. [CrossRef]

21. Cicero, A.F.; Derosa, G.; Pisciotta, L.; Barbagallo, C.; SISA-PUFACOL Study Group. Testing the Short-Term Efficacy of a Lipid-Lowering Nutraceutical in the Setting of Clinical Practice: A Multicenter Study. *J. Med. Food* **2015**, *18*, 1270–1273. [CrossRef] [PubMed]
22. Cicero, A.F.; Brancaleoni, M.; Laghi, L.; Donati, F.; Mino, M. Antihyperlipidaemic effect of a Monascus purpureus brand dietary supplement on a large sample of subjects at low risk for cardiovascular disease: A pilot study. *Complement. Ther. Med.* **2005**, *13*, 273–278. [CrossRef]
23. Demonty, I.; Ras, R.T.; van der Knaap, H.C.; Meijer, L.; Zock, P.L.; Geleijnse, J.M.; Trautwein, E.A. The effect of plant sterols on serum triglyceride concentrations is dependent on baseline concentrations: A pooled analysis of 12 randomised controlled trials. *Eur. J. Nutr.* **2013**, *52*, 153–160. [CrossRef] [PubMed]
24. Cicero, A.F.; Fogacci, F.; Bove, M.; Veronesi, M.; Rizzo, M.; Giovannini, M.; Borghi, C. Short-Term Effects of a Combined Nutraceutical on Lipid Level, Fatty Liver Biomarkers, Hemodynamic Parameters, and Estimated Cardiovascular Disease Risk: A Double-Blind, Placebo-Controlled Randomized Clinical Trial. *Adv. Ther.* **2017**, *34*, 1966–1975. [CrossRef] [PubMed]
25. Cicero, A.F.; Fogacci, F.; Morbini, M.; Colletti, A.; Bove, M.; Veronesi, M.; Giovannini, M.; Borghi, C. Nutraceutical Effects on Glucose and Lipid Metabolism in Patients with Impaired Fasting Glucose: A Pilot, Double-Blind, Placebo-Controlled, Randomized Clinical Trial on a Combined Product. *High. Blood Press Cardiovasc. Prev.* **2017**, *24*, 283–288. [CrossRef] [PubMed]
26. Palmieri, L.; Donfrancesco, C.; Giampaoli, S.; Trojani, M.; Panico, S.; Vanuzzo, D.; Pilotto, L.; Cesana, G.; Ferrario, M.; Chiodini, P.; et al. Favorable cardiovascular risk profile and 10-year coronary heart disease incidence in women and men: Results from the Progetto CUORE. *Eur. J. Cardiovasc. Prev. Rehabil.* **2006**, *13*, 562–570. [CrossRef]
27. Cicero, A.F.; Colletti, A. Combinations of phytomedicines with different lipid lowering activity for dyslipidemia management: The available clinical data. *Phytomedicine* **2016**, *23*, 1113–1118. [CrossRef]
28. Rosato, V.; Temple, N.J.; La Vecchia, C.; Castellan, G.; Tavani, A.; Guercio, V. Mediterranean diet and cardiovascular disease: A systematic review and meta-analysis of observational studies. *Eur. J. Nutr.* **2019**, *58*, 173–191. [CrossRef]
29. Cholesterol Treatment Trialists' (CTT) Collaboration. Efficacy and safety of more intensive lowering of LDL cholesterol: A meta-analysis of data from 170000 participants in 26 randomised trials. *Lancet* **2010**, *376*, 1670–1681. [CrossRef]
30. Cicero, A.F.; Fogacci, F.; Rosticci, M.; Parini, A.; Giovannini, M.; Veronesi, M.; D'Addato, S.; Borghi, C. Effect of a short-term dietary supplementation with phytosterols, red yeast rice or both on lipid pattern in moderately hypercholesterolemic subjects: A three-arm, double-blind, randomized clinical trial. *Nutr. Metab.* **2017**, *14*, 61. [CrossRef]
31. Baila-Rueda, L.; Pérez-Ruiz, M.R.; Jarauta, E.; Tejedor, M.T.; Mateo-Gallego, R.; Lamiquiz-Moneo, I.; de Castro-Orós, I.; Cenarro, A.; Civeira, F. Cosegregation of serum cholesterol with cholesterol intestinal absorption markers in families with primary hypercholesterolemia without mutations in LDLR, APOB, PCSK9 and APOE genes. *Atherosclerosis* **2016**, *246*, 202–207. [CrossRef] [PubMed]
32. EFSA Panel on Dietetic Products, Nutrition and Allergies (NDA). Scientific Opinion on the substantiation of health claims related to niacin and energy-yielding metabolism (ID 43, 49, 54), function of the nervous system (ID 44, 53), maintenance of the skin and mucous membranes (ID 45, 48, 50, 52), maintenance of normal LDL-cholesterol, HDL-cholesterol and triglyceride concentrations (ID 46), maintenance of bone (ID 50), maintenance of teeth (ID 50), maintenance of hair (ID 50, 2875) and maintenance of nails (ID 50, 2875) pursuant to Article 13 of Regulation (EC) No 1924/2006 on request from European Commission. *EFSA J.* **2009**, *7*, 1224. [CrossRef]

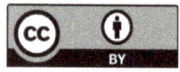

© 2020 by the authors. Licensee MDPI, Basel, Switzerland. This article is an open access article distributed under the terms and conditions of the Creative Commons Attribution (CC BY) license (http://creativecommons.org/licenses/by/4.0/).

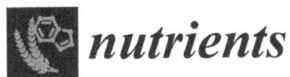

Article

Efficacy and Safety of Armolipid Plus®: An Updated PRISMA Compliant Systematic Review and Meta-Analysis of Randomized Controlled Clinical Trials

Arrigo F. G. Cicero [1,2,3,*], Cormac Kennedy [4], Tamara Knežević [5], Marilisa Bove [1,2], Coralie M. G. Georges [6], Agnė Šatrauskienė [7,8], Peter P. Toth [9,10] and Federica Fogacci [1,2,3]

1. Hypertension and Atherosclerosis Research Group, Medical and Surgical Sciences Department, Sant'Orsola-Malpighi University Hospital, 40138 Bologna, Italy; marilisa.bove@aosp.bo.it (M.B.); federica.fogacci@studio.unibo.it (F.F.)
2. IRCCS Azienda Ospedaliero-Universitaria di Bologna, 40138 Bologna, Italy
3. Italian Nutraceutical Society (SINut), 40138 Bologna, Italy
4. Department of Pharmacology and Therapeutics, Trinity College Dublin and St James Hospital, Dublin 8, Ireland; kennec30@tcd.ie
5. Department of Nephrology, Hypertension, Dialysis and Transplantation, University Hospital Centre Zagreb, 10000 Zagreb, Croatia; tknezev2@kbc-zagreb.hr
6. Department of Cardiology, Cliniques Universitaires Saint-Luc, Université Catholique de Louvain, 1200 Brussels, Belgium; coralie.georges@uclouvain.be
7. Faculty of Medicine, Vilnius University, LT-03101 Vilnius, Lithuania; agne.satrauskiene@santa.it
8. Vilnius University Hospital Santariškiu Klinikos, LT-08661 Vilnius, Lithuania
9. CGH Medical Center, Sterling, IL 61081, USA; peter.toth@cghmc.com
10. Cicarrone Center for the Prevention of Cardiovascular Disease, Johns Hopkins University School of Medicine, Baltimore, MD 21287, USA
* Correspondence: arrigo.cicero@unibo.it; Tel.: +39-512142224; Fax: +39-51390646

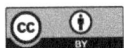

Abstract: Armolipid Plus® is a multi-constituent nutraceutical that claims to improve lipid profiles. The aim of this PRISMA compliant systematic review and meta-analysis was to globally evaluate the efficacy and safety of Armolipid Plus® on the basis of the available randomized, blinded, controlled clinical trials (RCTs). A systematic literature search in several databases was conducted in order to identify RCTs assessing the efficacy and safety of dietary supplementation with Armolipid Plus®. Two review authors independently identified 12 eligible studies (1050 included subjects overall) and extracted data on study characteristics, methods, and outcomes. Meta-analysis of the data suggested that dietary supplementation with Armolipid Plus® exerted a significant effect on body mass index (mean difference (MD) = -0.25 kg/m^2, $p = 0.008$) and serum levels of total cholesterol (MD = -25.07 mg/dL, $p < 0.001$), triglycerides (MD = -11.47 mg/dL, $p < 0.001$), high-density lipoprotein cholesterol (MD = 1.84 mg/dL, $p < 0.001$), low-density lipoprotein cholesterol (MD = -26.67 mg/dL, $p < 0.001$), high sensitivity C reactive protein (hs-CRP, MD = -0.61 mg/L, $p = 0.022$), and fasting glucose (MD = -3.52 mg/dL, $p < 0.001$). Armolipid Plus® was well tolerated. This meta-analysis demonstrates that dietary supplementation with Armolipid Plus® is associated with clinically meaningful improvements in serum lipids, glucose, and hs-CRP. These changes are consistent with improved cardiometabolic health.

Keywords: Armolipid Plus®; red yeast rice; berberine; nutraceutical; supplementation; lipids; blood pressure; fasting plasma glucose

1. Introduction

Atherosclerosis cardiovascular diseases (ASCVD) are the leading cause of mortality worldwide, and the main cause of death in persons under 75 years old in Western countries, with a huge social and economic impact [1]. Pooling data from 204 countries, the Global Burden of Disease (GBD) Study recently showed that prevalent cases of total CVD nearly doubled from 271 million in 1990 to 523 million in 2019, and the number of CVD deaths steadily increased from 12.1 million in 1990, reaching 18.6 million in 2019 [2].

High serum levels of low-density lipoprotein cholesterol (LDL-C) are the most important risk factor for the development of ASCVD [3]. The American Heart Association (AHA) 2016 update on heart disease and stroke statistics verified that only 75.7% of US children and 46.6% of US adults have total cholesterol (TC) within the advised ranges (< 170 mg/dL for untreated children and < 200 mg/dL for untreated adults), with comparable rates for other Western countries [4,5].

To reach the LDL-C target, the international guidelines recommend lifestyle changes and lipid-lowering therapy depending on the severity of dyslipidemia and global CV risk [6,7]. Specific lifestyle interventions for hypercholesterolemia include a diet low in saturated fat, moderate to high-intensity physical activity, smoking cessation, as well as weight loss for overweight and obese patients [8,9]. If maintained over the long term, these lifestyle modifications can reduce LDL-C by 5% to 15% and improve ASCVD risk [10]. However, patients unable to reach their target LDL-C goals through lifestyle interventions can consider using lipid-lowering nutraceuticals [11], as also suggested by the International Lipid Expert Panel [12].

Nutraceuticals with a detectable lipid-lowering effect can be divided into natural inhibitors of hepatic cholesterol synthesis, inhibitors of intestinal cholesterol absorption, and enhancers of the excretion of LDL-C on the basis of their mechanisms of action [12]. However, the lipid-lowering effect of most nutraceuticals occurs through multiple mechanisms. The possibility that they act synergistically on multiple stages of lipid-induced vascular damage makes them potential candidates for improving the lipid-lowering effects when used in combination with diet, medications, or other nutraceuticals [13].

Armolipid Plus® is a widely tested and used proprietary formulation of six naturally occurring substances containing red yeast extract (200 mg, corresponding to 3 mg of monacolin K), policosanols (10 mg), and berberine (500 mg), in addition to folic acid (0.2 mg), astaxanthin (0.5 mg), and coenzyme Q10 (2 mg), with a detectable effect on serum lipids, blood pressure (BP), fasting plasma glucose (FPG), and several markers of insulin resistance with a good safety profile [14].

Given the increasing number of good quality studies on this nutraceutical combination, the aim of our systematic review and meta-analysis was to evaluate the efficacy and safety of Armolipid Plus® on the basis of the available randomized, blinded, controlled clinical trials.

2. Materials and Methods

The study was designed according to guidelines in the 2009 preferred reporting items for systematic reviews and meta-analysis (PRISMA) statement [15], and was registered in the PROSPERO database (Registration number CRD42020212600). Due to the study design (meta-analysis), neither institutional review board (IRB) approval nor patient informed consent were required.

2.1. Search Strategy

PubMed, EMBASE, SCOPUS, Google Scholar, Web of Science by Clarivate, and ClinicaTrial.gov (accessed on 1 February 2021) databases were searched, with no language restriction, using the following search terms: "Armolipid Plus®" AND ("Cholesterol" OR "LDL" OR "Triglycerides" OR "Body mass index" OR "BMI" OR "Plasma Glucose" OR "Glycemia" OR "Insulin"). The wild-card term "*" was used to increase the sensitivity of the search strategy, which was limited to studies in humans. The reference list of identified papers was manually checked for additional relevant articles. In particular, additional searches for potential trials included the references of review articles on the topic of the meta-analysis and relevant abstracts from selected congresses. The literature was searched from inception to 3 February 2021.

All paper abstracts were screened by two reviewers (F.F. and A.F.G.C.) in an initial process to remove ineligible articles. The remaining articles were obtained in full text and assessed again by the same two researchers, who evaluated each article independently and carried out data extraction and quality assessment. Disagreements were resolved by discussion with a third party.

2.2. Study Selection Criteria

Original studies were included if they met the following criteria: (i) being a clinical trial with either a multicenter or single-center design, (ii) having an appropriate controlled design for Armolipid Plus®, (iii) investigating the effect of Armolipid Plus® on plasma lipids, (iv) testing the safety of Armolipid Plus®, and (v) reporting all the adverse events that occurred during the supplementation.

Exclusion criteria included the following: (i) lack of a control group for Armolipid Plus® administration, (ii) lack of blinding, (iii) lack of sufficient information about plasma lipids at baseline or follow-up, and (iv) lack of sufficient information about the prevalence and specification of adverse events. Studies were also excluded if they contained overlapping subjects with other studies.

2.3. Data Extraction

Data abstracted from the eligible studies were: (i) first author's name; (ii) year of publication; (iii) study design; (iv) main inclusion criteria and underlying disease; (v) treatment duration; (vi) study groups; (vii) number of participants in the active and control group; (viii) background lipid-lowering treatment; (ix) age and sex of study participants; (x) weight, body mass index (BMI), waist circumference, systolic BP (SBP), diastolic BP (DBP), TC, triglycerides (TG), high-density lipoprotein cholesterol (HDL-C), LDL-C, aspartate aminotransferase (AST), alanine aminotransferase (ALT), creatine phosphokinase (CPK), FPG, fasting plasma insulin (FPI), homeostatic model assessment for insulin resistance (HOMA-IR) and high sensitivity C reactive protein (hs-CRP) at baseline; and (xi) discontinuation of treatment and adverse events occurred during the trials. All data extraction and database typing were reviewed by the principal investigator (A.F.G.C.) before the final analysis, and doubts were resolved by mutual agreement among the authors.

2.4. Quality Assessment

A systematic assessment of risk of bias in the included studies was performed using the Cochrane criteria [16]. The following items were used: adequacy of sequence generation, allocation concealment, blind addressing of dropouts (incomplete outcome data), selective outcome reporting, and other probable sources of bias [17]. Risk-of-bias assessment was performed independently by 2 reviewers (F.F. and A.F.G.C.); disagreements were resolved by a consensus-based discussion.

2.5. Data Synthesis

Meta-analysis was entirely conducted using Comprehensive Meta-Analysis (CMA) V3 software (Biostat, NJ) [18].

Net changes in the investigated parameters (change scores) were calculated by subtracting the value at baseline from the one after intervention, in the active-treated group and in the control one. All values were collated as mean change from baseline. Standard deviations (SDs) of the mean difference were obtained as follows, as reported by Follman et al.: SD = square root $[(SD_{pre-treatment})^2 + (SD_{post-treatment})^2 - (2R \times SD_{pre-treatment} \times SD_{post-treatment})]$, assuming a correlation coefficient (R) = 0.5 [19]. If the outcome measures were reported in median and range (or 95% confidence interval (CI)), mean and SD values were estimated using the method described by Wan et al. [20]. The findings of the included studies were combined using a fixed-effect model or a random-effect model (using the DerSimonian–Laird method) and the generic inverse variance method based on the level of inter-study heterogeneity, which was quantitatively assessed using the Higgins index (I^2) [21]. For continuous parameters, effect sizes were expressed as absolute mean differences (MD) and 95%CI, standardized by the change score in SD. For treatment emergent adverse events, odd ratios (OR) and 95%CI intervals were calculated using the Mantel–Haenszel method [22]. A safety analysis was performed by excluding studies with zero events in both arms. If one or more outcomes could not be extracted from a study, the study was removed only from the analysis involving those outcomes. Adverse events were considered for the analysis only if they occurred in at least two of the included clinical trials.

In order to evaluate the influence of each study on the overall effect size, a sensitivity analysis was conducted using the leave-one-out method (i.e., removing one study at a time and repeating the analysis) [23]. Two-sided p-values ≤ 0.05 were considered statistically significant for all tests.

2.6. Publication Biases

Potential publication biases were explored using a visual inspection of Begg's funnel plot asymmetry, Begg's rank correlation test, and Egger's weighted regression test [24]. The Duval and Tweedie "trim and fill" method was used to adjust the analysis for the effects of publication biases [25]. Two-sided p-values < 0.05 were considered statistically significant.

3. Results

3.1. Flow and Characteristics of the Included Studies

After database searches were performed according to inclusion and exclusion criteria, 445 published articles were identified, and the abstracts were reviewed. Of these, 112 were excluded because they were not original articles. Another 314 were eliminated because they did not meet the inclusion criteria. Thus, 19 articles were carefully assessed and reviewed. An additional 7 studies were excluded because of a lack of a controlled design for Armolipid Plus® administration (n = 3) or lack of blinding (n = 4). Finally, 12 studies were eligible and included in the meta-analysis [26–37]. The study selection process is shown in Figure 1.

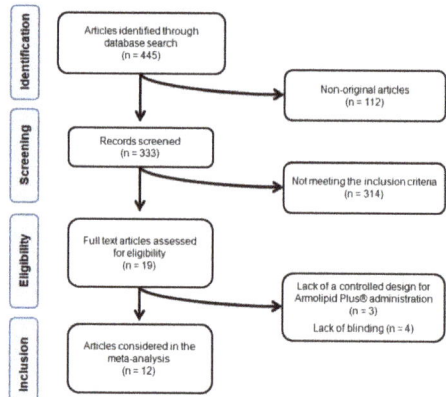

Figure 1. Flow chart of the number of studies identified and included in the systematic review.

Data were pooled from 12 clinical trials comprising 24 treatment arms, which included 1050 subjects, with 544 in the actively treated arm and 536 in the control one.

Eligible studies were published between 2010 and 2020. Follow-up periods ranged between 4 weeks and 12 months. All selected trials were designed with parallel groups and were multicenter [29,35,37] or single-center [26–28,30–34,36] clinical studies. Enrolled subjects were patients in primary prevention for CVD [28–30,32,36], patients with documented coronary artery disease (CAD) [33], with a metabolic syndrome [26,30,34–36], or with a good status of health [28,37]. The baseline characteristics of the evaluated studies are summarized in Tables 1 and 2.

Table 1. Main characteristics of the included clinical studies and baseline hemodynamic parameters of enrolled patients.

Author, Year	Study Design	Follow-Up	Main Inclusion Criteria	Study Group	Participants (n)	Background Lipid-Lowering Treatment (Percentage of Subjects)	Male (n (%))	Age (years; mean ± SD)	BMI (Kg/m²; mean ± SD)	Waist Circumference (cm; mean ± SD)	SBP (mmHg; mean ± SD)	DBP (mmHg; mean ± SD)
Affuso, 2012 [26]	Randomized, double-blind, placebo-controlled, parallel-group clinical study	18 weeks	Metabolic syndrome 18–65 years of age	Armolipid Plus®	29	Statins (28%)	20 (69)	53 ± 7	32.2 ± 4.6	110 ± 9	125 ± 13	78 ± 8
				Placebo	30	Statins (27%)	18 (60)	50 ± 11.9	34.7 ± 5.1	115 ± 13	125 ± 14	81 ± 8
Affuso, 2010 [27]	Randomized, double-blind, placebo-controlled, parallel-group clinical study	6 weeks	18–70 years of age TC > 220 mg/dL LDL-C > 130 mg/dL	Armolipid Plus®	25	None	13 (52)	55 ± 8	28 ± 3.8	NA	125 ± 13	78 ± 8
				Placebo	25	None	13 (52)	55 ± 7	28 ± 3.3	NA	125 ± 14	81 ± 8
Cicero, 2012 [28]	Randomized, double-blind, placebo-controlled, parallel-group clinical study	12 months	Primary prevention for CVD overweight	Armolipid Plus®	71	None	NA	NA	26.95 ± 0.86	NA	134.4 ± 6.2	86.3 ± 6.1
				Placebo	64	None		NA	24.17 ± 0.99	NA	133.2 ± 5.3	84.1 ± 6.8
D'Addato, 2017 [29]	Multicenter, randomized, double-blind, placebo-controlled, parallel-group clinical study	4 weeks	Primary prevention for CVD 18–75 years of age TC ≥ 200 mg/dL and ≤260 mg/dL LDL-C ≥ 115 mg/dL and ≤180 mg/dL	Armolipid Plus®	51	None	17 (33)	53.7 ± 11.6	24 ± 4	NA	NA	NA
				Placebo	51	None	17 (33)	49.7 ± 12.3	24.9 ± 4.6	NA	NA	NA
Galletti, 2019 [30]	Randomized, double-blind, placebo-controlled, parallel-group clinical study	24 weeks	Metabolic syndrome Left ventricular mass >48 g/m²⁷ for men and >44 g/m²⁷ for women 18–70 years of age	Armolipid Plus®	71	Statins (62%)	42 (59)	55.6 ± 8.9	29.4 ± 3.6	100.8 ± 9.3	130.6 ± 10.5	80.7 ± 8.1
				Placebo	70	Statins (63%)	37 (53)	55.6 ± 9.3	29.2 ± 3.5	100.3 ± 8.7	131.4 ± 10.6	81.6 ± 8
Gentile, 2015 [31]	Randomized, double-blind, placebo-controlled, parallel-group clinical study	8 weeks	Familial combined hyperlipidemia	Armolipid Plus®	15	None	(77)	44.1 ± 13	26 ± 2.8	92 ± 10.2	123 ± 12.3	77.9 ± 8.3
				Placebo	15	None			26.7 ± 2.8	97.3 ± 8.5	122.5 ± 9.2	78.1 ± 6.9
Gonnelli, 2014 [32]	Randomized, double-blind, placebo-controlled, parallel-group clinical study	24 weeks	Estimated 10-year CV risk <20% according to Framingham risk scoring 18–60 years of age BMI ≥ 19 Kg/m² and <30 Kg/m² LDL-C > 150 mg/dL	Armolipid Plus®	30	None	15 (50)	46.4 ± 9.7	26.9 ± 4.9	89.9 ± 10.9	120.1 ± 11.1	77.2 ± 7
				Placebo	30	None	14 (47)	46.4 ± 10.1	26.4 ± 4.1	88.7 ± 10.9	119.1 ± 19.7	75.2 ± 10

Table 1. Cont.

Author, Year	Study Design	Follow-Up	Main Inclusion Criteria	Study Group	Participants (n)	Background Lipid-Lowering Treatment (Percentage of Subjects)	Male (n (%))	Age (years; mean ± SD)	BMI (Kg/m²; mean ± SD)	Waist Circumference (cm; mean ± SD)	SBP (mmHg; mean ± SD)	DBP (mmHg; mean ± SD)
Marazzi, 2017 [33]	Randomized, single-blind, parallel-group clinical study	3 months	Documented CAD treated with PCI in the previous 12 months high-dose statin intolerance LDL-C > 100 mg/dL <50% reduction in LDL-C with low-dose statin treatment	Armolipid Plus® + low-dose statin	50	Statins (100%) Atorvastatin 5 mg (8%) Atorvastatin 10 mg (36%) Simvastatin 10 mg (14%) Simvastatin 20 mg (32%) Rosuvastatin 5 mg (10%)	26 (52)	69 ± 10	NA	NA	NA	NA
				Low-dose statin	50	Statins (100%) Atorvastatin 5 mg (8%) Atorvastatin 10 mg (34%) Simvastatin 10 mg (18%) Simvastatin 20 mg (32%) Rosuvastatin 5 mg (8%)	28 (56)	67 ± 12	NA	NA	NA	NA
Marazzi, 2011 [34]	Randomized, single-blind, placebo-controlled, parallel-group clinical study	12 months	>75 years of age TC > 200 mg/dL LDL-C > 160 mg/dL statin intolerance and refusal of other treatments for hypercholesterolemia	Armolipid Plus®	40	None	21 (53)	82.5 ± 4.4	NA	NA	NA	NA
				Placebo	40	None	20 (50)	82.5 ± 4.9	NA	NA	NA	NA
Mercurio, 2020 [35]	Randomized, double-blind, placebo-controlled, parallel-group clinical study	24 weeks	Metabolic syndrome echocardiographic evidence of left ventricular hypertrophy 18–70 years of age stable anti-hypertensive and lipid-lowering therapy over the past three months	Armolipid Plus®	79	Statins (55%)	43 (58)	55.6 ± 9	29.1 ± 3	NA	131 ± 11	81 ± 9
				Placebo	79	Statins (58%)	38 (54)	55.6 ± 9	29.3 ± 3	NA	131 ± 11	82 ± 8

Table 1. *Cont.*

Author, Year	Study Design	Follow-Up	Main Inclusion Criteria	Study Group	Participants (n)	Background Lipid-Lowering Treatment (Percentage of Subjects)	Male (n (%))	Age (years; mean ± SD)	BMI (Kg/m²; mean ± SD)	Waist Circumference (cm; mean ± SD)	SBP (mmHg; mean ± SD)	DBP (mmHg; mean ± SD)
Ruscica, 2014 [36]	Randomized, double-blind, placebo-controlled, cross-over clinical study	8 weeks	Primary prevention for CVD metabolic syndrome >18 years of age LDL-C ≥ 130 mg/dL and ≤170 mg/dL	Armolipid Plus® Placebo	30	None	23 (77)	55.4 ± 9.7	26.8 ± 2.4	96.3 ± 7.9 for men; 91.7 ± 5.1 for women	123 ± 12.3	80.7 ± 5.7
Sola, 2014 [37]	Randomized, double-blind, placebo-controlled, parallel-group clinical study	12 weeks	Primary prevention for CVD ≥18 years of age LDL-C ≥ 130 mg/dL and <190 mg/dL	Armolipid Plus® Placebo	51 51	None None	18 (35) 14 (28)	49.9 ± 11.6 52.4 ± 11.2	25.4 ± 4.1 28 ± 8.7	86.2 ± 11.8 90.4 ± 11.6	122.2 ± 18.1 123.8 ± 17.6	76.5 ± 12.2 76.8 ± 11.2

Expressed as median (interquartile range); BMI = body mass index; CAD = coronary artery disease; CHD = coronary heart disease; CV = cardiovascular; CVD = cardiovascular disease; DBP = diastolic blood pressure; LDL-C = low-density lipoprotein cholesterol; NA = not available; PCI = percutaneous coronary intervention; SBP = systolic blood pressure; SD = standard deviation; TC = total cholesterol.

Table 2. Baseline lipids, fasting plasma glucose, and markers of insulin resistance.

Author, Year	Study Group	TC (mg/dL; mean ± SD)	TG (mg/dL; mean ± SD)	HDL-C (mg/dL; mean ± SD)	LDL-C (mg/dL; mean ± SD)	FPG (mg/dL; mean ± SD)	FPI (mU/L; mean ± SD)	HOMA-IR (mean ± SD)	hs-CRP (mg/L; mean ± SD)
Affuso, 2012 [26]	Armolipid Plus®	209 ± 39	156 ± 76	42 ± 10	135 ± 7	103 ± 22	9 ± 4.2	3.2 ± 1.5	NA
	Placebo	197 ± 40	170 ± 74	46 ± 14	118 ± 39	85 ± 12	9 ± 6.9	2.7 ± 2.2	NA
Affuso, 2010 [27]	Armolipid Plus®	255 ± 29	57 ± 32	58 ± 18	176 ± 25	84 ± 12	NA	NA	NA
	Placebo	252 ± 31	65 ± 28	53 ± 14	171 ± 22	87 ± 12	NA	NA	NA
Cicero, 2012 [28]	Armolipid Plus®	218.3 ± 14.4	225.2 ± 42.7	38.6 ± 4.5	134.6 ± 15.2	109.6 ± 12	11.49 ± 4.34	3.2 ± 1.4	2.05 ± 0.31
	Placebo	213.5 ± 17	192.8 ± 44.4	39 ± 4.3	136 ± 18.9	92.2 ± 10.3	7.47 ± 3.14	1.7 ± 0.8	1.85 ± 0.43
D'Addato, 2017 [29]	Armolipid Plus®	234.6 ± 18	110.8 ± 41.5	65.1 ± 13.3	147.5 ± 16.3	NA	NA	NA	NA
	Placebo	235.6 ± 17.9	110.5 ± 41.9	70 ± 16.2	143.6 ± 15	NA	NA	NA	NA
Galletti, 2019 [30]	Armolipid Plus®	224.3 ± 44.7	151.3 ± 82.5	50.7 ± 11.9	132.9 ± 36.5	103.9 ± 14.5	15.7 ± 11.6	4.1 ± 3.2	1.85 ± 2.34
	Placebo	218.4 ± 38.2	159.6 ± 86.6	50.4 ± 12.1	128.4 ± 28.6	105.7 ± 17.9	16.3 ± 9	4.2 ± 2.4	1.35 ± 1.01
Gentile, 2015 [31]	Armolipid Plus®	228.8 ± 41.1	290.3 ± 104.3	40.8 ± 6.6	134.7 ± 46.5	91.5 ± 17.5	NA	NA	NA
	Placebo	241.9 ± 42.1	204.2 ± 80.9	38.2 ± 9.1	162.8 ± 41.2	93 ± 5.9	NA	NA	NA
Gonnelli, 2014 [32]	Armolipid Plus®	238.4 ± 26.9	132.1 ± 55.2	53.1 ± 13.2	162 ± 22.5	92.5 ± 8.8	NA	NA	NA
	Placebo	248.1 ± 32.4	119 ± 50.4	55.7 ± 14.5	165.8 ± 29	94.4 ± 10	NA	NA	NA
Marazzi, 2017 [33]	Armolipid Plus®	198 ± 9	177 ± 51	35 ± 4	127 ± 15	NA	NA	NA	NA
	Placebo	199 ± 11	176 ± 51	35 ± 4	129 ± 17	NA	NA	NA	NA
Marazzi, 2011 [34]	Armolipid Plus®	252 ± 23	179 ± 48	44 ± 12	172 ± 16	94 ± 6	7.2 ± 2.4	1.7 ± 0.6	NA
	Placebo	253 ± 19	179 ± 50	44 ± 8	173 ± 10	91 ± 7	6.5 ± 2.4	1.5 ± 0.6	NA
Mercurio, 2020 [35]	Armolipid Plus®	227 ± 44	160 ± 88	49 ± 11	138 ± 34	105 ± 16	NA	4.2 ± 3	NA
	Placebo	218 ± 40	151 ± 83	53 ± 13	124 ± 30	104 ± 16	NA	4 ± 3	NA
Ruscica, 2014 [36]	Armolipid Plus®	240 ± 31	216 (171, 284)*	40 ± 9	151 ± 24	88 ± 16	6 ± 4	1.3 ± 0.9	2 ± 1
	Placebo	240 ± 39	230 (173, 307)*	41 ± 7	150 ± 29	86 ± 18	6.4 ± 4.4	1.3 ± 1	2 ± 3
Solà, 2014 [37]	Armolipid Plus®	243.6 ± 24.4	107.2 ± 61.3	66.5 ± 21.2	155.7 ± 14.6	90.6 ± 9.3	8.2 ± 9.2	1.8 ± 2.6	NA
	Placebo	243.4 ± 19.5	115 ± 56	61.1 ± 14.1	159.3 ± 15.7	92.8 ± 10.3	7.5 ± 5.4	1.7 ± 1.3	NA

Expressed as median (interquartile range); FPG = fasting plasma glucose; FPI = fasting plasma insulin; HDL-C = high-density lipoprotein cholesterol; HOMA-IR = homeostatic model assessment for insulin resistance; hs-CRP = high sensitivity C reactive protein; LDL-C = low-density lipoprotein cholesterol; NA = not available; SD = standard deviation; TC = total cholesterol; TG = triglycerides.

3.2. Risk of Bias Assessment

Almost all of the included studies were characterized by sufficient information regarding sequence generation, allocation concealment, and personal and outcome assessments. All showed low risk of bias because of incomplete outcome data and selective outcome reporting. Details of the quality of bias assessment are reported in Table 3.

Table 3. Quality of bias assessment of the included studies according to the Cochrane guidelines.

First Author, Year	Sequence Generation	Allocation Concealment	Blinding of Participants, Personnel, and Outcome Assessment	Incomplete Outcome Data	Selective Outcome Reporting	Other Potential Threats to Validity
Affuso, 2012 [26]	L	L	L	L	L	U
Affuso, 2010 [27]	L	L	L	L	L	U
Cicero, 2012 [28]	L	L	L	L	L	L
D'Addato, 2017 [29]	L	L	L	L	L	L
Galletti, 2019 [30]	L	L	L	L	L	L
Gentile, 2015 [31]	L	L	L	L	L	U
Gonnelli, 2014 [32]	L	L	L	L	L	U
Marazzi, 2017 [33]	L	L	L	L	L	L
Marazzi, 2011 [34]	L	L	L	L	L	U
Mercurio, 2020 [35]	L	L	L	L	L	L
Ruscica, 2014 [36]	L	L	L	L	L	U
Solà, 2014 [37]	L	L	L	L	L	L

H = High risk of bias; L = Low risk of bias; U = Unclear risk of bias.

3.3. Effect of Armolipid Plus® on Anthropometric Measures, Blood Pressure, Serum Lipids, and Other Metabolic Parameters

Meta-analysis of the data suggested that Armolipid Plus® supplementation exerted a significant effect on BMI (MD = -0.25 kg/m^2, 95%CI($-0.43,-0.06$) Kg/m^2, $p = 0.008$; I^2 = 0%) (Figure 2) and serum levels of TC (MD = -25.07 mg/dL, 95%CI($-33.17,-16.97$) mg/dL, $p < 0.001$; I^2 = 87%), TG (MD = -11.47 mg/dL, 95%CI($-17.85,-5.08$) mg/dL, $p < 0.001$; I^2 = 34%), HDL-C (MD = 1.84 mg/dL, 95%CI(0.92,2.77) mg/dL, $p < 0.001$; I^2 = 0%), LDL-C (MD = -26.67 mg/dL, 95%CI($-33.76,-19.58$) mg/dL, $p < 0.001$; I^2 = 82%) (Figure 3), hs-CRP (MD = -0.61 mg/L, 95%CI($-1.13,-0.09$) mg/L, $p = 0.022$; I^2 = 47%) (Figure 4), FPG (MD = -3.52 mg/dL, 95%CI($-5.1,-1.94$) mg/dL, $p < 0.001$; I^2 = 49%) (Figure 5), without affecting weight (MD = -0.89 kg, 95%CI($-4.60,2.82$) kg, $p = 0.638$; I^2 = 0%), waist circumference (MD = -0.5 cm, 95%CI($-3.17,2.17$) cm, $p = 0.714$; I^2 = 0%) (Figure S1), SBP (MD = -0.57 mmHg, 95%CI($-3.2,2.06$) mmHg, $p = 0.670$; I^2 = 12%), DBP (MD = -0.89 mmHg, 95%CI($-2.61,0.83$) mmHg, $p = 0.312$; I^2 = 0%) (Figure S2), FPI (MD = -0.58 mU/L,

95%CI($-1.24, 0.09$), $p = 0.091$; $I^2 = 30\%$), and HOMA-IR (MD = -0.09, 95%CI($-0.44, 0.26$), $p = 0.599$; $I^2 = 61\%$) (Figure S3).

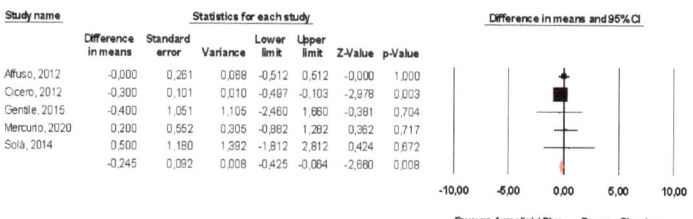

Figure 2. Forest plot displaying mean differences and 95% confidence intervals for the impact of the supplementation with Armolipid Plus® on BMI.

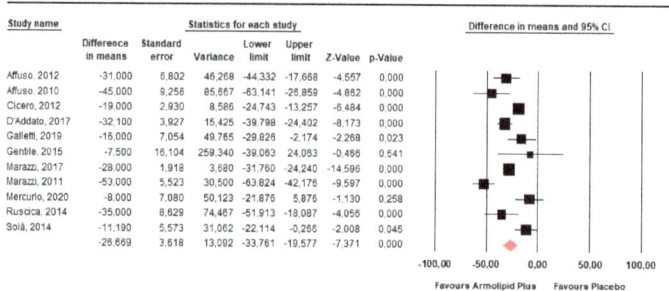

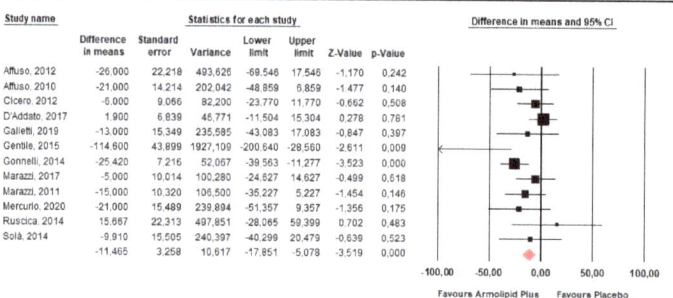

Figure 3. *Cont.*

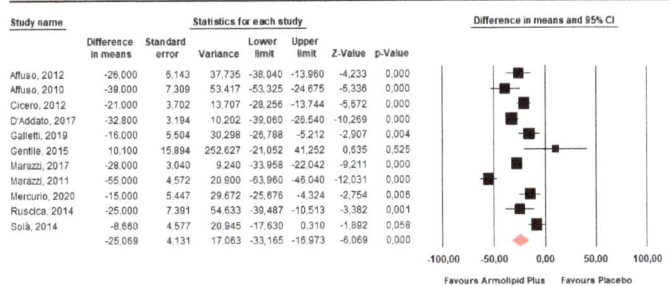

Figure 3. Forest plot displaying mean differences and 95% confidence intervals for the impact of the supplementation with Armolipid Plus® on serum levels of TC, TG, HDL-C, and LDL-C.

Figure 4. Forest plot displaying mean differences and 95% confidence intervals for the impact of the supplementation with Armolipid Plus® on serum levels of hs-CRP.

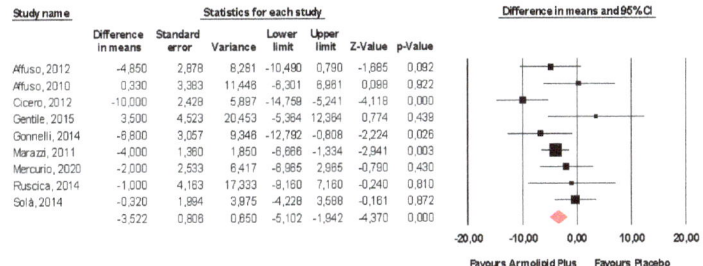

Figure 5. Forest plot displaying mean differences and 95% confidence intervals for the impact of the supplementation with Armolipid Plus® on FPG.

The effect sizes were robust in the leave-one-out sensitivity analysis and not mainly driven by a single study (data not shown).

A visual inspection of Begg's funnel plots did not show significant asymmetry, suggesting no potential publication bias for the effect of Armolipid Plus® on the efficacy outcomes (Figures S4–S7). This finding was confirmed by the results of Begg's rank correlation test and Egger's linear regression (Table 4).

The Duval and Tweedie trim-and-fill method identified three potentially missing studies on the left side of the funnel plot that resulted in the pooled effect size for DBP reaching statistical significance (Table 4).

Table 4. Assessment of publication bias on efficacy outcomes.

Outcomes	Adjustment with Duval and Tweedie's Trim-and-Fill Method				Begg's Rank Correlation Test	Egger's Linear Regression
	Number of Trimmed Studies	Adjusted Effect Sizes				
		MD	95% Confidence Interval		p-Value	p-Value
			Lower Bound	Upper Bound		
Weight	-	-	-	-	0.602	0.672
BMI	2	−0.262	−0.440	−0.085	1	0.174
Waist circumference	1	−0.819	−3.10	1.462	0.174	0.6
SBP	2	1.044	−1.287	3.374	0.624	0.485
DBP	3	−1.764	−3.192	−0.336	0.624	0.186
TC	1	−26.708	−29.212	−24.203	0.815	0.981
TG	2	−10.559	−16.861	−4.257	0.337	0.238
HDL-C	2	1.658	0.778	2.537	0.484	0.587
LDL-C	2	−29.049	−31.667	−26.432	0.392	0.478
FPG	2	−4.007	−5.521	−2.492	0.532	0.563
FPI	-	-	-	-	0.652	0.842
HOMA-IR	-	-	-	-	0.851	0.852

BMI = body mass index; DBP = diastolic blood pressure; FPG = fasting plasma glucose; FPI = fasting plasma insulin; HDL-C = high-density lipoprotein cholesterol; HOMA-IR = homeostatic model assessment for insulin resistance; LDL-C = low-density lipoprotein cholesterol; MD = mean difference; SBP = systolic blood pressure; TC = total cholesterol; TG = triglycerides.

3.4. Safety Analysis

Supplementation with Armolipid Plus® exerted a slight, though clinically insignificant, increase in serum levels of ALT (MD = 2.16 U/L, 95%CI(0.68,3.64) U/L, p = 0.004; I^2 = 0%) (Figure 6), without affecting AST (MD = 0.63 U/L, 95%CI(−0.96,2.21) U/L, p = 0.437; I^2 = 0%) or CPK (MD = 7.37 U/L, 95%CI(−1.20,15.93) U/L, p = 0.092; I^2 = 39%) (Figure S8).

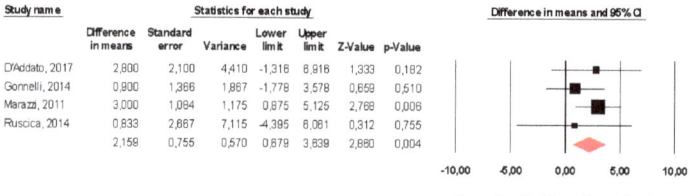

Figure 6. Forest plot displaying mean differences and 95% confidence intervals for the impact of the supplementation with Armolipid Plus® on serum levels of ALT.

Moreover, supplementation with Armolipid Plus® was not associated with increased risk of either musculoskeletal disorders (OR = 0.78, 95%CI(0.29,2.11), p = 0.618; I^2 = 0%) or gastrointestinal disorders (OR = 1.19, 95%CI(0.35,4.06), P = 0.786; I^2 = 0%) (Figure S9).

The effect sizes were robust in the leave-one-out sensitivity analysis and not mainly driven by a single study (data not shown).

A visual inspection of Begg's funnel plots did not show significant asymmetry, suggesting no potential publication bias for the effect of Armolipid Plus® on the safety outcomes (Figures S9–S13). This finding was confirmed by the results of Begg's rank correlation test and Egger's linear regression (Table 5).

Table 5. Assessment of publication bias on safety outcomes.

Safety Parameters	Adjustment with Duval and Tweedie's Trim-and-Fill Method				Begg's Rank Correlation Test	Egger's Linear Regression
	Number of Trimmed Studies	Adjusted Effect Sizes			*p*-Value	*p*-Value
		MD	95% Confidence Interval			
			Lower Bound	Upper Bound		
ALT	1	2.275	0.851	3.699	0.497	0.611
AST	1	0.583	−0.983	2.15	0.497	0.601
CPK	1	7.868	−0.365	16.101	0.174	0.552

Treatment-Emergent Adverse Events	Adjustment with Duval and Tweedie's Trim-and-Fill Method				Begg's Rank Correlation Test	Egger's Linear Regression
	Number of Trimmed Studies	Adjusted Effect Sizes			*p*-Value	*p*-Value
		OR	95% Confidence Interval			
			Lower Bound	Upper Bound		
Musculoskeletal disorders	-	-	-	-	1	0.759
Gastrointestinal disorders	1	1.014	0.321	3.201	0.602	0.951

ALT = alanine aminotransferase; AST = aspartate aminotransferase; CPK = creatine phosphokinase; MD = mean difference; OR = odds ratio.

The Duval and Tweedie trim-and-fill method yielded one potentially missing study on the right side of the funnel plot, increasing the pooled effect size for ALT, and one potentially missing study on the right side of the funnel plot, increasing the pooled effect size for CPK. In addition, Duval and Tweedie's trim-and-fill method yielded one potentially missing study on the left side of the funnel plot, decreasing the pooled effect size for AST, and one potentially missing study on the left side of the funnel plot, decreasing the estimated risk of gastrointestinal disorders (Table 5).

4. Discussion

According to our findings, dietary supplementation with Armolipid Plus® exerts a significant effect on BMI and serum levels of TC, TG, HDL-C, LDL-C, hs-CRP, and FPG. Importantly, it is not associated with an increased risk of musculoskeletal symptoms and gastrointestinal disorders, though it results in a slight, though clinically insignificant, increase in ALT serum levels.

To our knowledge, this is the first systematic review and meta-analysis to comprehensively and critically evaluate the existing body of evidence for the use of Armolipid Plus® in daily clinical practice. As a matter of fact, previous meta-analyses on this topic are outdated and not PRISMA compliant [38,39]. Moreover, they included clinical trials that were not adequately controlled for Armolipid Plus® supplementation and clinical studies with an observational design that finally led to not fully reliable results [40–44].

Armolipid Plus® is a dietary supplement widely used in clinical practice and the only combined lipid-lowering nutraceutical recommended by the International Lipid Expert Panel (ILEP) for the management of hypercholesterolemia in statin-intolerant patients [45]. In effect, red yeast rice at the dosage contained in Armolipid Plus® has been shown to be safe also following a recent large meta-analysis of 53 randomized controlled clinical trials enrolling 8535 participants overall [46]. Dietary supplementation with Armolipid Plus® in statin-intolerant patients previously treated with ezetimibe resulted in reductions of approximately 35% in LDL-C and 25% in TG [47], which was similar to results reported for moderate-intensity statins, according to the latest guidelines from the European Society of Cardiology (ESC) and the European Atherosclerosis Society (EAS) [48].

The lipid-lowering effect of red yeast rice (alone or combined with other lipid-lowering nutraceuticals) is well known, as it has been verified by several meta-analyses of randomized controlled clinical trials [49,50]. The interaction between red yeast rice and other natural products with different mechanisms of action, such as the other components of Armolipid Plus®, may have additive or synergistic lipid-lowering effects [51]. As a matter of fact, the inhibition of HMG-CoA reductase by monacolins contained in red yeast rice might be advantageously coupled with other nutraceuticals to enhance the hepatic uptake of cholesterol (berberine, soybean proteins), increase lipid excretion in the bowel (soluble fibers, plant sterols, glucomannan, probiotics), or induce LDL-C excretion (berberine, soy proteins, chlorogenic acid) [52,53]. Furthermore, several studies evaluated the efficacy and safety of red yeast rice in combination with policosanols, a mixture of aliphatic alcohols derived from purified sugar cane, even though the mechanism underlying their lipid-lowering effect is still being discussed [54,55]. Policosanols, together with berberine, may also be responsible for the reduction in FPG levels observed after dietary supplementation with Armolipid Plus® [56].

Although there are no trials showing that Armolipid Plus® reduces the risk of ASCVD events, some studies have shown benefits in terms of improved vascular function, as demonstrated by flow-mediated dilation [27] and carotid-femoral pulse wave velocity [57]. Absolute and relative risk reduction (RRR) in CV events with Armolipid Plus® is challenging to estimate based on the available short-term data. There is a linear association between LDL-C reduction and a decrease in ASCVD events, as reported originally by the CTT's(Cholesterol Treatment Trialists') meta-analyses of the statin trials where a 1 mmol/L (~39 mg/dL) LDL-C reduction was associated with a 21–23% RRR in CV events over five years [58]. Robust and growing evidence highlights that this linear association is observed regardless of the LDL lowering approach adopted, i.e., low-fat diet, anion exchange resins, ezetimibe, etc. [59]. On the basis of our findings, it is therefore plausible to expect a 14–15% ASCVD event reduction after long-term dietary supplementation with Armolipid Plus®.

Despite its strengths, this systematic review and meta-analysis has some limitations. One limitation is the heterogeneity for the effect size on TC and LDL-C, which was moderately high, proving that additional evidence is needed to establish the extent of cholesterol reduction that can be achieved following supplementation with Armolipid Plus®. In addition, we had to exclude a relatively large number of clinical trials not compliant with the inclusion criteria for this meta-analysis. The sample size on some laboratory and clinical outcomes was consequently reduced. In particular, some non-significant results (e.g., changes in weight and waist circumference) might be related to a low statistical power.

Nonetheless, the observed results are in line also with a large trial carried out in a setting of the general population involving 1751 volunteers but not included in the meta-analysis, as it did not meet our pre-specified inclusion criteria [42].

Other lipid-lowering nutraceutical combinations could exert a relevant lipid-lowering effect, but the data on Armolipid Plus® are currently most robust.

5. Conclusions

Pooling data from the available randomized controlled clinical studies, the current systematic review and meta-analysis provides data in support of the use of Armolipid Plus® in clinical practice as add-on treatment to lifestyle modifications for hypercholesterolemia in order to promote improved cardiometabolic health. Further studies to identify a benefit in terms of CV outcomes are required.

Supplementary Materials: The following are available online at https://www.mdpi.com/2072-6643/13/2/638/s1, Figure S1: Forest plot displaying mean differences and 95% confidence intervals for the impact of supplementation with Armolipid Plus® on weight and WC, Figure S2: Forest plot displaying mean differences and 95% confidence intervals for the impact of supplementation with Armolipid Plus® on SBP and DBP, Figure S3: Forest plot displaying mean differences and 95% confidence intervals for the impact of supplementation with Armolipid Plus® on FPI and HOMA-IR, Figure S4: Funnel plots detailing publication bias for the effect of supplementation with Armolipid Plus® on weight, BMI, and waist circumference, Figure S5: Funnel plots detailing publication bias for the effect of supplementation with Armolipid Plus® on blood pressure, Figure S6: Funnel plots detailing publication bias for the effect of supplementation with Armolipid Plus® on serum lipid concentrations, Figure S7: Funnel plots detailing publication bias for the effect of supplementation with Armolipid Plus® on glycemia and markers of insulin resistance, Figure S8: Forest plot displaying mean differences and 95% confidence intervals for the impact of supplementation with Armolipid Plus® on AST and CPK, Figure S9: Forest plots displaying the risk of treatment-emergent adverse events during supplementation with Armolipid Plus®, Figure S10: Funnel plot detailing publication bias for the effect of supplementation with Armolipid Plus® on serum concentrations of ALT, Figure S11: Funnel plot detailing publication bias for the effect of supplementation with Armolipid Plus® on serum concentrations of AST, Figure S12: Funnel plot detailing publication bias for the effect of supplementation with Armolipid Plus® on serum concentrations of CPK, Figure S13: Funnel plot detailing publication bias for risk of treatment-emergent adverse events during supplementation with Armolipid Plus®.

Author Contributions: Conceptualization, F.F. and A.F.G.C.; methodology, F.F. and A.F.G.C.; software, F.F.; validation, F.F. and A.F.G.C.; formal analysis, F.F.; investigation, F.F., M.B., P.P.T., and A.F.G.C.; data curation, F.F., M.B., and A.F.G.C.; writing—original draft preparation, F.F. and A.F.G.C.; writing—review and editing, C.K., T.K., M.B., C.M.G.G., A.Š., and P.P.T.; supervision, A.F.G.C. All authors have read and agreed to the published version of the manuscript.

Funding: This research received no external funding.

Institutional Review Board Statement: Ethical review and approval were waived for this study, due to the study design (meta-analysis).

Informed Consent Statement: Patient consent was waived due to the study design (meta-analysis).

Data Availability Statement: Data supporting findings of this analysis are available from the Corresponding Authors upon reasonable request.

Conflicts of Interest: A.F.G.C. served as consultant to Meda-Mylan and Sharper; F.F. served as consultant to Meda-Mylan and Neopharmed Gentili s.p.a. The other authors declare no conflict of interest.

References

1. World Health Organization (WHO). Cardiovascular Diseases. Available online: http://www.who.int/mediacentre/factsheets/fs317/en/ (accessed on 26 December 2020).
2. Roth, G.A.; Mensah, G.A.; Johnson, C.O.; Addolorato, G.; Ammirati, E.; Baddour, L.M.; Barengo, N.C.; Beaton, A.Z.; Benjamin, E.J.; Benziger, C.P.; et al. Global Burden of Cardiovascular Diseases and Risk Factors, 1990–2019. *J. Am. Coll. Cardiol.* **2020**, *76*, 2982–3021. [CrossRef]
3. Colantonio, L.D.; Bittner, V.; Reynolds, K.; Levitan, E.B.; Rosenson, R.S.; Banach, M.; Kent, S.T.; Derose, S.F.; Zhou, H.; Safford, M.M.; et al. Association of Serum Lipids and Coronary Heart Disease in Contemporary Observational Studies. *Circulation* **2016**, *133*, 256–264. [CrossRef]
4. Mozaffarian, D.; Benjamin, E.J.; Go, A.S.; Arnett, D.K.; Blaha, M.J.; Cushman, M.; Das, S.R.; De Ferranti, S.; Després, J.-P.; Fullerton, H.J.; et al. Heart Disease and Stroke Statistics—2016 Update: A Report from the American Heart Association. American Heart Association Statistics Committee, Stroke Statistics Subcommittee. *Circulation* **2016**, *133*, e38–e360. [CrossRef] [PubMed]
5. NCD Risk Factor Collaboration (NCD-RisC); Taddei, C.; Jackson, R.; Zhou, B.; Bixby, H.; Danaei, G.; Di Cesare, M.; Kuulasmaa, K.; Hajifathalian, K.; Bentham, J.; et al. National trends in total cholesterol obscure heterogeneous changes in HDL and non-HDL cholesterol and total-to-HDL cholesterol ratio: A pooled analysis of 458 population-based studies in Asian and Western countries. *Int. J. Epidemiol.* **2019**, *49*, 173–192. [CrossRef]
6. Wilson, P.W.F.; Polonsky, T.S.; Miedema, M.D.; Khera, A.; Kosinski, A.S.; Kuvin, J.T. Systematic Review for the 2018 AHA/ACC/AACVPR/AAPA/ABC/ACPM/ADA/AGS/APhA/ASPC/NLA/PCNA Guideline on the Management of Blood Cholesterol: A Report of the American College of Cardiology/American Heart Association Task Force on Clinical Practice Guidelines. *Circulation* **2019**, *139*, e1144–e1161. [CrossRef]
7. Zeitouni, M.; Sabouret, P.; Kerneis, M.; Silvain, J.; Collet, J.-P.; Bruckert, E.; Montalescot, G. 2019 ESC/EAS Guidelines for management of dyslipidaemia: Strengths and limitations. *Eur. Hear. J. Cardiovasc. Pharmacother.* **2020**, *77*. [CrossRef]
8. Piepoli, M.F.; Hoes, A.W.; Agewall, S.; Albus, C.; Brotons, C.; Catapano, A.L.; Cooney, M.-T.; Corrà, U.; Cosyns, B.; Deaton, C.; et al. 2016 European Guidelines on cardiovascular disease prevention in clinical practice. *Atherosclerosis* **2016**, *252*, 207–274. [CrossRef] [PubMed]

9. Arnett, D.K.; Blumenthal, R.S.; Albert, M.A.; Buroker, A.B.; Goldberger, Z.D.; Hahn, E.J.; Himmelfarb, C.D.; Khera, A.; Lloyd-Jones, D.; McEvoy, J.W.; et al. 2019 ACC/AHA Guideline on the Primary Prevention of Cardiovascular Disease: A Report of the American College of Cardiology/American Heart Association Task Force on Clinical Practice Guidelines. *Circulation* **2019**, *140*, e596–e646. [CrossRef]
10. Poli, A.; Barbagallo, C.M.; Cicero, A.F.; Corsini, A.; Manzato, E.; Trimarco, B.; Bernini, F.; Visioli, F.; Bianchi, A.; Canzone, G.; et al. Nutraceuticals and functional foods for the control of plasma cholesterol levels. An intersociety position paper. *Pharmacol. Res.* **2018**, *134*, 51–60. [CrossRef]
11. Cicero, A.F.G.; Colletti, A.; Bajraktari, G.; Descamps, O.; Djuric, D.M.; Ezhov, M.; Fras, Z.; Katsiki, N.; Langlois, M.; Latkovskis, G.; et al. Lipid-lowering nutraceuticals in clinical practice: Position paper from an International Lipid Expert Panel. *Nutr. Rev.* **2017**, *75*, 731–767. [CrossRef] [PubMed]
12. Patti, A.M.; Toth, P.P.; Giglio, R.V.; Banach, M.; Noto, M.; Nikolic, D.; Montalto, G.; Rizzo, M. Nutraceuticals as an Important Part of Combination Therapy in Dyslipidaemia. *Curr. Pharm. Des.* **2017**, *23*, 2496–2503. [CrossRef] [PubMed]
13. Cicero, A.F.G.; Fogacci, F.; Colletti, A. Food and plant bioactives for reducing cardiometabolic disease risk: An evidence based approach. *Food Funct.* **2017**, *8*, 2076–2088. [CrossRef] [PubMed]
14. Barrios, V.; Escobar, C.; Cicero, A.F.G.; Burke, D.; Fasching, P.; Banach, M.; Bruckert, E. A nutraceutical approach (Armolipid Plus) to reduce total and LDL cholesterol in individuals with mild to moderate dyslipidemia: Review of the clinical evidence. *Atheroscler. Suppl.* **2017**, *24*, 1–15. [CrossRef]
15. Moher, D.; Liberati, A.; Tetzlaff, J.; Altman, D.G. For the PRISMA Group Preferred reporting items for systematic reviews and meta-analyses: The PRISMA statement. *BMJ* **2009**, *339*, b2535. [CrossRef]
16. Higgins, J.; Green, S. *Cochrane Handbook for Systematic Reviews of Interventions*; Report Version 5.0.2.2009; John Wiley and Sons Ltd.: Chichester, UK, 2010.
17. Fogacci, F.; Ferri, N.; Toth, P.P.; Ruscica, M.; Corsini, A.; Cicero, A.F.G. Efficacy and Safety of Mipomersen: A Systematic Review and Meta-Analysis of Randomized Clinical Trials. *Drugs* **2019**, *79*, 751–766. [CrossRef] [PubMed]
18. Borenstein, M.; Hedges, L.; Higgins, J.; Rothstein, H. *Comprehensive Meta-Analysis Version 3*; Biostat: Englewood, NJ, USA, 2005; Volume 104.
19. Follmann, D.; Elliott, P.; Suh, I.; Cutler, J. Variance imputation for overviews of clinical trials with continuous response. *J. Clin. Epidemiol.* **1992**, *45*, 769–773. [CrossRef]
20. Wan, X.; Wang, W.; Liu, J.; Tong, T. Estimating the sample mean and standard deviation from the sample size, median, range and/or interquartile range. *BMC Med Res. Methodol.* **2014**, *14*, 1–13. [CrossRef]
21. Melsen, W.G.; Bootsma, M.C.J.; Rovers, M.M.; Bonten, M.J.M. The effects of clinical and statistical heterogeneity on the predictive values of results from meta-analyses. *Clin. Microbiol. Infect.* **2014**, *20*, 123–129. [CrossRef]
22. Haenszel, W.; Hon, N.B. Statistical approaches to the study of cancer with particular reference to case registers. *J. Chronic Dis.* **1956**, *4*, 589–599. [CrossRef]
23. Fogacci, F.; Banach, M.; Cicero, A.F.G. Resveratrol effect on patients with non-alcoholic fatty liver disease: A matter of dose and treatment length. *Diabetes Obes. Metab.* **2018**, *20*, 1798–1799. [CrossRef]
24. Fogacci, F.; Rizzo, M.; Krogager, C.; Kennedy, C.; Georges, C.M.; Knežević, T.; Liberopoulos, E.; Vallée, A.; Pérez-Martínez, P.; Wenstedt, E.F.; et al. Safety Evaluation of α-Lipoic Acid Supplementation: A Systematic Review and Meta-Analysis of Randomized Placebo-Controlled Clinical Studies. *Antioxidants* **2020**, *9*, 1011. [CrossRef]
25. Duval, S.; Tweedie, R. Trim and Fill: A Simple Funnel-Plot-Based Method of Testing and Adjusting for Publication Bias in Meta-Analysis. *Biometrics* **2000**, *56*, 455–463. [CrossRef]
26. Affuso, F. A nutraceutical combination improves insulin sensitivity in patients with metabolic syndrome. *World J. Cardiol.* **2012**, *4*, 77–83. [CrossRef]
27. Affuso, F.; Ruvolo, A.; Micillo, F.; Saccà, L.; Fazio, S. Effects of a nutraceutical combination (berberine, red yeast rice and policosanols) on lipid levels and endothelial function randomized, double-blind, placebo-controlled study. *Nutr. Metab. Cardiovasc. Dis.* **2010**, *20*, 656–661. [CrossRef]
28. Cicero, A.F.G.; De Sando, V.; Benedetto, D.; Cevenini, M.; Grandi, E.; Borghi, C. Long-term efficacy and tolerability of a multicomponent lipid-lowering nutraceutical in overweight and normoweight patients. *Nutrafoods* **2012**, *11*, 55–61. [CrossRef]
29. D'Addato, S.; Scandiani, L.; Mombelli, G.; Focanti, F.; Pelacchi, F.; Salvatori, E.; Di Loreto, G.; Comandini, A.; Maffioli, P.; DeRosa, G. Effect of a food supplement containing berberine, monacolin K, hydroxytyrosol and coenzyme Q10 on lipid levels: A randomized, double-blind, placebo controlled study. *Drug Des. Dev. Ther.* **2017**, *11*, 1585–1592. [CrossRef] [PubMed]
30. Galletti, F.; Fazio, V.; Gentile, M.; Schillaci, G.; Pucci, G.; Battista, F.; Mercurio, V.; Bosso, G.; Bonaduce, D.; Brambilla, N.; et al. Efficacy of a nutraceutical combination on lipid metabolism in patients with metabolic syndrome: A multicenter, double blind, randomized, placebo controlled trial. *Lipids Heal. Dis.* **2019**, *18*, 66. [CrossRef]
31. Gentile, M.; Calcaterra, I.; Strazzullo, A.; Pagano, C.; Pacioni, D.; Speranza, E.; Rubba, P.; Marotta, G. Effects of Armolipid Plus on small dense LDL particles in a sample of patients affected by familial combined hyperlipidemia. *Clin. Lipidol.* **2015**, *10*, 475–480. [CrossRef]
32. Gonnelli, S.; Caffarelli, C.; Stolakis, K.; Cuda, C.; Giordano, N.; Nuti, R. Efficacy and Tolerability of a Nutraceutical Combination (Red Yeast Rice, Policosanols, and Berberine) in Patients with Low-Moderate Risk Hypercholesterolemia: A Double-Blind, Placebo-Controlled Study. *Curr. Ther. Res.* **2015**, *77*, 1–6. [CrossRef] [PubMed]

33. Marazzi, G.; Campolongo, G.; Pelliccia, F.; Quattrino, S.; Vitale, C.; Cacciotti, L.; Massaro, R.; Volterrani, M.; Rosano, G. Comparison of Low-Dose Statin Versus Low-Dose Statin + Armolipid Plus in High-Intensity Statin-Intolerant Patients with a Previous Coronary Event and Percutaneous Coronary Intervention (ADHERENCE Trial). *Am. J. Cardiol.* **2017**, *120*, 893–897. [CrossRef]
34. Marazzi, G.; Cacciotti, L.; Pelliccia, F.; Iaia, L.; Volterrani, M.; Caminiti, G.; Sposato, B.; Massaro, R.; Grieco, F.; Rosano, G. Long-term effects of nutraceuticals (berberine, red yeast rice, policosanol) in elderly hypercholesterolemic patients. *Adv. Ther.* **2011**, *28*, 1105–1113. [CrossRef]
35. Mercurio, V.; Pucci, G.; Bosso, G.; Fazio, V.; Battista, F.; Iannuzzi, A.; Brambilla, N.; Vitalini, C.; D'Amato, M.; Giacovelli, G.; et al. A nutraceutical combination reduces left ventricular mass in subjects with metabolic syndrome and left ventricular hypertrophy: A multicenter, randomized, double-blind, placebo-controlled trial. *Clin. Nutr.* **2020**, *39*, 1379–1384. [CrossRef] [PubMed]
36. Ruscica, M.; Gomaraschi, M.; Mombelli, G.; Macchi, C.; Bosisio, R.; Pazzucconi, F.; Pavanello, C.; Calabresi, L.; Arnoldi, A.; Sirtori, C.R.; et al. Nutraceutical approach to moderate cardiometabolic risk: Results of a randomized, double-blind and crossover study with Armolipid Plus. *J. Clin. Lipidol.* **2014**, *8*, 61–68. [CrossRef]
37. Sola, R.; Valls, R.-M.; Puzo, J.; Calabuig, J.-R.; Brea, A.; Pedret, A.; Moriña, D.; Villar, J.; Millán, J.; Anguera, A. Effects of Poly-Bioactive Compounds on Lipid Profile and Body Weight in a Moderately Hypercholesterolemic Population with Low Cardiovascular Disease Risk: A Multicenter Randomized Trial. *PLoS ONE* **2014**, *9*, e101978. [CrossRef]
38. Pirro, M.; Mannarino, M.R.; Bianconi, V.; Simental-Mendía, L.E.; Bagaglia, F.; Mannarino, E.; Sahebkar, A. The effects of a nutraceutical combination on plasma lipids and glucose: A systematic review and meta-analysis of randomized controlled trials. *Pharmacol. Res.* **2016**, *110*, 76–88. [CrossRef]
39. Millán, J.; Cicero, A.F.; Torres, F.; Anguera, A. Effects of a nutraceutical combination containing berberine (BRB), policosanol, and red yeast rice (RYR), on lipid profile in hypercholesterolemic patients: A meta-analysis of randomised controlled trials. *Clín. Investig. Arterioscler.* **2016**, *28*, 178–187. [CrossRef] [PubMed]
40. Pirro, M.; Lupatelli, G.; Del Giorno, R.; Schillaci, G.; Berisha, S.; Mannarino, M.R.; Bagaglia, F.; Melis, F.; Mannarino, E. Nutraceutical combination (red yeast rice, berberine and policosanols) improves aortic stiffness in low-moderate risk hypercholesterolemic patients. *PharmaNutrition* **2013**, *1*, 73–77. [CrossRef]
41. Izzo, R.; De Simone, G.; Giudice, R.; Chinali, M.; Trimarco, V.; De Luca, N.; Trimarco, B. Effects of nutraceuticals on prevalence of metabolic syndrome and on calculated Framingham Risk Score in individuals with dyslipidemia. *J. Hypertens.* **2010**, *28*, 1482–1487. [CrossRef] [PubMed]
42. Trimarco, B.; Benvenuti, C.; Rozza, F.; Cimmino, C.S.; Giudice, R.; Crispo, S. Clinical evidence of efficacy of red yeast rice and berberine in a large controlled study versus diet. *Med. J. Nutrition. Metab.* **2011**, *4*, 133–139. [CrossRef] [PubMed]
43. Cicero, A.F.G.; Rovati, L.C.; Setnikar, I. Eulipidemic effects of berberine administered alone or in combination with other natural cholesterol-lowering agents: A single-blind clinical investigation. *Arzneimittelforschung* **2007**, *57*, 26–30. [CrossRef]
44. Pisciotta, L.; Bellocchio, A.; Bertolini, S. Nutraceutical pill containing berberine versus ezetimibe on plasma lipid pattern in hypercholesterolemic subjects and its additive effect in patients with familial hypercholesterolemia on stable cholesterol-lowering treatment. *Lipids Heal. Dis.* **2012**, *11*, 123. [CrossRef] [PubMed]
45. Banach, M.; Patti, A.M.; Giglio, R.V.; Cicero, A.F.; Atanasov, A.G.; Bajraktari, G.; Bruckert, E.; Descamps, O.; Djuric, D.M.; Ezhov, M.; et al. The Role of Nutraceuticals in Statin Intolerant Patients. *J. Am. Coll. Cardiol.* **2018**, *72*, 96–118. [CrossRef]
46. Fogacci, F.; Banach, M.; Mikhailidis, D.P.; Bruckert, E.; Toth, P.P.; Watts, G.F.; Reiner, Ž.; Mancini, J.; Rizzo, M.; Mitchenko, O.; et al. Safety of red yeast rice supplementation: A systematic review and meta-analysis of randomized controlled trials. *Pharmacol. Res.* **2019**, *143*, 1–16. [CrossRef]
47. Marazzi, G.; Campolongo, G.; Pelliccia, F.; Calabrò, P.; Cacciotti, L.; Vitale, C.; Massaro, R.; Volterrani, M.; Rosano, G. Usefulness of Low-Dose Statin Plus Ezetimibe and/or Nutraceuticals in Patients with Coronary Artery Disease Intolerant to High-Dose Statin Treatment. *Am. J. Cardiol.* **2019**, *123*, 233–238. [CrossRef] [PubMed]
48. Mach, F.; Baigent, C.; Catapano, A.L.; Koskinas, K.C.; Casula, M.; Badimon, L.; Chapman, M.J.; De Backer, G.G.; Delgado, V.; Ference, B.A.; et al. 2019 ESC/EAS guidelines for the management of dyslipidaemias: Lipid modification to reduce cardiovascular risk. *Atherosclerosis* **2019**, *290*, 140–205. [CrossRef]
49. Gerards, M.C.; Terlou, R.J.; Yu, H.; Koks, C.; Gerdes, V. Traditional Chinese lipid-lowering agent red yeast rice results in significant LDL reduction but safety is uncertain—A systematic review and meta-analysis. *Atherosclerosis* **2015**, *240*, 415–423. [CrossRef] [PubMed]
50. Zhao, S.P.; Liu, L.; Cheng, Y.C.; Shishehbor, M.H.; Liu, M.H.; Peng, D.Q.; Li, Y.L. Xuezhikang, an Extract of Cholestin, Protects Endothelial Function Through Antiinflammatory and Lipid-Lowering Mechanisms in Patients with Coronary Heart Disease. *Circulation* **2004**, *110*, 915–920. [CrossRef] [PubMed]
51. Cicero, A.F.G.; Fogacci, F.; Banach, M. Red Yeast Rice for Hypercholesterolemia. *Methodist Debakey Cardiovasc. J.* **2019**, *15*, 192–199. [PubMed]
52. Cicero, A.F.; DeRosa, G.; Borghi, C. Red Yeast Rice and Statin-Intolerant Patients. *Am. J. Cardiol.* **2010**, *105*, 1504. [CrossRef]
53. Cicero, A.F.; Fogacci, F.; Zambon, A. Red Yeast Rice for Hypercholesterolemia. *J. Am. Coll. Cardiol.* **2021**, *77*, 620–628. [CrossRef]
54. Varady, K.A.; Wang, Y.; Jones, P.J. Role of policosanols in the prevention and treatment of cardiovascular disease. *Nutr. Rev.* **2003**, *61*, 376–383. [CrossRef]

55. Guardamagna, O.; Abelló, F.; Baracco, V.; Stasiowska, B.; Martino, F. The treatment of hypercholesterolemic children: Efficacy and safety of a combination of red yeast rice extract and policosanols. *Nutr. Metab. Cardiovasc. Dis.* **2011**, *21*, 424–429. [CrossRef]
56. Liang, Y.; Xu, X.; Yin, M.; Zhang, Y.; Huang, L.; Chen, R.; Ni, J. Effects of berberine on blood glucose in patients with type 2 diabetes mellitus: A systematic literature review and a meta-analysis. *Endocr. J.* **2019**, *66*, 51–63. [CrossRef]
57. Pirro, M.; Francisci, D.; Bianconi, V.; Schiaroli, E.; Mannarino, M.R.; Barsotti, F.; Spinozzi, A.; Bagaglia, F.; Sahebkar, A.; Baldelli, F. NUtraceutical TReatment for hYpercholesterolemia in HIV-infected patients: The NU-TRY(HIV) randomized cross-over trial. *Atherosclerosis* **2019**, *280*, 51–57. [CrossRef] [PubMed]
58. Baigent, C.; Keech, A.C.; Kearney, P.M.; Blackwell, L.; Buck, G.; Pollicino, C.; Kirby, A.; Sourjina, T.; Peto, R.; Collins, R.; et al. Efficacy and safety of cholesterol-lowering treatment: Prospective meta-analysis of data from 90 056 participants in 14 randomised trials of statins. *Lancet* **2005**, *366*, 1267–1278. [CrossRef] [PubMed]
59. Silverman, M.G.; Ference, B.A.; Im, K.; Wiviott, S.D.; Giugliano, R.P.; Grundy, S.M.; Braunwald, E.; Sabatine, M.S. Association Between Lowering LDL-C and Cardiovascular Risk Reduction Among Different Therapeutic Interventions. *JAMA* **2016**, *316*, 1289–1297. [CrossRef] [PubMed]

MDPI
St. Alban-Anlage 66
4052 Basel
Switzerland
Tel. +41 61 683 77 34
Fax +41 61 302 89 18
www.mdpi.com

Nutrients Editorial Office
E-mail: nutrients@mdpi.com
www.mdpi.com/journal/nutrients

www.ingramcontent.com/pod-product-compliance
Lightning Source LLC
LaVergne TN
LVHW070154100526
838202LV00015B/1941